Public Health
and Social Justice

Public Health and Social Justice

Martin Donohoe

EDITOR

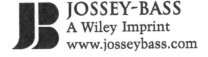

JOSSEY-BASS
A Wiley Imprint
www.josseybass.com

Published by Jossey-Bass
A Wiley Imprint
One Montgomery Street, Suite 1200, San Francisco, CA 94104-4594—www.josseybass.com

Jossey-Bass books and products are available through most bookstores. To contact Jossey-Bass directly call our Customer Care Department within the U.S. at 800-956-7739, outside the U.S. at 317-572-3986, or fax 317-572-4002.

Wiley also publishes its books in a variety of electronic formats and by print-on-demand. Some material included with standard print versions of this book may not be included in e-books or in print-on-demand. If the version of this book that you purchased references media such as CD or DVD that was not included in your purchase, you may download this material at http://booksupport.wiley.com. For more information about Wiley products, visit www.wiley.com.

Library of Congress Cataloging-in-Publication Data

Public health and social justice : a Jossey-Bass reader / Martin Donohoe, editor.—1st ed.
    p. ; cm.
  Includes bibliographical references and index.
  ISBN 978-1-118-08814-2 (pbk.); ISBN 978-1-118-22309-3 (ebk.); ISBN 978-1-118-23676-5 (ebk.); ISBN 978-1-118-26170-5 (ebk.)
  I. Donohoe, Martin, 1963-
  [DNLM: 1. Public Health—Collected Works.   2. Socioeconomic Factors—Collected Works.
3. Environmental Health—methods—Collected Works.   4. Health Education—Collected Works.
5. Health Status Disparities—Collected Works.   6. Social Justice—Collected Works. WA 30]
  362.1—dc23
                                                                    2012031837

Printed in the United States of America
FIRST EDITION
PB Printing   SKY10096108_011425

Contents

•••

PART I
Human Rights, Social Justice, Economics, Poverty, and Health Care

PART TWO
Special Populations

PART THREE
Women's Health

PART FOUR
Obesity, Tobacco, and Suicide by Firearms: The Modern Epidemics

PART FIVE
Food: Safety, Security, and Disease

PART SIX
Environmental Health

PART SEVEN
War and Violence

PART EIGHT
Corporations and Public Health

PART NINE
Achieving Social Justice in Health Care Through Education and Activism

•••

For my family

Introduction

Many of the rights described in the Universal Declaration of Human Rights, this collection's first and most important reading, were earlier enumerated by President Franklin Delano Roosevelt. In his penultimate State of the Union speech, Roosevelt called on Americans to work toward a new bill of rights, to complement the one laid out by the country's founding fathers. He said,

> True individual freedom cannot exist without economic security and independence. Necessitous men are not free men. People who are hungry and out of a job are the stuff of which dictatorships are made. ... We have accepted ... a second Bill of Rights under which a new basis of security and prosperity can be established for all regardless of station, race, or creed. Among these are: The right to a useful and remunerative job in the industries or shops or farms or mines of the Nation; the right to earn enough to provide adequate food and clothing and recreation; the right of every farmer to raise and sell his products at a return which will give him and his family a decent living; the right of every businessman, large and small, to trade in an atmosphere of freedom from unfair competition and domination by monopolies at home or abroad; the right of every family to a decent home; the right to adequate medical care and the opportunity to achieve and enjoy good health; the right to adequate protection from the economic fears of old age, sickness, accident, and unemployment; [and] the right to a good education. All of these rights spell security....We must be prepared to move forward, in the implementation of these rights, to new goals of human happiness and well-being.[1]

In many ways, our government and others around the world have failed, individually and collectively, to guarantee these rights. As such, social injustices abound, many of which have profound implications for public health. These include widespread poverty; social and economic inequalities; homelessness; environmental degradation; racism, classism, and sexism; war and other forms of violence; and increasing corporate control over basic resources.

This reader is designed to present an overview of the links between public health and social justice along with in-depth analyses of certain topic areas. It began as a collection of many of my own writings over the years, originally published in journals whose circulation is dwarfed by most news magazines and medical periodicals. As the project took shape, I decided to add writings (from peer-reviewed articles to newspaper articles to personal essays) that have influenced my personal philosophy and career development, affected me emotionally, and that I have used in my courses in medical humanities, public health, ethics, and women's rights. This reader is not meant to serve only as a comprehensive overview of the very broad area of public health and social justice, but also to provide an analysis of certain important areas and issues, some of which have not been addressed in other relevant, important collections.

From ancient times through the nineteenth century, medical (and nursing) training was carried out via the apprenticeship model, which was then replaced by a patchwork system of educational institutions of variable quality, offering nonstandardized curricula of varying length, which produced practitioners of varying quality. Following educator Abraham Flexner's important report on this uneven and often subpar system of medical education, early twentieth-century schools adopted the European model, and the medical curriculum was transformed into the one that still largely exists today, consisting of two preclinical years, followed by two clinical years, followed by an internship and residency in one's chosen field, with some undertaking further subspecialty fellowship training.

Prior to the adoption of Flexner's recommended changes, the fields of public health and medicine were intertwined. Regrettably, the new model of medical education had little room for public health and the latter field developed independently. Given the profound advances in basic sciences over the last century and the need for new health care providers to acquire an exponentially increasing knowledge base in physiology, biochemistry, and molecular biology, the social sciences were excluded from most curricula until the 1970s. Since the 1980s, ethics and medical humanities have gained some traction in medical education.

Over the last three to four decades, progressives have developed a strong voice to advocate for the disenfranchised and for inclusion of basic principles of public health and social justice in health professions training and practice. A seminal event was the 1978 conference organized by the World Health Organization (WHO) and the United Nations Children's Emergency Fund (now the United Nations Children's Fund, or UNICEF) at Alma Ata in the Soviet Union. The main product of this meeting was the Alma Ata Declaration, which defines health as a fundamental human right and "a state of complete physical, mental, and social well-being and not merely the absence of disease or infirmity."[2] The declaration emphasizes primary care and addresses many of the economic and social inequities that prevent the attainment of health for all. The declaration has inspired many movements, notably the People's

Health Movement (PHM). The PHM's charter lays out a vision for social justice in public health:

> Equity, ecologically sustainable development and peace are at the heart of our vision of a better world—a world in which a healthy life for all is a reality; a world that respects, appreciates and celebrates all life and diversity; a world that enables the flowering of people's talents and abilities to enrich each other; a world in which people's voices guide the decisions that shape our lives ...[3]

Programs to improve public health and social justice are carried out internationally by groups like the United Nations (UN) and WHO, nationally by entities such as the Centers for Disease Control and Prevention (CDC), and at all levels, locally to internationally, through treaties and by nongovernmental organizations, many of which are identified on the Public Health and Social Justice website (http://www.publichealthandsocialjustice.org or http://www.phsj.org).

Today public health is gaining traction in undergraduate,[4] medical, and nursing education but many efforts are incipient, underfunded, and subject to battles with basic science and clinical departments for curricular time and funding. Some programs involve only a few faculty members, and if these instructors switch institutions, the programs can dissolve. Even so, today major national and international medical organizations advocate for, and accreditation agencies require, training and evaluation in professionalism, including advocacy for the societal, economic, educational, and political changes that can ameliorate suffering and contribute to human well-being.[5]

Nevertheless, important topics in public health and social justice remain marginalized in most curricula taught in health professions training schools, including schools of medicine, nursing, and sometimes even public health. Public health students and professionals often work independently from health care providers, confronting the same health problems, each in their own, important ways, yet without the type of coordinated approach that would improve the health status of individuals and of the overall population.

This reader is designed for health professions students, health care providers, and public health professionals. It provides an exposé of injustices present in the United States and worldwide and an entrée into the lives of society's disenfranchised. I hope the readings contained herein will not only educate health care professionals about important social justice topics, but also motivate them to work collaboratively with each other, with their patients, with nongovernmental organizations, and through their elected officials, to achieve social justice and promote the health and welfare of the world's many peoples.

The reader should also be valuable for undergraduate and graduate students from a number of fields, including but not limited to ethics, sociology, anthropology, history, and philosophy, as well as to activists of all ages working to solve society's most pressing, and often most intractable, problems.

The reader is divided into nine sections:

- The first explores the relationship between public health and social justice, reviews the social determinants of health, lists fundamental human rights, and examines major sociopolitical institutions and trends that have contributed to a world of contradictions—where exorbitant wealth exists alongside desperate poverty and where some have access to boutique medical care while others die prematurely of easily preventable diseases—a world in which access to scientific information can be as limited as access to food, housing, and other basic needs.

- The second section covers special populations that suffer disproportionately from social injustices. These include the homeless; racial, ethnic, and sexual and gender minorities; the mentally ill; migrant farm workers; and prisoners.

- The third section focuses on women's health, particularly forms of individual and structural (or societal) violence against women (including social, educational, political, and legal marginalization, and impaired access to reproductive health services).

- The fourth section covers modern, noninfectious epidemics (obesity, tobacco smoking, and suicide by firearms), whose health care consequences involve enormous suffering and carry huge economic costs, but in which public health advocates have achieved significant successes.

- The fifth section covers food and agriculture, focusing on the pharmaceutical industry-promoted overuse of agricultural antibiotics by factory farms, the health and environmental risks of genetically modified foods, and dangers associated with the use of nonmedicinal hormones in food production.

- The sixth section explores the contributions of social injustice to environmental degradation and global warming; the health, environmental, and human rights consequences of floriculture and of diamond and gold mining; and the "greening" of our health care system.

- The seventh section focuses on war and violence, including economic and social costs; the medical impacts of Hiroshima; human subject experimentation under the Nazis (which raises numerous ethical questions for how contemporary research is conducted); and rape in war.

- The eighth section addresses the role of corporations in subverting, obfuscating, and repressing science in their quest for profit. It describes corporate activities that cause significant adverse consequences for public health. The chapters provide an overview of corporate policies; examine how corporate corruption of science affects workers and the environment; and critique the pharmaceutical industry, the use of unnecessary yet highly reimbursable screening tests, and the drug testing industry.

- The ninth and final section offers advice for health professionals, educators, patients, legislators, and concerned citizens who hope to improve awareness of social justice issues and change social policy. Essays cover the promotion of public understanding of population health; a common agenda for achieving social justice; examples of successful campaigns by activist-oriented groups against corporate malfeasance; the case for a single-payer, national health care plan; the education of medical trainees through immersion in their communities; and pedagogical approaches to teaching health professionals about social justice using great works of literature and photography. Successful campaigns and workable strategies for positive change are highlighted.

The struggle for social justice is a struggle for democracy and equality, which are critical to the survival of our country and indeed the world. The United States, for all its proclamations of moral leadership and support of just causes, has a disturbing history of domestic and international activities antithetical to freedom, peace, and justice. The increasing disparities between rich and poor in America portend societal dissolution and eventual collapse. Primo Levi has counseled, ''A country is considered the more civilized the more the wisdom and efficiency of its laws hinder a weak man from becoming too weak or a powerful one too powerful.''[6] Uncivilized countries eventually dissolve from within.

Advocating for the voiceless and promoting social justice can take many forms but all involve a willingness to speak out on behalf of the disenfranchised, in accordance with Nobel Prize–winning writer Günter Grass's admonition, ''The first job of a citizen is to keep your mouth open.''[7] It is best to start small, think globally and act locally, and join groups committed to solving problems about which you feel particularly passionate. When problems seem overwhelming, remember the African proverb, ''If you think you are too small to have an impact, try going to bed with a mosquito in your tent.'' Do not grow discouraged at what may seem an endless, uphill battle against powerful forces. No doubt those who fought against slavery and child labor and for women's suffrage faced daunting challenges, yet they ultimately succeeded. Keep in mind anthropologist Margaret Mead's encouraging observation, ''Never doubt that a small group of thoughtful, committed people can change the world. Indeed, it is the only thing that ever has.''[8]

Happily, a life spent in the pursuit of justice and service to others can be most satisfying. As Ralph Waldo Emerson recognized, "To know that even one life has breathed easier because you have lived, that is to have succeeded."[9] It is my hope that those who read this book come away with increased knowledge, inspiration, and a burning desire to achieve justice. Together we can create a better world for ourselves, our children, our children's children, and all the creatures of the world.

This Book and the Public Health and Social Justice Website

Physician-editor Gavin Yamey notes that many corporate publishing industry practices make it impossible for most people worldwide, particularly in low- and middle-income countries, to access the biomedical literature. This has important consequences for health care policy makers, practitioners, and ultimately patients. Yamey, acknowledging that knowledge is power, argues that access to scientific and medical knowledge is a human right. He presents an alternative publishing model, open access, a more socially responsive and equitable approach to knowledge dissemination.[10]

The publisher of this book has graciously allowed this reader to realize this model, and all the chapters in this collection that I wrote are available on the Public Health and Social Justice website at http://www.public healthandsocialjustice.org (or http://www.phsj.org). Moreover, almost all the other chapters reprinted herein are available elsewhere on the Internet.

In fact, all of my publications, as well as accompanying open-access slide shows (updated every six to twelve months), syllabi, and contributions from others working in related fields, can be found on the Public Health and Social Justice website (see http://www.publichealthandsocialjustice.org or http://www.phsj.org). (Note that the website's link addresses have "2007" in them.... this is because they were originally created then, and it does not designate when the most recent update occurred.) The site, which also contains links to hundreds of academic programs, publications, and progressive and activist groups, is always accepting new material. This book will be of greatest use to the reader who supplements the articles with the material present on the website.

Notes

1. Roosevelt, F. D. *State of the Union address.* January 11, 1944. Retrieved from http://www.presidency.ucsb.edu/ws/index.php?pid=16518.

2. Baum, F. Health for all now! Reviving the spirit of Alma Ata in the twenty-first century: An introduction to the Alma Ata Declaration. *Social Medicine,* 2007, *2*(1), 34–41. Retrieved from http://www.medicinasocial.info/index.php/social medicine/article/view/76/187.

3. *People's health movement: People's charter for health.* Retrieved from http://www .phmovement.org/sites/www.phmovement.org/files/phm-pch-english.pdf.

4. Association of Schools of Public Health. *Undergraduate public health learning outcomes model.* July 2011. Retrieved from http://www.asph.org/document .cfm?page=1085.

5. American Medical Association. *Declaration of professional responsibility: Medicine's social contract with humanity.* Retrieved from http://www.ama-assn.org /ama/upload/mm/369/decofprofessional.pdf; Earnest, M. A., Shale, L. W., & Federico, S. G. Physician advocacy: What is it and how do we do it? *Academic Medicine,* 2010, *85*(1), 63–67; Royal College of Physicians Policy Statement. *How doctors can close the gap: Tackling the social determinants of health through culture change, advocacy, and education.* Retrieved from http://www.sdu.nhs.uk/docu ments/publications/1279291348_jQjW_how_doctors_can_close_the_gap.pdf, and: http://www.rcplondon.ac.uk/professional-Issues/Public-Health/Documents/RCP -report-how-doctors-can-close-the-gap.pdf. *Global consensus for social accountability of medical schools.* December 2010. Retrieved from http://global healtheducation.org/resources/Documents/Both%20Students%20And%20Faculty /Global_Consensus_for_Social_Accountability_of_Med_Schools.pdf.

6. Levi, P. *Survival at Auschwitz* (New York: Simon and Schuster, 1996; originally published in 1958).

7. Hightower, J. In a time of terror, protest is patriotism. *Hightower Lowdown,* November 14, 2001. Retrieved from http://www.alternet.org/story/11924/.

8. Mead, M. Retrieved from http://www.quotedb.com/quotes/1821.

9. Emerson, R. W. *Success quotes, sayings, and thoughts.* Retrieved from http://www .inspirationalspark.com/success-quotes.html.

10. Yamey, G. Excluding the poor from accessing biomedical literature: A rights violation that impedes global health. *Health and Human Rights,* 2008, *10*(1), 21–42. Retrieved from http://hhrjournal.org/index.php/hhr/article/view/20/103.

Acknowledgments

This book owes its inspiration to a number of individuals who have shaped my life, supported my education, and opened my eyes to the many injustices facing our world, without closing them to the goodness within people and the possibilities for a better world. I hope that in my life and work I can live up to their examples.

My most significant influences have been my family. My father, Martin, and mother, Annette, provided unconditional love and tirelessly sacrificed to offer my brothers and me educational and cultural opportunities that allowed us to reach our full potential. Their parents in turn sacrificed to give them opportunities, such that within just two generations, a wood, coal, and ice salesman and a bookie, housewife, paper mill worker, and cook raised a mathematician and coloratura soprano, who then raised a physician, a CEO, and a teacher and screenwriter. My brothers, Pat and Paul, have always been my best friends, whose loyalty has been constant and whose own passion for education and justice have pushed me to try harder in my endeavors. My sisters-in-law, Michele and Holly, have also been influential and supportive, as has my extended family (Marie, Bob, Katherine, Nell, Tom, Kathleen, Mary, Nance, Peter, Walt, Sue, Kim, Kelly, Tina, Wayne, Trevor, Kirk, Dana, Brett, Justin, Josh, Melanie, Bonnie, George, Brett, Dana, Justin, Josh, and Melanie).

Edith (White) Achterman, Deborah Meyers, Hermione Loofs, Joan Lebow, Tracey Hyams, Karen Adams, and my daughter, Rachel, brought me much happiness, helped me to grow emotionally, and taught me compassion and myriad new ways of thinking about the world. This book is written with hope for the next generation, especially Rachel; my nephews, Ben, Aidan, and Emerson; and my niece, Paris.

Thanks also to Mario Pariante, the Willigs, the Wadmans, Heidi and Steve Bush, the Mularskis, Mohammad Ismail, D'Anne Rygg, Rob and Jutta Rygg, Linda and Betty Ward, John and Chenit Flaherty, Naseem Rakha, Chuck Sheketoff, Robin Larson, Mariano Torres (and all the staff in Waimea, Kauai), Don Baham, Safina Koreishi, Kari Skedsvold, Judy Rubino, and Patty Marshall.

Certain professors and colleagues have encouraged my development, from basic scientist to clinical researcher to clinician to teacher and public health advocate. Sherman Melinkoff, dean emeritus at UCLA, encouraged my love of literature and appreciation for the rich history of medicine. Drs. Harrison Frank and Andrew Ippoliti, my undergraduate and medical school research mentors, inspired a love of scientific inquiry and developed my ability to question the workings of the human body. Dr. Lee Miller, Dr. Marshall Wolf and many other physicians from the UCLA School of Medicine and the Department of Medicine at Brigham and Women's Hospital helped me to develop as a clinician. Dr. Richard Kravitz taught me about health policy and health services research. Dr. Michael Lacombe (with his wife, Maggie) has been particularly generous, influential, and supportive as a mentor and a dear friend. Dr. Hal Holman at Stanford gave the single most important piece of advice any educator has given me in that it led to a dramatic shift in my career plans. On beginning my fellowship training (generously funded by the Robert Wood Johnson Foundation), filled with uncertainty about what to do with my years of education and clinical training (health services research? medical humanities? public health? teaching? clinical medicine?), he told me to "go sit under a tree and read and think for a month." This led to a career in which I have aimed to reverse the early twentieth century schism between medicine and public health, introduce students to literature and history relevant to health care, and help to create practitioners not only skilled at treating individuals but also armed with the knowledge and passion to advocate for social, environmental, and economic justice and for the health of their communities and of the world.

In my professional career, major influences have been physician-activists and ethicist-educators including Matt Anderson, Andy Jameton, Peter White-house, Lanny Smith, Vic Sidel, Barry Levy, Bob Gould, Patrice Sutton, Catherine Thomasson, Martha Livingston, Josh Freeman, Bill Wiist, Nick Freudenberg, Rick North, Patch Adams, Oli Fein, Howard Waitzkin, Neil Arya, Shafik Dharamsi, Shelley White, Jonathan White, Sid Wolfe, Peter Lurie, Sue Daniel-son, Peter Sainsbury, Lynne Madden, Claire Robinson, Albert Hutter, John Pearson, Maye Thompson, Barbara Gottlieb, Fran Storrs, Charles Grossman, Rudi Nussbaum, Andy Harris, Kelly Campbell, Angela Crowley-Koch, Emma Sirois (and all my colleagues at Physicians for Social Responsibility—national and Oregon), Amy Hagopian, Claire Hooker, Federico Hewson, Paul Farmer, Jim Kim, Jared Diamond, Howard Frumkin, Vicente Navarro, Jim Dwyer, David Himmelstein, Steffie Woolhandler, Stephen Bezruchka, David Wallinga, and Lauri Andress. Other major influences on my thinking, without their knowing it, are Charles Dickens, Wendell Berry, Noam Chomsky, Howard Zinn, Carl Sagan, Ralph Nader, Barbara Ehrenreich, Michael Moore, Gret Palast, Eric Schlosser, Jon Stewart, Stephen Colbert, and other members of the progressive media. Thanks also to my clinical colleagues at Kaiser.

I would like to thank Matthew Anderson, Erica Frank, Martha Livingston, and Randall White, who provided thoughtful and constructive comments on the draft manuscript. Thanks also to Vicki Anderson, Ursula Snyder, and Peggy Kean of Medscape, and Cameron Madill and Hannah Ferber from Synotac.

Finally, I am grateful to my editors, Andy Pasternack, Seth Schwartz, and Kelsey McGee, who have been very supportive and generous with their time and expertise.

Most of my essays are a consequence of having my own eyes, brain, and spirit opened by these individuals to the issues I cover. Whatever is good and worthwhile is a product of their influence. Any errors, though unintentional, are entirely my own.

Martin Donohoe

The Editor

Martin Donohoe, MD, FACP, is adjunct associate professor in community health at Portland State University and senior physician in internal medicine at Kaiser Permanente. He serves on the social justice committee of Physicians for Social Responsibility and the board of advisors of Oregon Physicians for Social Responsibility (PSR), and was chief scientific advisor to Oregon PSR's Campaign for Safe Food.

He received his BS and MD from UCLA, completed his internship and residency at Brigham and Women's Hospital/Harvard Medical School, and was a Robert Wood Johnson Clinical Scholar at Stanford University.

Donohoe has taught courses in medical humanities, public health, social justice ethics, women's studies, and the history of medicine at UCLA, UCSF, Stanford, OHSU, Clark College, and Portland State. He writes and frequently lectures on literature and medicine and social justice in public health.

His slide shows, articles, and syllabi can be found at http://www.phsj.org or at http://www.publichealthandsocialjustice.org.

The Contributors

Leo Alexander, MD, was a psychiatrist, neurologist, educator, and author. He helped write the Nuremberg Code after World War II.

Dan E. Beauchamp was a professor of health policy at the School of Public Health at the University of North Carolina at Chapel Hill from 1972 to 1990 and also at the State University of New York at Albany from 1988 to 1998.

Stephen Bezruchka, MPH, is senior lecturer at the Department of Health Services, University of Washington School of Public Health.

Judith B. Bradford, PhD, is director of the Center for Population Research in LGBT health, cochair of The Fenway Institute in Boston.

Eleanor Cooney has published four novels. She lives in Mendocino, California.

Peter A. Clark, SJ, PhD, is the director of the Institute of Catholic Bioethics and a professor of medical ethics at Saint Joseph's University in Philadelphia, Pennsylvania.

Alice Fornari, EdD, is assistant professor, Department of Family and Social Medicine, Albert Einstein College of Medicine, Bronx, New York.

Hilary Goldhammer is with the Fenway Institute in Boston.

Victoria Gorski, MD, is assistant professor, Department of Family and Social Medicine, Albert Einstein College of Medicine, Bronx, New York.

David Hemenway, PhD, is an economist and director of the Harvard Injury Control Research Center and the Harvard Youth Violence Prevention Center in Cambridge, Massachusetts.

David U. Himmelstein, MD, FACP, is professor in the CUNY School of Public Health at Hunter College and visiting professor of medicine at Harvard Medical School. He is also a cofounder of Physicians for a National Health Program.

Andrew Jameton, PhD, is professor in the Department of Health Promotion, Behavioral, & Social Health Sciences, College of Public Health at the University of Nebraska Medical Center.

David S. Jones, MD, PhD, is the A. Bernard Ackerman Professor of the Culture of Medicine at Harvard University.

Lincoln Khasakhala, MBChB, is on staff at Department of Psychiatry, Nairobi University and Africa Mental Health Foundation, Nairobi, Kenya.

Safina Koreishi, MD, is a family physician at the Rosewood Family Health Center Yakima Valley Farmworkers Clinic.

Eliana Korin is senior associate, Department of Family and Social Medicine, Albert Einstein College of Medicine, Bronx, New York.

Stewart Landers is with John Snow, Inc., Boston, and the Massachusetts Department of Public Health, Boston.

Walter J. Lear was a prominent medical and public health administrator, political organizer and activist, and medical archivist and historian.

Barry S. Levy, MD, is a physician and a former president of the American Public Health Association.

Harvey J. Makadon, MD, is director of professional education and development at Fenway Institute in Boston, and with the Division of General Medicine and Primary Care, Beth Israel Deaconess Medical Center, Harvard Medical School, Boston.

Kenneth H. Mayer, MD, is medical research director and cochair of The Fenway Institute, Boston, and Miriam Hospital, Providence, Rhode Island.

Matthew Miller, MD, MPH, ScD, a general internist and medical oncologist, is currently the associate director of the Harvard Injury Control Research Center and an associate professor of health policy and injury prevention at the Harvard School of Public Health.

Peter Montague, PhD, is a historian and journalist and is currently executive director of Environmental Research Foundation, and serves on the board of the Science and Environmental Health Network.

Vicente Navarro, MD, DrPH, is a professor of health and social policy at the Johns Hopkins University. In Spain, he has been an extraordinary professor of economics in the Compentense University in Madrid, a professor of economics at the Barcelona University, and a professor of political and social sciences at the Pompeu Fabra University, where he directs the Public Policy Program jointly sponsored by the Pompeu Fabra University and the Johns Hopkins University.

Emmanuel M. Ngui, DrPH, is assistant professor of health disparities, The UW-Milwaukee Joseph J. Zilber School of Public Health.

Jennifer R. Niebyl, MD, is the head of the department of obstetrics and gynecology, University of Iowa Hospitals and Clinics, Iowa City.

David Nndetei, MD, PhD, is on staff at the Department of Psychiatry, Nairobi University and Africa Mental Health Foundation, Nairobi, Kenya.

Rick North is former project director of the Campaign for Safe Food, Oregon Physicians for Social Responsibility.

Philip Ozuah, MD, PhD, is professor and chair, Department of Pediatrics, Albert Einstein College of Medicine, Bronx, New York.

Matthew Power is a freelance print and radio journalist and a contributing editor at *Harper's Magazine*.

Carolyn Raffensperger, MA, JD, is executive director of the Science and Environmental Health Network.

Laura Weiss Roberts, MD, MA, serves as chairman and Katharine Dexter McCormick and Stanley McCormick Memorial Professor in the Department of Psychiatry and Behavioral Sciences at the Stanford University School of Medicine. She previously was the chairman and Charles E. Kubly Professor of Psychiatry and Behavioral Medicine at the Medical College of Wisconsin and professor and vice chair for administration in the Department of Psychiatry, the Jack and Donna Rust Professor of Biomedical Ethics, and the founder and director of the Institute of Ethics at the University of New Mexico.

Peter A. Selwyn, MD, MPH, is professor and chair, Department of Family and Social Medicine, Albert Einstein College of Medicine, Bronx, New York.

Victor W. Sidel, MD, is adjunct professor of public health at Weill Medical College of Cornell University. He was also chair of the Department of Social Medicine at Montefiore Medical Center and the Albert Einstein College of Medicine, Bronx, New York, and was appointed Distinguished University Professor of Social Medicine in 1984.

Ron Stall, PhD, MPH, is with the Graduate School of Public Health, University of Pittsburgh, as professor and chair, Department of Behavioral and Community Health Sciences and Department of Infectious Diseases and Microbiology.

Elanor Starmer is a special assistant at the US Department of Agriculture. She previously served as western region director at Food & Water Watch and a contributing writer at ethicurean.com.

A. H. Strelnick, MD, is professor, Department of Family and Social Medicine, Albert Einstein College of Medicine, Bronx, New York.

Debbie Swiderski, MD, is assistant professor, Department of Medicine, Albert Einstein College of Medicine, Bronx, New York.

Catherine Thomasson, MD, is executive director of the national organization Physicians for Social Responsibility (PSR), Washington, DC.

Janet M. Townsend, MD, is associate professor, Department of Family and Social Medicine, Albert Einstein College of Medicine, Bronx, New York.

Pamela Bea Wilson Vergun, PhD, was the translator and editor of *A Dimly Burning Wick* and is a sociologist and policy analyst.

Robert Vergun, PhD, provides education research and economic analysis for Portland Community College in Oregon.

David Wallinga, MD, MPA, is a senior advisor in science, food, and health at the Institute for Agriculture and Trade Policy, Minneapolis.

Robert Weissman, JD, is the president of Public Citizen.

Steffie Woolhandler, MD, MPH, FACP, is professor in the CUNY School of Public Health at Hunter College and visiting professor of medicine at Harvard Medical School. She is also a cofounder of Physicians for a National Health Program.

Public Health
and Social Justice

Part One

Human Rights, Social Justice, Economics, Poverty, and Health Care

In the wake of the Nazi atrocities of World War II, the newborn United Nations (UN) established a commission on human rights to enumerate the fundamental rights of mankind. This group completed the Universal Declaration on Human Rights, which was adopted by the UN in 1948. The thirty rights laid out in this seminal document form the basis for many subsequent national laws as well as international treaties and agreements. These rights grew out of numerous religious and political traditions, historical documents, and social movements. The declaration is the first chapter in this collection because the rights elaborated therein provide the foundation for all the social justice issues discussed in this reader.[1]

Chapter Two (by Dan E. Beauchamp) was originally presented at the American Public Health Association's annual meeting in 1975, yet it remains relevant today because it provides an ethical framework for the relationship between public health and social justice. The author defines justice as the fair and equitable distribution of society's benefits and burdens. He contrasts the dominant model of American justice, market justice, with its opposite, social justice. In the spirit of Rudolph Virchow (the father of social medicine, discussed in the reader's final chapter) and others, he emphasizes the right to health, prevention, collective action, and the importance of political struggle in achieving justice.

Chapter Three (by Vicente Navarro) provides an overview of the importance of class, race, and gender power relations within and between countries. The author argues that an alliance between the dominant classes of developed and developing countries is responsible for many of the neoliberal policies carried out by market-oriented countries and by global institutions such as the World Bank and the International Monetary Fund. These organizations, a product of the Bretton Woods Conference of 1944, are supposed to stabilize world economies while ensuring that aid to developing nations promotes sustainable economic growth and poverty reduction. Unfortunately, neoliberal policies have increased class divisions, damaged the environment, encouraged the profitable (for a few) privatization of public resources, and impeded the development of national health care programs and other public health interventions, subverting social justice and contributing to suffering and death. Navarro examines different governmental traditions in terms of their contributions to developing a public health infrastructure based on principles of social justice.

The next two chapters describe extremes of life faced by the bitterly poor and the über-rich. Matthew Power's evocative Chapter Four on trickle-down economics in a Philippine garbage dump documents the miserable, hard-scrabble existence of those who struggle to meet life's most basic needs while living and working atop a hundred-foot mountain of trash in a country where nearly half the population lives on less than two dollars a day. This is followed by Chapter Five (by Martin Donohoe), which describes the phenomenon of luxury (also known as concierge or boutique) health care, a relatively recent development currently available to the wealthiest citizens. Although most Americans live under a mediocre health care system that provides middling outcomes, our wealthiest citizens can take advantage of luxury care, often in clinics associated with academic medical centers. These centers are widely recognized as the arbiters of cost-effective medical testing, and have been the traditional providers to the poor and underserved. However, their concierge clinics often promote excessive, clinically unsupported testing, catering to patients' fears of unrecognized disease, which can lead to worse outcomes. Furthermore, while supporting luxury care clinics, many have limited their provision of services to the medically needy. Not covered in this chapter are other forms of "health care" available to the rich, such as transplant tourism (which often uses organs obtained through illegal and immoral means from the desperately poor). To learn more about luxury care, visit the luxury care/concierge care page of the Public Health and Social Justice website at http://phsj.org/luxury-care-concierge-care/.

Note

1. Leaning, J. (1997). Human rights and medical education: Why every medical student should learn the Universal Declaration of Human Rights. *BMJ*, 1997, *315*,1390–1391. Retrieved from http://www.bmj.com/content/315/7120/1390.full

Chapter 1

Universal Declaration of Human Rights

Preamble

Whereas recognition of the inherent dignity and of the equal and inalienable rights of all members of the human family is the foundation of freedom, justice and peace in the world,

Whereas disregard and contempt for human rights have resulted in barbarous acts which have outraged the conscience of mankind, and the advent of a world in which human beings shall enjoy freedom of speech and belief and freedom from fear and want has been proclaimed as the highest aspiration of the common people,

Whereas it is essential, if man is not to be compelled to have recourse, as a last resort, to rebellion against tyranny and oppression, that human rights should be protected by the rule of law,

Whereas it is essential to promote the development of friendly relations between nations,

Whereas the peoples of the United Nations have in the Charter reaffirmed their faith in fundamental human rights, in the dignity and worth of the human person and in the equal rights of men and women and have determined to promote social progress and better standards of life in larger freedom,

Whereas Member States have pledged themselves to achieve, in cooperation with the United Nations, the promotion of universal respect for and observance of human rights and fundamental freedoms,

Whereas a common understanding of these rights and freedoms is of the greatest importance for the full realization of this pledge,

Now, therefore,

The General Assembly,

Proclaims this Universal Declaration of Human Rights as a common standard of achievement for all peoples and all nations, to the end that every individual and every organ of society, keeping this Declaration constantly in mind, shall strive by teaching and education to promote respect for these rights and freedoms and by progressive measures, national and international, to secure their universal and effective recognition and observance, both among the peoples of Member States themselves and among the peoples of territories under their jurisdiction.

Article 1

All human beings are born free and equal in dignity and rights. They are endowed with reason and conscience and should act towards one another in a spirit of brotherhood.

Article 2

Everyone is entitled to all the rights and freedoms set forth in this Declaration, without distinction of any kind, such as race, colour, sex, language, religion, political or other opinion, national or social origin, property, birth or other status. Furthermore, no distinction shall be made on the basis of the political, jurisdictional or international status of the country or territory to which a person belongs, whether it be independent, trust, non-self-governing or under any other limitation of sovereignty.

Article 3

Everyone has the right to life, liberty and security of person.

Article 4

No one shall be held in slavery or servitude; slavery and the slave trade shall be prohibited in all their forms.

Article 5

No one shall be subjected to torture or to cruel, inhuman or degrading treatment or punishment.

Article 6

Everyone has the right to recognition everywhere as a person before the law.

Article 7

All are equal before the law and are entitled without any discrimination to equal protection of the law. All are entitled to equal protection against any discrimination in violation of this Declaration and against any incitement to such discrimination.

Article 8

Everyone has the right to an effective remedy by the competent national tribunals for acts violating the fundamental rights granted him by the constitution or by law.

Article 9

No one shall be subjected to arbitrary arrest, detention or exile.

Article 10

Everyone is entitled in full equality to a fair and public hearing by an independent and impartial tribunal, in the determination of his rights and obligations and of any criminal charge against him.

Article 11

1. Everyone charged with a penal offence has the right to be presumed innocent until proved guilty according to law in a public trial at which he has had all the guarantees necessary for his defence.
2. No one shall be held guilty of any penal offence on account of any act or omission which did not constitute a penal offence, under national or international law, at the time when it was committed. Nor shall a heavier penalty be imposed than the one that was applicable at the time the penal offence was committed.

Article 12

No one shall be subjected to arbitrary interference with his privacy, family, home or correspondence, nor to attacks upon his honour and reputation. Everyone has the right to the protection of the law against such interference or attacks.

Article 13

1. Everyone has the right to freedom of movement and residence within the borders of each State.
2. Everyone has the right to leave any country, including his own, and to return to his country.

Article 14

1. Everyone has the right to seek and to enjoy in other countries asylum from persecution.
2. This right may not be invoked in the case of prosecutions genuinely arising from non-political crimes or from acts contrary to the purposes and principles of the United Nations.

Article 15

1. Everyone has the right to a nationality.
2. No one shall be arbitrarily deprived of his nationality nor denied the right to change his nationality.

Article 16

1. Men and women of full age, without any limitation due to race, nationality or religion, have the right to marry and to found a family. They are entitled to equal rights as to marriage, during marriage and at its dissolution.

2. Marriage shall be entered into only with the free and full consent of the intending spouses.

3. The family is the natural and fundamental group unit of society and is entitled to protection by society and the State.

Article 17

1. Everyone has the right to own property alone as well as in association with others.

2. No one shall be arbitrarily deprived of his property.

Article 18

Everyone has the right to freedom of thought, conscience and religion; this right includes freedom to change his religion or belief, and freedom, either alone or in community with others and in public or private, to manifest his religion or belief in teaching, practice, worship and observance.

Article 19

Everyone has the right to freedom of opinion and expression; this right includes freedom to hold opinions without interference and to seek, receive and impart information and ideas through any media and regardless of frontiers.

Article 20

1. Everyone has the right to freedom of peaceful assembly and association.

2. No one may be compelled to belong to an association.

Article 21

1. Everyone has the right to take part in the government of his country, directly or through freely chosen representatives.

2. Everyone has the right to equal access to public service in his country.

3. The will of the people shall be the basis of the authority of government; this will shall be expressed in periodic and genuine elections which shall be by universal and equal suffrage and shall be held by secret vote or by equivalent free voting procedures.

Article 22

Everyone, as a member of society, has the right to social security and is entitled to realization, through national effort and international co-operation and in accordance with the organization and resources of each State, of the economic, social and cultural rights indispensable for his dignity and the free development of his personality.

Article 23

1. Everyone has the right to work, to free choice of employment, to just and favourable conditions of work and to protection against unemployment.

2. Everyone, without any discrimination, has the right to equal pay for equal work.

3. Everyone who works has the right to just and favourable remuneration ensuring for himself and his family an existence worthy of human dignity, and supplemented, if necessary, by other means of social protection.

4. Everyone has the right to form and to join trade unions for the protection of his interests.

Article 24

Everyone has the right to rest and leisure, including reasonable limitation of working hours and periodic holidays with pay.

Article 25

1. Everyone has the right to a standard of living adequate for the health and well-being of himself and of his family, including food, clothing, housing and medical care and necessary social services, and the right to security in the event of unemployment, sickness, disability, widowhood, old age or other lack of livelihood in circumstances beyond his control.

2. Motherhood and childhood are entitled to special care and assistance. All children, whether born in or out of wedlock, shall enjoy the same social protection.

Article 26

1. Everyone has the right to education. Education shall be free, at least in the elementary and fundamental stages. Elementary education shall be compulsory. Technical and professional education shall be made generally available and higher education shall be equally accessible to all on the basis of merit.

2. Education shall be directed to the full development of the human personality and to the strengthening of respect for human rights and fundamental freedoms. It shall promote understanding, tolerance and friendship among all nations, racial or religious groups, and shall further the activities of the United Nations for the maintenance of peace.

3. Parents have a prior right to choose the kind of education that shall be given to their children.

Article 27

1. Everyone has the right freely to participate in the cultural life of the community, to enjoy the arts and to share in scientific advancement and its benefits.

2. Everyone has the right to the protection of the moral and material interests resulting from any scientific, literary or artistic production of which he is the author.

Article 28

Everyone is entitled to a social and international order in which the rights and freedoms set forth in this Declaration can be fully realized.

Article 29

1. Everyone has duties to the community in which alone the free and full development of his personality is possible.

2. In the exercise of his rights and freedoms, everyone shall be subject only to such limitations as are determined by law solely for the purpose of securing due recognition and respect for the rights and freedoms of others and of meeting the just requirements of morality, public order and the general welfare in a democratic society.

3. These rights and freedoms may in no case be exercised contrary to the purposes and principles of the United Nations.

Article 30

Nothing in this Declaration may be interpreted as implying for any State, group or person any right to engage in any activity or to perform any act aimed at the destruction of any of the rights and freedoms set forth herein.

Chapter 2

Public Health as Social Justice

Dan E. Beauchamp

A nthony Downs has observed that our most intractable public problems have two significant characteristics. First, they occur to a relative minority of our population (even though that minority may number millions of people). Second, they result in significant part from arrangements that are providing substantial benefits or advantages to a majority or to a powerful minority of citizens. Thus solving or minimizing these problems requires painful losses, the restructuring of society and the acceptance of new burdens by the most powerful and the most numerous on behalf of the least powerful or the least numerous. As Downs notes, this bleak reality has resulted in recent years in cycles of public attention to such problems as poverty, racial discrimination, poor housing, unemployment or the abandonment of the aged; however, this attention and interest rapidly wane when it becomes clear that solving these problems requires painful costs that the dominant interests in society are unwilling to pay. Our public ethics do not seem to fit our public problems.

It is not sufficiently appreciated that these same bleak realities plague attempts to protect the public's health. Automobile-related injury and death; tobacco, alcohol and other drug damage; the perils of the workplace; environmental pollution; the inequitable and ineffective distribution of medical care services; the hazards of biomedicine — all of these threats inflict death and disability on a minority of our society at any given time. Further, minimizing or even significantly reducing the death and disability from these perils entails that the majority or powerful minorities accept new burdens or relinquish existing privileges that they presently enjoy. Typically, these new burdens or restrictions involve more stringent controls over these and other hazards of the world.

This somber reality suggests that our fundamental attention in public health policy and prevention should not be directed toward a search for new technology, but rather toward breaking existing ethical and political barriers to minimizing death and disability. This is not to say that technology will never again help avoid painful social and political adjustments. Nonetheless, only the technological Pollyannas will ignore the mounting evidence that the critical barriers to protecting the public against death and disability are not the barriers to technological progress—indeed the evidence is that it is often technology itself that is our own worst enemy. The critical barrier to dramatic reductions in death and disability is a social ethic that unfairly protects the most numerous or the most powerful from the burdens of prevention.

This is the issue of justice. In the broadest sense, justice means that each person in society ought to receive his due and that the burdens and benefits of society should be fairly and equitably distributed. But what criteria should be followed in allocating burdens and benefits: Merit, equality or need? What end or goal in life should receive our highest priority: Life, liberty or the pursuit of happiness? The answer to these questions can be found in our prevailing theories or models of justice. These models of justice, roughly speaking, form the foundation of our politics and public policy in general, and our health policy (including our prevention policy) specifically. Here I am speaking of politics not as partisan politics but rather the more ancient and venerable meaning of the political as the search for the common good and the just society.

These models of justice furnish a symbolic framework or blueprint with which to think about and react to the problems of the public, providing the basic rules to classify and categorize problems of society as to whether they necessitate public and collective protection or whether individual responsibility should prevail. These models function as a sort of map or guide to the common world of members of society, making visible some conditions in society as public issues and concerns, and hiding, obscuring or concealing other conditions that might otherwise emerge as public issues or problems were a different map or model of justice in hand.

In the case of health, these models of justice form the basis for thinking about and reacting to the problems of disability and premature death in society. Thus, if public health policy requires that the majority or a powerful minority accept their fair share of the burdens of protecting a relative minority threatened with death or disability, we need to ask if our prevailing model of justice contemplates and legitimates such sacrifices.

Market-Justice

The dominant model of justice in the American experience has been market-justice. Under the norms of market-justice people are entitled only to those valued ends such as status, income, happiness, etc., that they have acquired by fair rules of entitlement, e.g., by their own individual efforts, actions or abilities. Market-justice emphasizes individual responsibility, minimal collective action and freedom from collective obligations except to respect other persons' fundamental rights.

While we have as a society compromised pure market-justice in many ways to protect the public's health, we are far from recognizing the principle that death and disability are collective problems and that all persons are entitled to health protection. Society does not recognize a general obligation to protect the individual against disease and injury. While society does prohibit individuals from causing direct harm to others, and has in many instances regulated clear public health hazards, the norm of market-justice is still dominant and the primary duty to avert disease and injury still rests with the individual. The individual is ultimately alone in his or her struggle against death.

Barriers to Protection

This individual isolation creates a powerful barrier to the goal of protecting all human life by magnifying the power of death, granting to death an almost supernatural reality. Death has throughout history presented a basic problem to humankind, but even in an advanced society with enormous biomedical technology, the individualism of market-justice tends to retain and exaggerate pessimistic and fatalistic attitudes toward death and injury. This fatalism leads to a sense of powerlessness, to the acceptance of risk as an essential element of life, to resignation in the face of calamity, and to a weakening of collective impulses to confront the problems of premature death and disability.

Perhaps the most direct way in which market-justice undermines our resolve to preserve and protect human life lies in the primary freedom this ethic extends to all individuals and groups to act with minimal obligations to protect the common good. Despite the fact that this rule of self-interest predictably fails to protect adequately the safety of our workplaces, our modes of transportation, the physical environment, the commodities we consume or the equitable and effective distribution of medical care, these failures have resulted so far in only half-hearted attempts at regulation and control. This response is explained in large part by the powerful sway market-justice holds over our imagination, granting fundamental freedom to all individuals to be left alone—even if the "individuals" in question are giant producer groups with enormous capacities to create great public harm through sheer inadvertence. Efforts for truly effective controls over these perils must constantly struggle against a prevailing ethical paradigm that defines as threats to fundamental freedoms attempts to assure that all groups—even powerful producer groups—accept their fair share of the burdens of prevention.

Market-justice is also the source of another major barrier to public health measures to minimize death and disability—the category of voluntary behavior. Market-justice forces a basic distinction between the harm caused by a factory polluting the atmosphere and the harm caused by the cigarette or alcohol industries, because in the latter case those that are harmed are perceived as engaged in "voluntary" behavior. It is the radical individualism inherent in the market model that encourages attention to the individual's behavior and inattention to the social preconditions of that behavior. In the case of smoking, these preconditions include a powerful cigarette industry and accompanying social and cultural forces encouraging the practice of smoking. These social forces include norms sanctioning smoking as well as all forms of media, advertising, literature, movies, folklore, etc. Since the smoker is free in some ultimate sense to not smoke, the norms of market-justice force the conclusion that the individual voluntarily "chooses" to smoke; and we are prevented from taking strong collective action against the powerful structures encouraging this so-called voluntary behavior.

Yet another way in which the market ethic obstructs the possibilities for minimizing death and disability, and [provides] alibis [for] the need for structural change, is through explanations for death and disability that "blame the victim." Victim-blaming misdefines structural and collective problems of the entire society as individual problems, seeing these problems as caused by the behavioral failures or deficiencies of the victims. These behavioral explanations for public problems tend to protect the larger society and powerful interests from the burdens of collective action, and instead encourage attempts to change the "faulty" behavior of victims.

Market-justice is perhaps the major cause for our over-investment and over-confidence in curative medical services. It is not obvious that the rise of medical science and the physician, taken alone, should become fundamental obstacles to collective action to prevent death and injury. But the prejudice found in market-justice against collective action perverts these scientific advances into an unrealistic hope for "technological shortcuts" to painful social change. Moreover, the great emphasis placed on individual achievement in market-justice has further diverted attention and interest away from primary prevention and collective action by dramatizing the role of the solitary physician-scientist, picturing him as our primary weapon and first line of defense against the threat of death and injury....

Public Health Measures

I have saved for last an important class of health policies—public health measures to protect the environment, the workplace or the commodities we purchase and consume. Are these not signs that the American society is willing to accept collective action in the face of clear public health hazards?

I do not wish to minimize the importance of these advances to protect the public in many domains. But these separate reforms, taken alone, should be cautiously received. This is because each reform effort is perceived as an isolated exception to the norm of market-justice; the norm itself still stands. Consequently, the predictable career of such measures is to see enthusiasm for enforcement peak and wane. These public health measures are clear signs of hope. But as long as these actions are seen as merely minor exceptions to the rule of individual responsibility, the goals of public health will remain beyond our reach. What is required is for the public to see that protecting the public's health takes us beyond the norms of market-justice categorically, and necessitates a completely new health ethic....

Social Justice

The fundamental critique of market-justice found in the Western liberal tradition is social justice. Under social justice all persons are entitled equally to key ends such as health protection or minimum standards of income. Further, unless collective burdens are accepted, powerful forces of environment, heredity or social structure will preclude a fair distribution of these ends. While many forces influenced the development of public health, the historic dream of public health that preventable death and disability ought to be minimized is a dream of social justice. Yet these egalitarian and social justice implications of the public health vision are either still not widely recognized or are conveniently ignored....

Ideally, then, the public health ethic is not simply an alternative to the market ethic for health—it is a fundamental critique of that ethic as it unjustly protects powerful interests from the burdens of prevention and as that ethic serves to legitimate a mindless and extravagant faith in the efficacy of medical care. In other words, the public health ethic is a *counter-ethic* to market-justice and the ethics of individualism as these are applied to the health problems of the public....

This new ethic has several key implications which are referred to here as "principles": (1) controlling the hazards of this world, (2) to prevent death and disability, (3) through organized collective action, (4) shared equally by all except where unequal burdens result in increased protection of everyone's health and especially potential victims of death and disability.

These ethical principles are not new to public health. To the contrary, making the ethical foundations of public health visible only serves to highlight the social justice influences at work behind pre-existing principles.

Controlling the Hazards

A key principle of the public health ethic is the focus on the identification and control of the hazards of this world rather than a focus on the behavioral defects of those individuals damaged by these hazards. Against this principle it is often argued that today the causes of death and disability are multiple and frequently behavioral in origin. Further, since it is usually only a minority of the public that fails to protect itself against most known hazards, additional controls over these perilous sources would not seem to be effective or just. We should look instead for the behavioral origins of most public health problems, asking why some people expose themselves to known hazards or perils or act in an unsafe or careless manner.

Public health should—at least ideally—be suspicious of behavioral paradigms for viewing public health problems since they tend to "blame the victim" and unfairly protect majorities and powerful interests from the burdens of prevention. It is clear that behavioral models of public health problems are rooted in the tradition of market-justice, where the emphasis is upon individual ability and capacity, and individual success and failure.

Public health, ideally, should not be concerned with explaining the successes and failures of differing individuals (dispositional explanations) in controlling the hazards of this world . . . .

Prevention

Like the other principles of public health, prevention is a logical consequence of the ethical goal of minimizing the numbers of persons suffering death and disability. The only known way to minimize these adverse events is to prevent the occurrence of damaging exchanges or exposures in the first place or to seek to minimize damage when exposures cannot be controlled.

Prevention, then, is that set of priority rules for restructuring existing market rules in order to maximally protect the public. These rules seek to create policies and obligations to replace the norm of market-justice, where the latter permits specific conditions, commodities, services, products, activities or practices to pose a direct threat or hazard to the health and safety of members of the public, or where the market norm fails to allocate effectively and equitably those services (such as medical care) that are necessary to attend to disease at hand.

Thus, the familiar public health options:

1. Creating rules to minimize exposure of the public to hazards (kinetic, chemical, ionizing, biological, etc.) so as to reduce the rates of hazardous exchanges

2. Creating rules to strengthen the public against damage in the event damaging exchanges occur anyway, where such techniques (fluoridation, seatbelts, immunization) are feasible

3. Creating rules to organize treatment resources in the community so as to minimize damage that does occur since we can rarely prevent all damage

Collective Action

Another principle of the public health ethic is that the control of hazards cannot be achieved through voluntary mechanisms but must be undertaken by governmental or non-governmental agencies through planned, organized and collective action that is obligatory or non-voluntary in nature. This is for two reasons.

The first is because market or voluntary action is typically inadequate for providing what are called public goods. Public goods are those public policies (national defense, police and fire protection or the protection of all persons against preventable death and disability) that are universal in their impacts and effects, affecting everyone equally. These kinds of goods cannot easily be withheld from those individuals in the community who choose not to support these services (this is typically called the "free rider" problem). Also, individual holdouts might plausibly reason that their small contribution might not prevent the public good from being offered.

The second reason why self-regarding individuals might refuse to voluntarily pay the costs of such public goods as public health policies is because these policies frequently require burdens that self-interest or self-protection might see as too stringent. For example, the minimization of rates of alcoholism in a community clearly seems to require norms or controls over the substance of alcohol that limit the use of this substance to levels that are far below what would be safe for individual drinkers.

With these temptations for individual noncompliance, justice demands assurance that all persons share equally the costs of collective action through obligatory and sanctioned social and public policy.

Fair-Sharing of the Burdens

A final principle of the public health ethic is that all persons are equally responsible for sharing the burdens—as well as the benefits—of protection against death and disability, except where unequal burdens result in greater protection for every person and especially potential victims of death and disability. In practice this means that policies to control the hazards of a given substance, service or commodity fall unequally (but still fairly) on those involved in the production, provision or consumption of service, commodity or substance. The clear implication of this principle is that the automotive industry, the tobacco industry, the coal industry and the medical care industry—to mention only a few key groups—have an unequal responsibility to bear the costs of reducing death and disability since their actions have far greater impact than those of individual citizens.

Doing Justice: Building a New Public Health

I have attempted to show the broad implications of a public health commitment to protect and preserve human life, setting out tentatively the logical consequences of that commitment in the form of some general principles. We need, however, to go beyond these broad principles and ask more specifically: What implications does this model have for doing public health and the public health profession?

The central implication of the view set out here is that doing public health should not be narrowly conceived as an instrumental or technical activity. Public health should be a way of doing justice, a way of asserting the value and priority of all human life. The primary aim of all public health activity should be the elaboration and adoption of a new ethical model or paradigm for protecting the public's health. This new ethical paradigm will necessitate a heightened consciousness of the manifold forces threatening human life, and will require thinking about and reacting to the problems of disability and premature death as primarily collective problems of the entire society . . . .

Conclusion

The central thesis of this article is that public health is ultimately and essentially an ethical enterprise committed to the notion that all persons are entitled to protection against the hazards of this world and to the minimization of death and disability in society. I have tried to make the implications of this ethical vision manifest, especially as the public health ethic challenges and confronts the norms of market-justice.

I do not see these goals of public health as hopelessly unrealistic nor destructive of fundamental liberties. Public health may be an "alien ethic in a strange land." Yet, if anything, the public health ethic is more faithful to the traditions of Judeo-Christian ethics than is market-justice.

The image of public health that I have drawn here does raise legitimate questions about what it is to be a professional, and legitimate questions about reasonable limits to restrictions on human liberty. These questions must be addressed more thoroughly than I have done here. Nonetheless, we must never pass over the chaos of preventable disease and disability in our society by simply celebrating the benefits of our prosperity and abundance or our technological advances. What are these benefits worth if they have been purchased at the price of human lives?

Nothing written here should be construed as a per se attack on the market system. I have, rather, surfaced the moral and ethical norms of that system and argued that, whatever other benefits might accrue from those norms, they are woefully inadequate to assure full and equal protection of all human life.

The adoption of a new public health ethic and a new public health policy must and should occur within the context of a democratic polity. I agree with Professor Milton Terris that the central task of the public health movement is to persuade society to accept these measures.

Finally, it is a peculiarity of the word *freedom* that its meaning has become so distorted and stretched as to lend itself as a defense against nearly every attempt to extend equal health protection to all persons. This is the ultimate irony. The idea of liberty should mean, above all else, the liberation of society from the injustice of preventable disability and early death. Instead, the concept of freedom has become a defense and protection of powerful vested interests, and the central issue is viewed as a choice between freedom on the one hand and health and safety on the other. I am confident that ultimately the public will come to see that extending life and health to all persons will require some diminution of personal choices, but that such restrictions are not only fair and do not constitute abridgement of fundamental liberties, they are a basic sign and imprint of a just society and a guarantee of that most basic of all freedoms—protection against man's most ancient foe.

Chapter 3

What We Mean by Social Determinants of Health

Vicente Navarro

Introduction: Welcoming the WHO Commission on Social Determinants of Health

Thank you very much for inviting me to give the inaugural speech at the Eighth European Conference of the International Union of Health Promotion and Education, taking place in this beautiful setting in Turin, Italy.[1] Let me start by congratulating you on choosing as a major theme of this conference the social determinants of health. As you know, the WHO Commission on Social Determinants of Health has just published its long-awaited report. The report has, deservedly, created worldwide interest and within a few days has monopolized the health and medical news worldwide—with some notable exceptions such as the United States, where the report has barely been noticed in the media. I saluted the establishment of the WHO Commission and now applaud most of the recommendations in its report. But my enthusiasm for the report is not uncritical, and I will enlarge on this later in my presentation.

Let's start with some of the facts presented in the Commission's report, facts that should cause discomfort for any person committed to the health and quality of life of our populations, because the problems described in the report—how death and poor health are not randomly distributed in the world—are easily solvable. We know how to solve them. The problem, however, is not a scientific one. But before touching on this issue—the major theme of my talk—let's look at the facts.

To quote one statistic directly from the report: ''A girl born in Sweden will live 43 years longer than a girl born in Sierra Leone.'' The mortality differentials among countries are enormous. But such inequalities also appear within each country, including the so-called rich or developed countries. Again, quoting from the report: "In Glasgow, an unskilled, working-class person will have a lifespan 28 years shorter than a businessman in the top income bracket in Scotland." We could add here similar data from the United States. In East Baltimore (where my university, the Johns Hopkins University, is located), a black unemployed youth has a lifespan 32 years shorter than a white corporate lawyer. Actually, as I have documented elsewhere,[2] a young African American is 1.8 times more likely than a young white American to die from a cardiovascular condition. Race mortality differentials are large in the United States, but class mortality differentials are even larger. In the same study, I showed that a blue-collar worker is 2.8 times more likely than a businessman to die from a cardiovascular condition. In the United States, as in any other country, the highest number of deaths could be prevented by interventions in which the mortality rate of all social classes was made the same as the mortality rate of those in the top income decile. These are the types of facts that the WHO Commission report and other works have documented. So, at this point, the evidence that health and quality of life are socially determined is undeniable and overwhelming.

Changes in Political, Economic, and Social Contexts over the Past 30 Years

Before discussing the results and recommendations of the WHO Commission, I want to analyze the changes we have seen in the world over the past 30 years—changes in the social, political, and economic contexts in which mortality inequalities are produced and reproduced. The most noticeable changes are those that were initiated by President Reagan in the United States and by Prime Minister Thatcher in Great Britain in the late 1970s and early 1980s. During the period 1980–2008, we have seen the promotion of public policies throughout the world that are based on the narrative that (a) the state (or what is usually referred to in popular parlance as "the government") must reduce its interventions in economic and social activities; (b) labor and financial markets must be deregulated in order to liberate the enormous creative energy of the market; and (c) commerce and investments must be stimulated by eliminating borders and barriers to the full mobility of labor, capital, goods, and services. These policies constitute the *neoliberal* ideology.

Translation of these policies in the health sector has created a new policy environment that emphasizes (a) the need to reduce public responsibility for the health of populations; (b) the need to increase choice and markets; (c) the need to transform national health services into insurance-based health care systems; (d) the need to privatize medical care; (e) a discourse in which patients are referred to as *clients* and planning is replaced by *markets*; (f) individuals' personal responsibility for health improvements; (g) an understanding of health promotion as behavioral change; and (h) the need for individuals to increase their personal responsibility by adding social capital to their endowment. The past 30 years have witnessed the implementation of these policies and practices worldwide, including in the United States, in the European Union, and in international agencies such as the WHO. Such policies have appeared in the *Washington Consensus,* in the *Brussels Consensus,* and, indeed, in the WHO *Consensus,* as evidenced by the *WHO Report 2000* on health systems performance.[3,4]

The theoretical framework for development of these economic and social policies was the belief that the economic world order has changed, with a globalization of economic activity (stimulated by these policies) that is responsible for unprecedented worldwide economic growth. In this new economic and social order, states are losing power and are being supplanted by a new, worldwide market-centered economy based on multinational corporations, which are assumed to be the main units of activity in the world today. This theoretical scenario became, until recently, dogma, applauded by the *New York Times,* the *Financial Times,* the *Economist,* and many other media instruments that reproduce neoliberal establishments' conventional wisdom around the world.

While these organs of the financial establishment applaud the neoliberal scenario, there are those in the anti-establishment tradition (such as Susan George, Eric Hobsbawm, large sectors of the anti-globalization movement, and the World Social Forum, among others) that lament it. But they interpret the reality in the same way: that we are living in a globalized world in which the power of states is being replaced by the power of multinational corporations; the only difference is that while the establishment forces applaud globalization, the anti-establishment forces mourn it. The problem with this interpretation of reality is that both sides—the establishment and the anti-establishment forces—are wrong!

Look at the Practice, Not the Theory, of Neoliberalism

We need to analyze the ideological assumptions underlying these interpretations of current realities. To start with, contrary to the claims of neoliberal theory, *there has been no reduction of the public sector in most OECD countries.* In most countries, public expenditures (as percentage of gross national product [GNP] and as expenditures per capita) have grown. In the United States, the leader of the neoliberal movement, public expenditures increased from 34 percent of GNP in 1980, when President Reagan started the neoliberal revolution, to 38 percent of GNP in 2007; and they increased from $4,148 per capita in 1980 to $18,758 per capita in 2007. We have also seen that in most OECD countries, there has been an increase rather than a decrease in taxes as percentage of GNP: in the United States, an increase from 35 percent in 1980 to 39 percent in 2007; or, without payroll taxes, an increase from 32 percent in 1980 to 36 percent in 2007. Actually, under President Reagan, the United States saw an increase in federal public expenditures from 21.6 percent to 23 percent of GNP, while taxes increased not once, but twice. As a matter of fact, Reagan increased taxes for a greater number of people (in peace time) than any other US president. He reduced taxes for the top 20 percent of earners but increased taxes for everyone else. As John Williamson, the father of the neoliberal Washington consensus, wrote, "We have to recognize that what the US government promotes abroad, the US government does not follow at home."[5]

What we are witnessing in recent days, with active federal interventions to resolve the banking crisis created by deregulation of the banking industry, is just one more example of how wrong is the thesis that states are being replaced by multinationals! States are not disappearing. What we are seeing is not a reduction of state interventions, but rather a change in the nature of these interventions. This is evident if we look at the evolution of public federal expenditures. In 1980, the beginning of the neoliberal revolution, 38 percent of these expenditures went to programs targeted to persons, 41 percent to the military, and 21 percent to private enterprises. By 2007, these percentages had changed quite dramatically: expenditures on persons declined to 32 percent, military expenditures increased to 45 percent, and expenditures in support of private enterprises increased to 23 percent. And all of this occurred before the massive assistance now going to the banking community (as a way of resolving the financial crisis) as approved by the US Congress.

A similar situation is evident in the health care sector. We have seen further privatization of health services, with expansion of the role of insurance companies in the health sector supported by fiscal policies, from tax exemptions to tax subsidies that have increased exponentially. Similarly, the private management of public services has been accompanied by an increased reliance on markets, co-payments, and co-insurances. There has also been a massive growth of both public and private investment in biomedical and genetics research, in pursuit of the biological bullet that will resolve today's major health problems, with the main emphasis on the biomedical model—and all of this occurs under the auspices and guidance of the biomedical and pharmaceutical industry, clearly supported with tax money.

The Changing Nature of Public Interventions: The Importance of Class

A characteristic of these changes in public interventions is that they are occurring in response to changes in the distribution of power in our societies. Indeed, the changes have systematically benefited some groups to the detriment of others. Public interventions have benefited some classes at the expense of other classes, some races at the expense of others, one gender at the expense of the other, and some nations at the expense of other nations. We have seen a heightening of class as well as race, gender, and national tensions—tensions resulting from growing class as well as race, gender, and national inequalities. And I need to stress here the importance of speaking about class as well as race, gender, and national inequalities. One element of the postmodernist era is that class has almost disappeared from political and scientific discourse. Class analysis is frequently dismissed as antiquated, a type of analysis and discourse for "ideologs," not for serious, rigorous scientists. As class has practically disappeared from the scientific literature, it has been replaced by "status" or other less conflictive categories. The disappearance of class analysis and class discourse, however, is politically motivated. It is precisely a sign of class power (the power of the dominant class) that class analysis has been replaced by categories of analysis less threatening to the social order. In this new scenario, the majority of citizens are defined as middle class, the vast majority of people being placed between "the rich" and "the poor."

But classes do exist, and the data prove it. The two most important sociological scientific traditions in the western world are the Marxist and Weberian traditions, which have contributed enormously to the scientific understanding of our societies. Both traditions consider class a major category of power, and conflicts among classes a major determinant for change. To define class analysis as antiquated is to confuse antique with antiquated. The law of gravity is antique, but it is not antiquated. If you don't believe this, test the idea by jumping from a fourth floor window. And I am afraid that many analysts are jumping from the fourth floor. Forgetting or ignoring scientific categories carries a huge cost. One of them is an inability to understand our world.

Neoliberalism is the ideology of the dominant classes in the North and in the South. And the privatization of health care is a class policy, because it benefits high-income groups at the expense of the popular classes. Each of the neoliberal public policies defined above benefits the dominant classes to the detriment of the dominated classes. The development of these class policies has hugely increased inequalities, including health inequalities, not only between countries but within countries.

Another example of the cost of forgetting about class is that the commonly used division of the world into rich countries (the North) and poor countries (the South) ignores the existence of classes within the countries of the North and within the countries of the South. In fact, 20 percent of the largest fortunes in the world are in so-called poor countries. The wealthiest classes in Brazil, for example, are as wealthy as the wealthiest classes in France. The poor in Brazil are much poorer than the poor in France, but there is not much difference among the rich. And let's not forget that a young unskilled worker in East Baltimore has a life expectancy shorter than the average life expectancy in Bangladesh. There are classes in each country. And what has been happening in the world during the past 30 years is the forging of an alliance among the dominant classes of the North and South, an alliance that has promoted neoliberal policies that go against the interests of the dominated classes (the popular classes) of both North and South. There is an urgent need to develop similar alliances among the dominated classes of the North and South. As public health workers, we either can facilitate or obstruct the development of such alliances.

Class Alliances as Determinants of Non-Change

I became fully aware of this situation when I was advisor to the Unidad Popular government presided over by Dr. Salvador Allende in Chile. It was not the United States that imposed the fascist coup led by Pinochet (as was widely reported at the time). I was in Chile and could see what was happening. It was the *Chilean* economic, financial, and land-owning elites, the *Chilean* Church, the *Chilean* upper and upper-middle classes, and the *Chilean* army that rose up against the democratic government, in a fascist coup supported not by the United States (the United States is not a country of 244 million imperialists) but by the US federal government, headed by the highly unpopular President Nixon (who had sent the US Army to put down a general strike in the coal mining region of Appalachia). One should never confuse a country's people with its government. And this is particularly important in the United States: 82 percent of the population believes the government does not represent their interests, but rather the interests of the economic groups (in the United States called the *corporate class*) that dominate the behavior of the government.

I am aware of the frequently made argument that the average US citizen benefits from the imperialist policies carried out by the US federal government. Gasoline, for example, is relatively cheap in the United States (although increasingly less so). This, it is said, benefits the working class of the United States. But this argument ignores the heavy dependence of Americans on private transportation and the costs of this transportation for the popular classes, who would greatly benefit from (and would much prefer, according to most polls) public transportation, which is virtually non-existent in much of the country. It is an alliance between the automobile industry and the oil and gasoline industry that is responsible for the failure to maintain and develop public transportation. There is a lack of awareness outside the United States that the American working class is the first victim of the US economic and political system. The health sector is another example of this. No other working population faces the problems seen in the US health sector. In 2006, 47 million Americans did not have any form of health benefits coverage. And people die because of this. Estimates of the number of preventable deaths vary from 18,000 per year (estimated by the conservative Institute of Medicine) to a more realistic level of more than 100,000 (calculated by Professor David Himmelstein of Harvard University). The number depends on how one defines "preventable deaths." But even the conservative figure of 18,000 deaths per year is six times the number of people killed in the World Trade Center on 9/11. That event outraged people (as it should), but the deaths resulting from lack of health care seem to go unnoticed; these deaths are not reported on the front pages, or even on the back pages, of the *New York Times, Washington Post, Los Angeles Times,* or any other US newspaper. These deaths are so much a part of our everyday reality that they are not news.

But besides the problem of the uninsured, the United States has another major problem: the underinsured. One hundred and eight million people had insufficient coverage in 2006. Many believe that because they have health insurance, they will never face the problem of being unable to pay their medical bills. They eventually find out the truth, however—that their insurance is dramatically insufficient. Even for families with the best health benefits coverage available, the benefits are much less comprehensive than those provided as entitlements in Canada and in most E.U. countries. Paying medical bills in the United States is a serious difficulty for many people. In fact, inability to pay medical bills is the primary cause of family bankruptcy, and most of these families have health insurance. Furthermore, 20 percent of families spend more than 10 percent of their disposable income on insurance premiums and medical bills (the percentage is even higher for those with individual insurance: 53 percent). In 2006, one of every four Americans lived in families that had problems with paying medical bills. Most of them had health insurance. And 42 percent of people with a terminal disease worry about how they or their families are going to pay their medical bills. None of the E.U. countries face this dramatic situation.

The Situation in Developing Countries

The class dominance and class alliances existing in the world today are at the root of the problem of poverty. These alliances reproduce the exploitation responsible for that poverty and for the underdevelopment of health. Let me quote from a respectable source. The *New York Times,* in a rare moment of candor, analyzed poverty in Bangladesh, the "poorest country in the world." But, Bangladesh is not poor. Quite to the contrary. It is a rich country. Yet the majority of its people are poor, with very poor health and quality of life. As the *New York Times* reported:[6]

> The root of the persistent malnutrition in the midst of relative plenty is the unequal distribution of land in Bangladesh. Few people are rich here by Western standards, but severe inequalities do exist and they are reflected in highly skewed land

ownership. The wealthiest 16 percent of the rural population controls two-thirds of the land and almost 60 percent of the population holds less than one acre of property.... The new agricultural technologies being introduced have tended to favor large farmers, putting them in a better position to buy out their less fortunate neighbors. Nevertheless, with the government dominated by landowners—about 75 percent of the members of the Parliament hold land—no one foresees any official support for fundamental changes in the system.... Food aid officials in Bangladesh privately concede that only a fraction of the millions of tons of food aid sent to Bangladesh has reached the poor and hungry in the villages. The food is given to the government, which in turn sells it at subsidized prices to the military, the police, and the middle class inhabitants of the cities.

Finally, the *New York Times* concluded:

Bangladesh has enough land to provide an adequate diet for every man, woman and child in the country. The agricultural potential of this lush green land is such that even the inevitable population growth of the next 20 years could be fed easily by the resources of Bangladesh alone.

Let me repeat. It is not the North versus the South, it is not globalization, it is not the scarcity of resources—it is the power differentials between and among classes in these countries and their influence over the state that are at the root of the poverty problem. In most developing countries, the dominant land-owning class, which is in alliance with the dominant classes of the developed countries, controls the organs of the state. And historical experience shows that when the landless masses revolt against this situation to force a change, the dominant classes, of both South and North, unite to oppose change by any means available, including brutal repression. This is the history of populations that try to break with their state of health underdevelopment. And we are witnessing now the hostility in the mainstream media of the United States and of the European Union against governments like the Chavez government in Venezuela or the Evo Morales government in Bolivia that carry out reforms that affect the economic interest of those class alliances.

The Failure of Neoliberalism

Another assumption made in the neoliberal discourse is that the development of neoliberal policies has stimulated tremendous economic growth and improved populations' health and quality of life. Here again, the evidence contradicts this assumption. The average growth of real gross domestic product (GDP) per capita in Latin America was an impressive 82 percent during the period 1960–1980, but declined to 9 percent in the liberal period 1980–2000 and, further, to 1 percent in the period 2000–2005. This decline explains the rebellions against neoliberal policies when they were implemented in Latin

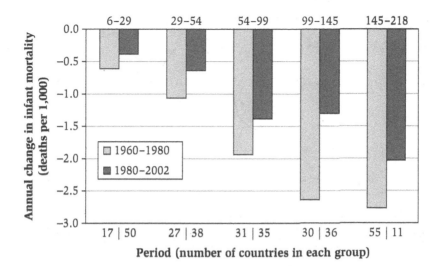

Figure 3.1. Infant Mortality Rate

Source: M. Weisbrot, D. Baker, and D. Rosnick. The scorecard on development: 25 years of diminished progress. *Int. J. Health Serv.* 36(2):211–234, 2006.

America. Regarding health indicators, as Figure 3.1 shows, for countries with similar levels of development at the starting point of the study period (e.g., in 1980 having the same level of development that others have in 1960), there was a much lower level of improvement in infant mortality during 1980–2002 than during 1960–1980. A similar situation appears in developed countries. In the United States, there has been a large increase in mortality differentials and a steady deterioration in the health benefits coverage of the population. One million people have lost health benefits coverage every year in that country over the last ten years.

The Social Situation in Europe

Let's now look at what has been happening in the European Union—what has been happening in the labor market, unemployment, salaries, working conditions, social protections, social benefits, and business profits in the E.U. 15. We'll focus on the E.U. 15 here because these countries have been in the European Union for the longest time and thus exposed to E.U. policies for the longest periods.

Figure 3.2 shows how unemployment has increased in the E.U. 15 since the early 1970s, coinciding with the development of policies aimed at establishing the European Union. Notice that Europe had lower unemployment than the United States during the period 1960–1980, and much larger unemployment in the period 1980–2003.

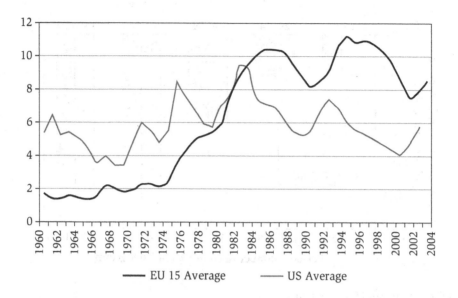

Figure 3.2. Unemployment: Evolution of Unemployment (as Percentage of Population), Average of the European Union 15 (Black, Lower Left to Upper Right) and United States (Gray), 1960–2003

Source: Annual Macroeconomic Database (AMECO), European Commission.

In Figure 3.3 we see how labor compensation (which includes compensation for work, social protection of workers, contributions to retirement allowances, and self-employment), as a percentage of the national income in the E.U. 15, declined during the period 1975–2005. That reduction took place even though the number of workers increased. Moreover, it was independent of the economic cycle.

Figure 3.4 shows how intensity and stress at work increased in practically all E.U. 15 countries. On average, the percentage of workers living under pressure increased from 32 percent in 1991 to 45 percent in 2005. A consequence in the workplace is that work-related illness also increased.

The rate of growth of social public expenditures, as shown in Figure 3.5, also decreased during the period 1990–2004. And Table 3.1 shows how social benefits (sickness insurance compensation, occupational accident compensation, and unemployment insurance) declined in all countries during the period 1975–1995. The Anglo-Saxon liberal countries (Australia, Canada, United States, Ireland, New Zealand, and United Kingdom) saw the largest cuts in benefits, followed by the Christian democratic countries and the social democratic countries; the reduction was not linear, with some cuts more accentuated in some social democratic countries than in liberal countries. But, in all the E.U. 15 countries, social benefits declined.

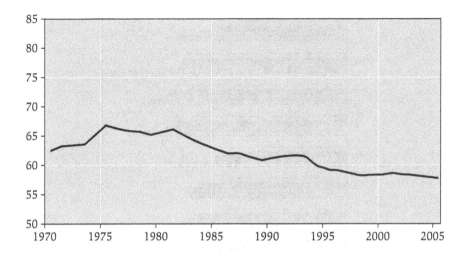

Figure 3.3. Salaries: Percentage of Labor Compensation in National Income in E.U. 15, 1970–2005. Total Compensation for Work, Including Social Protection of Workers, Contributions to Retirement Allowance, and Self-Employment

Source: OECD estimates, using OECD Economic Outlook database.

As these figures and table show, the conditions of work and of social benefits coverage for the working class and other sectors of the popular classes have deteriorated, in stark contrast to the exuberant profits enjoyed by the employer class. From 1999 to 2006, profits increased 33.2 percent in the E.U. 15 and 36.6 percent in the Eurozone. Labor costs, however, increased only 18.2 percent.

In summary, then, during the years of establishing the E.U. 15, there were increased capital incomes, decreased workers' incomes, increased salary inequalities, increased fiscal regressivity, decreased social benefits, and decreased social protections—all resulting in an increase in social inequalities. And this has been accompanied by an increased percentage of the population that considers the income inequalities excessive (78 percent, the largest percentage since World War II). It is also worth noting that a growing number of people in the working and popular classes believe that the deterioration of their social situation is due to the public policies developed as a consequence of establishment of the European Union. Are they right in their beliefs?

What Explains the Anti-European Mood Among Europe's Working Classes?

To answer this question, we must first look at the reasons given by the European establishment—the *Brussels Consensus*—for the growth of unemployment in the E.U. 15. The E.U. establishment has attributed the increased

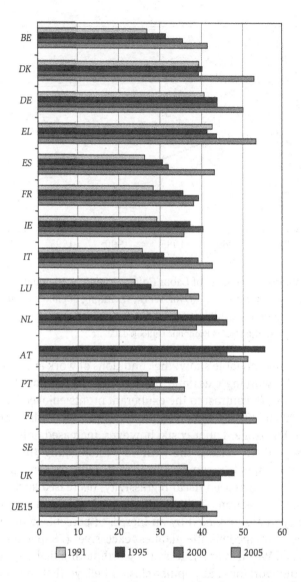

Figure 3.4. Work Intensity: Evolution of Work Intensity (Percentage of Population Working Under Stressful Conditions), E.U. 15, 1991–2005. Countries, from Top to Bottom: Belgium, Denmark, Germany, Greece, Spain, France, Ireland, Italy, Luxembourg, Netherlands, Austria, Portugal, Finland, Sweden, United Kingdom, and E.U. 15. For Each Country, Bars Represent, from Top to Bottom, 1991, 1995, 2000, 2005.

Note: 1991 data for Austria, Finland, and Sweden are not included because they were not part of the European Union in 1991.

Source: Eurofound.

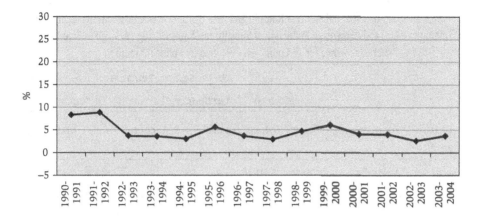

Figure 3.5. Social Protection: Decrease of the Rate of Change (Percent) in Public Social Expenditure per Capita, E.U. 15, 1990–2004

Source: Eurostat (online access July 25, 2007).

unemployment to three factors: (a) excessive regulation of the labor markets, (b) excessive generosity of social benefits, and (c) excessive public expenditures. Consequently, the E.U. establishment has (a) deregulated labor markets; (b) restrained and/or reduced public expenditures—an example, among many others, is the declaration by Pedro Solbes, for many years the commissioner of Economic and Monetary Affairs of the E.U. 15, now Minister of Economy of the socialist government in Spain, that "the policy that I am most proud of is not to have increased public expenditures in Spain," a declaration made in the country with the lowest public expenditures (after Poland) in the E.U. 15; and (c) reduced social benefits, which has reached its maximum expression in the proposal to increase the allowable working time to more than 65 hours per week.

These policies have been instituted within the framework of the monetary policies established in the Stability Pact, which requires austerity in public expenditures, and the European Central Bank policies of prioritizing the control of inflation over economic growth and job creation. In the United Kingdom (the first country that developed those policies, under Thatcher), a consequence of these policies has been a slowing down of the rate of mortality decline for all age groups, as shown in Figure 3.6.

Components of a National Health Program: What Should It Contain?

Clearly, the traditional responses of medical care institutions to all of these realities are completely insufficient. Medical care does indeed provide more

Table 3.1. Social Benefits: Substitution Rates in Sickness Insurance, Occupational Accident, and Unemployment, and Percentage Reduction of Substitution Rates During 1975–1995 (Five-Year Periods)—Data for 16 Countries, Classified by Political Tradition

		Social Security Program					
		Sickness		Occupational accident		Unemployment	
Political tradition	Country	Level	Reduction	Level	Reduction	Level	Reduction
Liberal	Australia	48.4	-10.1^a	—	—	48.4	-10.1^a
	Canada	62.9	-15.4^a	—	—	72.7	-13.1^a
	USA	—	—	—	—	59.8	-12.8^a
	Ireland	56.3	-33.5^c	64	-31.5^c	56.3	-34.9^c
	New Zealand	57.5	-34.7^c	94.3	-16^a	57.5	-25^a
	United Kingdom	63.4	-43.1^a	71.6	-51.3^a	63.4	-39.9^a
Christian democratic	Germany	100	0	100	0	74.3	-6.4^a
	Austria	99.2	-4.6^c	100	-3.4^c	47.4	-10.1^c
	Belgium	91.9	-0.3^a	100	-3.7^a	76	-28.1^b
	France	55.7	-6.8^a	66.8	0	41.1	-7.2^c
	Italy	68.1	0	74.1	0	66.8	-23.8^b
	Netherlands	84.7	-14.7^b	84.7	-14.7^b	81.6	-13.2^b
Social democratic	Denmark	74.7	-21.4^b	74.7	-21.4^b	81.9	-24.5^a
	Finland	86.1	-10.3^d	100	0	59.1	-5^d
	Norway	55	0	55	0	73.5	-10^a
	Sweden	90.3	-13.8^c	92.6	-21.8^c	77.1	-7.3^d

Source: W. Korpi and J. Palme. New politics and class politics in the context of austerity and globalization: Welfare state regress in 18 countries, 1975–95. *American Political Science Review* 97(3):425–446, 2003.
Note: Years of last maximum: $a = 1975$, $b = 1980$, $c = 1985$, $d = 1990$.

care than cure. The major causes of mortality—cancer and cardiovascular diseases—will not be solved through medical interventions. Medical institutions take care of individuals with these conditions and improve their quality of life, but they do not resolve these (or most other) chronic problems. Disease prevention and health promotion programs primarily based on behavioral and lifestyle interventions are also insufficient. We have plenty of evidence that

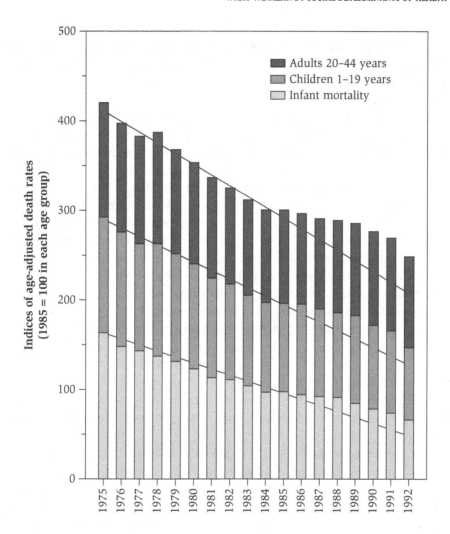

Figure 3.6. Indices Showing Changes in Death Rates Among Young Adults, Children, and Infants (Male and Female Combined), England and Wales, 1975–1992.

Source: R. G. Wilkinson, *Unhealthy Societies,* Figure 5.10, Routledge, 1996.

programs aimed at changing individual behavior have limited effectiveness. And understandably so. Instead, we need to broaden health strategies to include political, economic, social, and cultural interventions that touch on the *social* (as distinct from the *individual*) determinants of health. These interventions should have the empowerment of people as their first objective. Thus, a national health policy should focus on the structural determinants of health and should have as its primary components political, economic, social, and cultural health policy interventions, focusing on (a) public policy to encourage participation and influence in society, (b) economic and social determinants, (c) cultural determinants, (d) working life interventions, (e) environmental and consumer protection interventions, (f) secure and favorable conditions during childhood and adolescence and during retirement, and (g) health care interventions that promote health.

Let me stress that empowering people is of paramount importance. We are witnessing on both sides of the Atlantic, in the United States and in the European Union, a crisis of democracy. The representative institutions are widely perceived as controlled and instrumentalized by the dominant economic and financial groups in society. In the United States, confidence in the political establishment (referred to as "Washington"), perceived as captive to the corporate class, is at an all-time low. All political candidates in the 2008 presidential primaries, even John McCain, presented themselves as anti-Washington. A similar situation is occurring in the E.U. 15, where in country after country the working classes are clearly rejecting the European project that has been constructed by economic and financial groups with a minimum of democratic participation. It is not just that France, the Netherlands, and Ireland have rejected the European Constitution, but polls also show that the working classes of Denmark, Sweden, Germany, and many other countries are against the Constitution. An extremely important and urgent public health project is to recover the representativeness of political institutions and make them accountable to the large sectors of the population that have been disenfranchised—which leads me, finally, to my critique of the WHO Commission's report.

As I mentioned at the beginning of this talk, I saluted the establishment of the WHO Commission on the Social Determinants of Health and welcome its analysis and recommendations. As a matter of fact, I wish the Commission could receive the Nobel Prize in Medicine, or the Peace Prize, for its work. It has produced a solid, rigorous, and courageous report, and it goes a long way in denouncing the social constraints on the development of health. The report's phrase "social inequalities kill" has outraged conservative and liberal forces, which find the narrative and discourse of the report too strong to stomach.

And yet, this is where the report falls short. It is not *inequalities* that kill, but *those who benefit from the inequalities* that kill. The Commission's studious avoidance of the category of power (class power, as well as gender, race, and national power) and how power is produced and reproduced in political institutions is the greatest weakness of the report. It reproduces a widely held practice in international agencies that speaks of policies without touching on politics. It does emphasize, in generic terms, the need to redistribute resources, but it is silent on the topic of whose resources, and how and through what instruments. It *is profoundly apolitical, and therein lies the weakness of the report.*

My comments here, I should note, are not so much a critique of the Commission's report as a criticism of the WHO—and other such international agencies, for that matter. These agencies always have to reach a consensus, and consensus always gives the most powerful the power of veto. Any conclusion or subject or terminology that may offend the powerful groups seated at the table, who have to approve the report, must be dropped. The Commission's report goes very far in describing how inequalities are killing people. But we know the names of the killers. We know about the killing, the process by which it occurs, and the agents responsible. And we, as public health workers, must denounce not only the process, but the forces that do the killing. The WHO will never do that. But as public health workers we can and must do so. It is not enough to define disease as the absence of health. Disease is a social and political category imposed on people within an enormously repressive social and economic capitalist system, one that forces disease and death on the world's people.

Recall that it was Chadwick, one of the founders of public health, who, as Commissioner of the Board of Health of Great Britain in 1848–1854, declared that the poorer classes of that country were subject to steady, increasing, and sure causes of death: "The result [of the social situation] is the same as if twenty or thirty thousand of these people were annually taken out of their wretched dwelling and put to death." A century and a half later, millions of people, in both the North and the South, are put to death in just this way. And we know the economic, financial, and political forces responsible for this. And we have to denounce them by name.

It was Engels who, in his excellent public health work on the conditions of the British working class, showed the incompatibility between the capitalist economic system and the health and working conditions of working people. And it was Virchow who, in response to the outraged dismissal as too political of his recommendations to improve the population's health—by redistributing the land, water, and property of Germany—by the city fathers (the owners of the land, water, and property), responded: "Medicine is a social science and politics is nothing more than medicine on a large scale."[7] What we, as public health workers, need to do is to act as agents, including political agents, for change. I hope you agree.

Thank you very much for your attention.

Notes

1. This keynote address was given at the Eighth IUHPE European Conference on September 9, 2008, in Turin, Italy, and was originally published in *IUHPE—Global Health Promotion*, Vol. 16, No. 1, 2009, SAGE Publications.

2. Navarro, V. Race or class versus race and class: Mortality differentials in the US. *Lancet* 336:1238–1240, 1990.

3. Navarro, V. Assessment of the World Health Organization Report 2000. *Lancet* 356:1598–1601, 2000.

4. Navarro, V. World Health Report 2000: Responses to Murray and Frenk. *Lancet* 357:1701–1702; discussion, 1702–1703, 2001.

5. Williamson, J. *What Washington Means by Policy Reform.* Institute for International Economics, Washington, DC, 1990.

6. *New York Times*, September 12, 1992.

7. Virchow, R. Die medizinische Reform, 2. In: H. E. Sigerist, *Medicine and Human Welfare*, 93, 1941.

Chapter 4

The Magic Mountain

Trickle-Down Economics in a Philippine Garbage Dump

Matthew Power

The traffic in Quezon City—blaring, belching, scarcely moving—seems to be in a permanent state of rush-hour gridlock. Quezon, population 2.2 million, is the largest of the seventeen municipalities that form the megalopolis of greater Manila. Chrome-clad Jeepneys, the chopped and airbrushed descendants of WWII army jeeps pressed into public service, engage in a slow-motion chariot race with motorized tricycles, oxcarts laden with scrap metal, and passengerless bicycle rickshaws. A knot of metal and rubber binds every intersection. Ragged children dart between vehicles at lights, selling cigarettes with one hand and huffing gasoline-soaked rags with the other. The tinted windows and air-conditioning of the odd SUV create a bubble of sorts for its occupants, keeping the dusty pre-monsoon swelter and the pleas of the riffraff at bay, but do nothing at all to speed them along. The children, hair coppery with protein deficiency, paw like cats against the windows, studiously ignored by passengers a few inches away. Above it all, the chubby, smiling visage of Quezon's mayor, Feliciano "Sonny" Belmonte, beams down with paternal warmth from an enormous billboard, the base of which, strung with wash, has been converted into a tidy home by enterprising squatters.

Nearly half of all Filipinos live on less than two dollars a day, and metropolitan Manila, which in its poverty, enormity, utter squalor, and lack of services, perfectly represents the catastrophic twenty-first-century vision of the megacity as most of the world's poor will experience it. I am crowded in the back of a taxi with the photographer Misty Keasler and Klaid Sabangan, our guide and translator. Our driver, a Filipino named Johnny Ramone, blasts seventies singer-songwriter standards on his radio and is not in the least dismayed by the vehicular quagmire we're navigating as we wind our way toward the Payatas dump.

Like most of the outside world, I had first heard of Payatas, the fifty-acre dumpsite on Quezon City's northern boundary, when it flashed briefly across headlines in July 2000. Little else besides people dying in great numbers on a slow news day will bring notice to a place like this. After weeks of torrential rains spawned by a pair of typhoons, a hundred-foot mountain of garbage gave way and thundered down onto a neighborhood of shanties built in its shadow. The trash, accumulated over three decades, had been piled up to a 70-degree angle, and the rain-saturated mountain had collapsed. Hundreds of people were killed, buried alive in an avalanche of waste. That most of the victims made a living scavenging from the pile itself rendered the tragedy a dark parable of the new millennium, a symptom of the 1,000 social and economic ills that plague the developing world. I knew that the scavengers had continued living and working at the site even after the disaster, and, thinking there was some human truth to be dug from underneath the sorry facts, I wanted to see Payatas for myself.

Johnny Ramone squeaks his taxi through a gap, and we turn right down a narrow street between rows of tin-roofed shacks, alleys crowded with fruit sellers sitting by heaps of oranges and flapping roosters straining against their tethers. Junk shops line the street, their proprietors living among house-high piles of bottles and sacks of aluminum cans clouded by flies. A parade of dripping garbage trucks jounces along the potholed street, workers clinging to the roofs and young boys chasing after them hoping something salvageable might fall off.

As we come over a rise, my first glimpse of Payatas is hallucinatory: a great smoky-gray mass that towers above the trees and shanties creeping up to its edge. On the rounded summit, almost the same color as the thunderheads that mass over the city in the afternoons, a tiny backhoe crawls along a contour, seeming to float in the sky. As we approach, shapes and colors emerge out of the gray. What at first seemed to be flocks of seagulls spiraling upward in a hot wind reveal themselves to be cyclones of plastic bags. The huge hill itself appears to shimmer in the heat, and then its surface resolves into a moving mass of people, hundreds of them, scuttling like termites over a mound. From this distance, with the wind blowing the other way, Payatas displays a terrible beauty, inspiring an amoral wonder at the sheer scale and collective will that built it, over many years, from the accumulated detritus of millions of lives.

Behind a broad desk, Colonel Jameel Jaymalin looks pressed and combed despite the crushing heat and the bouquet of decomposing municipal waste that drifts in on the breeze. He seems happy in his position, lord of a fiefdom offered tribute by some 450 garbage trucks a day, many of which idle at the entrance gate outside his office as we speak. The colonel recites a history of the site and the government's efforts to clean things up following the disaster in 2000. Thirty years ago, Payatas had been a ravine surrounded by rice paddies and farming villages shaded over with the remnants of the rainforest canopy. As Manila rebuilt in the postwar decades, a great migration from the countryside to the city ballooned the population from 1.5 million in 1950 to nearly 15 million today.

By the 1970s, low-lying Payatas, on the anarchic fringe of a massive city, began by dint of gravity and convenience to be used as a dumping ground. Truckloads of household waste gathered up by sanitation privateers from across the city were poured into the ravine. The site also became infamous as a body dump during the gang wars that raged across the city's slum districts, fought out with spears, machetes, poison arrows, and homemade guns called *sumpak*. Creeks were filled in and the topography shifted; a hill began to grow, accruing layer upon layer and combed over by a population of 10,000 scavengers, junk-shop operators, and garbage brokers who followed the metropolis's waste stream wherever it led. Absent any government oversight, a city of shanties grew up around, and on, the dump. The entire local economy was built on a sort of Trash Rush. By 2000, the Payatas dump was 130 feet high, taller than anything in the surrounding landscape, a dormant and unstable volcano waiting for chance and gravity to run their course.

After the July rains and the collapse, after what bodies that could be recovered had been buried and the television crews went away, there was still enormous political pressure on the Quezon City government to do something about conditions at the site. At first the dump was closed, but the absence of an alternative meant that garbage piled up around the city. Despite the dump's dangers, the scavengers and the dumping cartels wanted Payatas reopened, and within months that is exactly what happened. By year's end the national government had passed an extraordinarily ambitious, if almost completely unenforceable, law called the Ecological Solid Waste Management Act [ESWMA], which called for all open dumps in the country to be closed and replaced with sealed sanitary landfills. According to the act, Payatas was supposed to close by February 16 of this year. When I point out to the colonel that it is now March, and there are several hundred loaded garbage trucks idling outside his door, he admits that, yes, there have been some unavoidable delays in locating a new site. But he insists there have been profound changes at the dump. Payatas is a flagship project: we can go see for ourselves. "Just please don't take pictures of the children."

The colonel hands us off to Rafael Saplan, the dump's chief engineer, who shows us a series of maps and charts illustrating his master plan. Saplan tells me that except for the absence of a liner to prevent waste from contaminating the groundwater, the dump has been largely converted into a sanitary landfill. "It would take 3,000 trucks a day eleven years to cart all this garbage to a new engineered landfill," Saplan tells me. The steep face of the pile, which had been nearly vertical before the collapse, has been recontoured to a more stable 40 degrees, and terraced steps have been cut into it to prevent slides. Toxic leachate, the heavy metal-laced liquid that percolates down through compressed garbage, is collected and pumped back into the pile. Deep-rooted vetiver grass has been planted to control erosion, and a system of I.D. cards has been created to document scavengers. No workers under fourteen are allowed.

Saplan is working on a pilot project to mine the millions of cubic feet of methane produced by the pile's decay every year, some of which is pumped into a one-megawatt gas generator. The ultimate goal is to build a generating station that could provide electricity to around 2,000 local households for a decade. The government would even be able to receive emissions credits for the methane project under the Kyoto Protocol. And then the site could be turned into an eco-park, maybe even a golf course. In the meantime, the actor Martin Sheen—who spent more than a year in the Philippines filming *Apocalypse Now*—has built a child-care center at the foot of the pile where the scavengers' children can splash in a wading pool while their parents work above. It looks good on paper: a beneficent, progressive government doing what it can to deal with a huge, toxic, public-health headache. I mention to Klaid that the ESWMA seems like an incredibly forward-thinking piece of legislation. He laughs. "Yes, but in the Philippines the law is only a suggestion."

With laminated passes given to us by one of the colonel's aides, we walk through the gate and down the hill. Truck after truck rumbles by, piled high with household and commercial waste from across Quezon. In the tropical heat the smell of rot and smoke is everywhere; it seeps into the pores and clings to the back of your throat. Our clothes soak through with sweat. We cut through a maze of narrow alleys filled with uniformed school kids and men playing billiards, dogs collapsed under the shade of the feltless tables. The neighborhood architecture is cobbled together out of chicken wire, cinder blocks, rusted tin. One rooftop is made entirely out of liberated street signs. Klaid leads us down a narrow trail through the jungle, which in places still edges the slum. We walk across a narrow bamboo bridge and up a steep hill, where a group of people—mothers with babies, men with arms crossed—sit in the shade of a military-style tent, in which a cooking class is under way.

At the foot of the hill lies a half-acre of vegetables: beautifully tended rows of lettuce, tomatoes, carrots, squash, corn. A few people rest under a giant star-apple tree by a small creek. A pregnant woman with a little boy works her way down a row of tomato plants, pulling weeds. Tropical butterflies flit about. It would be an utterly rural and bucolic scene if it weren't for the rusty jumble of houses that begin at the field's edge, towered over by the gray hill of Payatas. The rumble of the bulldozers and the trucks circling the road up its side is a dull grind, and periodically a plastic bag caught in an updraft drifts toward us and descends, delicate as a floating dandelion seed, into the branches of the trees.

"These are all *mangangalahigs,* the scavengers from the local community," Klaid tells me. *Mangangalahig* means something like "chicken-scratcher," after the way the scavengers pick through the trash. For the last six months, with money from the Consuelo "Chito" Madrigal Foundation, funded by one of the Philippines' wealthiest families, Klaid has been running an organic-gardening training program to classes of twenty at a time. Each student was given a plot of land to use and basic instruction.

Klaid, goateed, pierced, with a baby face and a shaved head, looks like a cherubic interpretation of a pirate. He picked up his nickname as a teenage street break-dancer with his partner "Bonny." An idealist who struggled for years in his former job at the United Nations Human Settlements Program, he jumped at the chance to do community work without the bureaucratic red tape. "That's why I left the U.N.," he tells me. "I said, 'For three years I've been hearing you talk, and set paradigms, and talk about frameworks and structures, and not one house has been built.' What we are doing here is the very essence of what the U.N. is trying to do, but they are limited by bureaucracy and internal politics."

When the class lets out, Klaid introduces me to one of the students, Ronald Escare, a stocky, grinning man with a ponytail tucked under a Mickey Mouse hat who goes by the nickname Bobby. Bobby has scavenged in Payatas for eight years, and he is just about to start his afternoon shift. Among the many new rules implemented by the government, the vast and chaotic population of *mangangalahigs* has been divided into work groups, each with a scheduled shift and a specific assignment of truck numbers whose contents they are allowed to pick over. We pull on knee-high gum boots and walk along a dusty path through the shanties to the dump entrance, trailed by a group of giggling children. On the street by the main gate, perhaps fifty yards from Martin Sheen's drop-off center (the wading pool empty, the children absent), a teenage boy tends to a large pile of burning wires, poking them periodically with a stick, his T-shirt pulled up over his nose and mouth. It is a halfhearted attempt to filter out the carcinogenic smoke, laden with dioxins and furans, which are released when insulation is burned off to sell the copper wire for scrap.

Bobby turns out to be a one-man commodities board of the latest scrap prices. "Red copper, 150 pesos a kilo at junk shop," he tells me. "I sell at factory, no junk shop. Two hundred pesos." His derisive laugh suggests that anyone who does not cut out the middleman in these transactions is a sucker. He gestures at the burning tangle of wire with his kalahig, the tool used by all the scavengers to dig through the trash. The kalahig is an L-shaped steel spike, perhaps eighteen inches long, with a wooden handle and a needle-sharp point. With a practiced flick of the wrist, Bobby demonstrates how to spear a can on the ground and deposit it into the sack he has slung over his shoulder. When I tell Bobby that aluminum cans in the States can be redeemed for the astronomical equivalent of two pesos each, he gives me a look of unalloyed wonder, as if I'd announced that the streets in America are made of chocolate.

We wave the colonel's passes at the guard, a city employee wearing a fluorescent orange T-shirt emblazoned with the word ENFORCER. On the back it bears the message "environmentally friendly" in lowercase script. He waves us through after exacting a toll of a couple cigarettes. On a steep path up the hillside, a line of dusty scavengers, finishing their daytime shifts, stumble down with bulging plastic sacks on their heads. The smell increases as we climb, a miasma of rotting food and burning tires, but before long my sense of smell, apparently defeated, ceases to register the full force of the stench. The ground underneath our boots is spongy, and as we climb, black rivulets of leachate flow down the access road. A black puddle releases methane bubbles like a primordial swamp, and the ground itself shakes when a loaded truck rumbles by. A road cut reveals a gray cross section of oozing agglomerate, shredded plastic bags the only recognizable remnants in the hyper-compressed pile.

The colonel's dreams of a grass-covered return to nature at Payatas seem far off as we ascend through the decades-old strata of the pile. Garbage dumps are far from inert. As rainwater percolates down through the pile and organic matter decays, a continuous and unpredictable biochemical reaction occurs, leaching toxins from the various plastics, metals, and organic compounds. The "slow smokeless burning of decay" is a process of centuries: ancient Roman dumps produce leachate to this day. Newsprint can remain legible for decades. Beneath its surface, Payatas is a roiling and poisonous pressure cooker, and any plan to cover it with a green mantle will ultimately have to come to terms with what is buried there.

Trying hard not to slip back down the rancid surface of the pile, we finally clamber to the top. The highest point in the landscape, the "active face" of the Payatas dump, is a broad plain of trash, extending to a false horizon so that it seems to contain the entire world. Unlike the gray muck of the mountain's sides, the summit is a riot of torn-open, primary-colored plastic bags in festive profusion, like a Mardi Gras parade hit by a cluster bomb. A line of trucks rumbling up the road drops load upon load, which are sifted and pushed to the edges as the hill grows skyward. The quaking geology of trash beneath our feet is laid down layer by layer, and covered daily with truckloads of dirt, as Bobby explains: *lupa, basura, lupa, basura*—earth, garbage, earth, garbage—in sedimentary gradations, building an utterly man-made landscape. Could they be read, the layers at Payatas—like Mesolithic middens of oyster shells or the trash heaps of Pompeii—might unravel to a future archaeologist some mystery of the millions of vanished lives whose leavings made this mountain.

Hundreds of scavengers, brandishing kalahigs and sacks, faces covered with filthy T-shirts, eyes peering out like desert nomads through the neck holes, gather in clutches across the dump. Gulls and stray dogs with heavy udders prowl the margins, but the summit is a solely human domain. The impression is of pure entropy, a mass of people as disordered as the refuse itself, swarming frantically over the surface. But patterns emerge, and as trucks dump each new load with a shriek of gears and a sickening glorp of wet garbage, the scavengers surge forward, tearing open plastic bags, spearing cans and plastic bottles with a choreographed efficiency. The intense focus and stooped postures of the *mangangalahigs'* bodies recall a post-agricultural version of Millet's *Gleaners*. We stand by the side of a fresh pile and watch as it is worked over with astonishing speed. A kalahig slits open a bag as if it were a fish, garbage entrails spilling out, and with a series of rapid, economical movements, anything useful is speared and flicked into a sack to be sorted later. The ability to discern value at a glimpse, to sift the useful out of the rejected with as little expenditure of energy as possible, is the great talent of the scavenger.

Cleanliness is relative here. After filling a sack with slop for his pigs—melon rinds, cold spaghetti, some congealed fried chicken at the bottom of a takeout bag—Bobby plunges his greasy hands into a rotting watermelon to clean them off, and then wipes them down with a moldering orange, grinning. He points out the different grades of plastic and their market prices as he walks us around a new heap being combed over by a group of his friends. The group's leader is a striking transvestite with the given name Romeo Derillo, self-christened Camille. Hand on hip, calling out orders to her crew and twirling a kalahig like a majorette, she somehow manages an unassailable glamour while standing knee-deep in a freshly dumped load from one of Manila's huge new shopping malls. This is premium garbage, so she has ordered all kalahigs sheathed, and the valuable plastic bottles are pulled out by hand. One worker collects nothing but drink straws; another, hundreds of plastic cups. Compact discs catch the sunlight like iron pyrite in a slag heap. A boy runs past, shouting with joy, holding aloft a pair of beat-up roller skates he's just salvaged. A bulldozer rumbles by, the ground quivering, trailing a bloody-looking garland of McDonald's ketchup packets from its rear axle.

Camille, like a great many of the Filipinos who find themselves working in Payatas, came here from the hinterlands of central Luzon island as a teenager. The economic choice between farming in the countryside (all fortunes the whim of the monsoon, of landowners, of the market price of rice or bananas) and mining the wealth of the metropolis's waste was not a difficult one. "In Payatas, they make a better living than they could ever hope to in the countryside,'' Klaid tells me. Bobby's 50 percent premium (when he cuts out the junk-shop middlemen) means he can make 150 pesos a day; about three dollars, which is 50 percent higher than the Philippine median.

The existence of "garbage slums," where the desperately poor find their economic niche amid the dumping grounds of municipal waste, is by no means a solely Filipino phenomenon. In his terrifying, magisterial work *Planet of Slums,* Mike Davis cites Beirut's Quarantina, Khartoum's Hillat Kusha, Calcutta's Dhapa, and Mexico City's enormous Santa Cruz Meyehualco as a few of the more egregious examples of this new urban form. Only in the last decade, since it eclipsed Manila's notorious Smokey Mountain (closed by the government in 1995), has the garbage slum in Payatas reached its apogee. Household and industrial trash has become for the world's poor a more viable source of sustenance than the agriculture and husbandry that has supported civilization since the first cities sprang up in the Fertile Crescent.

Occupying a niche like the bacteria and fungi that break down organic wastes in a forest and feed them back into the energy cycle, scavengers have existed in large cities at least since the Industrial Revolution. Victorian London, for instance, had an elaborately structured recycling system, with every subgroup filling its adapted role in the vast city's digestive tract. Night-soil men gathered human waste from privies and sold it as fertilizer. Pure finders gathered dog shit for use in the tanning of hides. Small children called *mudlarks* scoured the tidal flats along the Thames looking for bits of rope or lumps of coal, and bone grubbers dispatched animal skeletons to the rag-and-bone shops. The advent of plastics in modern industry has changed what the *mangangalahigs* are gathering up, but it hasn't altered their key role in the ecosystem of the city.

Even within the economic bottom-feeding of Payatas there is a self-imposed hierarchy, a funhouse mirror of larger societal inequalities. Scavengers unaffiliated with organized groups are called *ramblistas,* or "ramblers." Like hyenas skulking around a pride of lions at a kill, *ramblistas* circle outside the groups working the newest piles, picking over the dregs. The *paleros,* boys who work on the trucks themselves, making collection rounds of neighborhoods, are in a better position, snatching up the choicest bits before they even reach the dump. Some of the trucks we had seen had huge bags hanging on their sides, and the *paleros* were grabbing what they could from their load and squirreling it away. Before entering the gate by the colonel's office, a truck will pull up in front of one of the junk shops, and the paleros heft their day's take onto a scale, dividing up the money to supplement their 50 peso wage. The jumpers, usually small boys who climb aboard moving trucks and shovel valuable items overboard, have been banned from the dump proper under the new regulations, but that has only pushed them outside the gates. I had spotted them waiting at intersections, where they climb under the tarps of unguarded and idling trucks and grab whatever they can.

Just to the side of the several-acre spot where the trucks are dropping new loads sits a cluster of shacks and lean-tos, shaded by ragged tarps. "That's the food court," says Klaid, "just like the mall." And it is just like the mall, save perhaps the oversight of health inspectors. Small cook stoves heat tea and bubbling pots of stew. For a few pesos the scavengers can get lunch here instead of hiking down to the bottom of the hill. Klaid purchases a balut, a fertilized duck egg that has developed for two weeks before being hard-boiled. It is a Filipino delicacy, and with a gold-toothed grin he makes a show of cracking the shell, slurping the juice, and swallowing the fetal duck whole.

Wandering from pile to pile, calling out, *"Piyesa! Piyesa!"* (Parts! Parts!), are brokers of electronic and computer components, a new and lucrative category of waste. I ask Bobby what's worth the most, and he replies without hesitating, "Epson." An empty refillable printer cartridge in working condition can go for as much as 350 pesos. Bobby knows the prices for all these, too: Monitor, 50 pesos. Motherboard, 30. Circuit boards for 25 a kilo, to be melted down for trace amounts of gold. Pentium chips, if the pins can be straightened, 50. A boy approaches the brokers with a scuffed-up printer cartridge, which they glance at before rejecting. It is a buyer's market, and the general sentiment among everyone I talk to is that business has been getting worse.

A year ago, say Bobby and his friends, a *ramblista* might have made 1,000 pesos a week. Now she'll be lucky to glean 600. Most of the best pickings are intercepted en route or diverted to other dumpsites. I ask Bobby what he'll do if Payatas finally closes down. He shrugs, smiles. His five-months-pregnant wife is working as a *ramblista* a few yards away. "I'll go to Montalban," he says. Klaid tells me that this is the new dumpsite even farther out in the countryside. Many scavengers have already moved there. The enormous waste stream of Manila shifts like the mouth of a river, and wherever it spreads its rich alluvial fan the *mangangalahigs* and *paleros* and *ramblistas* will follow.

The impulse to gamble, the faint hope that the dump might offer up a buried treasure, becomes a kind of religion to the thousands of scavengers. Payatas, which in the 2000 collapse had shown itself capable of taking everything away, can offer up extraordinary bounty. I ask Bobby what is the greatest thing he has ever heard of being found. A Rolex, 65,000 pesos in a box, gold teeth, a half-burned hundred-dollar bill. There are dangers, too: some boys once found a hand grenade and, not realizing what it was, blew themselves up. Just last week Bobby found a huge Styrofoam box containing a 150-pound swordfish, still frozen solid. His group hacked it up on the spot and took it home. He thinks the *paleros* must have grabbed it by accident from outside a restaurant. "Sometimes they don't know what they throw away," he says.

Having come here expecting to see a violent and irrational struggle for existence, I begin to find something reassuring about the efficient dignity with which the *mangangalahigs* go about their work. Bobby tells me that with the new system of collectives, the scavengers share profits within their groups, which leads to more cooperation in the gleaning process, and many participate in a local savings program, from which they can draw small loans. The scavengers seem less victims than rational economic actors, skilled and highly organized laborers who actually provide a sort of public service.

The sun is sliding fast toward the horizon, and we pick our way back down the hill as the next shift's workers begin to make their way up. They will work long into the night, as long as the trucks keep coming, lighting their way with homemade miner's lamps of taped-together batteries. Walking down through the village, I notice several shrines to St. Anthony, the patron saint of poor people and seekers of lost objects, decorated with plastic bottle-ends cut into festive blossoms.

Day after day we return to Payatas, climbing around the pile to talk to people or wandering through the surrounding neighborhoods. There are actually two peaks in the topography of trash here: the newer one, where some 1,300 tons of municipal waste are dumped a day; and the older one, site of the 2000 collapse, which was graded and closed shortly thereafter. That part of the dump now houses Saplan's methane-generation project. We pass an outflow pipe coming out of the pile's base next to a small creek. A steady flow of espresso-black leachate, the poison distillate of millions of tons of putrescent garbage, pours out, running downhill directly into the creek, which joins the flow of the toxic Pasig River as it winds through the heart of the metropolis to Manila Bay.

Below a bridge that spans the creek, a group of half-naked boys stand in the gray water up to their waists, rinsing out hundreds of plastic garbage bags, which they bundle up in great bales. Another boy stomps down a truckload of plastic cups that resembles a hay wain. The bag-washers in the river have set alight a pile of waste plastic, which flickers and pops as it sends a black plume across the shacks and frames the scene in Hadean shades. They look up at me, laughing, calling out: "Hey Joe!" "Hey Joe, you're my father!" Laughing and splashing around as they work, the boys are scarcely aware of the health risks to which they and all the scavengers of Payatas are subjecting themselves. Tuberculosis is epidemic, made worse by air pollution and overcrowding. Tetanus, asthma, and staph infections are common. There are a few medical charities that visit, but regular care is rare. Bobby says he's lost three of his children to illness in Payatas: nine years, six years, and three months, "from the methane." He tells me this matter-of-factly, as if he were reciting the market prices of aluminum cans. Personal tragedy is a commodity worth very little in Payatas.

We wander through warrens of shacks, built on blocks to weather the monsoon. The soot-covered houses seem half destroyed, and the people next to the dump don't own the land they live on. Squatters' shacks overhang the banks of the Pasig River, which has been turned into a vast cloaca for the city's waste and yearly rises above its banks to sweep away the most vulnerable settlements. Manila has a severe monsoon, and informal housing among the slum population leaves tens of thousands living in flood-prone, cramped, disease-ridden squalor. Even in the worst locations, or on the periphery where the city fades away into the rice fields and swamps, there is always the threat of a more powerful economic force that can edge squatters out from whatever place they've taken as theirs. They are haunted everywhere by the bulldozers of progress.

Time and again in Manila, huge slums have been emptied to avoid the unwanted notice of the outside world. Imelda Marcos was notorious for clearing out tens of thousands of slum dwellers in the mid-1970s before the arrival of the Miss Universe pageant, the visit of President Gerald Ford, and an IMF–World Bank meeting. Not to be outdone, her nominally democratic successor Corazon Aquino reportedly evicted 600,000 squatters during her presidency. When prices rise and landowners want to clear shantytowns from their property, one of the favored methods in Manila is arson, known as ''hot demolition.'' A popular technique involves releasing a rat or cat soaked in kerosene and set alight into a settlement, where the terrified creature can start dozens of fires before it dies.

We cut across the narrow valley between the two hills and cross a ditch into the neighborhood that was once known as Lupang Pangako: the Promised Land. This spot, Klaid tells me, is where the hill came down. A woman named Ruth Manadong, sweeping her alley a few yards from the edge of the dump, points us to the exact spot. She and her eight-year-old nephew escaped, climbing the slope behind their house as the saturated garbage surged down like lava. They later returned, she tells me, but were driven away from the site by restive ghosts rattling their windows, knocking pots over in the kitchen, visiting nightmares into fitful attempts at sleep. She does not look up as she tells this to Klaid. She points us down the alleyway, where steps lead to a concrete patio and a memorial on which several hundred names are inscribed: Abalos. Villeno. George. Whole extended families were wiped out in the putrid wave of mud and plastic. No one will ever know for sure how many were swallowed up. More than two hundred bodies were pulled out, but the flow had filled in the ravine thirty feet deep in places, utterly shifting the landscape and making a full recovery impossible.

Not thirty yards from the memorial, a group of mud-covered workers are digging a deep trench into the collapsed hillside. At first I think they are a work detail digging for remains, to give a proper burial to the nameless dead still buried in the site. Klaid speaks with one of them in Tagalog and then explains, ''When the dump was first being piled up, the value of aluminum was so low that people didn't collect it for scrap. So they're digging out twenty-year-old cans from the site of the collapse.'' By the dictates of the open market the decades-old layers of trash were now a relatively rich ore, regardless of the fact that the abandoned tailings the workers now sifted through were laced with their own dead. In a sense, it is all a matter of how quickly one is buried alive in the garbage: in a few terror-filled moments or by the slow measure of a lifetime's labor.

One Sunday Bobby meets us at a McDonald's in Quezon, where we pile into a motorcycle taxi with a sidecar and bump and rattle down pothole-covered streets into the heart of the slum. Bobby's wife is working a *ramblista* shift today, and women don't often come where we are going. Pulling up into a dusty, open courtyard, we are met by the suspicious stares of a hundred men who are gathered around a squared-off enclosure of rusted sheet metal. Sunday mornings in Quezon are for church or for cockfights, and we have come for the latter.

Men hold their prize birds under their arms, smoothing their feathers, whispering to them quietly, running their fingers down the long green tails as though through a lover's hair. The wall around the enclosure is chest-high and crowded three-deep with spectators. Bobby and I climb up on a corner post, a boy scrambling between my legs to look over. Two scarred men with poorly rendered tattoos enter the dusty ring through a gate, their birds' heads tucked under their armpits to calm them. A hulking man with a notepad stands in the center, sweat running in rivulets down his face, and starts calling out odds in Filipino, waving a splay-fingered hand at the crowd like a magician casting a spell. Surging against the barrier, the sidelines erupt with bets being placed, peso notes held high, men shoving and yelling to get closer to the edge of the ring, sizing up the competitors.

The man taking the bets is called the Cristo—the Christ—and, like an auctioneer, his skill is to build the bidding to a fever pitch. Fistfuls of pesos change hands, odds are given, supplications are made to the heavens. Cockfighting is called *sabong* in Filipino, and as many as 10 percent of Filipinos are active participants in this billion-dollar industry. In some slum economies, as much as a fifth of the average income is redistributed through gambling, and, as with state lotteries in the United States, the poorest people in the Philippines are those most likely to gamble on birds. They are also the primary consumers of *shabu*, a local variety of methamphetamine, and *rugby*, a generic term for glues and solvents with addictive fumes.

Holding the roosters feet up, a handler—Bobby tells me this is often his job—removes the leather sheath from the curved, razor-sharp, three-inch spur tied to the right leg of each bird. The men in the pit clear out a space at the center, giving a wide berth to the cocks, which have been known to kill unlucky bystanders with their spurs. The handlers draw the birds close enough to peck at each other and then back off, repeating this three times before dropping the agitated birds to the ground. The effect is instantaneous and explosive: a blur of color, a broad fan of bright green neck feathers, and a flapping of wings as the birds leap upon each other, lunging with the spurs faster than the eye can follow, seeming to become a single chaotic being. The crowd erupts in cheers, faces contorted, eyes bulging, screaming for their favorites. Bobby, utterly in his element, is swept up in the fervor, pounding against the sheet metal and yelling with the throng. In and out of the ring is a scene of pure, animal aggression, unapologetic and unself-conscious.

As the roosters flail in the dust, the men left in the ring leap to stay out of the way of the flashing surgical steel blades. A bird flaps high into the air and brings a blade straight into the feathers of its opponent's back. Blood flies out in an arc, spattering the barrier. Another lunge and a wing is broken, splayed out on the ground as the injured cock drags itself upright, still lunging after its opponent with the working half of its body. A handler picks both up and swings them together for a last desperate round, trying to stoke whatever smoldering fury they still possess. The crowd leans in, cackling and leering, as the cocks are thrown together. One bird manages to get on top of the other and, even with a broken wing, methodically plunges its spur to the hilt three times in its opponent's throat, just beneath the green fan of neck feathers. Both birds flap weakly, kick, and lie still, breasts pulsing, eyes wide. The Cristo picks them both up, and bright blood drips steadily from a beak, turning black in the dust. The birds are drawn together once more but are too weak to be provoked. The Cristo drops the dying loser onto the blood-caked ground and holds the dying winner aloft. The crowd howls. The whole fight has lasted perhaps twenty seconds.

Around the outside of the pit, money changes hands in an exchange of gloating and recrimination at the defeated rooster. With little ceremony, a man carries the loser, still breathing, out of the pit, and lays it across a bloodstained log, where another man with a cleaver hacks off the spur leg with one swing. A boy unties the steel spur from the severed leg and passes it to the next contestant. The bird is plunged headfirst into a can of water boiling on a trash pile, and it flaps once in the water but within a few moments is defeathered and handed to the victor, a trophy for the soup pot on top of his winnings. The champion bird has its spur untied, and just as quickly is whisked off to the "doctor," who sits on a log near the ring. With a needle and thread and packets of powdered antibiotics, the doctor patches the bird up, probing gashes with a finger for internal bleeding before sewing them up. After a month on the mend the rooster will be back in the pit.

In the afternoon we return to the garden. Bobby, back to earth after the glories of the cockpit, sets to work on his neat rows of tomato plants, watering and pulling weeds alongside his wife, who has finished her shift on the dump. If Payatas closes down, as the colonel has promised, Bobby has no interest in finding a new career. As a scavenger he makes his own hours, he works when it pleases him, and, even with the slowdown at the dump, he earns enough to live. The gardening project is a good diversion, and he'll get food and a bit of income from what he's growing. There's a certain irony, which I point out to Klaid, in retraining migrants who have fled the countryside to be farmers again. "It's true," he replies. "There's no opportunity out there. The city is attractive. For a farmer, life on a dumpsite is comparatively easy. This is not a question of quality of life, but a question of survival."[1]

So what does the garden really do? I ask. "It gives them a place to be quiet, to be patient. To garden instead of gamble. I was a community organizer for ten years, and it did nothing because I tried to save the world. People would get transferred to something even worse, a place with no work and no services, beyond the edge of everything. With this project we decided that if we could reach one person at a time, on an individual level, then it is a huge step."

Whether the garden, whatever it brings to the lives of the scavengers, will even continue to exist is an open question. The property is owned by the Madrigals, but there are many who think the most valuable use of the land would be to build housing for the poor, and that a garden is, at best, a quaint diversion. Ging Gonzales, one of the members of the foundation's board, says as much to me as we are driving through Quezon's traffic to a meeting with Sonny Belmonte, the mayor whose face graces the better part of the city's billboards. "How many children could we send to school for the money we are spending on the garden?" she asks me. "The problem is knowing what is the most efficient means of helping."

When we arrive at his office, Belmonte, as smiley in person as he is on billboards, is receiving hundreds of visitors, interest groups from across his enormous slice of the metropolis. Belmonte sits down with us for a few minutes as Klaid clicks through a slide show about the garden project. "This might be a good thing," says the mayor, in a noncommittal way. "Maybe it will give them skills to take back to the provinces with them." In his rapidly expanding city, an exodus of the poorest newcomers would relieve Belmonte of an enormous social headache. I ask him when Payatas is really going to close. "Now we are hoping for January 2007." A few days later, Belmonte and several other metropolitan Manila mayors are named in a lawsuit by environmental groups for failing to close Payatas and other dumpsites. But no amount of arguing, for or against, seems likely to change the fundamental facts on the ground: every single day, 7,000 tons of metropolitan Manila's household garbage must go somewhere. "If you think Payatas is bad," one of the mayor's aides tells me, "you should go see Pier 18."

Pier 18, on the industrial shorefront of Manila's north harbor, lies half-obscured behind a row of shanties that line a frontage road. We inch our way there, in a solid stream of truck traffic, as the cumulonimbus clouds piled over the western rim of the bay unleash a hot downpour. The low-lying road through the Navotas slum fills with knee-deep puddles in a few minutes. The squatter settlements creep right up to the edge of the road, and even the five-foot-wide median has been littered with squatters' scrap-wood shacks and split-bamboo chicken coops, constant traffic within inches on either side. Passing trucks throw up bow wakes, and waves travel along the narrow alleyways, surging right into the ground floors of the houses. Flotsam butts up against rotted walls, and children splash through the muck, lifting their soaked shirts. Several huts are roofed with the stolen signboards of political candidates, and it seems that the sheltering placards provide a far more tangible benefit to the poor than any unachievable campaign promises printed upon them.

The rain passes, and we get out of the taxi and walk past a sign that reads "Pier 18 North Harbor." Pier 18 is an enormous transfer station the size of several football fields where hundreds of trucks from across Manila dump their daily loads to be picked over and consolidated before being shipped out to Montalban. Hundreds of scavengers, a great many of them small children, swarm over the pile, swinging kalahigs wildly as each new load is dumped. Trucks plow in and out through the site, and several times I see children, boots suctioned by the mud, nearly fall beneath their wheels. Jumpers scramble up onto the loads and surf the waves of trash as they slide out of the tilting truck beds. Stray dogs and pigs rove over the piles, rooting out rotting food.

I speak to an eight-year-old boy named Gerald, who has a raw gash over his right eye from the swinging trap door of a truck. I ask him where he lives, and he points across the lake of mud to a row of tarp-covered shacks right on the edge of the pier. His parents work here, too, and he comes every day after school. He turns and runs as a new pile gets dropped, very nearly getting plowed under by a bulldozer, and squirms his way to the top of the pile with the adults, filling his sack with shocking speed. People follow behind the bulldozers, spearing anything of value churned up by their treads. Teenage boys burn strings of Christmas lights in an old suitcase. There are no rules, no I.D.s, no flagship social programs or green reclamation, no sense that there is anyone managing or overseeing this chaos. It is the Darwinian free market in its purest and most ruthless form. To witness this makes all the beneficence of the Madrigals and the economic development programs of the World Bank seem like so much well-intentioned folly.

But even in this swampy hell there is a degree of remove, of levity. At the edge of the pier, under a tin roof, a karaoke machine is running, the words spooling out on a screen beneath a shot of a beautiful girl walking on a beach. A young girl in rubber boots, covered with mud, grabs the microphone and starts singing a Filipino pop song in a cracked but totally heartfelt voice. The *mangangalahigs* have distilled survival, and even joy, down to an essence. That life prevails here is a testament to what can be endured; in the midst of squalor, laughter and karaoke can still be heard. Even the landscape insistently offers up signs of regeneration: when we leave the pier, there is a dim rainbow bent over the piled housing of Navotas. North of the slum, the fenced-off dumpsite of Smokey Mountain lies dormant and abandoned, after ten years its slopes already beginning to be reclaimed by grass and shrubs.

On our last day in Payatas, we accept an invitation to stay at the house of Nanay Remy, a frail, toothless woman of seventy-three, her face half-paralyzed by a stroke. She lives in a 500-square-foot compound with twenty-four family members and still works as a *ramblista* on the pile every day. Dozens of rusty box springs fence off the compound, and inside are several neat huts and a small garden, which Remy planted after her training at Madrigal. As I talk with Bobby and Klaid, Remy serves a feast of fried fish and rice and salad from her garden plots. She has lived in Payatas for fifteen years and doesn't have a clue where they'll all go if the dump closes down. She wants to stay together with her people. The family is the core of Filipino society, and population numbers are often discussed in terms of families rather than individuals. She has two of her tiny, wide-eyed grandchildren in her lap. Their mother, a *shabu* addict, has abandoned them, and Remy feeds them with her fingers as she retells the history of her life: the evacuation from the Visayas islands during the war, the years squatting in the Tondo slum, a husband lost to drink, children and grandchildren raised, the endurance of a long life here. Her story isn't a plea for pity, and she isn't asking for anything except what the trash heap offers up.

Remy has cleared out one of her bamboo and sheet-metal huts for us. I lie on the hard floor, listening as the evening crows of a dozen roosters echo through the village, doomed some Sunday to be called to the pit by the Cristo. At the open window the equatorial darkness falls like a curtain, and across the creek the mountain of the dumpsite rears black beneath a net of stars. Against the silhouette of the garbage mountain, a faint line of lights works its way upward. They are the homemade headlamps of the night shift tracing their way up the pile. Reaching the top, they spread themselves out, shining their lights on the shifting ground to begin their search. Beneath the wide night sky those tiny human sparks split and rearrange, like a constellation fallen to earth, as if uncertain of what hopeful legend they are meant to invoke.

Note

1. A farmer from the provinces who makes his way to Payatas probably won't realize that he's part of the largest migration in human history. More than 1.3 million people abandon their lives in the countryside every week, and sometime this year, according to the U.N., more than half of the global population will live in cities for the first time, up from 3 percent two hundred years ago. A billion will live in slums like Payatas.

Chapter 5

Family Medicine Should Encourage the Development of Luxury Practices

Negative Position

Martin Donohoe

Mankind has become so much one family that we cannot ensure our own prosperity except by ensuring that of everyone else.

Bertrand Russell

Introduction

Luxury care—also known as *boutique medicine, concierge care, retainer practice, executive health care,* and *premium practice*—has been flourishing over the last few years in the United States (US) and, to a lesser extent, other parts of the western world.[1-3] I will use these terms interchangeably and, focusing on the US experience,* argue that the concept of luxury care is antithetical to sound science, to public health, and to fundamental ethical principles of modern medical care. As such, family medicine, indeed medicine as a profession, should not promote the development of luxury care.

---

*Data on specific programs come from their websites and promotional brochures unless otherwise noted.

Luxury Primary Care Clinics

Concierge clinics began in 1996 when the former team doctor for the National Basketball Association's Seattle Supersonics founded MD2. Since then, MD2 has grown, as have other groups like MDVIP and Platinum Health Service LLC.

In retainer practices, patients are charged an average fee of between $2,000 and $4,000.

At luxury clinics, patients are indulged with perks. These include valet parking, escorts and plush bathrobes; seating in oak-paneled rooms lined with fine art and outfitted with televisions, computer terminals and fax machines; buffet meals with herbal tea; and saunas and massages.[1-3] Subspecialty referral appointments occur on the same day as the general physical exam. Vaccines in short supply elsewhere are readily available. Physicians are available by cell phone or pager year-round; some doctors will even make house calls. Waiting times for an initial appointment are short, and patient-physician ratios are between 10 and 25% of typical managed care levels.[1-3]

In general, two or more full-time clinicians staff luxury primary care clinics, with many subspecialists available for immediate referral appointments. The only published study of the costs and benefits of executive physicals evaluated the Bank One in-house program, which is ironically much more evidence-based in its selection of tests than the programs offered by academic medical centers.[4] At a cost of $400 per exam for executives earning at least $125,000 per year, participants in this voluntary program had fewer short-term disability days and decreased overall medical costs over a 3-year period.[4] However, the cost of this exam was significantly lower than the typical cost of an executive physical.

Between 5 and 10% of the nation's nearly 3,000 nonprofit hospitals are experimenting with boutique health care service models.[5] Marketing for luxury primary care clinics is directed at the heads of successful small and large companies.[1] In addition to obtaining full reimbursement for services (patients are responsible for what insurance does not cover), hospitals hope these high-level managers will steer their companies' lucrative health care contracts towards the institution and its providers. Some programs give discounted rates in exchange for a donation to the hospital.

Luxury primary care clinics cater to "busy executives" who "demand only the best" from their physicians.[1-3] Patients who work two jobs on an hourly pay scale and must find child care each time they return for a diagnostic test or subspecialty appointment would be offended by these clinics' promotional materials, which imply that high-level executives are busier and lead more hectic lives than other patients and thus require same-day service. In fact, it is the lower socioeconomic status workers/patients who have the worst health outcomes and most need efficient, comprehensive health care.[1,6]

Corporate clients for executive health programs include tobacco companies, organizations with extensive histories of environmental pollution, pharmaceutical companies (whose egregiously inflated profits and lack of true innovation contribute to health care disparities), and health insurers (whose own policies increasingly limit the coverage of sick individuals).[1,2,7] Interestingly, a substantial proportion of university presidents serve on the boards of directors of such companies.[8]

Patients come from the US and abroad. Most of the patients are asymptomatic, fairly healthy, and come from upper management. Thus they are disproportionately white men, based on data from one executive health program;[4] on the fact that women, who make up 46% of the US work force, hold less than 2% of senior-level management positions in Fortune 500 companies;[9] and on the lower socioeconomic status of non-Caucasians. Some programs offer a package of evaluation and testing benefits to upper management employees, raising questions of patient confidentiality when the employer directly purchases clinical services for these employees.

A recent national survey found that retainer-practice physicians have much smaller patient panels (898 vs. 2,303 patients) and care for fewer African Americans, Hispanics, and Medicaid patients than do non-retainer-practice physicians.[10] Physicians who converted to a retainer practice kept an average of only 12% of their former patients.[10] Most retainer physicians conducted charity care (although the nature and amount of such care is unknown), and many continued to see some non-retainer patients.[10] Another survey found that physicians converting from non-concierge to concierge care reduced their patient panels from an average of 2,716 to an average of 491 patients.[1] Their daily workload decreased from 26 to 10 patients.[10] Once physicians are established in concierge practices, they make substantially more money than non-concierge physicians.[12]

Boutique doctors often cite the desire for greater autonomy and more independence in decision making (less paperwork, fewer prior authorizations), increased time to spend with their families or on altruistic endeavors, and the satisfaction of getting to know their patients more intimately. Such motivations are understandable, even laudable, and an unfortunate consequence of the current US health care system. Even so, increased financial compensation is likely an important factor for some concierge physicians.

Luxury Primary Care Clinics and Academic Medical Centers

Most training in professional ethics, as well as the development and teaching of evidence-based practice guidelines, occurs in medical schools and at teaching hospitals. These institutions, historically the providers of last resort for the poor and destitute, have been particularly hard hit by the financial crisis affecting health care in the US. Reasons include high costs associated with medical training, a disproportionate share of complex and/or uninsured patients, erosion of their infrastructure, shrinking funds, and the closing of public hospitals.[1,6,13-16] Insurance companies and the US government have been unwilling to adequately compensate teaching hospitals for their losses.[17]

To survive financially, academic medical centers have been forced to compete with more efficient private and community hospitals. Owing to limited success, teaching hospitals have undertaken two initiatives to improve their competitive financial edge: (1) development of luxury primary care (or executive health) clinics and (2) active recruitment of wealthy foreigners as patients. [For more detail on the latter strategy, see note 1.]

While the exact number of academic medical centers sponsoring luxury primary care clinics is not known, the list includes many well-known US medical schools and teaching hospitals.**[1,2] Approximately 3,000 individuals visit the Mayo Clinic each year for executive health physicals, 3,500 go to the Cleveland Clinic, and 1,950 are seen at Massachusetts General Hospital.[1]

Some academic institutions participate in the Executive Health Registry, which provides services to 150 corporations and 10,000 traveling executives worldwide. Executive Health Exams, International has a nationwide network of 600 health care providers who perform 25,000 exams per year. While this company is not affiliated with any specific academic medical center, many of its providers have academic appointments.

No data are available on the participation of medical students and residents in luxury primary care clinics at teaching hospitals. Little to nothing is publicly known about start-up costs, degree of profitability, or whether financial resources from these clinics are diverted to other programs, and if so what programs. My experience calling and then sending a very brief questionnaire to the heads of ten clinics associated with major programs, and receiving only one response, suggests that institutions may be reluctant to divulge such information.

Other Forms of Boutique Medical Care

Other trends in boutique medical care include the proliferation of VIP floors in medical centers; the rise of specialty hospitals; medi-spas providing alternative

---

**Institutions include Massachusetts General Hospital, Johns Hopkins, New York Presbyterian, University of Pennsylvania, University of California–San Francisco, Stanford, University of Miami, Vanderbilt, Wake Forest, Washington University, Emory, Georgetown, George Washington, University of California–Irvine, Ohio State, Bowman Gray, Duke, Mayo Clinic, Northwestern, Cleveland Clinic, Oregon Health and Science University, Virginia Mason (affiliated with the University of Washington), Cedars-Sinai (affiliated with the University of California–Los Angeles), and others.

or cosmetic services in luxurious surroundings; professional sports contracts; travel medicine clinics that stock vaccines and provide preventive health information and accessories for exotic destinations; second opinion and e-consulting services provided via the Internet; and practices which sell health and nutritional products.[2]

As a medical student in the late 1980s, I remember visiting patients on the penthouse VIP ward. I was distressed to observe that some, but not all, faculty spent much more time with patients on that ward than with their other charges. The behavior of a few physician-teachers bordered on the obsequious. One such ward, Mount Sinai Hospital's Eleven West, is supervised by managers who typically have a background in the hotel industry. It offers private rooms, higher nurse-patient ratios, luxurious décor, and gourmet meals. Operated since 1993, it currently generates profits of more than $1 million annually on about $2.5 million in revenue.[5]

Despite an ever-widening socioeconomic gap in access to health care and in response to increasing privatization, China and other Asian countries have likewise built VIP floors and sometimes entire VIP hospitals.[18] Wealthy Westerners have received care in these institutions, sometimes to avoid publicity.

Since 1990, over 100 specialty hospitals have opened in the US, primarily offering cardiac, surgical, and orthopedic procedures.[19,20] An 18-month moratorium on construction of new facilities expired last year. These hospitals adversely impact nearby community hospitals, as they tend to cherry pick younger, healthier, and wealthier patients and avoid the costs of providing traditionally money-losing emergency services.[19,20] Patient selection likely accounts for their slightly better outcomes. These hospitals have been criticized for avoiding the ban on physician self-referral to institutions in which they have a financial stake and for inadequate provider coverage.[19,20] The American Hospital Association and the Federation of American Hospitals have vigorously opposed the development of these facilities.[19]

One example of a medi-spa involves Wellpoint, the largest US health benefits company, which has joined Dole Food Company, Inc. and Four Season Hotels and Resorts to develop "Wellbeing Institutes" in California and Hawaii.

Historically, professional sports teams would hire the most qualified physicians to treat their athletes. Today hospitals and medical groups pay teams for the exclusive right to treat their high-salaried players, a marketing ploy designed to encourage non-professional athletes with high income but lesser abilities to visit their clinics.[21] For example, the New York University-Hospital for Joint Diseases pays baseball's New York Mets more than $1 million a year, and Houston's Methodist Hospital (affiliated with Baylor University) pays baseball's Astros and football's Texans $2 million annually.[21]

Meanwhile, low cost "boutique" clinics are burgeoning. Walmart, CVS, Rite Aid, Piggly Wiggly, and other supermarket and pharmacy chains have opened walk-in clinics, staffed largely by nurse practitioners, to treat minor acute illnesses for fees of $30 to $65.[22] Such retail mini-clinics do not constitute true primary care, cannot guarantee coordination with patients' other providers, and the uninsured may utilize such quickie checkups as a substitute for the thorough, life- and cost-saving interventions that a more complete evaluation would provide.

Barriers to and Legal Risks of Boutique Medicine

The proliferation of boutique practices has spawned boutique health care law firms, which help doctors to navigate the legal requirements and avoid the legal risks of practice transformation. The development of boutique practices has also led to consulting and practice management companies catering to luxury care. Physicians in retainer practice have their own organization, the American Academy of Private Physicians (http://www.aapp.org/), formerly known as the Society for Innovative Practice Design, and before that as the American Society of Concierge Physicians.

Legal risks of operating boutique practices in the US include violation of Medicare regulations, the False Claims Act, provider agreements with private insurance companies, state insurance laws, and the anti-kickback statute and other laws prohibiting payments to induce patient referrals, along with liability for the abandonment of existing patients.[23] Medicare regulations prohibit charging Medicare beneficiaries for services covered by Medicare.[23] A majority of recently surveyed concierge physicians found the Medicare guidelines unclear and insufficient.[11] Nearly three-quarters continued to participate in Medicare, while one-fifth had opted out.[11]

Some hospitals have used economic credentialing to deny hospital privileges to physicians practicing concierge care. Certain states have investigated the payment mechanisms of concierge practices.[24] New Jersey prevents insurers from contracting with physicians who charge extra fees for their services.[24] New York State's Department of Health prohibits concierge medicine for enrollees in health maintenance organizations.[24] At the federal level, the Equal Access to Medicare Act has not moved beyond Congressional committee discussions.

Problems Associated with Luxury Medical Care

Erosion of Science

There is no evidence documenting a higher quality of care in concierge practices, and little data support the clinical- or cost-effectiveness of many tests offered to their asymptomatic clients. Examples include percent of body fat measurements, chest X-rays in smokers and non-smokers aged 35 and older to screen for lung cancer, electron-beam computed tomography (CT) scans and stress echocardiograms looking for evidence of coronary artery disease, and abdominal-pelvic ultrasounds to screen for ovarian or liver cancer.[1] Other examples such as mammography starting at age 35 and genetic testing are also controversial. Ironically, this over-testing occurs despite the well-documented underutilization of validated, beneficial interventions in both uninsured and insured patients.[25]

While clients pay for these procedures, technicians and equipment time are diverted to produce immediate results. Since patients jump the queue in the radiology and phlebotomy suites,[1] tests may be delayed on other patients with more appropriate and urgent needs.

False-positive results may lead to further unnecessary investigations, additional costs (and increased profits), and heightened anxiety. Multiple tests increase the likelihood of false positive results. Nevertheless, some people's need for reassurance is so strong that they will pay exorbitant amounts of money for such testing, and companies have sprung up to meet this demand. For example, Biophysical 250 charges $3,400 "to screen for hundreds of diseases and conditions ... including cancer, cardiovascular disease, metabolic disorders, autoimmune disease, viral and bacterial disease and hormonal imbalance" (http://www.biophysicalcorp.com/).

In 2002, one year after television talk show host Oprah Winfrey underwent a full-body screening CT scan, 32 million Americans paid up to $1,000 apiece for this test.[26] A 2004 survey of 300 Americans found that 85% would choose a full-body CT scan over $1,000 cash. These scans can deliver a radiation dose nearly 100 times that of a typical mammogram.[26] A single scan exposes the patient (victim?) to a level of radiation linked to increased cancer mortality in low-dose atom bomb survivors from Hiroshima and Nagasaki.[26] Receiving such scans annually would substantially increase one's lifetime risk of malignancy.[26]

On the other hand, true positive results can lead to the over-diagnosis of conditions that would not have become clinically significant, leading to further risky interventions and possibly impairing future insurability.[1]

The use of clinically unjustifiable tests erodes the scientific underpinnings of medical practice and sends a mixed message to trainees and patients about when and why to utilize diagnostic studies.[27] It also runs counter to physicians' ethical obligations "to contribute to the responsible stewardship of health care resources."[28] Some might argue that if patients are willing to pay for a scientifically unsupported test, they should be allowed to do so. However, such a "buffet" approach to diagnosis over-medicalizes care and makes a mockery of evidence-based medicine.

Erosion of Professional Ethics

The general public contributes substantially, through state and federal taxes, to the education and training of new physicians.[17] Even so, many physicians who staff luxury primary care clinics limit their practices to the wealthiest fraction of our citizenry.[1,2] Given their investment in the training of physicians, the public might find it hard to accept physicians limiting their practices to the wealthy. They might also object to physicians refusing to care for Medicaid or Medicare patients. On the other hand, medical students incur significant debt by the end of their education. As doctors, they might justify limiting their practices to the wealthy by claiming a right to freely choose where they practice and for whom they care (within limits, since they cannot, for instance, refuse to care for acquired immunodeficiency virus [HIV] syndrome patients solely on the basis of their HIV seropositive status or African-Americans solely on the basis of their race).

Similarly, medical centers might justify sponsoring luxury primary care clinics via a utilitarian argument if income from these ventures cross-subsidizes indigent care or teaching programs. One economic analysis suggests that an average 600-bed luxury hospital in a city of one million people with average incomes could generate, with profit margins of 30 to 55% as much as $6 million in incremental annual profit, which could be used to cross-subsidize research or other patient care activities.[29] Nevertheless, there are few publicized instances of cross-subsidization. Virginia Mason's (University of Washington's) Dare Center uses a portion of its approximately $650,000 annual profit to offset the cost of caring for the uninsured and money-losing community programs;[5] Tufts New England Medical Center's Pratt Diagnostic Clinic intends to begin transferring roughly $350,000 to $400,000 to the institution's money-losing primary care practice in 2006;[5] and the two VIP medical wards at one Chinese hospital in Hong Kong cross-subsidize some uncompensated care.[18] Nevertheless, such arrangements do not promote equality and solidarity, and hospitals can use other ways that display beneficence and social justice to attempt to improve their financial circumstances.

The American Medical Association (AMA) believes that, with appropriate safeguards (e.g., physicians ensuring ongoing care for their former patients when converting to luxury primary care practices), luxury primary care diversifies health care delivery. The AMA also believes that increasing the choices available to health care purchasers should increase the total amount of health care available to the entire population,[30] a variation of former president Ronald Reagan's failed "trickle down" economic theory of the 1980s.

Some comments regarding the state of contemporary health care will hopefully illuminate how luxury care will not solve current problems, but rather magnify existing inequities and injustices. The trend toward luxury primary care has been occurring at a time of increasing injustice in health care in the US and worldwide, and during a period of increasing dissatisfaction and cynicism among patients, practicing physicians, and trainees. Today 47 million Americans lack health insurance.[17] Millions more are underinsured, remain in "dead-end" jobs to maintain their health insurance, or go without needed prescriptions because of skyrocketing drug prices. The proportion of physicians providing charity care has declined over the last decade.[31] The development of luxury care has diverted attention from these issues without improving health outcomes at the population level.

Despite spending a larger proportion of its gross domestic product on health care than any other westernized nation, the US ranks near the bottom among such nations in life expectancy and infant mortality, and 20–25% of its children live in poverty.[7,25] Disparities have grown in wealth, access to care, and morbidity and mortality between rich and poor.[6,7,25] Racial inequalities in processes and outcomes of care persist, some seemingly explainable only by racism or poverty (itself in part a consequence of past and present racism).[32] Differences between developed and developing nations, in terms of financial, economic, environmental and health-related resources, have further widened and are especially dramatic.[7,33] For instance, hunger kills as many individuals in two days as died during the atomic bombing of Hiroshima, one billion people lack access to clean drinking water, and three billion lack adequate sanitation services.[7,33]

The profit motive at the root of America's capitalist economic system has driven, to some extent, the increase in luxury practices. The increasing role played by for-profit corporations in causing and perpetuating worldwide social injustice which exacerbates health disparities is mirrored in the pernicious influence of for-profit entities (health maintenance organizations [HMOs], hospital systems, and pharmaceutical and biotechnology companies) on the American health care system.[34] In the US, investor-owned firms have come to dominate renal dialysis, nursing home care, inpatient psychiatric and rehabilitation facilities, and HMOs.[35] They are likewise acquiring a significant share of acute care hospitals, outpatient surgical centers, home care agencies, and even hospices.[35] Services such as billing, auditing, transcription, and radiograph interpretation are being outsourced to the developing world. For-profit health care entities have been widely cited for higher death rates, lower quality of care, and higher administrative costs.[35]

Luxury care will not solve, and will likely worsen, other problems with America's ailing health care system. For instance, patient and physician dissatisfaction with many aspects of our current fragmented health care system is growing.[34-36] Basic preventive services at recommended frequencies are commonly missed or delayed owing to time and financial constraints.[4,25] Investigators have already described erosion of professionalism, about which physicians and the public have expressed concern, such as some doctors offering varied levels of testing and treatment for a given illness, depending on a patient's ability to pay.[37,38] Despite strong desire among patients to discuss out-of-pocket costs, such discussions take place infrequently, which contributes to high degrees of noncompliance with more expensive medications.[39]

Our failure to provide universal coverage could lead some desperate patients to lie, for example, by not disclosing a worrisome personal or family medical problem in order to obtain insurance or by exaggerating symptoms to obtain needed care. Physicians may be more likely to recommend services for insured rather than uninsured patients,[38] and a sizeable minority of physicians admit to "gaming the system" by manipulating reimbursement rules so their patients can receive care that the doctors perceive is necessary.[40] Moreover, increasing numbers of US patients are traveling abroad for heavily discounted, non-cosmetic, surgical procedures.[41]

Meanwhile, many medical students and residents display increasingly cynical attitudes as their training progresses; some educators have expressed concern about the adequacy of students' humanistic and moral development.[42] Contemporary ethics training tends to address inadequately the socioeconomic, cultural, occupational, environmental, and psychological contributors to the health of individuals and populations.[43,44]

Interest in primary care among medical students has been declining for much of the past decade.[45] Young physicians are leaving general internal medicine much faster than the subspecialties of internal medicine.[45] Increasing numbers of physicians have stopped seeing patients with certain types of insurance, complain of fatigue and burnout, and feel that medicine has lost its soul. Some are even leaving the profession. The proportion of US physicians providing charity care has declined from 76% in 1996–97 to 68% in 2004–05.[31]

Do Physicians Receive Luxury Care?

To some degree many physicians have access to a form of special care for themselves and their families. Doctors can curbside their colleagues, write their own prescriptions (within limits), and sometimes see specialists whose skills they have observed directly. They can (and do) take drug samples intended for indigent patients,[46] and tend to get more attentive, personalized care than the average non-physician patient.

On the other hand, the nature of the fragmented US system of health care insurance means that such special treatment is frequently not possible. As a result of changing my employment status four times over the last ten years, I have had four different primary care physicians under three different health plans. My family has mostly been covered by doctors outside the hospital system in which I work. I have waited as long as anyone else for emergency care and for routine medical and dental appointments, my choice of providers is limited, and I receive no special discount on a limited and changing array of covered pharmaceuticals.

Furthermore, it is not clear that, when physicians do get special care, it is better care. Self-treatment is ill-advised, and VIP care carries risks of both under-treatment and over-treatment. Moreover, such care violates the concept of fairness.

Solutions

Academic institutions have begun to heed the call of educators and policy makers to improve training in, and the practice of, professionalism in medicine.[47-49] Medical organizations have called for an increased emphasis on professionalism and ethical practice, and for empathic and equal provision of care to all individuals, despite their insurance status, financial resources, or race.[50]

On the other hand, many training programs have adopted teaching models like "The One-Minute Preceptor," which despite its laudable learner-centered emphasis capitulates to decreasing visit lengths and the inadequate time available for student and resident teaching. As such, trainees might focus less on patient-centered care, which requires taking the time to understand the social, cultural, economic, and religious contributors to patients' beliefs about their health and their abilities to respond to illness. We need to capture the interest and excitement of disillusioned trainees and practitioners, but yielding to methodologies that devalue talking with patients and reimbursement schemes that reward procedural skills far more generously than diagnostic acumen is not the proper approach.

Medical schools and professional societies have been relatively quiet on the subject of luxury primary care, no doubt in part to avoid drawing attention to their support of profitable enterprises which illuminate existing inequities in health care. Promoting luxury care in the face of current inequities perpetuates unscientific practice and erodes fundamental ethical principles of medicine such as equity and justice.

For teaching institutions to sponsor concierge care will engender even greater cynicism among student-doctors and the general public. Instead of continuing to promote an overt, two-tiered system of care, medical schools should renounce the measure of the marketplace as their dominant standard or value,[51] divert their intellectual and financial resources to more equitable and just investments in community and global health, and implement curricular changes designed to encourage trainees to find constructive solutions to the problems caused by our market-based health care system.[17] Closing some academic medical centers and/or consolidating redundant educational and clinical programs in nearby teaching hospitals may save money, which can be diverted toward indigent care programs. Academic medical centers can become more competitive by reducing costs (e.g., through quality improvement programs, improving governance and decision making, and augmenting philanthropic contributions).[14] Increasing alliances with industry could provide needed funds, but risk undue corporate influence on academic institutions' agendas. Patient input into systems changes, such as increasing the flexibility of appointment scheduling, could increase satisfaction and compliance and improve outcomes.

Physicians must educate the public and policy makers about the important roles they play in research, education, and patient care, particularly in terms that are relevant to individuals and their families.[13] These ideas should be convincingly communicated to business leaders, government representatives, and purchasers of health care,[13] particularly by deans, hospital presidents, department chairs, and division chiefs. In turn, legislators should provide increased funding for the education and training of future physicians and for the continued health of these vital institutions.

Some might argue that food and shelter are as important as (if not more important than) health care, and that physicians are no more obligated to work for equitable and universal health care coverage than builders are to lobby for universal housing and farmers for food subsidies for the poor. I disagree. Article 25 of the Universal Declaration of Human Rights, adopted in 1948 by the United Nations' General Assembly, states, "Everyone has the right to a standard of living adequate for the health and well-being of himself and of his family, including food, clothing, housing and medical care and necessary social services, and the right to security in the event of unemployment, sickness, disability, widowhood, old age or other lack of livelihood in circumstances beyond his control."[52] Leaving aside powerful arguments in favor of food and housing for all, which would in turn improve the overall health and welfare of the populace, physicians do have an obligation, borne of their privileged status, the public's investment in their training, and their roles as stewards of the public's health, to be politically active and ensure that our leaders provide for the sickest among us. This is especially true now, when fewer scientists hold positions of authority than in times past and when scientific truths have been deliberately obfuscated by the well-funded and sophisticated public relations and lobbying campaigns of those with a vested interest in profiting from the provision of a basic human right like health care.

Role models for physician activism include Rudolph Virchow, Thomas Hodgkin, Margaret Sanger, Albert Schweitzer, Florence Nightingale, and innumerable individuals who labor, often anonymously, in support of the disenfranchised. Virchow argued that many diseases result from the unequal distribution of civilization's advantages.[53] He asserted the moral un-neutrality of medicine, and wrote, "If medicine is really to accomplish its great task, it must intervene in political and social life."[53]

Furthermore, hospitals must be especially wary of corporate contracts which limit academic freedom and the dissemination of research findings vital to the public's health. Health care organizations should divest themselves of stock holdings in harmful products such as tobacco and advocate for strong laws and treaties to curb tobacco use and obesity, major contributors to morbidity and mortality.[54] They should develop strong policies regarding conflict of interest, especially surrounding the biotechnology and pharmaceutical industries. They should avoid associations with, and divest from, corporations whose business practices harm human health and/or violate human rights,[7,33,54-56] as well as companies which conduct business in countries with oppressive human rights agenda.[7,33,55-57] Finally, they should support evidence-based humanitarian interventions and work toward solutions to poverty.

Achieving Health Care Equity

The Future of Family Medicine report[58] echoes statements of the American College of Physicians[59] and other doctors' groups in calling for universal access. Unfortunately, all their proposals leave in place our inefficient, wasteful, patchwork, mixed private and public system.

Some individuals advocate consumer-directed health plans, including medical savings accounts, yet fail to recognize that the average person lacks the factual data, research time, and choices needed to make a fully informed decision regarding coverage of current or future illnesses.[60] Cost-sharing leads to adverse outcomes for many people who cannot afford necessary care. Such individuals avoid preventive care, delay needed care, and are noncompliant with medications even when small co-payments are imposed.[60]

Analyses show that the US, the only industrialized nation without national health insurance, can afford a single payer health care system. Such a system would be more efficient and effective than our current non-system and have significant advantages for patients, physicians, and businesses.[61] Such a system is supported by a majority of students, residents, faculty, and medical school deans[62] and was endorsed by the American College of Surgeons in the early 1990s.

Conclusion

Family medicine should not only withhold support for the development of luxury practices, but also vigorously oppose them, especially in academic medical centers. Family medicine should support a single payer health care system in the US and greater equity in health care delivery worldwide.

Acknowledgment

The author thanks Rachel Adams for excellent research assistance.

Notes

1. Donohoe MT. Luxury primary care, academic medical centers, and the erosion of science and professional ethics. *J Gen Intern Med*. 2004;19:90–94.

2. Weber DO. For sale: Body scans, boutique care and second opinions. *The Physician Executive* 2003(March/April):10–16.

3. Brennan TA. Luxury primary care—market innovation or threat to access? *N Engl J Med*. 2002;346:1165–1168.

4. Burton WN, Chen, CY, Conti DJ, Schultz AB, Edington DW. The value of the periodic executive health examination: Experience at Bank One and summary of the literature. *J Occup Environ Med*. 2002;44:737–744.

5. Costa L. High end healthcare: Though they have their opponents, boutique-style services can subsidize care for the poor. *Stanford Social Innovation Rev*. 2005(Spring):50–52. http://csi.gsb.stanford.edu/high-end-healthcare. Accessed March 13, 2006.

6. Lynch JW, Kaplan GA, Pamuk ER, Cohen RD, Heck KE, Balfour JL, et al. Income inequality and mortality in metropolitan areas of the United States. *Am J Public Health* 1998;88:1074–1080.

7. Donohoe MT. Causes and health consequences of environmental degradation and social injustice. *Soc Sci Med*. 2003;56:573–587.

8. Kniffin K. Serving two masters: University presidents moonlighting on corporate boards. *Multinational Monitor* 1997;18. www.multinationalmonitor.org/hyper/mm1197.05.html. Accessed May 24, 2006.

9. Donohoe MT. Individual and societal forms of violence against women in the United States and the developing world: An overview. *Curr Women's Health Reports* 2002;2:313–319.

10. Alexander GC, Kurlander J, Wynia MK. Physicians in retainer practice: A national survey of physician, patient, and practice characteristics. *J Gen Intern Med*. 2005;20:1079–1083.

11. United States Government Accountability Office. *Physician services: Concierge care characteristics and considerations for Medicare*. Washington, DC: United States Government Accountability Office, 2005. http://www.gao.gov/new.items/d05929.pdf.

12. Fleck C. Want your doctor to pamper you? Pay extra. *AARP Bulletin* 2004(October). www.aarp.org/bulletin/yourmoney/a2004-11-11-boutique.html/?print. Accessed April 10, 2006.

13. Pardes H. The future of medical schools and teaching hospitals in the era of managed care. *Acad Med*. 1997;72:97–102.

14. Blumenthal D, Weissman JS, Griner PF. Academic health centers on the front lines: Survival strategies in highly competitive markets. *Acad Med*. 1999;74:1037–1049.

15. White KL, Connelly JE. The medical school's mission and the population's health. *Ann Intern Med*. 1991;115:968–972.

16. Staff. Report warns decrease in public hospitals poses threat to health. *The Nation's Health* 2005(October):10.

17. Wolfe SM. The destruction of medicine by market forces: Teaching acquiescence or resistance and change? *Acad Med.* 2002;77:5–7.

18. Cong Y, Linying H, Dwyer J. The VIP floors (case study). *Hastings Cent Rep.* 2005;35:16–17.

19. Iglehart JK. The emergence of physician-owned specialty hospitals. *N Engl J Med.* 2005;352:78–84.

20. Bristol N. Physician-owned specialty hospitals in the USA. *Lancet* 2005;366:193–194.

21. Pennington B. A sports turnaround: the team doctors now pay the team. *New York Times* 2004(May 14). www.nytimes.com/2004/05/18/sports/othersports/18DOCT.html. Accessed May 21, 2004.

22. Kher U. Get a checkup in aisle 3. *TIME* 2006(March 20):52–53.

23. Goldstein SM. The legal risks of boutique medicine. *Sacks Tierney Healthcare Law* 2003(July). www.sackstierney.com/articles/boutique.htm. Accessed April 11, 2006.

24. Linz AJ, Haas PF, Fallon F, Metz RJ. Impact of concierge care on healthcare and clinical practice. *JAOA.* 2005;105:515–520.

25. Donohoe MT. Comparing generalist and specialty care: Discrepancies, deficiencies, and excesses. *Arch Intern Med.* 1998;158:1596–1608.

26. Gupta S. Danger: Body scans. *TIME* 2004(September 13):105.

27. Cohen JJ. Missions of a medical school: A North American perspective. *Acad Med.* 1999;74(suppl.):S27–S30.

28. American College of Physicians. Ethics manual. *Ann Intern Med.* 1998;128:576–594.

29. Gordian MA, Mango PD. A consumer view of boutique health care. *The McKinsey Quarterly* 2004(1). www.mckinseyquarterly.com/article_print.aspx?L2=12&L3=61&ar=1395. Accessed April 11, 2006.

30. Mauney FM. Report of the council on medical service of the American Medical Association: Special physician-patient contracts. *CMS Report* 9-A-02, 2002:1–5. http://www.google.com/url?sa=t&rct=j&q=mauney%20fm.%20report%20of%20 the%20council%20on%20medical%20service%20of%20the%20american%20 medical%20association%3A%20special%20physician-patient%20contracts &source=web&cd=1&ved=0CCMQFjAA&url=http%3A%2F%2Fwww.ama-assn .org%2Fresources%2Fdoc%2Fcms%2Fcms902.doc&ei=Bd -aT42vNKfhiALVsPTHDg&usg=AFQjCNFPoR81s2tS1IYsRcCWtfLEu26aKA.

31. Cunningham PJ, May JH. A growing hole in the safety net: Physician charity care declines again. *Center for Studying Health System Change* 2006(March).

http://www.rwjf.org/files/research/TR%2013%20
-%20Charity%20Care%20FINAL.pdf. Accessed May 17, 2006.

32. Epstein AM, Ayanian JZ. Racial disparities in medical care. *N Engl J Med.* 2001;344:1471–1473.

33. Donohoe MT. Roles and responsibilities of health professionals in confronting the health consequences of environmental degradation and social injustice: education and activism. Monash Bioethics Review, 2008;27(Nos. 1 and 2):65-82.

34. Himmelstein D, Woolhandler S, Hellander I. *Bleeding the patient: The consequences of corporate health care.* Monroe, ME: Common Courage Press, 2001.

35. Woolhandler S, Himmelstein DU. The high costs of for-profit care. *CMAJ.* 2004;170:1814–1815.

36. Joos SK, Hickam DH, Borders LM. Patients' desires and satisfaction in general medicine clinics. *Public Health Rep.* 1993;108:751–759.

37. Weiner S. "I can't afford that!" Dilemmas in the care of the uninsured and underinsured. *J Gen Intern Med.* 2001;16:412–418.

38. Alexander GC, Casalino LP, Meltzer DO. Patient-physician communication about out-of-pocket costs. *JAMA.* 2003;290:953–958.

39. Mort EA, Edwards JN, Emmons DW, Convery K, Blumenthal D. Physician response to patient insurance status in ambulatory care clinical decision-making: Implications for quality of care. *Med Care* 1996;34:783–797.

40. Wynia MK, Cummins DS, VanGeest JB, Wilson IB. Physician manipulation of reimbursement rules for patients: Between a rock and a hard place. *JAMA.* 2000;283:1858–1865.

41. Kher U. Outsourcing your heart. *TIME* 2006(May 29):44–47.

42. Branch WT. Supporting the moral development of medical students. *J Gen Intern Med.* 2000;15:503–508.

43. Sugarman J. (ed.). *Ethics in primary care.* New York: McGraw-Hill, 2000.

44. Sulmasy DP, Dwyer M, Marx RR. Knowledge, confidence, and attitudes regarding medical ethics: How do faculty and housestaff compare. *Acad Med.* 1995;70:1038–1040.

45. Sox HC. Leaving (internal) medicine. *Ann Intern Med.* 2006;144:57–58.

46. Westfall JM, McCabe J, Nicholas RA. Personal use of drug samples by physicians and office staff. *JAMA.* 1997;278:141–143.

47. Rothman DJ. Medical professionalism—focusing on the real issues. *N Engl J Med.* 2000;342:1284–1286.

48. Donohoe MT. Exploring the human condition: Literature and public health issues. In: Hawkins AH, McEntyre MC (eds.), *Teaching literature and medicine.* New York: Modern Language Association, 2000.

49. Brennan T. for the Project of the American Board of Internal Medicine Foundation, American College of Physicians-American Society of Internal Medicine Foundation,

and the European Foundation of Internal Medicine. Medical professionalism in the new millennium: A physician charter. *Ann Intern Med.* 2002;136:243–246.

50. Pellegrino ED, Relman AS. Professional medical associations: Ethical and practical guidelines. *JAMA.* 1999;282:984–986.

51. Souba WW. Academic medicine and the search for meaning and purpose. *Acad Med.* 2002;77:139–144.

52. United Nations. Universal Declaration of Human Rights. www.un.org/Overview/rights.html. Accessed July 11, 2006.

53. Donohoe MT. Advice for young investigators: Historical perspectives on scientific research. *Adv Health Sci Educ.* 2003;8:167–171.

54. Donohoe MT. Cigarettes: The other weapons of mass destruction. *Medscape Ob/Gyn and Women's Health* 2005;10(1). Posted April 5, 2005. www.medscape.com/viewarticle/501586.

55. Donohoe MT. GE—bringing bad things to life: Cradle to grave health care and the alliance between General Electric Medical Systems and New York–Presbyterian Hospital. *Synthesis/Regeneration* 2006(Fall);41:31–33.

56. Donohoe MT. Flowers, diamonds, and gold: The destructive human rights and environmental consequences of symbols of love. *Human Rights Quarterly* 2008;30:164–82.

57. Donohoe MT. War, rape and genocide: Never again? *Medscape Ob/Gyn and Women's Health* 2004;9(2). Posted October 22, 2004. www.medscape.com/viewarticle/491147.

58. Martin JC, Avant RF, Bowman MA, Bucholtz JR, Dickinson JR, Evans KL, et al. The future of family medicine: A collaborative project of the family medicine community. *Ann Fam Med.* 2004;2(suppl. 1): S3–S32.

59. American College of Physicians. Where we stand: Access to care. www.acponline.org/hpp/menu/access.htm. Accessed May 12, 2006.

60. Geyman JP. Family medicine and health care reform. *Am Fam Physician* 2005;72:752–755.

61. *Proposal of the physicians' working group for a single-payer national health insurance.* Physicians for a National Health Program. http://www.pnhp.org/PDF_files/Physicians%20ProposalJAMA.pdf. Accessed May 13, 2006.

62. Simon SR, Pan RJD, Sullivan AM, Clark-Chiarelli N, Connelly MT, Peters AS, Singer JD, et al. Views of managed care: A survey of students, residents, faculty, and deans at medical schools in the United States. *N Engl J Med.* 1999;340:928–936.

Part Two

Special Populations

This section covers certain special populations that by virtue of poverty and housing status, race, sexuality, mental illness, gender identity, citizenship, occupational status, and criminal justice system involvement suffer disproportionately and face unique challenges. Worldwide many individuals could be classified as "special populations," such as those who lack housing, clean water, sanitation, adequate food, employment with fair wages, and equal rights regardless of gender, sexual preference, race, or migrant status. These populations are also covered in other sections.

Chapter Six (by Martin Donohoe) covers homelessness, a persistent problem for which society has failed to provide adequate solutions, instead relying on a patchwork of poorly funded services provided by overworked and underpaid yet highly committed individuals.

Chapter Seven (by Safina Koreishi and Martin Donohoe) describes the plight of a group even less visible than the homeless: the migrant and seasonal farm workers whose dangerous, underpaid, often-abusive labor puts food on our tables daily.

Chapter Eight (by David S. Jones) reviews persistent health disparities among Native Americans, whose victimization began with the arrival of Christopher Columbus. The explorer's log entry on meeting the Arawaks of the Bahamas was, "They ... brought us ... many ... things .... They willingly traded everything they owned.... They do not bear arms.... They would make fine servants .... With fifty men we could subjugate them all and make them do whatever we want."[1] This encounter led to European colonization of the Americas and the decimation of native populations by smallpox and other diseases for which they lacked immunity. Then followed the US government's westward expansion, which forced Native Americans onto smaller and smaller plots of less-than-ideal land. These factors, along with attempts to destroy their culture by "westernizing" them, have contributed to numerous economic and health disparities, which persist despite access to government-funded health care.

Chapter Nine (by Peter A. Clark) provides a historical, ethical, and policy analysis of how contemporary prejudices within the medical profession against African Americans affects doctors and patients. From the legacy of slavery to the abuses of the Tuskegee syphilis study to the ongoing quest for civil rights, African Americans have suffered numerous injustices. These include income and educational disparities, higher levels of unemployment and criminal justice system involvement, neighborhoods subject to an inordinate number of toxic waste dumps (environmental racism), and persistent overt and subtle discrimination (e.g., in housing, "driving while black," etc.). They face higher levels of poverty,[2] unemployment,[3] and uninsurance,[4,5] than Caucasians; have higher maternal and infant mortality;[6] receive fewer diagnostic tests and undergo fewer therapeutic procedures;[7] and face shorter life expectancies and suffer from higher death rates for most diseases.[8] Whereas medical advances averted 176,633 deaths between 1991 and 2000, equalizing the mortality rates of whites and African Americans would have averted 686,202 deaths.[9]

Chapter Ten (by Kenneth H. Mayer, Judith B. Bradford, Harvey J. Makadon, Ron Stall, Hillary Goldhammer, and Stewart Landers) discusses methods for defining and measuring a highly marginalized population, sexual and gender minorities, also known as lesbian, gay, bisexual, and transgendered individuals. The authors review the health care needs of this group and the societal and structural barriers they face in obtaining needed care and services (including stigmatization). They conclude by offering suggestions for creating a healthier environment for these minorities through research, education, and culturally appropriate programs.

Chapter Eleven (by Emmanuel M. Ngui, Lincoln Khasakhala, David Ndetei, and Laura Weiss Roberts) addresses the global burden of mental disorders, with particular attention to developing nations. The authors cover the scope of mental illness and the relationship of mental disorders to health inequalities and economic development. They describe the extent of stigmatization of and discrimination against the mentally ill, the ethical principles relevant to mental health inequalities between people and between nations, and the absence of adequate and quality mental health services in many nations. They offer a public health approach to combatting mental health disparities, which includes the integration of mental and physical health into primary care.

Chapter Twelve (by Martin Donohoe) analyzes the health and welfare of those incarcerated in our jails and prisons, explores the prison-industrial complex, criticizes the criminal justice system for its failure to rehabilitate convicts, and critiques the death penalty.

These chapters paint a bleak picture of the situation facing marginalized populations, yet all include descriptions of people and programs involved in countering the consequences of marginalization as well as suggestions for activism. Further information regarding the topics in this part can be found on the following pages of the Public Health and Social Justice website: homelessness at http://phsj.org/homelessness/; migrant farm workers at http://phsj.org/migrant-and-seasonal-farm-worker-health/; race, ethnicity, and culture at http://phsj.org/race-ethnicity-and-culture/; homosexuality and human rights at http://phsj.org/homosexuality-and-human-rights/; and the criminal justice system at http://phsj.org/the-criminal-justice-system/.

Notes

1. Zinn, H. *A people's history of the United States* (New York: Harper Collins, 1995), 1.

2. US Census. *Income, poverty, and health insurance coverage in the US, 2009.* Retrieved from http://www.census.gov/prod/2010pubs/p60-238.pdf.

3. Bureau of Labor Statistics. *Table A-2: Employment status of the civilian population by race, sex, and age,* January 7, 2011. Retrieved from http://www.bls.gov/news.release/empsit.t02.htm.

4. Kaiser Family Foundation. *Worker's health insurance coverage by race and ethnicity, 2009.* Retrieved from http://facts.kff.org/chart.aspx?cb=60&sctn=174&ch=1911. US Census, ibid.

5. US Census. *Income, poverty and health insurance coverage in the US, 2009.* Available at http://www.census.gov/newsroom/releases/archives/income_wealth/cb10-144.html#tablec.

6. Centers for Disease Control and Prevention. Health disparities and inequalities report, US 2011. *Morbidity and Mortality Weekly Report,* January 14, 2011. Retrieved from http://www.cdc.gov/mmwr/pdf/other/su6001.pdf.

7. Ibid.

8. Ibid.

9. Woolf, S. H., Johnson, R. E., Fryer, G. E., Fust, G., & Satcher, D. The health impact of resolving racial disparities: An analysis of US mortality data. *American Journal of Public Health,* 2004, *94,* 2078–2081. Retrieved from http://ajph.aphapublications.org/cgi/reprint/94/12/2078.

Chapter 6

Homelessness in the United States

History, Epidemiology, Health Issues, Women, and Public Policy

Martin Donohoe

Introduction

This article discusses the recent history and current etiologies of homelessness in the United States, presents information regarding homeless persons and their health problems, and describes steps healthcare providers can take to care for homeless patients and to try to overcome the social problem of homelessness. Although most issues relevant to homelessness affect both men and women, homeless women's unique circumstances and health problems will be emphasized when relevant.

Background and Recent History

The United States is a signatory to the Universal Declaration of Human Rights. Article 25(1) of this document states: "Everyone has the right to ... food, clothing, *housing* and medical care and necessary social services" [emphasis mine].[1] The explicit nature of the nation's societal contract to meet the housing needs of its citizens is spelled out in the Housing Act of 1949, which stipulates the "realization as soon as feasible of the goal of a decent home ... for every American family."[2] In 1968, The Fair Housing Act made discrimination on the basis of race in the housing market illegal. Regrettably, neither the Universal

Declaration nor these landmark laws have solved the problem of homelessness, nor of substandard housing and racial profiling by sellers and realtors.[3]

In the United States, de-institutionalization of the mentally ill— unaccompanied by promised outpatient psychiatric and social services—led to a large increase in the homeless, mentally ill population in the late 1970s. The number of homeless grew in the 1980s as housing and social service cuts increased. This was in part a consequence of the transfer of federal dollars to a huge military buildup (including the spectacularly wasteful and unsuccessful "Star Wars" strategic missile defense initiative) and consequent large budget deficits. Fortunately, public compassion soared, and in 1986, 5 million Americans joined hands across the country to raise money for homeless programs (May 25, 1986, Hands Across America). In 1987, the McKinney Act authorized millions of dollars for housing and hunger relief.

Epidemiology

Almost 20 years later, homelessness is largely ignored by the mainstream press and the general public, and the numbers affected continue to grow. Over 7% of persons living in the United States have been homeless (defined as sleeping in shelters, the street, abandoned buildings, cars, or bus and train stations) at some point in their lives.[4] Homelessness rates have increased over each of the past 2 decades. An estimated 2.5 to 3.5 million people now experience homelessness each year.[5,6] Approximately half are families with children, the fastest-growing segment of the homeless population.[5,6] In 1 study,[7] youth had a 1-year rate of homelessness of at least 1 night of 7.6%.

Although 20% of homeless persons maintain full- or part-time jobs,[8] only 5% are privately insured, often through COBRA.[9] The majority of homeless adults are not eligible for Medicaid in most states, and are also not eligible for Medicare. Approximately 23% of homeless persons (and from 3.1% to 4.4% of homeless women) are veterans of the armed services, yet only 57% have received healthcare services through the VA system, where long waits for care exist.[10]

Because they usually lack health insurance, homeless persons tend not to get adequate preventive care and appropriate routine management of such chronic illnesses as hypertension, heart disease, diabetes, and emphysema. They tend to visit emergency rooms for acute illnesses.[11] Besides lack of health insurance, other barriers to care include denial of health problems; the pressure to fulfill competing nonfinancial needs, such as those for food, clothing, and temporary shelter; and misconceptions, prejudices, and frustrations on the part of health professionals.[12] When hospitalized, the average length of stay of a homeless individual, in 1 study,[13] was 4.1 days, or 36% longer than that of low-income, non-homeless individuals, even after adjustment for differences in the rates of substance abuse and mental illness and other clinical and demographic characteristics. The cost of the additional hospital days per discharge ranged from $2,414 to $4,094 (1992–1993 dollars).

Homeless adults have an age-adjusted mortality rate nearly 4 times that of the general population; their average life span is shorter than 45 years.[14] Homeless women 18 to 44 years of age are between 5 and 31 times more likely to die than women in the general population.[15] Homeless women older than age 44 are only 1 to 2 times as likely to die, and are healthier than their male counterparts.[15] However, homeless women in their mid-fifties are as physiologically aged as housed women in their seventies and are afflicted to a similar degree with chronic diseases, yet they do not qualify for elderly housing assistance.[8]

Homeless women are more likely than homeless men to have experienced childhood sexual abuse and/or foster care and adult partner abuse.[16] More than 50% of all homeless women and children become homeless as a direct result of fleeing domestic violence.[17] The availability of domestic violence shelter beds in the United States is poor; up to 70% to 80% of women, and 80% of children, are turned away on any given night in major cities.[17] Shelters are woefully underfunded; some do not allow children. Average length of stay at a US shelter is 14 days; most allow a 30-day maximum stay.[17] Ironically, women fleeing domestic violence are often not counted in studies of homelessness since they are considered to have a home (albeit unlivable) or are staying temporarily in shelters.

Health Problems of the Homeless

On average, homeless adults have 8 to 9 concurrent medical illnesses.[18] The homeless commonly suffer from dermatologic conditions (e.g., skin lice, scabies, eczema, and allergic rashes), respiratory infections, tooth decay, foot problems (e.g., trench foot, tinea pedis), vision disturbances, sexually transmitted infections (STIs), and trauma. Functional limitations, substance abuse, and mental illness (particularly depression, schizophrenia, posttraumatic stress disorder, and personality disorders) are very common. Mental illness is reported in 30% of homeless persons, and in 50% to 60% of homeless women.[8] The usual chronic diseases, such as hypertension, diabetes, and asthma, are quite prevalent and difficult to manage. Preventive tests are underutilized because of time and funding constraints[5] and because patients tend to present with acute care needs that require immediate attention. Homeless children frequently suffer from respiratory, ear, and skin infections, failure to thrive, developmental delay, and face neglect and abuse.[19]

STIs are common among homeless girls and women, a function of limited access to reproductive health services, prostitution, and survival sex (i.e., sex in exchange for food, drugs, or temporary shelter). Twenty-six percent of female street youths (28% of male street youths and 10% of shelter youths) report having participated in survival sex, which is associated with older age, more days away from home, victimization, criminal behaviors, substance use, suicide attempts, STIs, and pregnancy.[20] Homeless women have a pregnancy rate about twice the national rate.[16] HIV rates are higher than in the general population, which has been attributed to higher prevalence of intravenous drug use, STIs, prostitution, survival sex, and limited access to condoms.[5]

Unique aspects of homelessness that contribute to hard-to-manage medical and psychiatric illness include enhanced vulnerability to crime and violence; prolonged standing; excessive outdoor exposure; infectious disease transmission due to overcrowding; high risk of being robbed of medication; limited access to water for showers, dental care, and personal hygiene; inability to follow complex treatment and home care regimens; lack of privacy; and social isolation.[8] Those with language barriers—particularly those who lack citizenship and work long hours under dangerous conditions—such as homeless migrant and seasonal farm workers, face particular challenges and are often afraid to access even emergency care.[21,22]

The Future

Given the growing budget deficit, spiraling military costs of the wars in Iraq and Afghanistan, increasing wealth disparities between rich and poor (supported by the regressive tax cuts of the current administration), and job loss spurred in part by outsourcing, the problem of homelessness is likely to continue to grow. Regrettably, the president's budget for fiscal year 2005 calls for cutting federal housing assistance.

Suggestions for Healthcare Providers and Social Activists

Those providing care to homeless patients should familiarize themselves with the unique medical, psychological, economic, cultural, and social problems of this group; treat them with the same respect and empathy accorded other patients; be predictable and available; listen carefully to their life stories; avoid a judgmental attitude; empower patients; provide qualified translators when necessary; simplify medical regimens; schedule frequent follow-up visits; be familiar with local substance abuse programs and social service agencies; and learn how to enroll patients in Medicaid.[8]

Healthcare providers should lobby policy makers for increased funding for housing, mental health and substance abuse treatment, primary healthcare (ideally under a single payer system), and case management services for the homeless. Anti-vagrancy laws should be repealed. A living wage, indexed locally to the cost of housing, should replace the current minimum wage. Disability benefits for those who are unable to work should be adequate to prevent them from becoming homeless. Exclusionary zoning ordinances should be overturned, and businesses should be encouraged to invest in the revitalization of low-income neighborhoods, to counter trends toward abandonment on one hand and gentrification on the other.

Measures to educate women and to improve their legal and political status and access to reproductive health services should be vigorously advanced.[23-26] Medical and nursing school faculty should enlighten students to the problems of the homeless (and increase their compassion and combat negative stereotypes[27]) through lectures, literature by and about the homeless,[28-31] and via required rotations in clinics serving the homeless. Academic medical centers in particular need to renew their commitment to the homeless and underserved, instead of worsening our 2-tiered system of healthcare by developing and marketing luxury primary care clinics for the wealthy.[32] As a country and as a profession, we possess the resources to provide quality healthcare and social services to the homeless, and to transition them into temporary and even permanent housing. What we require is the communal vision and political will to accomplish this.

Notes

1. Universal Declaration of Human Rights. Adopted and proclaimed by the United Nations General Assembly on December 10, 1948. Available at http://www.un.org/en/documents/udhr/. Accessed June 16, 2004.

2. Freeman L. America's affordable housing crisis: A contract unfulfilled. *Am J Publ Hlth.* 2002;92:709–712.

3. Pintcoff W. No place to call home: America's housing crisis. *Dollars and Sense* 2000:24–25, 45–47.

4. Link BG, Susser E, Stueve A, et al. Lifetime and five-year prevalence of homelessness in the United States. *Am J Publ Hlth.* 1994;84:1907–1912.

5. Levy BD, O'Connell JJ. Health care for homeless persons. *N Engl J Med.* 2004;350:2329–2332. Abstract.

6. Isaacs SL, Knickman JR, eds. *To improve health and health care.* Volume 7. San Francisco: Jossey Bass; 2004:199.

7. Ringwalt CL, Greene JM, Robertson M, McPheeters M. The prevalence of homelessness among adolescents in the United States. *Am J Publ Hlth.* 1998;88:1325–1329.

8. Means RH. *A primary care approach to treating women without homes.* Available at http://www.ncbi.nlm.nih.gov/pubmed/11547264.

9. National Health Care for the Homeless Council. *Mainstreaming health care for homeless people.* Available at http://www.nhchc.org/wp-content/uploads/2011/10/Mainstreaming-Health-Care-for-Homeless-People.pdf.

10. Gamache G, Rosencheck R, Tessler R. Overrepresentation of women veterans among homeless women. *Am J Publ Hlth.* 2003;93:1132–1136.

11. Kushel MB, Perry S, Bangsberg D, et al. Emergency department user among the homeless and marginally housed: Results from a community-based study. *Am J Publ Hlth.* 2002;92:778–784.

12. Stark L. Barriers to health care for the homeless. In: Jahiel RI, ed. *Homelessness: A prevention-oriented approach.* Baltimore: Johns Hopkins University Press; 1992.

13. Salit SA, Kuhn EM, Hartz AJ, et al. Hospitalization costs associated with homelessness in New York City. *N Engl J Med.* 1998;338:1734–1740. Abstract.

14. Hibbs JR, Benner L, Klugman L, et al. Mortality in a cohort of homeless adults in Philadelphia. *N Engl J Med.* 1994;331:304–309. Abstract.

15. Cheung AM, Hwang SW. Risk of death among homeless women: A cohort study and review of the literature. *Can Med Assoc J.* 2004;170:1243–1247.

16. Robrecht LC, Anderson DG. Interpersonal violence and the pregnant homeless woman. *J Obstet Gyn Neonat Nurs.* 1998;27:684–691.

17. Jensen RH. Domestic violence facts. *Ms.* 1994;V(2):44–51.

18. Breaky WR, Fischer PJ, Kramer M, et al. Health and mental health problems of homeless men and women in Baltimore. *JAMA.* 1989;262:1352–1357. Abstract.

19. Usatine RP, Gelberg L, Smith MH, Lesser J. Health care for the homeless: A family medicine perspective. *Am Fam Physician* 1994:139–146.

20. Greene J, Ennett ST, Ringwalt CL. Prevalence and correlates of survival sex among runaway and homeless youth. *Am J Publ Hlth.* 89:1406–1409.

21. Donohoe MT. Trouble in the fields: Effects of migrant and seasonal farm labor on women's health and well-being. *Medscape Ob/Gyn and Women's Health.* Available at: http://www.medscape.com/viewarticle/470445. Posted March 4, 2004.

22. Hansen E, Donohoe MT. Health issues of migrant and seasonal farm workers. *J Health Care Poor Underserv.* 2003;14:153–164.

23. Donohoe MT. Violence and human rights abuses against women in the developing world. *Medscape Ob/Gyn and Women's Health* 2003;8(2). Available at http://www.medscape.com/viewarticle/464255. Posted November 26, 2003.

24. Donohoe MT. Causes and health consequences of environmental degradation and social injustice. *Soc Sci Med.* 2003;56:573–587. Abstract.

25. Donohoe MT. Individual and societal forms of violence against women in the United States and the developing world: An overview. *Curr Women's Hlth Rep.* 2002;2:313–319.

26. Donohoe MT. Teen pregnancy: A call for sound science and public policy. *Z Magazine* 2003;16:14–16.

27. Ugarriza DN, Fallon T. Nurses' attitudes toward homeless women: A barrier to change. *Nurs Outlook.* 1994;42:26–29. Abstract.

28. Donohoe MT. Exploring the human condition: Literature and public health issues. In: Hawkins AH, McEntyre MC, eds. *Teaching literature and medicine.* New York: Modern Language Association; 2000.

29. Donohoe MT, Danielson S. A community-based approach to the medical humanities. *Medical Education* 2004;38:204–217. Abstract.

30. Lars Eighner. *Travels with Lizbeth.* New York: St. Martin's Press; 1993.

31. Wolf KA, Goldfader R, Lehan C. Women speak: Healing the wounds of homelessness through writing. *Nursing Hlth Care Perspect Community* 1997;18:74–78.

32. Donohoe MT. Luxury primary care, academic medical centers, and the erosion of science and professional ethics. *J Gen Int Med.* 2004;19:90–94.

Chapter 7

Historical and Contemporary Factors Contributing to the Plight of Migrant Farmworkers in the United States

Safina Koreishi
Martin Donohoe

Introduction

American consumers rely on the labor of migrant and seasonal farmworkers, many of whom work for large agricultural corporations, to put food on our tables.[1] Immigration practices and policies dictate the extent to which migrant farmworkers have access to governmental health and social services. Even though their jobs involve significant occupational hazards, the majority of migrant farmworkers are ineligible for government services, and employers generally do not provide these workers with health insurance.[1] Migrant farmworkers also face food insecurity, poor housing conditions, impaired access to education for their children, and even human rights violations. This chapter begins with a description of migrant farmworkers, then progresses to a historical discussion of immigration and labor laws in order to help the reader understand the present-day plight of the migrant farmworker. The chapter also describes the workplace conditions, human rights violations, and lack of social services which migrant farmworkers confront every day in order to survive in an ever-expanding global marketplace.

Migrant Agricultural Labor in the United States Today

A migrant farmworker is ''an individual whose principal employment is in agriculture on a seasonal basis, and who, for purposes of employment, establishes a temporary home.''[1] Approximately 1.6 million migrant farmworkers work on American soil, harvesting fruits and vegetables for American consumers, as well as for export, thus contributing to the American economy.[2] While the majority of migrant farmworkers are Mexican, others come from countries such as Guatemala and the Dominican Republic, with smaller numbers from other parts of Latin America, Asia, Canada, and Europe.[3]

An estimated 70% of migrant farmworkers (or 24% of all farmworkers) are undocumented, and the majority live below the poverty line.[3,4] Their wages, relative to those of the leaders of the large corporate agribusiness operations which employ them, mirror the widening gap seen throughout US industries between management and labor. While on average farmworkers in the US earn $7,500 per year, Archer Daniels Midland, the world leader in production of soy meal, corn, wheat, and cocoa, reaped $1.7 billion in profits in 2003, and its chief executive officer, Allen G. Andreas, made a salary of over $2.9 million. Dole, the world's largest producer of fruit and vegetables, made $4.8 billion in revenues in 2003.[5]

Migrant farmworkers provide an essential service and perform jobs that many Americans are unwilling to do. Throughout the 20th century, the US government and corporations have collaborated to make it possible to use farmworkers as cheap laborers, claiming that their policies decrease the cost of food, yet resulting in huge profits for American corporations.

History of Immigration and Labor Laws

Agriculture's reliance on immigrant labor dates back to indentured servitude and slavery, both of which were critical to the economic development of the New World. In the 17th century, the colonies utilized indentured servants as an important source of labor. Indentured servants were afforded some rights, but as demands for labor grew, so did their cost. In order to maintain low wages, employers looked to slavery to fill their labor shortage. Unlike indentured servants, slaves were involuntary immigrants who lacked any rights of citizenship.[6]

After slavery was abolished in the 19th century, the US agricultural industry began to use Mexican workers as a source of cheap labor.[7] Because of a shortage of farmworkers during World War I, Congress passed the Immigration and Nationality Act in 1917, creating a legal pathway for 73,000 Mexican workers to enter the United States.[7] As a result of this legislation, many Mexicans continued to come to the United States to find work even after the war. Then, in a reversal of policy brought on by job losses during the Great Depression, the Immigration and Naturalization Service worked with Mexican authorities to deport approximately 40,000 Mexican Americans.

To address agricultural labor shortages during World War II, Mexico and the US partnered to create the Bracero program in 1943. This program allowed Mexicans to temporarily work in the American agricultural industry. Mexican laborers were required to return home after working for a given amount of time.[7] During the economic boom that followed World War II, President Eisenhower expelled 1.5 million Mexican farmworkers, 60% of whom were legal residents, through "Operation Wetback."[4]

Even so, between 1942 and 1964 nearly 5 million workers came to the US to help the labor shortages. The Bracero program continued until 1964, when Congress authorized the H-2 A visa program, designed to bring temporary low-wage workers into the United States.[22] The H-2 A visa program continues today, allowing foreign nationals to enter the US for temporary agricultural work and requiring that they return to their home country after a given amount of time. Many of these workers over-stay this time period, thus becoming "undocumented" immigrants. In addition, other undocumented immigrants enter the US without a work visa.

There are many common myths regarding migrant farmworkers, both documented and undocumented. One myth is that they are taking advantage of the American system by "free riding," and as such constitute a "drain on the economy."[6,8] In fact, evidence shows that all immigrants (documented and undocumented combined) contribute to the US economy in proportion to their share of the population.[6,9] Undocumented workers provide important services through their labor and pay state income, excise, and property taxes as well as federal Social Security and Medicare taxes.[10] A 2007 study by the Oregon Center for Public Policy (OCPP) estimated that undocumented immigrants contribute between $66 and $77 million in property taxes, state income taxes, and excise taxes annually in Oregon.[10] While undocumented immigrants in other cities and states contribute the same amount or more to the local and state economy than they receive in local and state benefits, in other locales, state and local government spending on undocumented immigrants exceeds the cost of state and local services.[8-12] Since undocumented workers are ineligible for most federal benefits, this shortfall is balanced by their contributions through Social Security and Medicare taxes (which are, however, not always distributed in proportion to a state's share of undocumented immigrants). The Social Security Administration estimates that nationwide, undocumented workers contribute $7 billion in Social Security taxes and $1.5 billion in Medicare taxes annually.[8] On average, the National Research Council estimates each undocumented immigrant will contribute approximately $80,000 more per capita over his or her lifetime than he or she will consume in governmental services.[8] Such workers also contribute to the economy through rental payments and by purchasing goods and services (e.g., food, clothing, and utilities). Nevertheless, they are able to access few public, tax-funded social benefits, such as supplemental security income and disability, food stamps, housing assistance, and free legal representation. Elderly undocumented immigrants rarely qualify for Medicare benefits.[8] Though undocumented immigrant children are provided free public education until high school (which accounts for a large percentage of the higher costs attributed to undocumented immigrants in those areas in which a shortfall exists), they are ineligible for federal student loans, and are therefore less likely to be able to afford burgeoning college tuition costs.[8]

A second myth is that undocumented immigrants take American jobs.[8] In fact, US unemployment rates have little to do with immigration and have more to do with neo-liberal "free-trade" policies that have effectively encouraged American companies to outsource manufacturing and service sector jobs to countries with lower wages, fewer taxes, and more lax environmental and occupational health and safety standards. It is difficult to outsource farming, so instead corporations have found a way to import cheap labor. Furthermore, many corporations support policies that create domestic inequalities, including unfair immigration rules designed to provide a continuous stream of vulnerable workers willing to labor for lower wages than unionized American employees (while simultaneously opposing unions).[8] Employers who lay off undocumented immigrants will not see their unemployment insurance (UI) tax rates increase since the undocumented immigrants cannot collect UI benefits, whereas employers whose workers receive UI benefits may see their state UI tax rate increase in the future.[10]

After American unions organized to improve working conditions and enforce labor regulations, corporations began to outsource manufacturing operations to developing countries. Because American agricultural industries could not feasibly relocate to developing countries, large agricultural corporations began to support the importation of "Third World" human labor. The ability of these corporations to continue to reap large profits is dependent on maintaining the secondary status of undocumented farmworkers.[6] Neo-liberal "free-trade" policies and the desire to increase (or at least maintain) profitability have had many deleterious effects on society, including deteriorating human rights conditions on American farms.[13] Many large food corporations have consolidated under the pressures of globalization. They subsequently underpay their growers and maintain poor working conditions in order to achieve a competitive advantage in the global food market. This situation has led to forced labor, beatings, sweatshop conditions, and modern-day slavery, which will be discussed in further detail following.[13]

The present-day situation regarding undocumented immigrants in this country is complex and controversial, and fair and just immigration reform is essential. President Barack Obama has proposed a plan for "immigration amnesty," which would benefit up to 20 million undocumented immigrants who are currently in the United States by allowing them to obtain a green card. His plan would also increase border control and create incentives for undocumented immigrants to "come out of the shadows," in order to earn the opportunity to become citizens. President Obama has also called for greater penalties for employers who hire undocumented immigrants.[14]

Social and Working Conditions of Migrant Farmworkers

Relevant International Standards

The International Labor Organization (ILO), created in 1919 at the end of World War I, formulates labor standards and basic rights for workers and works to promote social justice in the work place. The ILO stresses freedom of association, the right to organize, collective bargaining, and the abolition of forced labor. In 2006, they adopted a plan to give a fair deal to the millions of migrant workers throughout the world, which addresses issues such as abusive practices, specific job risks, and safety.[15]

The 1948 Universal Declaration of Human Rights states, "Everyone has the right to a standard of living adequate for the health and well-being of oneself and one's family, including food, clothing, housing, and medical care."[16] Though many countries have adopted this declaration, the United States government still does not view health care and many other social services as rights for immigrants to this country[16] (or, for that matter, for native-born persons). This regressive position perpetuates the precarious circumstances faced by undocumented farmworkers, who are already vulnerable in terms of occupational and environmental dangers, poverty, language barriers, lack of transportation, and educational, legal, and political marginalization.

Evolution of Federal and State Policy

Foreign guest workers temporarily working in the US agricultural industry are vulnerable and subject to workplace violations.[2] During the 1950s and 1960s the American government started to pay attention to the plight of farmworkers. In the early 1950s, the Public Health Service expanded its focus to include community and preventive health care for migrant farmworkers, and in 1954, the Surgeon General created the Migrant Health Unit to carry out research regarding the health of this population. In 1955, spurred by presidential committee reports on poor conditions in work camps, Congress extended social security benefits to migrant workers.[7] As a result of growing awareness of the poor working conditions and poor health of migrant farm workers, John F. Kennedy passed the Migrant Health Act in September 1962. This act authorized governmental grants to pay for migrant health centers.[7]

On Thanksgiving Day in 1960, the documentary *Harvest of Shame* by Edward R. Murrow aired on television.[7] This heightened public awareness of, and sympathy towards, the plight of farmworkers. Soon thereafter, Caesar Chavez, a Mexican-American labor leader and civil rights activist who founded the National Farmworkers Association, led farmworker labor strikes in California.* As a result of these strikes, in 1966 Congress amended the Fair Labor and Standards Act to require a minimum wage for farmworkers.[7] In 1970, the Occupational Safety and Health Administration was created to develop safety standards for all workers, including farmworkers. Nevertheless, violations of workers' rights continue. In 1983, Congress passed the Migrant and Seasonal Agricultural Workers Protection Act, which required employers to disclose employment conditions and wages to the government and to ensure that if housing was provided, it met certain standards.[7]

As discussed previously, it is legal to employ a foreign farmworker for a defined amount of time, after which these same workers immediately become "illegal" residents of the United States. In the past two decades there has been an increasing focus on undocumented immigrants, and an increasing amount of legislation has been passed to penalize them and those who employ them. In 1986, Congress passed the Immigration Reform and Control Act (IRCA). While providing amnesty for some undocumented immigrants and a path towards legalization for certain agricultural seasonal workers and immigrants, this law penalizes those who employ undocumented workers, and makes it illegal to knowingly hire undocumented immigrants. To circumvent IRCA, farm employers began to hire subcontractors to provide them with undocumented workers. Farmworkers continued to be placed in a vulnerable, powerless position. Though there are minimal laws in place to protect farmworkers against employer abuse, no laws exist to protect them from a "middleman." The lack of regulations covering subcontractors has led to deteriorating conditions in the workplace and to further farmworker disempowerment.[7]

Both the Illegal Immigration Reform and Immigrant Responsibility Act ("Immigration Reform Act") of 1996 and the Personal Responsibility and Work Opportunity Reconciliation Act ("Welfare Reform Act") of 1996 have restricted immigrants' access to public services.[7] The Immigration Reform Act bans legal immigrants from receiving Medicaid for five years after entering the country. The act also requires family members who sponsor relatives to pledge that they will help to keep the immigrant above 125% of the federal poverty line, thereby exceeding eligibility requirements for governmental support. The

---

*Thanks to a Campaign by the United Farm Workers and others, the Texas School Board recently shelved a proposal to eliminate all textbook references to Hispanics, including Cesar Chavez, since the conquest of Mexico in the early 16th century. The proposal was sadly ironic, given that Hispanics will soon comprise the majority of Texas schoolchildren. See United Farm Workers and the update on Cesar Chavez and the Texas history book situation. Available at http://www.ufw.org/_board.php?mode=view&b_code=hotissue&b_no=5861. Accessed January 23, 2010.

Welfare Reform Act denies both undocumented and legal immigrants public benefits such as food stamps, Aid to Families with Dependent Children, and Supplemental Security Income if they came to the US after August 22, 1996. In 2005, Congress passed the Deficit Reduction Act, which requires immigrants to show proof of citizenship when applying for Medicaid.[17] The Children's Health Insurance Program Reauthorization Act (CHIPRA) of 2009 expanded the State Children's Health Insurance Program (CHIP) and now covers children of legal immigrants without the previously required five year waiting period. However, undocumented immigrant children will continue to be ineligible for the program.[18]

The legislative measures of the past two decades have restricted public services to all immigrants, including farmworkers, and are in stark contrast to the increasing international focus on human rights endorsed by the United Nations.[19] Large agribusiness and other employers of farm laborers have lobbied to prevent effective labor and immigration law enforcement in the workplace. For such employers, it is advantageous to hire vulnerable undocumented workers who will work hard, often in short contract cycles, without challenging unfair or illegal treatment.[2]

Violations of Social and Working Conditions

The United States has relied on cheap agricultural labor since its inception, and has used concepts of racism and non-citizenship to perpetuate the second class status of its farmworkers.[4] When migrant farmworkers leave their families to come to work in America, they are vulnerable, speak little to no English, and are often willing to work for little pay in order to support themselves and their loved ones back home. In 2006, Mexican remittances were $23 billion, almost all of which was from Mexican farmworkers in the United States. Remittances make up approximately 13% of the average Mexican family's income.[20] Without such remittances, Mexico would face even greater poverty, which in turn would stimulate further emigration to the US and an increased need for US foreign aid to alleviate the social unrest and crime (including drug crime) that poverty fosters.

Farm employers often take advantage of their employees' disadvantaged state, reaping benefits from farmworkers' labor without providing fair treatment in return. The United Nations Commission on Human Rights claims that the US government violates the rights of migrant farmworkers and contributes to the propagation of modern-day slavery by denying them the right to unionize, as granted by the National Labor Relations Act.[13] In addition, many safety and fair pay regulations are minimally enforced in this population. The Coalition of Immokalee Workers (CIW) recently described "systematic violations of the human rights outlined in Articles 1, 2, 3, 4, 6, 7, 8, 10, 20, 22, 23, 24, 25, 26 and 28 of the Universal Declaration of Human

Rights" by agricultural employers, such as Taco Bell (a subsidiary of Yum! Brands).[13] They claimed that employers and their contractors have forced agricultural workers in Florida to labor under poor conditions, with little or no pay, and with the threat of debt, deportation, and violence as weapons of control.[13] According to a statement written by the Robert F. Kennedy Memorial Center for Human Rights, on behalf of the National Economic and Social Rights Initiative and the CIW, in Florida, inhumane working conditions are widespread:

> Sweatshop conditions in the fields are pervasive; violence and various forms of intimidation are common; and wages have plummeted while slavery has become more prevalent. Workers are pushed into severe poverty and dangerous working conditions, including up to 14 hour days for wages significantly below the official poverty rate.[13]

Though outlawed almost 150 years ago in the United States, there have been six recent slavery court cases brought against growers in Florida. In one of these, Judge Moore of the Southern District Court of Florida decried "corporate individuals who are ... sophisticated in the ways in which they can victimize the undocumented immigrants coming to the United States."[13]

To address slavery and deteriorating human rights among migrant farmworker populations, we must uncover the roots of discrimination and work to redress its consequences.[13]

Health Care Issues Related to Undocumented Migrant Farmworkers and Their Children

Migrant farmworkers have worse health outcomes than other workers in the United States, and often lack access to needed health care. Even those who are legal residents often receive only emergency medical care.[21] Medical needs include detection, treatment, and control of infectious diseases such as HIV and tuberculosis; maternal and child health care (including pregnancy care and immunizations); recognition, treatment, and prevention of pesticide poisoning; and prevention and management of chronic health conditions, such as heart disease, diabetes, and cancer.[22] Communicable disease prevention is relevant to the health of other farmworkers as well as to that of the general public.

Presently, some uninsured migrant farmworkers and their families obtain medical care through migrant health centers, which receive grants from the federal government. Though these clinics provide an important service, they cover only 12–15% of this population.[22] Migrant farmworkers also can receive emergency health care through emergency Medicaid, and hospitals must comply with the Emergency Medical Treatment and Labor Act (EMTALA) when treating this population. EMTALA requires emergency rooms to diagnose, treat, and stabilize all persons presenting for care and prevents patient "dumping" (i.e., transferring unstable persons who lack insurance to other institutions). Emergency care and hospitalization is less cost-effective, and certainly less optimal from a clinical perspective, than preventive care.

Children of undocumented farmworkers may work in agriculture starting at age twelve. Because of their migratory nature, children experience frequent moves and interrupted schooling. They (and their parents) encounter daily degrading and demeaning epithets (from being called "illegal" persons or hateful, demeaning racial slurs), which can impact their self-esteem and psychological development. Their lives are affected greatly by the immigration status and experiences of their parents.[22,23] Families are often torn apart by Immigration Customs Enforcement raids. Almost 30,000 people are currently being held in administrative detention for alleged violations of immigration law, an increase of almost 50% since 2005.[24] Such centers have been cited for substandard medical care.[24]

Undocumented children who come to the United States with their parents are excluded from non-emergency health care (except immunizations), unless they are able to be seen at a migrant health center, or a safety-net clinic, all of which are unable to meet the growing demand to provide services to uninsured patients (both documented citizens and undocumented immigrants). Even children who are born in the United States, and therefore eligible for governmental insurance, are often not enrolled in insurance plans because of language barriers, inadequate assistance in completing necessary paperwork, and parents' fears of deportation.[25] Though immigrant children use less ambulatory and emergency services, when emergency services are used, the amount spent is more than that spent on non-immigrant children. This may indicate that immigrant children are sicker when accessing emergency care since they were denied cheaper, upstream preventive health measures that could have been provided in the outpatient setting.[26] Furthermore, such children are more susceptible to pesticide exposure and toxicity as well as communicable and respiratory diseases, which have both short- and long-term health consequences.

There is a common myth that US public health insurance programs are overburdened with immigrants.[6,8] This is not true since undocumented immigrants are ineligible for federal services other than emergency Medicaid, and even emergency care is underutilized because of barriers such as transportation, low wages, and fears of deportation. However, twenty-one states have started using state-only funds to cover pregnant women and immigrant children.[8] This is a cost-effective measure since mothers who receive inadequate prenatal care are more likely to give birth to children with medical problems, and their children immediately become US citizens at birth, making them eligible for government-funded health care through Medicaid.

In 1994, voters passed California proposition 187 [which was later struck down by the State Supreme Court], making undocumented immigrants ineligible for all medical services except for emergency services. In addition, it required health care providers to report suspected undocumented persons to the Immigration and Naturalization Service. In a study assessing the effect of this law on the medical system, Fenton et. al.[27] found that proposition 187 resulted in a shift of mental health visits from the outpatient setting to crisis services, which are more expensive. Patients may have failed to access outpatient services or to fill their prescriptions secondary to fear of deportation.[27]

Conclusions and Call to Action

In the United States, we take our ability to buy cheap food and other items for granted. Very few people question where their food comes from, where their clothes are made, or the conditions under which those providing such items labor. Large corporations have been a party to the unjust nature of the agricultural industry, striving to keep costs down and profits up.[7] There are many grassroots organizations, both nationally and in Oregon, that are addressing important issues pertaining to migrant farmworkers. The Coalition of Immokalee Workers (CIW) recently began the "Fair Food: Field to Table" campaign, which promotes fair treatment for farmworkers and a more socially just food system.[28] The American Civil Liberties Union has launched the "Immigrants Rights' Project," which focuses on expanding the rights of immigrants, and addressing discrimination against them.[29] Founded in 1962 by Cesar Chavez, the United Farm Workers is a farmworkers' union that fights for the rights of farmworkers, including advocating for immigration reform.[30]

In Oregon, Oregon Health and Science University's Center for Research on Occupational and Environmental Toxicology studies pesticide exposures and, through its "Reducing Pesticide Exposure in Minority Communities" program, focuses on improving the health of migrant agricultural workers.[31] The Washington-based organization Yakima Valley Farm Workers Clinic runs several safety-net, migrant health clinics throughout Washington and Oregon, providing comprehensive health care to underserved patients, both documented and undocumented, with a mission to "improve the quality of life for the farm workers, the underserved and others as we work to strengthen the health of our communities."[32] Others have tried to raise awareness regarding the injustices experienced by farmworkers in a country that "was founded on the principle that all people are born with an unalienable right to freedom."[33] The box lists specific actions which can be taken to improve the health of migrant farmworkers.

What Can Be Done to Improve the Health of Migrant Farmworkers?

- Create a stronger public health infrastructure

  - Enroll more health care providers to work with underserved populations
  - Employ more community outreach workers
  - Train bilingual and bicultural health care providers
  - Encourage alternative health care delivery methods (e.g., "health care vans")
  - Implement more advanced information tracking systems that can be networked among clinicians
  - Increase preventive health services such as dental care, family planning, accident prevention, and detection and control of chronic diseases
  - Broaden legislation and protection through improved US Department of Labor, Occupational Safety and Health Administration, and Environmental Protection Agency standards to eliminate overcrowded and unsanitary living conditions and workplace hazards and exposures
  - Create a system of universal access to care

- Improve education among migrant farmworkers and health care providers

  - Educate migrant farmworkers about prevention, detection, and treatment at their homes, workplaces, or community centers
  - Include migrant health care in medical, nursing, dental, and public health school curricula
  - Improve physician recognition, management, and reporting of pesticide-related illnesses

---

Source: Adapted from Hansen E, and Donohoe M. Health issues of migrant and seasonal farmworkers. *J Healthcare Poor Underserved* 2003;14:153–163.

These issues are not unique to the United States as rural agricultural laborers throughout many countries experience human rights violations and adverse health consequences resulting from their work. Collecting accurate data is paramount to informing change, and official government data are often corrupted. In Argentina, the non-governmental organization South Watch helped to reveal the inaccuracies in "official data" regarding the extent to which rural agricultural workers experience work-related health problems. As Maria Silva noted, reassuring yet inaccurate data can create an "official silence," leading many to underestimate the hardships farmworkers suffer and remain ignorant of the reality of their situation.[34]

Since these problems are germane to most countries, it would benefit farmworkers everywhere for activists and governments to collaborate across national lines. Through independent research, educational campaigns, and consumer actions designed to raise public and professional awareness and effect change, the United States and other countries can hopefully move toward a more just and equitable system based on international labor and human rights standards. Such a system would provide safe working conditions (including all necessary safety equipment to avoid exposure to pesticides and herbicides); a fair, living wage; adequate housing; comprehensive social services; and quality medical care to undocumented workers who contribute to society, even if they are not legal residents. Ideally such a system would also involve a return to smaller, family and cooperative farms where organic methods are employed to encourage soil and water conservation and limit environmental pollution.[35-37]

Notes

1. Arcury T, Quandt S. Delivery of health services to migrant and seasonal farmworkers. *Ann Rev Publ Hlth.* 2007;28:345–363.

2. Farmworker Justice website. http://www.fwjustice.org/. Accessed June 12, 2009.

3. Suro R. *Survey of Mexican migrants, part two.* Pew Hispanic Center. June 5, 2005. Available at http://pewhispanic.org/reports/report.php?ReportID=46. Accessed January 23, 2010.

4. Hastings M. Legalizing farm workers: A shared necessity. December 10, 2009. Available at http://maribelhastings.com/analisis/archive/legalizing_farm _workers_a_shared_necessity/. Accessed December 29, 2009.

5. Ahn C, with Moore M, Parker N. *Migrant farmworkers: America's new plantation workers.* Food First. Institute for Food and Development Policy. March 31, 2004. Available at http://www.foodfirst.org/node/45. Accessed December 29, 2009.

6. Chomsky A. *"They take our jobs." And 20 other myths about immigration.* Boston: Beacon Press; 2007.

7. National Center for Farmworker Health, Inc. *About America's farmworkers.* Available at http://www.ncfh.org/?sid=36. Accessed June 12, 2009.

8. King M. *Immigrants in the US health care system: Five myths that misinform the American public.* June 7, 2007. Available at http://www.americanprogress.org/issues/2007/06/immigrant_health_report.html. Accessed June 12, 2009.

9. Fiscal Policy Institute. *Immigrants and the economy: Contributions of immigrant workers to the country's 25 largest metro areas.* December 2009. Available at http://www.fiscalpolicy.org/ImmigrantsIn25MetroAreas_20091130.pdf. Accessed January 24, 2010.

10. Oregon Center for Public Policy. *Undocumented immigrants are taxpayers too: Issue brief.* April 2006. Available at http://www.ocpp.org/media/uploads/pdf/2012 /01/iss20120125UndocumentedTaxpayers_fnl.pdf. Accessed January 25, 2012.

11. Immigration Policy Center. *Assessing the economic impact of immigration at the state and local level.* August 18, 2009. Available at http://www.immigrationpolicy .org/just-facts/assessing-economic-impact-immigration-state-and-local-level. Accessed January 24, 2010.

12. Congressional Budget Office. *The impact of unauthorized immigrants on the budgets of state and local governments.* December 2007. Available at http://www.cbo.gov /ftpdocs/87xx/doc8711/12–6Immigration.pdf. Accessed January 24, 2010.

13. Economic and Social Council, Subcommission on Human Rights. 57th session, item 6(b) of the provision agenda, July 15, 2005.

14. US Immigration Amnesty. *Immigration amnesty.* Available at http://www .usamnesty.org/. Accessed January 30, 2010.

15. The International Labor Organization. *Press release.* http://www.ilo.org/global /about-the-ilo/lang--en/index.htm. Accessed January 5, 2010.

16. *The universal declaration of human rights.* Adopted and proclaimed by General Assembly resolution 217 A (III) of December 10, 1948. Available at http://www.un .org/Overview/rights.html. Accessed February 10, 2009.

17. Gold R. *Immigrants and Medicaid after welfare reform.* The Guttmacher Report on Public Policy. May 2003. Available at http://www.guttmacher.org/pubs/tgr/06/2 /gr060206.html. Accessed January 8, 2010.

18. The Kaiser Commission on Medicaid and the Uninsured. Children's Health Insurance Program Reauthorization Act of 2009. February 2009. Available at http://www .kff.org/medicaid/upload/7863.pdf. Accessed February 12, 2009.

19. Beck C. *Migrant farm workers under the new regime.* Available at http://www.wcl .american.edu/hrbrief/v5i1/html/migrant.html. Accessed February 11, 2009.

20. Mexico: Migrants, emigration, economy. *Migrant News.* April 2007. Available at http://migration.ucdavis.edu/MN/more.php?id=3275_0_2_0. Accessed May 15, 2009.

21. Villarejo D. The health of US hired farm workers. *Ann Rev Publ Hlth.* 2003;24: 175–193.

22. Hansen E, Donohoe M. Health issues of migrant and seasonal farmworkers. *J Healthcare Poor Underserved* 2003;14:153–163.

23. Ku L. Improving health insurance and access to care for children in immigrant families. *Amb Peds.* 2007;7:412–420.

24. Editors. Inadequate health care for migrants in the USA. *Lancet* 2009;373:1053.

25. Kullgren J. Restrictions on undocumented immigrants' access to health services: The public health implications of welfare reform. *Am J Publ Hlth.* 2003;93:1631–1633.

26. Mohanty S, Woolhandler S, Himmelstein D, Pati S, Carrasquillo O, Bor D. Health care expenditures of immigrants in the United States: A nationally representative analysis. *Am J Publ Hlth.* 2005;95:1431–1436.

27. Fenton J, Catalano R, Hargreaves W. Data watch: Effect of proposition 187 on mental health service use in California: A case study. *Hlth Aff.* 1996;15:189–190.

28. *Coalition of Immokalee Workers: Campaign for fair food.* Available at http://ciw -online.org/101.html. Accessed December 29, 2009.

29. American Civil Liberties Union: About the Immigrants Rights' Project. Available at http://www.aclu.org/immigrants-rights/about-aclus-immigrants-rights-project. Accessed January 29, 2010.

30. United Farm Workers website. Available at http://www.ufw.org/. Accessed January 30, 2010.

31. Center for Research for Occupational and Environmental Toxicology. Available at http://www.ohsu.edu/xd/research/centers-institutes/croet/research/minority-fam.cfm. Accessed January 30, 2010.

32. Yakima Valley Farm Workers Clinic website. Available at http://www.yvfwc.com/. Accessed January 30, 2010.

33. The White House. Office of the Press Secretary. *Presidential proclamation—National Slavery and Human Trafficking Prevention Month.* Available at http://www.whitehouse.gov/the-pressoffice/presidential-proclamation-national-slavery-and-human-trafficking-prevention-month. Accessed January 5, 2010.

34. Silva, MA. Poverty and health in Argentina. *Social Medicine* 2009;4:98–108.

35. Donohoe MT. Factory farms, antibiotics, and anthrax. *Z Magazine* 2003(January):28–30. Available at http://zmagsite.zmag.org/Jan2003/donohoe0103.shtml. Accessed January 24, 2010.

36. Donohoe MT. Genetically modified foods: Health and environmental risks and the corporate agribusiness agenda. *Z Magazine* 2006(December):35–40. Available at http://zmagsite.zmag.org/Dec2006/donohoe1206.html. Accessed January 24, 2010.

37. Donohoe MT. Roles and responsibilities of health professionals in confronting the health consequences of environmental degradation and social injustice: Education and activism. *Monash Bioethics Review* 2008;27(nos. 1 and 2):65–82.

Chapter 8

The Persistence of American Indian Health Disparities

David S. Jones

The Indian Health Service faced a daunting challenge when it was established in 1955. Indian populations living in rural poverty suffered terribly from disease. Tuberculosis continued to thrive, and infant mortality reached 4 times the national average. During the past 50 years, the IHS has improved health conditions dramatically, but disparities persist—American Indians continue to experience the worst health conditions in the United States. Although this persistence is striking, it is even more striking that the disparities have existed not for 50 years but for 500 years. From the earliest years of colonization, American Indians have suffered more severely whether the prevailing diseases were smallpox, tuberculosis, alcoholism, or other chronic afflictions of modern society.

The history of these disparities provides perspective on many vexing problems of contemporary American Indian health policy. European and American observers have offered a diverse range of causes to explain Indian susceptibility, from the providential theories of Puritan colonists to emphasis on environment, behavior, genetics, or socioeconomic status. How did American Indians and their observers evaluate these long lists of potential causes and determine which were most important or meaningful? Observers have offered a similarly diverse range of responses, from attempts that relieved disparities through health care to efforts that ignored or even exacerbated them. How did political and economic interests shape their choices?

The history also raises questions about the actual causes of the disparities. Health disparities have persisted, even as the underlying disease environment has changed. Do American Indians have intrinsic susceptibilities to every disease for which disparities have existed? Or does the history of disparity after disparity suggest that social and economic conditions have played a more powerful role in generating Indian vulnerability to disease? Understanding the histories of health disparities may explain the complex reactions they provoke and why efforts with the best intentions have fallen short.

Encounters and Epidemics

American Indians struggled with ill health even before Europeans arrived. Although pre-Columbian populations were spared the ravages of smallpox, measles, influenza, and many other infections, they did not inhabit a disease-free paradise. Careful analyses of skeletal remains have revealed many diseases, including tuberculosis and pneumonia.[1] Whereas some populations, such as those of coastal Georgia or Brazil, enjoyed excellent health, many American Indian groups stretched their environments past the limits of sustainability. From the arid southwest to the crowded urban centers of Mexico and Peru, malnutrition, disease, and violence kept life expectancies below 25 years of age. Health disparities also existed within populations, such as the complex stratified societies of Mesoamerica and the Andes.[2] Moreover, paleoanthropologists have documented widespread evidence of worsening malnutrition and disease during the years before Europeans arrived. Baseline ill health made American Indians vulnerable to European diseases.[3]

Colonization made matters worse. Mortality increased soon after the arrival of Christopher Columbus, and it quickly reached catastrophic proportions. Estimates of pre-contact American populations vary between 8 and 112 million (2 to 12 million for North America), and estimates of total mortality range from 7 to 100 million.[4] Whatever the exact numbers, the mortality was unprecedented and overwhelming. Hispaniola, the first region subjected to Spanish conquest, foretold the fate of other areas: the Arawak population decreased from as many as 400,000 in 1496 to 125 in 1570.[5] Every new encounter brought new epidemics. Smallpox, measles, influenza, and malaria (and possibly hepatitis, plague, chickenpox, and diphtheria) spread into Mexico and Peru during the 16th century, New France and New England during the 17th century, and throughout North America and the Pacific islands during the 18th and 19th centuries. Populations often decreased by more than 90% during the first century after contact. As recently as the 1940s and 1960s, new highways and new missionaries brought pathogens to previously isolated tribes in Alaska and Amazonia.[6]

News of the devastation reached Europe rapidly. In 1516, Peter Martyr condemned Spanish brutality but acknowledged that many Indians died from "newe and straunge diseases." The combined impact of abuse and disease was horrifying: "They were once rekened to bee above twelve hundreth thousande heades: But what they are nowe, I abhorre to rehearse."[7] The English first encountered such mortality during their early efforts to colonize North Carolina and Maine. In 1585, Thomas Hariot witnessed epidemics among the Roanok: wherever the English visited, "the people began to die very fast."[8] In 1616, Richard Vines wintered with the Pemaquid in Maine. The local tribes "were sore afflicted with the Plague, for that the Country was in a manner left void of inhabitants."[9] Although its diagnosis remains unclear (smallpox? chicken pox? hepatitis?), the epidemic decimated the coast from Maine to Cape Cod and allowed colonists to move into abandoned Indian villages.[10] Another epidemic, likely smallpox, struck in 1633.[11] Wherever the English went, they saw evidence of mortality. According to William Bradford, the victims "not being able to bury one another, their skulls and bones were found in many places lying still above the ground where their houses and dwellings had been, a very sad spectacle to behold." Bradford estimated overall mortality at 95%.[12] Others guessed it was even higher.[13]

The mortality was not completely one-sided. Half of the Plymouth colonists died during the first winter.[14] Of 6,000 colonists sent to Jamestown between 1607 and 1624, only 1,200 remained in 1625.[15] Despite their own mortality, explorers and colonists marveled at disparities in disease susceptibility. When they remained healthy while the Roanok succumbed, the English wondered whether they should credit the odd epidemic to a recent comet, an eclipse, or a "speciall woorke of God for our sakes."[16] Although Vines and his crew shared winter cabins with the dying Pemaquid, "(blessed be GOD for it) not one of them ever felt their heads to ake."[17] When English colonists nursed American Indians suffering from smallpox in Connecticut in 1633, "by the marvelous goodness and providence of God, not one of the English was so much as sick."[18] By the late 17th century, it was clear that Indian and European populations had followed different trajectories. While the English thrived, northeastern Indians declined, victims of disease, displacement, and warfare.[19] As a New York missionary described in 1705, "the English here are a very thriving growing people, and ye Indians quite otherwise, they wast away & have done ever since our first arrival among them (as they themselves say) like Snow agt. ye Sun."[20]

Colonial Precedents

The mortality amazed European colonists. Their responses illustrate many themes that occurred repeatedly as Europeans, and then Americans, witnessed the ongoing health problems among American Indians. As already seen, providential explanations came quickly to Puritan minds. John Winthrop, for example, wrote that "Gods hand hath so pursued them, as for 300 miles space, the greatest parte of them are swept awaye by the small poxe."[21] But providence coexisted with many natural explanations. Although disparities in health status eventually contributed to the formation of modern ideas of racial difference, the colonists did not initially see any intrinsic differences between English and Indian bodies.[22] Philip Vincent, a leader of the English forces during the Pequot War, concluded that "we had the same matter, the same mold. Only art and grace have given us that perfection which yet they want, but may perhaps be as capable thereof as we."[23] Believing that English and Indian bodies shared the same vulnerabilities, colonists often explained Indian epidemics in the same ways that they explained their own diseases. The environment could support both health and disease, with cold winters causing aches and congestions and hot summers bringing fevers and fluxes. Starvation threatened both groups. New foods were just as dangerous. William Wood observed that when the Massachusett changed "their bare Indian commons for the plenty of England's fuller diet, it is so contrary to their stomachs that death or a desperate sickness immediately accrues, which makes so few of them desirous to see England."[24]

During these initial years of encounter between colonists and American Indians, providential and natural explanations appeared side by side. Early modern writers experienced a world in which all events had natural and spiritual causes simultaneously. This synergy of meaning and mechanism provided solace in a bewildering world, reassuring colonists that everything happened according to God's will. However, the different explanations often existed in tension. When fleeing Massachusett conspirators died in 1623, their leader, Ianough, feared that "the God of the English was offended with them, and would destroy them in his anger." Edward Winslow had a more practical explanation: "Through fear they set little or no corn, which is the staff of life, and without which they cannot long preserve health and strength."[25] Daniel Gookin described similar debates about the deaths of Indian students at Harvard College. Some "attributed it unto the great change upon their bodies, in respect of their diet, lodging, apparel, studies; so much different from what they were inured to among their own countrymen." Others saw the deaths as "severe dispensations of God," either because "God was not pleased yet to make use of any of the Indians to preach the gospel" or because Satan "did use all his strategems and endeavors to impede the spreading of the christian faith."[26] In these cases, the colonists did not find integrated synergy of providence and natural mechanism. Instead, they struggled to choose between them.

These debates make a crucial point: providential explanation was not simply the reflexive response of God-fearing colonists. Rather, colonial writers considered many different explanations: providence, environment, nutrition, behavior, and physical differences. Thus, they could emphasize the most meaningful or useful explanations. Their choices reflected local economic and political pressures. English leaders, for instance, had to justify their right to settle lands already inhabited by American Indians. King James I cited the epidemic-induced depopulation: "Those large and goodly Territoryes, deserted as it were by their naturall Inhabitants, should be possessed and enjoyed by such of our Subjects and People."[27] Many of Winthrop's most forceful statements of providential interpretation occurred when he argued in favor of English colonization. He believed smallpox "cleered our title to this place."[28] After all, "if God were not pleased with our inheriting these parts, why did he drive out the natives before us? And why dothe he still make roome for us, by deminishinge them as we increace?"[29] The English used disparities in health status to convince themselves that their mission in America was righteous.

The English were not alone in trying to turn the epidemic disparities to political advantage. Many Indian groups, at least according to their English chroniclers, were quick to see potential benefits. When the English did not succumb to epidemics that devastated the Roanok, Ensenore and other local elders concluded that the English controlled disease. Hoping to exploit this power, they asked the English to unleash the disease against their tribal enemies.[30] Hobbamock, a counselor to Wampanoag chief Massasoit, made a similar request of the Plymouth colonists: "Being at varience with another Sachem borderinge upon his Territories, he came in solemne manner and intreated the Governour, that he would let out the plague to destroy the Sachem, and his men who were his enemies."[31] Hobbamock and Ensenore hoped that English control over disease would make them powerful allies.

Some Indians also used the disparities in intratribal politics. Squanto, who learned to speak English when he was kidnapped by English explorers in 1614, realized that he could become an influential translator and mediator when the Plymouth colonists arrived in 1620. Believing that his position would be stronger if the Wampanoag feared the English, he manipulated the tribe's fear of disease. He told Hobbamock that the English stored plague in barrels, which they "could send forth to what place or people we would, and destroy them therewith, though we stirred not from home." When Hobbamock confronted the English about this, Squanto's ruse was exposed. Massasoit nearly had him executed.[32]

In some cases, American Indians engaged Europeans in debates about the etiologies of epidemics. The Jesuits, for instance, introduced smallpox and other ill-defined fevers when they arrived in Quebec in 1625. By 1637, 50% of the Huron had died. The Huron asked the Jesuits "why so many of them died, saying that since the coming of the French their nation was going to destruction."[33] The Jesuits, like the English, attributed the epidemics to a range of factors, including the hardship of Huron lives, Huron religious practices, and contagion. The Huron, who were suspicious of French intent, feared that the French "had a secret understanding with the disease" and could spread disease by a "crafty demon" concealed in a musket, "bewitched" cloaks, or poisoned water.[34] Although the French denied Huron allegations of deliberate infection, they did admit their culpability for the epidemics. As Hierosme Lalemant wrote, "Where we were most welcome, where we baptized most people, there it was in fact where they died the most."[35] Within this first generation of colonization in North America, both Indians and Europeans struggled to understand the devastation. Their responses echoed their own perspectives and interests.

Smallpox and the Moral Life

As European settlers moved into the North American interior, each new encounter triggered a new wave of epidemic decimation. Smallpox struck again and again throughout the 17th and 18th centuries. It reached the northwestern plains by the 1780s and the Pacific Northwest by 1802.[36] A particularly virulent outbreak struck the upper Missouri valley in 1837. It afflicted the tribes "with terror never before known, and has converted the extensive hunting grounds, as well as the peaceful settlements of those tribes, into desolate and boundless cemeteries." Between 10,000 and 150,000 Sioux, Mandan, Blackfeet, Arikara, and Assiniboine died. Abandoned villages covered the plains: "No sounds but the croaking of the raven and the howling of the wolf interrupt the fearful silence."[37] Although smallpox dominates the accounts of Indian mortality, observers also described alcoholism, syphilis, and many other fevers and fluxes.

Fur traders, soldiers, missionaries, and settlers followed their ancestors' lead and offered a range of explanations for the American Indians' susceptibility to smallpox. Although less prevalent, providence persisted. In 1764, Thomas Hutchinson abandoned his usual skepticism of Puritan mythology: "Our ancestors supposed an immediate interposition of providence in the great mortality among the Indians to make room for the settlement of the English. I am not inclined to credulity, but should not we go into the contrary extreme if we were to take no notice of the extinction of this people in all parts of the continent."[38] Most observers, however, emphasized destructive Indian behaviors: indifference to cleanliness, foreign diets, reckless use of sweat baths, and the "vicious and dissolute life" caused by alcohol.[39] According to George Catlin, these factors, and not "some extraordinary constitutional susceptibility," explained the smallpox mortality.[40]

Amid the diversity of potential explanations, the emphasis on behavior played a useful role. Although less overtly theological than providential explanations, behavioral theories had clear moral utility: disease became a tool of moral exhortation. According to missionaries, if vice brought disease to American Indians, then acceptance of Christian morality and lifestyles would bring them health. These arguments targeted white audiences as well. It was, after all, whites who had introduced American Indians to alcohol and other sinful behaviors. Catlin warned his readers that the legacy of white influence on Indian populations, "an unrequited account of sin and injustice," would haunt all Americans on judgment day.[41] American Indians shared this anger. When an Ioway delegation visited London during the 1840s, an English minister demanded that the Ioway acknowledge smallpox as divine punishment. Their war chief had a quick reply: "If the Great Spirit sent the small pox into our country to destroy us, we believe it was to punish us for listening to the false promises of white men. It is a white man's disease, and no doubt it was sent among White people to punish them for their sins."[42]

Tuberculosis, Extinction, and the Civilizing Process

Into the early 19th century, many European and American observers dismissed Catlin's concerns and argued that American Indians had brought mortality on themselves. This position became increasingly untenable during the 19th century. As contact between white and American Indian societies increased, it became obvious that federal policies adversely affected Indian health. The reservation system, which was imposed between the 1830s and the 1870s, transformed patterns of morbidity and mortality. Smallpox, measles, cholera, malaria, venereal diseases, and alcoholism remained common but were reportedly mitigated by government physicians with vaccination, fumigation, and quarantine.[43]

These problems, however, were dwarfed by tuberculosis. Consumption and scrofula had been present but rare among American Indians for centuries.[44] They quickly became the leading cause of death, especially on the Dakota reservations, where they dominated annual mortality reports, often causing half of all deaths.[45] Physician Z. T. Daniel believed that "it is practically the only disease that causes their large death rate."[46] Although the burden of disease had shifted from acute to chronic infections, the disparities persisted. The surgeon general reported that the consumption hospitalization rate for Indian soldiers in 1892 was more than 10 times the rate for white soldiers.[47] Sioux mortality from tuberculosis alone exceeded the mortality rates from all causes in most major cities.[48]

Observers had little difficulty explaining the prevalence of tuberculosis among the Sioux. Many blamed the reservation system and the terrible living conditions imposed on the confined tribes. Damp, poorly ventilated log cabins and inadequate government rations set the tribes up for disaster. However, as had happened before, they also were quick to blame the Sioux for specific behaviors, from unhygienic cooking to religious dances, pipe smoking, and cigarettes that made bad conditions worse.[49] O. M. Chapman stated these punitive sentiments most clearly: "The excessive mortality is but the sum total of all these influences combined—is the measure of their transgressions."[50]

A broad consensus accepted these problems as the proximate causes of Sioux tuberculosis. The crucial debates of the late 19th century instead confronted

the ultimate causes of the disparities in health status, specifically the roles
of racial differences and socioeconomic conditions. Ideas of racial hierarchy
were firmly entrenched in the national consciousness. Influential works, such
as Josiah Nott and George Gliddon's *Types of Mankind*, argued that although
American Indians had once thrived in America, they could neither compete
nor coexist with "Caucasians": "It is as clear as the sun at noon-day, that in
a few generations more the last of these Red men will be numbered with the
dead."[51] Some doctors saw these theories as compelling explanations for the
disparities in mortality. Daniel believed that Indians could only be saved by
mixing with other groups: they will "die everywhere they go, of tuberculosis,
until the race is so thoroughly crossed by 'foreign blood' that it will stamp out
the tubercle bacillus, and when that is done the Indian race in its original purity
will be no more."[52] For those who believed that extinction was inevitable, the
reservation system became little more than palliative care for a dying race.[53]

Other observers rejected these pessimistic visions and argued that the
outbreak of tuberculosis was not the inevitable result of hereditary inferiority.
Rather, it was the contingent product of the difficult transition from primitive
life to civilization. Physicians who observed the Sioux before and after their
confinement saw how quickly the native health of the Sioux deteriorated.
George Bushnell, for example, observed Sioux prisoners who were brought
to live among Sioux already settled on a reservation in 1881. He described
"scrofulous youths from the Agency, their fleshless limbs fully clad, looking
on wistfully at the dances of the warriors in the summer twilight ... revealing
in many instances a magnificent physique and a boundless vitality, which
contrasted cruelly with the listless aspect of some of their spectators."[54]

Although they knew that reservations had fueled tuberculosis, many
physicians and officials maintained their faith in the fundamental value of
civilization. Tuberculosis existed not because the civilizing process was wrong
but because it had been implemented badly. Indians were "reduced to the condition of paupers, without food, shelter, clothing, or any of those necessaries
of life which came from the buffalo; and without friends, except the harpies,
who, under the guise of friendship, feed upon them."[55] The government had
to intervene: "We have no right to assume that they are a race given over to
God to destruction, and we have less right to doom them ourselves."[56] Health
would be restored when the government enabled the Indians to enjoy the full
benefits of white civilization.

Persistent Disparities

Faith that civilization would eventually bring health to the American Indians
prevailed in the debate about the ultimate causes of tuberculosis. Some
government officials committed themselves to improving reservations through

education, economic reform, and health care. However, their paternalistic policies, which were based on the assumed superiority of white culture and religion, rarely led to improvement and often made matters worse. Medical campaigns, for example, suffered from inadequate funding. Commissioner of Indian Affairs T. J. Morgan compared the salaries paid to government physicians in the Army, Navy, and IHS and divided these sums by the populations served. He then calculated a crude estimate of how the government valued people: $21.91 per soldier, $48.10 per sailor, and $1.25 per Indian.[57]

The enthusiasm of the Progressive era brought new interest and new funding to the problem of Indian tuberculosis. During the International Congress on Tuberculosis in 1908, Commissioner of Indian Affairs Francis E. Leupp identified tuberculosis as "the greatest single menace to the Indian race."[58] President William Taft committed the government to new action. Congress responded in 1912 with an emergency appropriation of $12,000. The Bureau of Indian Affairs (BIA) organized campaigns against tuberculosis, trachoma, infant mortality, house flies, alcoholism, and tooth decay.[59] Annual appropriations grew steadily and reached $350,000 by 1917. That year, for the first time in more than 50 years, more Indians were born than died. Physician George Kober celebrated the progress: "Thanks to the progress of medical science and the splendid humanitarian efforts of our Government, a noble race of people has been snatched from the very jaws of death."[60] The 1921 Snyder Act strengthened the mandate for government action, and congressional appropriations continued to grow: $596,000 in 1925, $2,980,000 in 1935, $5,730,000 in 1945, and $17,800,000 in 1955.[61]

Disparities, however, persisted. Tuberculosis mortality in 1925 was 87/100,000 among the general population, 603/100,000 among Indians overall, and 1,510/100,000 among Arizona Indians.[62] During World War II, between 10% and 25% of Navajo soldiers and workers had to be returned to the reservation because of active tuberculosis.[63] Postwar surveys confirmed the problem: in 1947, tuberculosis mortality among Arizona Indians (302.4/100,000) dwarfed both the rate among Indians in general (200/100,000) and the national population (30/100,000).[64] The problem was not confined to tuberculosis. Incidence among the Navajo exceeded that of the general population by a factor of 15.8 for tuberculosis, 101.6 for pneumonia, and 1,163 for trachoma.[65] The Navajo also had the country's highest infant mortality rate.[66]

Explanations for the persistent tuberculosis disparities followed the framework of the late 19th century. Environmental theories were common; the new challenge was to explain how tuberculosis could thrive in the arid southwest, where the climate was recommended for many convalescing white patients. Physicians who were still critical of American Indian cultures found much to blame in Navajo living conditions: "Benefits to health from an outdoor life are over-balanced by the ill effects of overcrowding, lack of sanitary provisions, and the poverty which leads to a poor, inadequate supply of food."[67] They moved easily from blaming the conditions of poverty to emphasizing behaviors that the Navajo adopted while living in those conditions. Both the healthy and the sick expectorated freely without disinfecting their sputum. The Navajo ate meals irregularly and prepared food poorly. Intemperance, apathy, indolence, and hopelessness all weakened the people. No one sought proper medical attention. As physician Sydney Tillim complained, they lacked "intelligence in all things medical."[68]

The Navajo expressed both interest and skepticism in these explanations. When Manuelito Begay, a prominent medicine man and a member of the Navajo Tribal Council, saw a microscope slide of the tubercle bacillus, he was impressed but not convinced of its relevance: "They tell me that it is inflicted by a person coughing in your face—that is the way you get tuberculosis in your system. Right away I disagree with it. A person should not be that weak to be susceptible to a man's cough."[69] Other Navajo also scoffed at medical explanations of tuberculosis. One woman argued that if infected sputum sowed tuberculosis within Navajo homes, then chickens, which constantly pecked at the infected dirt floors, should have been devastated by the disease.[70]

White doctors shared Begay's puzzlement about the specific causes of Navajo susceptibility. Ill-defined genetic explanations remained popular. In 1923, the New Mexico State Department of Health went so far as to assert an ongoing process of natural selection: "Resistant race has not been bred as yet. Now undergoing process of weeding out the nonresistant strains."[71] Genetic explanations were used just as easily to explain the surprisingly low incidence of noninfectious diseases among the Navajo, including hypertension, cancer, heart disease, and baldness.[72] Most doctors, however, rejected genetic determinism. The National Tuberculosis Association argued in 1923 that "tuberculosis attacks without any racial preference."[73] Studies found that "the character of tuberculous lesions, as determined roentgenologically, is not significantly different from that observed among the white population."[74] Although the reservations clearly suffered severely from tuberculosis, "identical" epidemics existed among populations "living under like conditions among people of the White and Yellow races."[75] These writers believed that socioeconomic conditions, when severe enough, could destroy the health of any population.

Fighting Poverty with Medical Technology

The different explanations had clear implications for American Indian health policy. Whereas New Mexico officials seemed content to allow natural selection to solve the tuberculosis problem, most government officials accepted the causal role of economic nondevelopment and believed that health could only come from improvements in socioeconomic conditions. This became especially clear when a postwar economic recession struck the Navajo and Hopi reservations. Congressional investigators were shocked by what they found: "So long as the Navajos remain on the barren wasteland on which they live, without communities, roads, water, sanitation, or the opportunity to earn a living wage, they must continue to live in squalor and disease."[76] Congress responded in 1950 with a $90,000,000 program for the long-range rehabilitation of the Navajo and Hopi.[77] This intensive program for the Navajo and Hopi reservations paralleled postwar political interest in international economic development. In each case, policy makers believed that the disparities in health status between developed and developing populations arose from disparities in socioeconomic conditions. Improved health could be achieved most fundamentally by economic development.

Although economic development remained the ultimate goal, health officials realized that it could not be achieved easily or quickly enough. They wanted to find ways to improve the health of underdeveloped populations living in rural poverty. One clear problem, which was highlighted in a 1950 American Medical Association report, was the inadequacy of existing health services on the reservations.[78] Annie Wauneka, who led the health committee of the Navajo Tribal Council, agreed during her testimony to Congress: "We think there is no real health program. If there is, we haven't heard about it or seen it. And our sick people are paying for it."[79] Emboldened by postwar optimism and by faith in new technologies, such as penicillin, isoniazid, and DDT, health officials believed that they would be able to improve health conditions, even in the absence of economic changes. Walsh McDermott's "Health Care Experiment at Many Farms" put this question to the test.[80] After choosing a remote area of the Navajo Reservation, McDermott's team of doctors, anthropologists, and social scientists worked closely with Wauneka and other Navajo leaders to reduce morbidity and mortality in the absence of socioeconomic reforms. They found that their treatment programs controlled tuberculosis but had little impact on the other leading causes of morbidity and mortality, especially childhood diarrhea and pneumonia. These failures surprised the researchers: "When one considers our pre-experiment expectations, soundly grounded in the conventional wisdom, these results were clearly disappointing."[81] Entrenched disparities in health status did not yield easily to medical technology.

McDermott's work was part of a broader effort to reform health care on the reservations. Frustrated by the continuing failures of the BIA to relieve health disparities, Congress moved the medical services from the BIA to the Public Health Service, thus creating the Indian Health Service [IHS] in 1955.[82] The IHS conducted an initial health survey and found wide disparities in health status and health services between Indians and the general population. Among American Indians, total mortality was 20% higher, infant mortality was 3 times higher, life expectancy was 10 years lower, and infectious diseases and accidents were more prevalent; however, heart disease and cancer were less common.[83]

Health conditions remained bad into the 1970s: life expectancy was two thirds the national average, and the incidence of infant mortality (1.5 times), diabetes (2 times), suicide (3 times), accidents (4 times), tuberculosis (14 times), gastrointestinal infections (27 times), dysentery (40 times), and rheumatic fever (60 times) also were above the national average. As a result, the Navajo Tribal Council articulated a new vision of Indian health self-determination and attempted to build its own medical school: "The day will arrive when a more effective health-care delivery system utilizing Indian professionals will replace the current system. The day will arrive when the American Indian will determine what his own health standards and services should be."[84] For Wauneka, the "paramount objective" was clear: "The care by Indians of our peoples' health."[85]

The Navajo did not succeed in obtaining funding to establish an independent medical school. However, the IHS steadily increased the participation and the leadership of Indian health professionals within the IHS. It continued to combat health disparities, and by 1989, it claimed great success, arguing that its efforts since 1955 had reduced tuberculosis by 96%, infant mortality by 92%, pulmonary infections by 92%, and gastrointestinal infections by 93%. Although parity with the general population had not been achieved, the gap had been narrowed.[86] However, as they have done for centuries, the disparities survived.

IHS data from the late 1990s showed higher mortality rates among American Indians and Alaskan Natives compared with the general population for most leading causes of mortality: heart disease (1.2 times), accidents (2.8 times), diabetes (4.2 times), alcohol (7.7 times), suicide (1.9 times), and tuberculosis (7.5 times). Only with cancer, the second-leading cause of death, was American Indian mortality not greater than that of the general population. Furthermore, these disparities all widened between 1995 and 1998.[87]

Congress and the IHS continue to work to improve conditions on the reservations. The 1975 Indian Self-Determination and Indian Assistance Act (Public Law 93–638) and the 1976 Indian Health Care Improvement Act renewed the government's commitment to Indian health and gave the tribes more control over their health care services.[88] Working with an annual budget of nearly $3,000,000,000, the IHS now provides services to 1.6 million people in 35 states.[89] However, as has been true since the 19th century, per capita expenditures remain far below those in the general population: $1,351 for Indians compared with $3,766 for the general population overall.[90] Casinos have brought wealth to a small number of tribes, but Indian gaming could prove to be catastrophic for Indian health if public perception of American Indians as gambling moguls dissolves the obligation felt by Congress to provide care for them.[91]

Conclusions

Disparities in health status between American Indians and Europeans and Americans have been recognized for 5 centuries. Many observers have felt that the existence of disparities is fundamentally wrong. Such moral outrage has motivated centuries of attempts to relieve them. How have disparities been able to persist? How have they been allowed to persist? Several things are clear.

First, there are striking patterns in attempts to account for the distribution of health and disease. Explanations have spanned a remarkable range of possible etiologies, including religion, diet, living conditions, climate, cultural practices, racial differences, and socioeconomic status. No single explanation has defined the phenomena of disease so clearly that other explanations have been precluded. Many of the explanations have persisted throughout the centuries, although their specific details and meanings have changed. Invocations of providence, for example, gave way to genetic determinism as the most common argument for inevitable disparity. Emphasis has also shifted, with religious explanations dominating initially but then giving way to behavioral, genetic, and socioeconomic explanations. Such a trajectory, however, is only a coarse approximation. Far more striking has been the persistence of the diversity of explanations over time.

Second, the enduring existence of an abundance of possible explanations has allowed observers to emphasize the most meaningful or useful understandings of disease. Needing land, colonists saw Massachusett depopulation as a gift of land. Wanting absolution for the destruction of Indian societies, federal officials saw Sioux tuberculosis as proof of Indians' inevitable demise. These choices could have been constrained by the plausibility of different explanations. Instead, persistent inadequacies in health data for American Indians have often prevented the establishment of clear consensus about the etiology of diseases and disparities. This has allowed observers to exercise considerable discretion in their assessments and has opened a large window for ideology to influence health data, theories, and policies.

Third, choices about explanations have reflected observers' attitudes about a fundamental question: where should responsibility for disparities be assigned? Although some observers blamed personal choices, others argued that Indian diseases were the product of the disrupted social conditions of colonization. Responsibility can fall on the sick (e.g., victims of genetic susceptibility) or the healthy (e.g., misguided architects of the reservation system), or it can be transferred to an outside authority (e.g., God's providence). These assignments have crucial implications for health policy.

Health disparities have been seen as proof of a natural order that can be exploited for observers' benefit, and they have been seen as markers of social injustice that observers must remedy. The shifting balance between these ideological poles contributed to the enormous heterogeneity of past federal Indian health policies. Furthermore, because disparities in health status parallel disparities in wealth and power, responses necessarily involve decisions to deploy or withhold economic and political resources. Policy makers have had to balance Indian health with other priorities and obligations of the federal government, including land acquisition, military needs, resource development, or questions about Indian sovereignty.

The tensions about responsibility and appropriate response appear in current debates about the genetics of health disparities. Researchers have proposed that American Indians have genetic susceptibilities to many diseases, from alcoholism to virgin-soil epidemics or Pima diabetes.[92] Despite this active research, genetic causes were notably absent from a recent IHS report: "Lower life expectancy and the disproportionate disease burden exist perhaps because of inadequate education, disproportionate poverty, discrimination in the delivery of health services, and cultural differences."[93] What generates the controversy surrounding genetic theories of health disparities? By focusing on biological origins, genetic theories naturalize disparities and reduce the shame and stigma associated with behavioral or cultural explanations. But this can be problematic. By introducing an aura of inevitability, genetic arguments reduce the obligation to intervene and prevent or reduce disparities. More practical concerns also contribute. Current interest in molecular genetics makes research into the genetics of disparities a safe bet for researchers in need of grants and publications. In contrast, genetic explanations can be a dead end for policy makers, especially when compared with the many interventions suggested by explanations that emphasize socioeconomic conditions or access to health care.[94]

Debates about the genetic origins of health disparities raise 1 last question. Empowered by the Human Genome Project, researchers hope to find genes for every disease and disparity. However, as more and more genetic links are proposed for American Indian ill health, the overall argument becomes harder to sustain. Disparities among American Indians have existed whether the prevailing diseases were acute infections (e.g., smallpox and measles), chronic infections (e.g., tuberculosis), or the endemic ailments of modern society (e.g., heart disease, diabetes, alcoholism, and depression). Recent trends suggest that disparities in cancer might also emerge. Is it conceivable that American Indians have genetic vulnerabilities to every class of human disease?

The existence of disparities regardless of the underlying disease environment is actually a powerful argument against the belief that disparities reflect inherent susceptibilities of American Indian populations. Instead, the disparities in health status could arise from the disparities in wealth and power that have endured since colonization.[95] Such awareness must guide ongoing research and interventions if the disparities in health status between American Indians and the general population are ever to be eradicated.

Acknowledgments

This research was supported in part by a grant from the Medical Scientist Training Program, National Institutes of Health; the Graduate School of Arts and Sciences, Harvard University; and the Program in Science, Technology, and Society, Massachusetts Institute of Technology.

I would like to thank Allan Brandt, Arthur Kleinman, David Barnes, Stephen Kunitz, and Ted Brown for their suggestions. Adele Lerner and James L. Gehrlich provided invaluable assistance at the New York Weill Cornell Medical Center Archives.

Notes

1. Howard S. Russell, *Indian New England Before the Mayflower* (Hanover: University of New Hampshire Press, 1980), 35, 104–105; Douglas H. Ubelaker, "Patterns of Demographic Change in the Americas," *Human Biology* 64 (June 1992): 364; Clark Spencer Larsen, "In the Wake of Columbus: Native Population Biology in the Postcontact Americas," *Yearbook of Physical Anthropology* 37 (1994): 109–154.

2. For discussions of the poor-health of pre-Columbian populations, see the many excellent chapters in Richard S. Steckel and Jerome C. Rose, *The Backbone of History: Health and Nutrition in the Western Hemisphere* (Cambridge, UK: Cambridge University Press, 2002). For a detailed discussion of 1 urban population, see Rebecca Storey, *Life and Death in the Ancient City of Teotihuacan: A Modern Paleodemographic Synthesis* (Tuscaloosa: University of Alabama Press, 1992), 253–266.

3. Larsen, "In the Wake of Columbus," 109–154; Rebecca Storey, Lourdes Marquez Morfin, and Vernon Smith, "Social Disruption and the Maya Civilization of Mesoamerica: A Study of Health and Economy of the Last Thousand Years," in Steckel and Rose, *Backbone of History*, pp. 283–306; Douglas H. Ubelaker and Linda A. Newson, "Patterns of Health and Nutrition in Prehistoric and Historic Ecuador," in Steckel and Rose, *Backbone of History*, pp. 343–375; S. Ryan Johansson and Douglas Owsley, "Welfare History on the Great Plains: Mortality and Skeletal Health, 1650 to 1900," in *Backbone of History*, ed. Steckel and Rose, pp. 524–560; Steckel and Rose, "Patterns of Health in the Western Hemisphere," in *Backbone of History*, pp. 563–579.

4. Henry F. Dobyns, "Estimating Aboriginal American Population: An Appraisal of Techniques with a New Hemispheric Estimate," *Current Anthropology* 7 (October 1966): 395–416; Ubelaker, "Patterns of Demographic Change in the Americas," 361–379; Michael H. Crawford, *The Origins of Native Americans: Evidence from Anthropological Genetics* (Cambridge, UK: Cambridge University Press, 1998), 33–39; David Henige, *Numbers from Nowhere: The American Indian Contact Population Debate* (Norman: University of Oklahoma Press, 1998).

5. "Estimates of the Precontact Population of Hispanola Have Ranged Between 60,000 and nearly 8,000,000." Noble David Cook, *Born to Die: Disease and New World*

Conquest, 1492–1650 (Cambridge, UK: Cambridge University Press, 1998), 22–23. The best available evidence has narrowed the range to between 100,000 and 400,000. Massimo Livi-Bacci, "Return to Hispanola: Reassessing a Demographic Catastrophe," *Hispanic American Historical Review* 83 (2003): 3–51.

6. Dean R. Snow and Kim M. Lanphear, "European Contact and Indian Depopulation in the Northeast: The Timing of the First Epidemics," *Ethnohistory* 35 (Winter 1988): 17; David E. Stannard, "Disease and Infertility: A New Look at the Demographic Collapse of Native Populations in the Wake of Western Contact," *Journal of American Studies* 24 (1990): 325–350; John W. Verano and Douglas H. Ubelaker, ed., *Disease and Demography in the Americas* (Washington, DC, Smithsonian Institution Press1992); Linda A. Newson, "The Demographic Collapse of Native Peoples of the Americas, 1492–1650," *Proceedings of the British Academy* 81 (1993): 247–288; Stephen J. Kunitz, *Disease and Social Diversity: The European Impact on the Health of Non-Europeans* (New York: Oxford University Press, 1994); Robert McCaa, "Spanish and Nahuatl Views on Smallpox and Demographic Catastrophe in Mexico," *Journal of Interdisciplinary History* 25 (Winter 1995): 429; Crawford, *The Origins of Native Americans*, 41–49.

7. Peter Martyr, *The Decades of the Newe Worlde* (1516), trans. Richard Eden (1555), in *The First Three English Books on America*, ed. Edward Arber (Birmingham: Nabu Press1885), 172, 199.

8. Thomas Hariot, *A Briefe and True Report of the New Found Land of Virginia* (1588; Ann Arbor, MI: Edward Brothers, 1931), F.

9. Ferdinando Gorges, *A Briefe Narration of the Originall Undertakings of the Advancement of Plantations into the Parts of America* (1658), in *Sir Ferdinando Gorges and his Province of Maine*, ed. James Phinney Baxter, vol. 19 (1890; New York: Burt Franklin, 1967), 19.

10. Arthur E. Speiss and Bruce D. Speiss, "New England Pandemic of 1616–1622: Cause and Archaeological Implication," *Man in the Northeast* 34 (1987): 71–83; Timothy L. Bratton, "The Identity of the New England Indian Epidemic of 1616–19," *Bulletin of the History of Medicine* 62 (Fall 1988): 351–383.

11. Sherburne F. Cook, "The Significance of Disease in the Extinction of the New England Indians," *Human Biology* 45 (September 1973): 485–508; Ann F. Ramenofsky, *Vectors of Death: The Archeology of European Contact* (Albuquerque: University of New Mexico Press, 1987); Dean R. Snow, "Microchronology and Demographic Evidence Relating to the Size of Pre-Columbian North American Indian Populations," *Science* 268 (June 16, 1995): 1601–1604.

12. William Bradford, *Of Plymouth Plantation, 1620–1647*, ed. Samuel Eliot Morison (New York: Alfred A. Knopf, 1979), 87, 270.

13. John White, for instance, wrote that "the Contagion hath scarce left alive one person in a hundred." White, *The Planters Plea* (1630), in *Tracts and Other Papers*, ed. Peter Force, vol. 2 (1836; New York: Peter Smith, 1947), 14.

14. Bradford to Thomas Weston, 1621, in Bradford, *Of Plymouth Plantation*, 95.

15. Karen Ordahl Kupperman, "Apathy and Death in Early Jamestown," *Journal of American History* 66 (June 1979): 24–40.

16. Hariot, *A Briefe and True Report*, F2.

17. Gorges, *Briefe Narration,* 19:19.

18. Bradford, *Of Plymouth Plantation,* 271.

19. Cook, "The Significance of Disease," 485–508; James D. Drake, *King Philip's War: Civil War in New England, 1675–1676* (Amherst: University of Massachusetts Press, 1999), 169–174.

20. Mr. Moor to the Secretary of the Society for the Propagation of the Gospel in Foreign Parts, 13 Nov. 1705, quoted in John Duffy, "Smallpox and the Indians in the American Colonies," *Bulletin of the History of Medicine* 25 (July–August 1951): 326.

21. John Winthrop to Simonds D'Ewes, 21 July 1634, in *Winthrop Papers,* ed. Malcolm Freiberg, vol. 3 (Boston: Massachusetts Historical Society, 1943), 171–172.

22. Compare Joyce Chaplin, "Natural Philosophy and an Early Racial Idiom in North America: Comparing English and Indian Bodies," *William and Mary Quarterly* 54 (1997): 230, 244; Chaplin, *Subject Matter: Technology, the Body, and Science on the Anglo-American Frontier, 1500–1676* (Cambridge: Harvard University Press, 2001), 8–9, 22–23, 158–197, 244–276, 319–323; and David S. Jones, *Rationalizing Epidemics: Meanings and Uses of American Indian Mortality Since 1600* (Cambridge: Harvard University Press, 2004), 39, 136–137.

23. Philip Vincent, *A true relation of the late batell fought in New-England, between the English and the Pequet Salvages* (1638), in *Collections of the Massachusetts Historical Society,* 3rd series, vol. 6 (Boston: American Stationers' Company, 1837), 34.

24. William Wood, *New England's Prospect* (1634), ed. Alden T. Vaughan (Amherst: University of Massachusetts Press, 1977), 82.

25. Edward Winslow, *Good Newes from New England* (1624), in *Chronicles of the Pilgrim Fathers of the Colony of Plymouth, from 1602 to 1625,* ed. Alexander Young, 2nd ed. (Boston: Charles C. Little and James Brown, 1844), 346.

26. Daniel Gookin, *Historical Collections of the Indians in New England, c. 1680* (1792; [n.p.]: Towtaid, 1970), 53–54.

27. Quoted in Gorges, *Briefe Narration,* 19:25–26n315.

28. Winthrop to D'Ewes, July 21, 1634, 3:172.

29. Winthrop to John Endecott, January 3, 1634, in *Winthrop Papers,* 3:149.

30. Hariot, A *Briefe and True Report,* F–F2.

31. Thomas Morton, *New English Canaan* (1632), in *Tracts and Other Papers,* ed. Peter Force, vol. 2 (1836; New York: Peter Smith, 1947), 71.

32. Winslow, *Good Newes from New England,* 291–292; John Smith, *The Generall History of Virginia, New-England, the Summer Iles* (1624), in *The Complete Works of Captain John Smith (1580–1631),* ed. Philip L. Barbour (Chapel Hill: University of North Carolina Press, 1986), 2:451; Bradford, *Plymouth Plantation,* 99; Morton, *New English Canaan,* 71.

33. For background, see Bruce G. Trigger, *The Children of Aataentsic: A History of the Huron People to 1660* (1976; Montreal: McGill-Queen's University Press, 1987). For Huron questioning, see Paul le Jeune, *Relation of What Occurred in New France in 1637,* August 31, 1637 (1638), in *The Jesuit Relations and Allied Documents: Travels*

and *Explorations of the Jesuit Missionaries in New France, 1610–1791*, ed. Reuben Gold Thwaites, 73 vols. (Cleveland: The Burrows Brothers Company, 1896–1901), 11:193.

34. Hierosme Lalemant, "Relation of What Occurred in the Mission of the Hurons," in *Jesuit Relations*, 19:93, 19:97; Paul le Jeune, "Relation of What Occurred in New France in 1637," in *Jesuit Relations*, 12:87; le Jeune, "Letter to the Father Provincial," 1637, in *Jesuit Relations*, 12:237.

35. Lalemant, "Relation of 1640," 19:93.

36. John Duffy, "Smallpox and the Indians in the American Colonies," *Bulletin of the History of Medicine* 25 (July–August 1951): 324–341; Russell Thornton, *American Indian Holocaust and Survival: A Population History Since 1492* (Norman: University of Oklahoma Press, 1987), 91–94.

37. "New Orleans, June 6, 1838," in Hannibal Evans Lloyd, "Translator's Preface," in Alexander Philip Maximilian, *Travels in the Interior of North America, in Early Western Travels, 1748–1846*, ed. Reuben Gold Thwaites, 32 vols. (Cleveland: Arthur H. Clark Company, 1904–1906), 22:33, 35. Mortality estimates: John James Audubon, in *Audubon and His Journals*, ed. Maria R. Audubon, 2 vols. (New York: Charles Scribner's Sons, 1897), 2:47; Henry R. Schoolcraft, *Information Respecting the History, Condition and Prospects of the Indian Tribes of the United States*, 6 vols. (Philadelphia: Lippincott, Grambo & Company, 1851–1857), 1:257–258, 6:486.

38. Thomas Hutchinson, *The History of the Colony of Massachusetts-Bay, 1628–1691* (Boston: Thomas & John Fleet, 1764), 35n.

39. For one example, see John Heckewelder, *An Account of the History, Manners, and Customs of the Indian Nations Who Once Inhabited Pennsylvania and the Neighbouring States* (1819), revised ed. (Philadelphia: Historical Society of Pennsylvania, 1876), 221–223.

40. George Catlin, *Illustrations of the Manners, Customs, and Condition of the North American Indians*, 10th ed. (London: Henry G. Bohn, 1866), 2:257.

41. Catlin, *Illustrations of the Manners, Customs, and Condition*, 2:256.

42. Quoted in George Catlin, *Catlin's Notes of Eight Years Travel and Residence in Europe* (London: Published by the author, 1848), 2:41. Contemporaries and historians have criticized Catlin for his lack of objectivity. For examples, see Audubon, in *Audubon and His Journals*, 2:10, 2:27; Hiram Martin Chittenden, *American Fur Trade of the Far West* (New York: Francis P. Harper, 1902), 37.

43. For control of acute epidemics, see Jones, *Rationalizing Epidemics*, 119–121. For lists of other diseases, see James R. Doolittle, *Conditions of the Indian Tribes* (Washington, DC: Government Printing Office, 1867), 4–5; W. T. Hughes, in *Annual Report of the Commissioner of Indian Affairs, 1877* (Washington, DC: Government Printing Office, 1877), 74.

44. Ales Hrdlicka, *Tuberculosis Among Certain Indian Tribes of the United States* (Washington, DC: Government Printing Office, 1909); Hans L. Reider, "Tuberculosis Among American Indians of the Contiguous United States,"

Public Health Reports 104 (November–December 1989): 654; Virginia Morell, "Mummy Settles TB Antiquity Debate," *Science* 263 (March 24, 1994): 1686–1687.

45. For examples, T. M. Bridges, in *Annual Report of the Commissioner of Indian Affairs, 1893* (Washington, DC: Government Printing Office, 1893): 286; James R. Walker, in *Annual Report of the Commissioner of Indian Affairs, 1901* (Washington, DC: Government Printing Office, 1902), 367; in O. M. Chapman, in *Annual Report of the Commissioner of Indian Affairs, 1906* (Washington, DC: Government Printing Office, 1907), 364.

46. Z. T. Daniel, in *Annual Report of the Commissioner of Indian Affairs, 1894* (Washington, DC: Government Printing Office, 1895), 290.

47. *Report of the Surgeon-General of the Army to the Secretary of War, 1892* (Washington, DC: Government Printing Office, 1892), 48.

48. T. M. Bridges, in *Annual Report of the Commissioner of Indian Affairs, 1895* (Washington, DC: Government Printing Office, 1896), 288.

49. Frederick Treon, "Medical Work Among the Sioux Indians," *Journal of the American Medical Association* 10 (February 25, 1888): 224–227; Treon, "Consumption Among the Sioux Indians," *Cincinnati Lancet-Clinic* 23 (August 10, 1889): 148–154; A. B. Holder, "Papers on Diseases Among Indians," *Medical Record* (New York) 42 (13 August, 17 September, 24 September 1892): 177–182, 329–331, 357–361; Z. T. Daniel, in *Annual Report of the Commissioner of Indian Affairs, 1903* (Washington, DC: Government Printing Office, 1904), 318.

50. O. M. Chapman, in *Annual Report of the Commissioner of Indian Affairs, 1904* (Washington, DC: Government Printing Office, 1905), 342.

51. J. C. Nott and George R. Gliddon, *Types of Mankind* (1854; Miami: Mnemosyne, 1969), 69.

52. Daniel, in *Annual Report, 1894*, 290.

53. S. N. Clark, "Memoranda: Importance of the Inquiry," in "Are the Indians Dying Out? Preliminary Observations Relating to Indian Civilization and Education," in *Annual Report of the Commissioner of Indian Affairs, 1877*, 494. See also George M. Fredrickson, *The Black Image in the White Mind: The Debate on Afro-American Character and Destiny, 1817–1914* (Hanover, NH: University Press of New England for Wesleyan University Press, 1971, 1987), 77, 159, 220–255.

54. George E. Bushnell, A *Study in the Epidemiology of Tuberculosis, with Especial Reference to Tuberculosis of the Tropics and of the Negro Race* (New York: William Wood and Company, 1920), 159–160.

55. Richard Irving Dodge, *Our Wild Indians: Thirty-Three Years' Personal Experience among the Red Men of the Great West* (1882; New York: Archer House, 1959), 296.

56. S. R. Riggs to John Eaton, August 27, 1877, quoted in Clark, "Memoranda: Importance of the Inquiry," 515.

57. T. J. Morgan, in *Annual Report of the Commissioner of Indian Affairs, 1890* (Washington, DC: Government Printing Office, 1890), xxi. For a parallel discussion of how the policies of the Canadian government exacerbated the health problems of the aboriginal peoples of Canada, see Mary-Ellen Kelm, *Colonizing Bodies:*

Aboriginal Health and Healing in British Columbia, 1900–50 (Vancouver: UBC Press, 1998); Maureen K. Lux, *Medicine That Walks: Disease, Medicine, and Canadian Plains Native People, 1880–1940* (Toronto: University of Toronto Press, 2001).

58. Francis E. Leupp, quoted in Francis Paul Prucha, *The Great Father: The United States Government and the American Indians* (Lincoln: University of Nebraska Press, 1984), 2:848.

59. William H. Taft, "Special Message to Congress," in *Annual Report of the Commissioner of Indian Affairs, 1912* (Washington, DC: Government Printing Office, 1913), 17–19. See also Diane Therese Putney, "Fighting the Scourge: American Indian Morbidity and Federal Policy, 1897–1928" (PhD Dissertation, Marquette University, 1980); Francis Paul Prucha, *The Great Father: The United States Government and the American Indians* (Lincoln: University of Nebraska Press, 1984), 2:850–855; Robert A. Trennert, *White Man's Medicine: Government Doctors and the Navajo, 1863–1955* (Albuquerque: University of New Mexico Press, 1998), 74–75, 136–138.

60. George M. Kober, George E. Bushnell, Joseph A. Murphy, Albert B. Tonkin, William H. Baldwin, and Hoyt E. Dearholt, in *Tuberculosis Among the North American Indians* (Washington, DC: Government Printing Office, 1923), 42.

61. US Public Health Service, *Health Services for American Indians*, Public Health Service Publication No. 531 (Washington, DC: Government Printing Office, 1957), 90–92; US Public Health Service, *The Indian Health Program of the US Public Health Service* (Washington, DC: US Department of Health, Education, and Welfare, 1966), 18–19; Jeff Henderson, "Native American Health Policy: From US Territorial Expansion to Legal Obligation," *JAMA*. 265 (May 1, 1991): 2272; Abraham B. Bergman, David C. Grossman, Angela M. Erdich, John G. Todd, and Ralph Forquera, "A Political History of the Indian Health Service," *Milbank Quarterly* 77 (1999): 591.

62. Herbert A. Burns, "Tuberculosis in the Indian," *American Review of Tuberculosis* 26 (July–December 1932): 498–499.

63. James R. Shaw, quoted in Bergman and others, "A Political History of the Indian Health Service," 577–578.

64. Fred T. Foard, "Health Services for the North American Indians," *Medical Woman's Journal* 571 (November 1950): 12.

65. J. Nixon Hadley, "Health Conditions Among Navajo Indians," *Public Health Reports* 70 (September 1955): 835.

66. J. A. Krug, *The Navajo: A Long Range Program for Navajo Rehabilitation* (Washington, DC: US Government Printing Office, 1948), 6.

67. Sydney J. Tillim, "Medical Annals of Arizona: Health Among the Navajos," *Southwestern Medicine* 20 (August 1936): 277.

68. Tillim, "Medical Annals of Arizona: Health Among the Navajos," *Southwestern Medicine* 20 (October 1936): 391. For other examples, see Isaac W. Brewer, "Tuberculosis Among the Indians of Arizona and New Mexico," *New York Medical*

Journal 84 (1906): 981–982; Kober and others, *Tuberculosis Among the North American Indians,* 29–37; Ralph M. Alley, "Tuberculosis Among Indians," *Diseases of the Chest* 6 (February 1940): 45.

69. Manuelito Begay, quoted in "Minutes of the Navajo Tribal Council," February 12, 1954, Walsh McDermott Papers, New York Weill Cornell Medical Center Archives, Box 11, Folder 7, p. 10; see also Kurt Deuschle, "Tuberculosis Among the Navajo: Research in Cross-Cultural Technologic Development in Health," *American Review of Respiratory Diseases* 80 (1959): 201.

70. Deuschle, "Tuberculosis Among the Navajo," 201.

71. New Mexico State Department of Health, quoted in Kober and others, *Tuberculosis Among the North American Indians,* 31.

72. For example, see Irvine H. Page, Lena A. Lewis, and Harvey Gilbert, "Plasma Lipids and Proteins and Their Relationship to Coronary Disease Among Navajo Indians," *Circulation* 13 (May 1956): 675–679.

73. Kober and others, *Tuberculosis Among the North American Indians,* 4.

74. J. G. Townsend, Joseph D. Aronson, Robert Saylor, and Irma Parr, "Tuberculosis Control Among the North American Indians," *American Review of Tuberculosis* 45 (1942): 46.

75. J. Arthur Myers, "Editorial: Tuberculosis Among American Indians," *Diseases of the Chest* 16 (1949): 248.

76. Frank S. French, James R. Shaw, and Joseph O. Dean, "The Navajo Health Problem, Its Genesis, Proportions and a Plan for Its Solution," *Military Medicine* 116 (June 1955): 453.

77. "An Act to Promote the Rehabilitation of the Navajo and Hopi Tribes of Indians and a Better Utilization of the Resources of the Navajo and Hopi Indian Reservations, and for Other Purposes," *Public Law* 474, United States Code, 81st Cong., 2nd sess., 1950, pp. 44–45. See also Stephen J. Kunitz, *Disease Change and the Role of Medicine: The Navajo Experience* (Berkeley: University of California Press, 1983), 26–43.

78. Lewis J. Moorman, "Tuberculosis on the Navaho Reservation," *American Review of Tuberculosis* 61 (1950): 589.

79. Annie Wauneka, Written Statement, November 2, 1953, read in the US Senate, in "Hearings on HR 303: An Act to Transfer the Maintenance and Operation of Hospital and Health Facilities for Indians to the Public Health Service," May 28–29, 1954, in Congressional Hearings, Senate, Interior and Insular Affairs, 83rd Cong., 2nd sess., 1953–1954, vol. 14, 83 S1085–10, p. 43.

80. Walsh McDermott, Kurt Deuschle, John Adair, Hugh Fulmer, and Bernice Loughlin, "Introducing Modern Medicine in a Navajo Community: Physicians and Anthropologists Are Cooperating in This Study of Changing Patterns of Culture and Disease," *Science* 131 (January 22, 1960): 197–205, 280–287; John Adair and Kurt Deuschle, *The People's Health: Medicine and Anthropology in a Navajo Community* (New York: Meredith Corporation, 1970); Walsh McDermott, Kurt Deuschle, and

Clifford R. Barnett, "Health Care Experiment at Many Farms," *Science* 175 (January 7, 1972): 23–31.

81. McDermott, "Draft of Chapter II," undated, in *Walsh McDermott Papers*, Box 11, Folder 6, p. 12. See also McDermott and others, "Health Care Experiment at Many Farms," 25–27; John Adair, Kurt Deuschle, and Clifford Barnett, with a chapter by Barnett and David L. Rabin, *The People's Health: Medicine and Anthropology in a Navajo Community*, 2nd ed. (Albuquerque: University of New Mexico Press, 1988), 157–159. See also David S. Jones, "The Health Care Experiment at Many Farms: The Navajo, Tuberculosis, and the Limits of Modern Medicine, 1952–1962," *Bulletin of the History of Medicine* 76 (Winter 2002): 749–790.

82. "An Act to Transfer the Maintenance and Operation of Hospital and Health Facilities for Indians to the Public Health Service, and for Other Purposes," Public Law 568, United States Code, 83rd Cong., 2nd sess., 1954; Stephen J. Kunitz, "The History and Politics of US Health Care Policy for American Indians and Alaskan Natives," *American Journal of Public Health* 86 (October 1996): 1465.

83. USPHS, *Health Services for American Indians*, 39–57, 230–232.

84. Navajo Health Authority, "Position Paper," *Walsh McDermott Papers*, Box 11, Folder 1, p. 5.

85. Wauneka to Elliot Richardson, July 1, 1971, in Navajo Health Authority, "Capsules of Navajo Health History," in "Summary of Program Components," c. 1974, *Walsh McDermott Papers*, Box 11, Folder 1, p. 19. See also Jones, *Rationalizing Epidemics*, 218–222. For the political background, see Bergman and others, "A Political History of the Indian Health Service," 575, 588.

86. US Public Health Service, *Indian Health Service: A Comprehensive Health Care Program for American Indians and Alaska Natives* (Washington, DC: US Department of Health and Human Services, 1989), v, 16–22.

87. Indian Health Service, "Facts on Indian Health Disparities," September 2002, downloaded from http://info.ihs.gov/health/health_index.asp.

88. Jeff Henderson, "Native American Health Policy: From US Territorial Expansion to Legal Obligation," *JAMA*. 265 (May 1, 1991): 2272–2273; Kunitz, "US Health Care Policy for American Indians," 1464–1473; Joseph G. Jorgensen, "Comment: Recent Twists and Turns in American Indian Health Care," *American Journal of Public Health* 86 (October 1996): 1362–1364.

89. IHS, "Facts on Indian Health Disparities."

90. Indian Health Service, "Year 2001 Profile," at http://www.ihs.gov /publicinfo/publicaffairs/pressreleases/press_release_2001/fy%202001%20ihs%20 profile.pdf.

91. Joan Stephenson, "For Some American Indians, Casino Profits Are a Good Bet for Improving Health Care," *JAMA*. 275 (June 19, 1996): 1783–1785; Marsha F. Goldsmith, "First Americans Face Their Latest Challenge: Indian Health Care Meets State Medicaid Reform," *JAMA*. 275 (June 19, 1996): 1786–1788; "Special Report: Indian Casinos," *Time Magazine* 160 (December 8, 2002): 44–58.

92. For alcohol, see Peter C. Mancall, *Deadly Medicine: Indians and Alcohol in Early America* (Ithaca: Cornell University Press, 1995), 1–10; James B. Waldram, *Revenge of the Windigo: The Construction of the Mind and Mental Health of North American Aboriginal Peoples* (Toronto: University of Toronto Press, 2004), 134–143, 165–166. For virgin soil epidemics, see Alfred W. Crosby, "Virgin Soil Epidemics as a Factor in the Aboriginal Depopulation in America," *William and Mary Quarterly* 33 (April 1976): 289–299; David S. Jones, "Virgin Soils Revisited," *William and Mary Quarterly* 60 (October 2003): 703–742. For Pima diabetes, see http://diabetes.niddk.nih.gov/dm/pubs/pima/index.htm.

93. IHS, "Facts on Indian Health Disparities."

94. Stephen J. Kunitz, "The Evolution of Disease and the Devolution of Health Care for American Indians," in *The Changing Face of Disease: Implications for Society,* ed. N. Mascie-Taylor, J. Peters, and S. T. McGarvey (New York: CRC Press, 2004), 153–169.

95. For the connections between wealth disparities and health disparities, see "Health and Wealth," *Daedalus* 123 (Fall 1994), 1–216; Robert G. Evans, Morris L. Barer, and Theodore R. Marmor, ed., *Why Are Some People Healthy and Others Not? The Determinants of Health of Populations* (New York: Aldine de Gruyter, 1994); Richard Wilkinson, *Unhealthy Societies: The Afflictions of Inequality* (London: Routledge, 1996); Norman Daniels, Bruce Kennedy, and Ichiro Kawachi, eds., *Is Inequality Bad for Our Health?* (Boston: Beacon Press, 2000).

Chapter 9

Prejudice and the Medical Profession

A Five-Year Update

Peter A. Clark

O ver the past decades the mortality rate in the United States has decreased and life expectancy has increased. Yet a number of recent studies have drawn Americans' attention to the fact that racial and ethnic disparities persist in health care. It is clear that the US health care system is not only flawed for many reasons including basic injustices, but also may be the cause of both injury and death for members of racial and ethnic minorities.

In 2002, an Institute of Medicine (IOM) report requested by Congress listed more than 100 studies documenting a wide range of disparities in the United States health care system. This report found that people belonging to racial and ethnic minorities often receive lower quality of health care than do people of European descent, even when their medical insurance coverage and income levels are the same as that of the latter.[1] A second study, whose results appeared in the *New England Journal of Medicine,* found that although African Americans and members of other ethnic minorities make up a growing percentage of Americans infected with the virus that causes Acquired Immunodeficiency Syndrome (AIDS), they are seriously underrepresented in clinical trials of new treatments for the disease. African Americans and Hispanics, the researchers discovered, were roughly half as likely as whites to participate in HIV treatment trials and about half as likely to receive experimental medicines.[2] This occurs at a time when HIV is spreading among African Americans at a higher rate than among whites.

A third study, in the *Archives of Internal Medicine*, found that African Americans were far less trusting than whites of the medical establishment, and of medical researchers in particular. African Americans were 79.2% more likely to believe that someone like them would be used as a guinea pig without his or her consent, versus 51.9% of whites surveyed. This study also found that 62.8% of African Americans (versus 38.4% of whites) believe that physicians often prescribed medication as a way of experimenting on people without consent.[3]

These studies only confirmed what many in the minority community had known for years—that racism, whether explicit or subtle, is alive and well in some members of the medical profession.[4] It is clear that a subtle, perhaps unconscious, form of racism is just as harmful as expressed hatred and bigotry because it affects the medical care of human beings. Although the IOM study found that most health care providers were well intentioned, the study cited "indirect evidence" that physicians' decisions were influenced by their perceptions of race.[5]

As a result of these studies, new initiatives were proposed and immediate action was taken to address these serious racial and ethnic disparities. Progress has been made in several areas since the original 2002 report. However, five years later, the 2007 National Healthcare Disparities Report (NHDR) reported that overall, disparities in quality and access for minority groups and poor populations have not been reduced since the original report. The three key themes that have emerged from this report are the following: (1) overall, disparities in health care quality and access are not getting smaller; (2) progress is being made, but many of the biggest gaps in quality and access have not been reduced; and (3) the problem of persistent uninsurance is a major barrier to reducing disparities.[6]

Unless measures are taken to address this racism, unless a new sense of trust is established between the medical professionals and racial and ethnic minorities, these injustices will continue to deepen and expand, and more lives will be placed in jeopardy. This chapter advocates for a comprehensive, multi-level, culturally relevant strategy that contains interventions that target individuals, communities, and the nation as a whole. This entails understanding the causes of racism that exist by some in the medical profession, identifying practical interventions that address racism in individuals, communities, and the nation as a whole, and forming partnerships that will work to develop a new sense of trust between members of the medical establishment and the minority communities.

The purpose of this chapter is fourfold: first, to give a historical context to this sense of mistrust for the medical establishment by racial and ethnic minorities, with focus on the African American community; second, to show the impact of the historical context on the present-day situation; third, to give an ethical analysis of why these injustices in the medical profession must be addressed and corrected; and fourth, to present some practical strategies and reforms on how to address the present racial and ethnic disparities in health care.

Historical Context

The Conspiracy Motif

The oral folklore tradition is deeply rooted in the African American heritage. For generations, a wide variety of negative stories have circulated within the community about the medical profession and public health programs. In 1972, when the tragedy of the Tuskegee Syphilis Study was revealed publicly, news spread rapidly throughout the African American community.[7] The truth was bad enough, but the problem was compounded as this information spread by word of mouth, and exaggerations and rumors intertwined with the truth. Today, in the African American community, and many other minority communities, the Tuskegee story is a major part of childhood folklore passed down by family members for the purpose of preparing present and future generations to deal with the harsh realities of life. By contrast, in the white community, very few have heard of the Tuskegee Syphilis Study, and even fewer have been affected by it.

Those who study folklore make a distinction between rumor and legend. A rumor is "a specific proposition for belief, passed along from person to person, usually by word of mouth without secure standards of evidence being present."[8] A legend "is a narrative account set in the recent past and containing traditional motifs that is told as true."[9] Since certain accounts incorporate modern motifs as well as traditional ones, most folklorists and social scientists now use the designation "contemporary legend" to describe "unsubstantiated narratives with traditional themes and modern motifs that circulate orally (and sometimes in print) in multiple versions and that are told as if they are true or at least plausible."[10] Drawing a clear distinction between rumor and contemporary legend is not always possible.[11] This chapter attempts to make this distinction and demonstrate the ways in which rumors and contemporary legends have affected, first, the oral folklore tradition of the African American community and, second, its relationship to the medical establishment.

The ethnologist Patricia A. Turner identifies two distinct but recurrent "motifs of danger" that have influenced the African American community in its distrust of the medical establishment and public health programs. The first is what she calls the *conspiracy motif*. The conspiracy motif suggests the existence of an organized plot by the "powers that be" against African Americans—a plot that first threatens individual black persons and then is translated into animosity toward the whole race and minorities in general. Turner traces the history of the conspiracy theory from the European involvement in the slave trade of black Africans to the contemporary "powers that be," including the Federal Bureau of Investigation (FBI), the Central Intelligence Agency (CIA), the Food and Drug Administration (FDA), the Centers for Disease Control (CDC), various branches of the armed services, commercial interests, and the medical and health establishments. This motif was dominant from the beginning of slavery in the United States through the late 19th century, but it also appeared in subtle ways during the past century, starting with the Tuskegee Syphilis Study.[12]

Turner's second motif of danger is the *contamination motif,* which she sees as dominant in the 20th century and continuing into the early years of the 21st century. Turner uses "contamination" to refer to "any item in which the physical well-being of individual black bodies is being manipulated for racist reasons."[13] This motif can be seen in some black views of contemporary medical and public health efforts; at times the motif coincides with the themes of genocide and conspiracy as discussed later in the chapter. An examination of these two motifs in an historical context will reveal why suspicion and distrust of the medical establishment and public health programs is reasonable on the part of African Americans. In many ways these two motifs focus on the trust issue from two different perspectives. The conspiracy motif's perspective focuses on the perceptions of African Americans, and the contamination motif's perspective focuses on actual disparities and on the behavior of physicians. Both perspectives lead to misinformation and misperceptions, which has caused ambiguity about and confusion and even mistrust of the medical profession. Such suspicion and distrust is the basis of African Americans' reluctance—and sometimes outright refusal—to participate in new clinical drug trials for AIDS and other experimental treatments.

Medicine has never been an entirely value-free discipline. It has inevitably reflected and reinforced the beliefs, values, and power dynamics of the society at large. As such, it has been influenced by race and racism directly and in subtle ways.[14] Evidence of this fact can be seen in the use of medical theories to justify slavery. Physicians in slaveholding cultures believed that black people possessed peculiar physiological and anatomical features that justified their enslavement. These medical theories not only reinforced the societal attitudes that black people were inferior—something less than human—but also justified the use of blacks for medical experimentation and dissection.[15] This is not to say that poor whites were not abused in the United States; rather, the point is that blacks were used more often and with greater disregard because of their race.[16]

In the antebellum South, black bodies were used by medical schools for teaching purposes. As the ideas of the "Paris school" of hospital medicine reached the United States, physicians who ran medical schools began to realize that they had to have human specimens.[17] Medical students need living people to study in order to learn anatomy, recognize and diagnose diseases, treat conditions requiring surgery, and try out new ideas and techniques. They also need dead bodies to perform the autopsies that help them confirm diagnoses and understand the effects of disease on the human body.[18] In the 30 years preceding the Civil War, southern medical schools fiercely competed with each other for new students, which put additional pressure on the schools to have an abundant supply of clinical materials.[19] This need for human specimens, both living and dead, was first met by placing various advertisements in local newspapers. The following ad, for example, which appeared in the *Charleston Mercury* between 1837 and 1839, announced the establishment of a special clinic for the treatment of blacks:

> Surgery of the Medical College of South Carolina, Queen Street—The faculty inform their professional brethren, and the public that they have established a Surgery, at the Old College, Queen Street, For The Treatment of negroes, which will continue during the session of the College, say from first November to the fifteenth of March ensuing. The object of the faculty, in opening this Surgery, is to collect as many interesting cases, as possible, for the benefit and instruction of their pupils—at the same time they indulge the hope, that it may not only prove an accommodation, but also a matter of economy to the public. They would respectfully call the attention of planters living in the vicinity of the city, to this subject; particularly such as may have servants laboring under Surgical diseases. Such persons of color as may not be able to pay for Medical advice, will be attended to gratis, at stated hours, as often as may be necessary. The faculty takes this opportunity of soliciting the co-operation of such of their professional brethren, as are favorable to their subjects.[20]

Such advertisements led both blacks and poor whites to fear mistreatment in southern hospitals.[21] They believed that, if admitted to such institutions, they would either be treated as experimental guinea pigs or allowed to die so that autopsies could be conducted on them. The evidence that this fear contributed to blacks and poor whites being mistreated in southern hospitals proves that this situation was real and not imagined.

After the Civil War, the absence of anatomical laws providing for the legal acquisition of human bodies led the medical profession to resort to illegal means of procuring cadavers. Bodies were illegally obtained by exhumation from graveyards, or bought or stolen before they could be buried; in some cases people were murdered so that their corpses could be sold to medical schools. Of the three methods, grave robbing was the most popular.[22] The term "night doctor" became well known in these years, especially in the black community. Its name was derived from the fact that victims were sought only at night, and it applied to both medical students and to professional grave robbers who sold stolen bodies to physicians for medical research.[23] The appearance of "night doctors" coincided with the post-Reconstruction era, when blacks were migrating to industrial centers from about 1880 to the end of the First World War.[24] The folklorist Gladys-Marie Fry contends that "many blacks are convinced that Southern landowners fostered a fear of 'night doctors' in the post-Reconstruction period in order to discourage the migration of blacks from rural farming areas to Northern and Southern urban centers."[25] Her theory appears to be historically well founded after examining the body of evidence from the post-Reconstruction era. However, some evidence indicates that "night doctors" did in fact play a major role in the procurement of black bodies for medical purposes.[26]

The oral folklore tradition of African Americans concerning "night doctors" is widespread, testifying to the influence that this belief in their existence had on blacks during this time. Stories of the "night doctors" are still told in the African American community, and historical research suggests that many may be true. It is estimated that, in those years, about 5,000 cadavers were dissected each year in the United States and that at least a majority were procured illegally.[27] By the 1920s, passage of anatomy acts eliminated body snatching in most parts of the United States, but it did not substantially alter the social origins of the supply of cadavers for medical schools.[28]

The oral folklore tradition of "night doctors" and the unethical practice of medical schools in obtaining cadavers for autopsies and bodies for experimentation not only fostered a fear of the medical establishment among African Americans that has been handed down through the centuries, but also reinforced societal attitudes toward racism. From 1619 until the early 1900s, it appears that the "powers that be" in the United States were often involved in a form of conspiracy against African Americans, both individually and corporately.[29] African Americans were degraded, threatened, and physically and emotionally abused by many in the medical profession. As a result, many African Americans today, aware of what occurred in previous times through oral folklore, have an innate mistrust of the medical establishment. With the advent of the 20th century, the influence of racism on the attitudes and values of medical professionals did not end, but became more subtle. The motif of conspiracy was replaced, for the most part, by the motif of contamination. Issues of trust and mistrust became intertwined with issues of bias and prejudice. The focus changed from the perceptions of African Americans to actual disparities and the behavior of physicians and the medical profession.

The Contamination Motif: A Form of Genocide

In the late 19th and early 20th centuries, many medical and public health journals began to focus on the problem of syphilis among African Americans.[30] Racist assumptions and stereotypes still existed within the medical establishment. Blacks were viewed as inferior, and this continued to justify using black bodies in ways that white bodies would have never been used. The predominantly white medical establishment maintained that "intrinsic racial characteristics such as excessive sexual desire, immorality, and overindulgence caused black people to have high rates of syphilis.... Physicians also pointed to alleged anatomical differences—large penises and small brains—to explain disease rates."[31] These racist assumptions became the basis for the initiation of the Tuskegee Study of Untreated Syphilis in the Negro Male.

In 1932 the United States Public Health Service initiated a study on African American men with syphilis in Macon County, Alabama, to determine the natural course of untreated, latent syphilis in black males. The study comprised 399 syphilitic men as well as 201 uninfected men who served as the control group. These subjects were recruited from churches and clinics throughout Macon County and were led to believe they would receive free meals and "special free treatment" for what was called "bad blood," in addition to burial insurance. In reality, however, they were enrolled in this study without informed consent. The infected men were neither informed that they had syphilis—a disease known to cause mental illness and death—nor treated for it. In fact, the researchers, in order to study the disease's natural course, withheld the standard treatment of mercury and arsenic compounds from the infected men. In 1947 when penicillin was determined to be an effective treatment for syphilis, this too was withheld. The treatment these men actively received came in the form of placebos.

The Tuskegee Syphilis Study was a covert medical research study. However, it was widely known in medical circles because articles about it were published in major medical journals, such as the *Southern Medical Journal* and the *Archives of Internal Medicine*.[32] As late as 1969, a committee at the federally operated CDC examined the study and agreed to allow it to continue. Not until 1972, when the first accounts of this study appeared in the press, did the Department of Health, Education and Welfare (HEW) terminate the experiment. At that time, 74 of the test subjects were still alive; at least 28, but perhaps more than 100, had died directly from advanced syphilitic lesions.[33] (In 1980 HEW was renamed the Department of Health and Human Services; the CDC was renamed the Centers for Disease Control which, in 1992, then became the Centers for Disease Control and Prevention.) For many in the African American community, news of the study confirmed what they had long suspected: that the medical profession and the federal government used various forms of contamination to commit genocide.

Stories about the motif of contamination, as a form of genocide, continued to spread in the African American community throughout the 20th century. There are many in the African American community who believe that condom distribution was part of a government plan to reduce the number of black births.[34] This belief became more credible when the contraceptive device Norplant became available.[35] Following its legalization, stories began to circulate that inner-city African American women on welfare were being forced to use this contraceptive device. Such stories intensified when various editorial writers and public policy makers began to suggest that "welfare mothers" be required to have the device implanted as a condition for further benefits.[36] Additional fertility-related measures, such as the sterilization statutes adopted by many states in the 1970s, also helped perpetuate this notion of genocide in the African American community. By the late 1920s, two dozen states, led by California, passed laws authorizing the sterilization of habitual prison inmates, and residents of mental institutions.[37] Tending to reinforce the notion is the finding that a direct correlation exists between the race of a patient and the availability of certain procedures.[38] Various medical studies have shown that certain procedures, such as renal transplants, hip and knee replacements, and gastrointestinal endoscopy, are less likely to be performed on blacks. However, blacks are more likely to undergo other procedures such as hysterectomies, bilateral orchiectomies, and the amputation of lower limbs.[39] These findings, coming from reputable medical journals, have only increased African American cynicism concerning members of the medical establishment.

Present-Day Concerns

Genetic screening and public immunization programs have also raised suspicions in the African American community. The sickle cell anemia screening programs of the 1970s created misinformation, confusion, and fear.[40] Inadequate planning and preparation by the medical profession and public health officials, and a failure to educate the American public on the difference between being a carrier versus having the disease, resulted in unnecessary stigma and discrimination. Ultimately this confusion and misinformation led to great suspicion in the African American community that this was another form of genocide.[41] The same has been true of public immunization campaigns. Especially widespread is the fear that certain drugs may be experimental and thus potentially toxic. Inoculations have been suspected of being vehicles for the introduction of experimental substances or infectious agents into the minority communities. Even today, health fairs and "immunization days" sponsored by community-based clinics sometimes cause concern among African American and other minority parents.[42] This fear has been fanned by the circulation in minority communities by books such as Curtis Cost's *Vaccines Are Dangerous: A Warning to the Black Community*, which describes vaccination as "purposely injecting loathsome filth from a diseased animal directly into the crystal-clear blood streams of our precious children."[43] As a result of this book, diagnostic tuberculosis (TB) skin testing has often been refused, because it involves injecting tuberculin material directly under the skin. Some believe that the test is intended to give TB rather than detect it.[44] Such misinformation has greatly contributed to the "legacy of mistrust" of some members of the medical establishment in the African American and other minority communities.

In the later part of the 20th century, the contamination theory has also been associated with the AIDS epidemic. Indeed, many believe that AIDS was conceived as a deliberate plot to exterminate African Americans and other minorities.[45] In a 1990 survey conducted by the Southern Christian Leadership Conference, 35% of the 1,056 black church members who responded believed that AIDS was a form of genocide.[46] A rumor found consistently among African Americans is that the AIDS virus was created in the CIA laboratory. According to such rumors, the virus is either a biological warfare experiment that was tried out on African Americans and Haitians or biological warfare intended to diminish the African and Haitian population.[47] These rumors, along with other factors, have contributed to the increase in HIV infections in the African American community. According to the Centers for Disease Control, although African Americans make up only 13% of the United States population, they account for almost half the estimated number of HIV/AIDS diagnoses made during 2006.[48]

In a 2002 study by Dr. Allen Gifford et al., it has been shown that even though African Americans and other minorities make up a growing percentage of Americans infected with HIV/AIDS, these minority groups are underrepresented in clinical trials studying new treatments for this disease.[49] Analysis of the findings of their nationally representative sample found that an estimated 14% of adults receiving care for HIV infection participated in a medical trial or study; 24% had received experimental medications; and 8% had tried and failed to obtain experimental treatment. According to multivariate models, non-Hispanic blacks and Hispanics were less likely to participate in trials than non-Hispanic whites (odds ratio for participation among non-Hispanic blacks, 0.50 [95% confidence interval, 0.28 to 0.91]; odds ratio among Hispanics, 0.58 [95% confidence interval, 0.37 to 0.93]) and to have received experimental medications (odds ratios, 0.41 [95% confidence interval, 0.32 to 0.54] and 0.56 [95% confidence interval, 0.41 and 0.78], respectively).[50] These findings confirm

that there are disparities among racial and ethnic groups in the rate of study enrollment, as others have observed in selected populations of patients with HIV or inferred from the racial and ethnic composition of particular cohorts; moreover these findings suggest that such disparities persisted up to four years after the National Institutes of Health issued guidelines for increasing enrollment of members of minority groups .... The effects of race or ethnic group were seen even within socioeconomic strata, remained apparent after multivariate adjustment for the level of education, and seemed to be present in all aspects of access to research.[51]

Although the authors did not pinpoint a single reason for the racial disparities, they believe there is less awareness and more widespread negative attitude about clinical research and experimental medications in minority communities. "Black persons may interpret informed consent procedures as 'liability waivers' for researchers to do little to protect patients," they write.[52]

Distrust of the medical professionals by minority groups was further confirmed in another study. In this study, researchers analyzed data from 527 African American and 382 white respondents to a national telephone survey on participation in clinical research. African Americans, this study found, were more likely than white respondents (41.7% to 23.4%) to expect their physicians to give less than a full explanation to research participation; they were also more likely (45.5% to 38.8%) to believe their physicians would expose them to unnecessary risks. African American respondents were in general more distrustful than white respondents.[53]

It is clear that minority communities in general and the African American community specifically exhibit a general attitude of mistrust toward some members of the medical profession. But there also exists some degree of mistrust of minority communities by physician-researchers. Researchers tend to "purposely avoid recruiting marginalized populations (such as members of minority groups, substance abusers, or homeless persons) to clinical trials because they believe that poor compliance is common in these groups."[54] Some could argue that this avoidance itself may be a form of racism. Studies have shown that many of these supposed compliance obstacles are probably surmountable and, more important, have not in many cases predicted poor compliance.[55] This lack of trust on the part of researchers, which has a long history, contributes to the disparities seen in the medical care provided to members of racial and ethnic minority groups. If physicians do not believe that the patient will be compliant, then it is less likely that the physician will prescribe the needed drugs. In some cases, physicians see this as a way of not wasting our limited medical resources. Only through the building of trust will patients be involved in care, adhere to recommended treatment, and willingly participate in clinical research increase.[56]

Underrepresentation of minorities in clinical research trials can be a matter of life and death for minority patients. In a study conducted by the Chronic Disease Prevention & Control Research Center at Baylor College of Medicine, Goldberg and Weinberg et al. found that between 1995 and 1999, blacks, Asian Pacific Islanders, Hispanics, and Native Americans together made up for less than 10% of patients included in new cancer drug trials. "Underrepresentation of this sort leads to results that do not account for a host of factors—genetic, cultural, racial, religious, linguistic, as well as variables related to age and gender—that could have a huge impact on how well new drugs do in the real world."[57] This report led to numerous discussions about how clinical trials are conducted, but until practical steps are taken to address these issues, the quality of evidence will be undermined.

Impact of the 2007 National Healthcare Disparities Report

The March 2002 Institute of Medicine Report showed that racial and ethnic minorities received a lower quality health care than whites, even when their insurance and income were the same as whites. The authors wrote:

> Even among the better-controlled studies, the vast majority indicated that minorities are less likely than whites to receive needed services, including clinically necessary procedures. These disparities exist in a number of disease areas, including cancer, cardiovascular disease, HIV/AIDS, diabetes, and mental illness, and are found across a range of procedures, including routine treatments for common health problems.[58]

The study found that patients' attitudes, such as their preferences for treatment, do not vary greatly according to race and so cannot explain racial and ethnic disparities in health care. In addition, the authors wrote, "There is considerable empirical evidence that well-intentioned white physicians who are not overtly biased and who do not believe that they are prejudiced typically demonstrate unconscious implicit negative racial attitudes and stereotypes. Both implicit and explicit stereotypes significantly shape interpersonal interactions, influencing how information is recalled and guiding expectations and differences in systematic ways."[59]

Since the original report, some progress has been made in key conditions that disproportionately affect minority populations. However, the 2007 National Healthcare Disparities Report summarizes the many areas where little to no progress has been achieved at reducing disparities. Success has been seen in four core areas:

1. The disparity between black and white hemodialysis patients with adequate dialysis was eliminated in 2005.

2. The disparity between Asians and whites who had a usual primary care provider was eliminated in 2004.

3. The disparity between Hispanic and non-Hispanic whites and between people living in poor communities and people living in high-income communities for hospital admissions for perforated appendix was eliminated in 2004.

4. Significant improvements were observed in childhood vaccinations for most priority populations.[60]

Other improvements among core measures include the following: children who received recommended vaccines among blacks, Asians, and Hispanics; new AIDS cases for blacks and Hispanics; tuberculosis treatment for foreign-born Asians; nursing home residents who developed pressure sores; adults who can sometimes or never get care as soon as they wanted and prenatal care for pregnant women; and for the poor, people under the age of 65, with health insurance. These findings show some progress in decreasing disparities, and each racial and ethnic group showed improvements in some areas. However, not all improvements closed the gap between these groups and reference groups.[61]

Despite these successes, there remain big disparities in the quality documented since the initial report. These disparities include the following:

1. Blacks had a rate of new AIDS cases 10 times higher than whites.

2. Asian adults age 65 and over were 50% more likely than whites to lack immunization against pneumonia.

3. American Indians and Alaska Natives were twice as likely to lack prenatal care in the first trimester as whites.

4. Hispanics had a rate of new AIDS cases over 3.5 times higher than that of non-Hispanic whites.

5. Poor children were over 28% more likely than high-income children to experience poor communication with their health care providers.[62]

Besides these areas listed in the 2007 report, there are other areas of concern. Blacks are more likely than whites to suffer severe, untreated, and disabling depression.[63] In a retrospective study of Atlanta hospitals between 1998 and 2004, researchers found that uninsured and Medicaid-insured patients, and those from ethnic minorities, had substantially increased risks of presenting with advanced-stage cancers at diagnosis. This means they are more likely to endure excruciating, and often more expensive, treatments, and they are more likely to die from cancer.[64]

A recent study confirms that black Americans continue to distrust medical research and clinical trials. Powe et al. found that minorities are 200% more likely to perceive harm coming from participating in research. This study provides direct evidence of why fewer blacks participate in cardiovascular prevention trial research. Failure to participate in clinical trials for conditions that affect blacks disproportionately and knowing that blacks often respond differently to medications will only perpetuate health disparities.[65] A National Institutes of Health survey released in 2005 — whose data had been compiled from a range of trials and research over two decades — found that minorities are actually willing to volunteer at the same rate as whites, but are not asked as often. It is interesting to note that an earlier research study by Thomas LaVeist and colleagues at the Johns Hopkins Bloomberg School of Public Health found that few blacks had heard of the Tuskegee experiment, and even fewer knew accurate facts. The researchers argue that the Tuskegee study plays only a modest role in producing distrust. Instead, they contend that the following reasons account for blacks' low participation in clinical trials: economic barriers, attending lower-quality health care facilities, time off to participate, difficulty getting appointments, negative experiences in the medical system, and the complexity of required procedures such as consent forms.[66]

Prejudice may play a role in disparities regarding health care for African Americans, but the issue of race and culture may be more important in achieving treatment goals. In another, more recent study by Thomas Sequist et al. in the *Archives of Internal Medicine*, the investigators found that African American patients often had worse outcomes than white patients regarding the treatment for diabetes mellitus. In the review of 4,556 white patients and 2,258 African American patient charts, treated by 90 physicians, researchers found that 57% of white patients were able to control their cholesterol, as compared to only 45% of African American patients; 47% of whites and 39% of African Americans achieved optimal hemoglobin levels. The researchers found that racial discrepancies applied to physicians across the board. They found that 30–40% of the discrepancies could be attributed to differences in patients' sex, income, insurance, and rates of obesity. However, the majority seemed to stem from the patient-physician relationship. The researchers found that a lot of diabetes care revolves around lifestyle changes, such as in diet and exercise levels. The problem is that physicians tend to promote a one-size-fits-all approach which does not account for individual needs and differences. For example, counseling African American and Latino patients with diabetes to lower carbohydrate intake by cutting rice from their diets may not be a realistic strategy if rice is an important staple for the family. Fruits and vegetables may be a part of one person's culture but not another's culture. This study attributed the differences less to overt racism than to a systematic failure to tailor treatments to patient's cultural norms.[67]

Research suggests that health care providers' diagnostic and treatment decisions, as well as their feelings about patients, are influenced by patients' race or ethnicity.[68] This has led to actual health disparities among minorities, especially the African American community. What is becoming clear is that a link exists among issues of trust, culture, race, and actual disparities in health care. The factual discussion of actual disparities shows that a substantial portion of medical disparities are due to physician bias and prejudice whether explicit or subconscious. However, some of these disparities are also due to the misinformation and mistrust that has been documented in this section. This distrust has had a critical impact on the physician-patient relationship. In many ways these subtle issues of distrust may have a greater impact on medical disparities in the African American community than many would have expected. Little is being done to address issues like cross-cultural education on medical professionals, increasing the number of minority physicians, and addressing the myths and rumors that persist in the African American community. Issues of explicit and subconscious racism among medical professionals, which can be the result of myths and rumors in the African American community, must be addressed from both a medical and ethical perspective.

Ethical Analysis

The evidence is quite compelling that racial and ethnic disparities in health care contribute to disparities in care for minorities in the United States. David Satcher, M.D., the former United States Surgeon General, argues that this evidence correlates with persistent health disparities in the burden of illness and death. Satcher writes,

> Compared with their white counterparts, black babies are twice as likely to die during their first year of life, and American Indian babies are 1.5 times as likely. The rate of diabetes among Native Americans is three to five times higher than the rest of the American population, and among Hispanics it is twice as high as in the majority population. Although constituting only 11% of the total population in 1996, Hispanics accounted for 20% of new tuberculosis cases. Also, women of Vietnamese origin suffer from cervical cancer at nearly five times the rate of white women.[69]

Satcher contends that although these disparities result from complex interactions among genetic variations, environmental factors, and specific health behaviors, there is also reason to believe that race and ethnicity play a major role.[70] This is certainly a medical problem, but it is also an ethical problem for all Americans. To allow race and ethnicity and issues of mistrust to play any role in providing health care to our fellow Americans goes against the basic principles of ethics. I will argue that—according to the ethical principles of respect for persons, beneficence/nonmaleficence, and justice—action must be taken immediately to address these concerns and counteract any form of racism that may be present in the medical profession, whether explicit or subconscious, and to also address any mistrust that exists in the African American community.

Respect for Persons

This principle incorporates two ethical convictions: first, that persons should be treated as autonomous agents; second, that persons with diminished autonomy are entitled to protection. The principle of respect for persons thus divides into two separate moral requirements: the requirement to acknowledge autonomy and the requirement to protect those with diminished autonomy.[71] The physician-patient relationship is a covenant that is based on mutual trust. It is a fiduciary relationship that is based on honesty. The bond of trust between a physician and patient is vital to the diagnostic and therapeutic process. Edmund Pellegrino, M.D., and David Thomasma, Ph.D., both of whom have written extensively in this area, argue that among the obligations that arise from the physician-patient relationship is technical competence: "The act of the medical professional is inauthentic and a lie unless it fulfills the expectation of technical competence."[72] Patients, that is, should be able to expect their physicians to have the technical skills to assess and manage their medical conditions.

Unfortunately, as discussed previously, racial and ethnic minorities believe their medical conditions are not being assessed or managed by physicians in the same way that the medical conditions of white patients are being assessed and managed. All five Institute of Medicine reports make it clear that disparities between whites and minorities exist in a number of disease areas.[73] Giselle Corbie-Smith, M.D., and her colleagues found that African Americans were "more likely to believe that their physicians would not explain research fully or would treat them as part of an experiment without their consent."[74] This was confirmed by research done by Neil Powe, M.D., and his colleagues at Johns Hopkins University Medical Center. They found that blacks were more reluctant than whites to take part in medical studies because they feared being improperly used as guinea pigs.[75] Medical abuses have come to light through the oral tradition of minority groups and published reports. Some minorities believe that their physicians cannot be trusted, that physicians sometimes use them as guinea pigs for experiments, and that they are sometimes not offered the same medical procedures that whites are offered, even though they have the same clinical symptoms. It appears that the technical competence of some physicians is being compromised by the impediment of prejudice and bias.

These concerns directly relate to the issue of informed consent. Patients have the right to be informed about the advantages and disadvantages of any medical treatment, experimental or otherwise, and about any viable alternatives as well. Research has shown that, in many cases, racial and ethnic minorities cannot give informed consent because they have not been informed of all their available treatment options. As stated previously, violations of informed consent by medical professionals have been documented and, in some cases, have been widely publicized. In fact, past and present injustices against minorities, both factual and perceived, have sometimes led them to interpret informed consent procedures as "liability waivers" for researchers, doing nothing for the former and freeing the latter from the risk of possible lawsuits.[76] One basic aspect of the principle of respect for persons is that a person should never be treated simply as a means to an end. When a caregiver fails to give his or her patient all relevant information concerning risks and benefits, or inform him or her of all possible treatment options, or purposely withholds "standard of care" treatment, or declines to recruit minorities for medical trials because he or she believes that poor compliance is common among them, then that caregiver is using patients as a means rather than an end. As a result of both explicit and subtle prejudice and bias by some medical professionals, minority patients suffer needlessly. This prejudice clearly violates the ethical principle of respect for persons. Minority patients' autonomy, the basic respect they deserve as human beings, is being violated because they are allowed to endure pain, suffering, and even death when such hardships could be alleviated.

Beneficence/Nonmaleficence

The principle of beneficence involves the obligation to prevent, remove, or minimize harm and risks and to promote and enhance the good of a person. Beneficence includes nonmaleficence, which prohibits the infliction of harm, injury, or death upon others. In medical ethics this principle has been closely associated with the maxim *Primum non nocere* ("Above all do no harm"). Allowing a person to endure pain and suffering that could be managed and relieved violates the principle of beneficence because one is not preventing harm and, therefore, not acting in the best interest of the patient. The duty to act in the patient's best interest must override a physician's or researcher's self-interest. Clinical researchers are aware that their work should involve diverse populations of patients. "Race, sex, and other socio-demographic factors can influence the course of disease, the response to treatment, the types of toxic effects, and health related behavior, and the degree of diversity can therefore affect the generalizability of the results," write A. L. Gifford and colleagues, the researchers in a study showing that African Americans and Hispanics were half as likely as whites to participate in HIV treatments trials and about half as likely to receive experimental medicines.[77] This lack of participation is caused by, first, minority's distrust of some medical professionals and, second, the tendency of physician-researchers to avoid recruiting minorities because they believe poor compliance is common in these groups.[78] As a result, blacks have, in absolute numbers, outnumbered whites in new AIDS diagnoses and deaths since 1996; since 1998, they outnumbered whites in people living with AIDS.[79] Because of their failure to become involved in clinical trials for new treatments, blacks and Hispanics have long been disproportionately affected by the AIDS epidemic. This has been suggested to be the basis of a cause/effect relationship regarding the spread of HIV/AIDS in the African American community. The stereotyping by researchers and physicians of racial and ethnic minorities (assuming, for example, that they are more likely to abuse drugs, comply improperly with treatment, and neglect follow-up care) may contribute to higher death rates and lower survival rates among minorities than among whites suffering from illnesses of comparable severity.

The recent 2008 Johns Hopkins University study by Powe and colleagues confirms this earlier research:

1. 24% of black Americans reported that their doctors would not fully explain research participation to them, versus 13% of whites.

2. 72% of black Americans said doctors would use them as guinea pigs without their consent, versus 49% of whites.

3. 35% of black Americans said doctors would ask them to participate in research even if it could harm them, versus only 16% of whites.

4. 8% of black Americans more often believed they could less freely ask questions of doctors, compared to 2% of whites.

5. 58% of black Americans said doctors had previously experimented on them without consent, compared to 25% of whites.[80]

Physicians have, as moral agents, an ethical responsibility to treat their patients in a way that will maximize benefits and minimize harms. Failure to adequately assess and manage medical conditions, for whatever reason, is not in the best interest of the patient.

Statistics from the American Cancer Society show that regardless of their insurance status, black and Hispanic patients still had an increased risk of having advanced-stage disease—typically stage III or IV—at diagnosis when compared with white patients. African American patients were less likely than white patients to receive therapy for cancers of the lung, breast, colon, and prostate regardless of the stage of their cancer.[81] Blacks are over 10 times as likely as whites to be diagnosed with AIDS and 15% less likely than whites to being admitted to the hospital for pediatric gastroenteritis. Uninsured black women were also less likely to have a mammogram in the past 2 years (44.2% compared with 76.3% for privately insured black women).[82]

It is clear, after reviewing these statistics and identifying the biases and stereotyping that exists among some medical professionals, that disparities in US health care expose minority patients to unnecessary risks, including possible injury and death. Physicians have a moral responsibility to do what is good for their patients. Should a physician be impeded in the exercise of his or her reason and free will because of prejudice or bias, then that physician has an ethical responsibility to overcome said impediment or transfer the patient to another physician, one who will do what is demanded by the basic precepts of medicine—that is, to seek the patient's good. It is also important that if mistrust due to rumor and myth is the cause of medical disparities, then leaders in the minority communities have an ethical responsibility to address this information. Correct information about vaccinations, HIV/AIDS, clinical trials for cancer, etc., must be disseminated in the minority communities. Allowing ignorance about these issues to prevail can become a matter of life and death. Failure to recognize prejudices, biases, and cultural differences and to address misinformation and distrust is a failure not only of the test of beneficence, but may also be a failure of the test of nonmaleficence.

Justice

This principle recognizes that each person should be treated fairly and equitably and be given his or her due. The principle of justice can be applied to this situation in two ways. First, inequality concerning adequate health care for all Americans is well documented. For years this inequality was attributed to socioeconomic causes, which led to a lack of access to health care. With the publication of the IOM reports, it is apparent that subtle racial and ethnic prejudice and differences in quality of health plans are also among the reasons why even insured members of minorities receive inferior care. Prejudice and negative racial and ethnic stereotypes may be misleading physicians, medical researchers, and other health care professionals. Whether such bias is explicit or unconscious, it is a violation of the principle of justice. It has been documented that members of minority groups are not receiving the same standard of care that whites are receiving, even when they have the same symptoms. This is a blatant disregard of the principle of justice.

Second, the principle of justice also pertains to the fair and equitable allocation of resources. It has been documented that members of minorities are less likely than whites to be given appropriate cardiac medicines or undergo coronary bypass surgery. They are less likely to receive kidney transplants or the best diagnostic tests and treatments for cancer. They are also less apt to receive the most sophisticated treatments for HIV. Americans espouse the belief that all men and women are equal. If we truly believe it, then we should insist that all men and women must, whatever their race or ethnicity, receive equal medical treatments and resources. Denying certain minorities these medical treatments—when whites receive them as standard care—is an unjust allocation of resources and violates a basic tenet of justice. Physicians and medical researchers have an ethical obligation to use available resources fairly and to distribute them equitably. Failure to do so is ethically irresponsible and morally objectionable. To compromise the basic ethical foundations upon which medicine stands is not only destructive for minority patients but for society as a whole.

Strategies and Reforms

Racial and ethnic disparities in health care continue to be documented. The root causes are multiple and diverse: a long history of discrimination; lack of access to high-quality, affordable health care; too few educational and professional opportunities; unequal access to safe, clean neighborhoods; and, in some African Americans, a lingering mistrust of the medical community.[83] This problem is not going to disappear. Much has been written about the failure of health care professionals and medical institutions to address this issue, but simple rhetoric without significant reform will accomplish nothing. Immediate changes that address the issues of racial and ethnic disparities directly and concretely are needed. To accomplish this task, we must initiate, and in some cases follow through with, the following initiatives.

First, society should undertake research that allows it to understand the causes of racial and ethnic prejudice and the ways that prejudice affects health care. We already know some of the causes: poverty, lack of access to quality health services, environmental hazards in homes and neighborhoods, and scarcity of effective prevention programs tailored to the needs of specific communities.[84] However, we need more research that focuses on the unconscious biases that seem to pervade the medical establishment. An example of such an initiative is the Federal Collaboration in Health Disparities Research (FCHDR) that has been developed by the Centers for Disease Control and Prevention, in collaboration with the Office of Public Health and Science's Office of Minority Health, and co-sponsored by AHRQ. FCHDR identifies and supports research priorities for cross-agency collaboration to hasten the elimination of health disparities, and identifying priority research topics on health disparities was one of its primary outcomes in 2006. Through FCHDR, federal partners have formed subject matter expert groups around four initial research topic areas for collaboration: obesity, built environment (which includes homes, schools, workplaces, parks and recreation areas, business areas, transportation systems, etc.), mental health care, and comorbidities. These priorities represent opportunities for federal agencies and other partners to collaborate on innovative research.[85]

Second, there is a need to educate both medical professionals and patients. Medical professionals need to become more aware of the subtle forms of prejudice that impact their medical decisions. Patients need to learn how to be more active and better informed in their decisions concerning medical treatment. The education of health care professionals on cultural and racial issues should begin in medical school and continue throughout their careers. It should focus on the fact that racial and ethnic disparities exist and on the ways they can be identified and confronted. The IOM has recommended cross-cultural education programs that, first, enhance health care professionals' awareness of how cultural and social factors influence health care and, second, provide methods for obtaining, negotiating, and managing this information clinically. "Cross-cultural education can be divided into three conceptual approaches," write the authors of the IOM report. These approaches focus, respectively, on the following: *attitudes* (cultural sensitivity/awareness approach), *knowledge* (multicultural/categorical approach), and *skills* (cross-cultural approach), and has been taught using a variety of interactive and experiential methodologies. Research to date demonstrates that training is effective in improving provider knowledge of cultural and behavioral aspects of healthcare and building effective communication strategies.[86]

Cross-cultural education can be done in medical schools, for interns and residents during their training, and for attending physicians as continuing medical education courses. On an individual basis, each physician should follow the recommendation of the American Medical Association: "Physicians should examine their own practices to ensure that racial prejudice does not affect clinical judgment in medical care."[87] Only through self-examination and continuing objective education will medical professionals be able to identify and conquer racial and ethnic bias and prejudice.

To educate the public, real and meaningful partnerships must be created between medical professionals and communities. Partnerships involving schools, churches, faith-based organizations, and civic and local groups are the key to creating trust with the minority communities. But such efforts cannot be seen as one-time events; they must be part of an ongoing process that involves engagement, dialogue, and feedback.[88] Medical professionals must engage target communities through mechanisms such as advisory boards, free medical screening for various illnesses, health fairs, public education lectures, etc. In these engagements they must conduct a dialogue that ensures open and honest communication and mutual respect. Such sessions will, on one hand, allow medical professionals to inform the public about the need for medical screening and clinical research, and, on the other, allow the public to voice its concerns about certain diseases, research protocols, new medications, and other matters.

Dialogue and transparency of this kind will provide the feedback that gives both medical professionals and the public the ability to listen to each other's concerns through periodic evaluations, reviews, and open forums. Only through honest and effective communication will trust be fostered and patients come to feel that they have some control in their health care decision-making. Hopefully, this honest communication will also help dispel any myths circulating in the minority communities about certain diseases, medications, experiments, and similar issues. Health care professionals must always be seen as advocates for all people. Only then will patients' involvement in care, adherence to recommended treatment, and willingness to participate in clinical research increase.[89]

Third, there needs to be collaboration and partnerships among interested parties from academia, industry, government, philanthropy, the corporate sector, and the community to reduce racial and ethnic health disparities. The Health Disparities Roundtable, for example, was convened in 2006 under the co-sponsorship of the Office of Minority Health and AHRQ and also in partnership with the Institute of Medicine. Its purpose is to generate action and engage interested parties in a collaboration and partnership that focuses on research and policy discussions. The committee addresses topics such as the following: effective cultural competency techniques and cross-cultural education in health care settings; strategies to expand and strengthen research to develop effective treatments for those diseases that disproportionately affect minority populations; educational strategies to end health disparities; strategies to develop and promote increased minority representation in medicine and health professions; and the causes of health and health care disparities and their best solutions.[90]

Fourth, one way to foster a sense of trust with the minority communities is to offer every citizen adequate health care coverage. Marcia Angell, former editor of the *New England Journal of Medicine,* believes that the United States needs a national "single-payer" system that would eliminate unnecessary administrative costs, duplication, and profits. She has proposed extending Medicare to the entire population. "Medicare is, after all, a government-financed single-payer system embedded within our private, market based-system" she writes. "It's by far the most efficient part of our health-care system, with overhead costs of less than 3 percent, and it covers virtually everyone over the age of 65."[91] Offering all Americans adequate health care coverage would be a significant step in building a sense of trust with the minority communities, who would benefit the most from this initiative. In addition, offering access to the same quality of health services for all Americans would help to eliminate the disparities that exist today.

Fifth, efforts should be made to increase the number of minority doctors. Recent statistics show that "[m]inorities, including African Americans, Asian Americans, Hispanics and American Indians, account for just 9% of the nation's doctors."[92] More specifically, "some 12% of the American population is Black, but only 4% of physicians are Black."[93] Increasing the number of minority doctors would both increase the trust factor between minorities and the medical establishment, and it would also assist in the communication and cultural issues between patients and physicians.

Sixth, the IOM study also suggests that physicians should rely on "evidence-based guidelines" to determine what care should be given to patients. Adherence to such guidelines, if made known to patients, could help dispel any fears that minority patients have regarding inferior care due to their race or ethnicity.

Seventh, to improve health care among the minority populations, there is a need to follow Martin Luther King Jr.'s example of grass-roots efforts and organize accordingly. This means organizing church by church and health fair by health fair to persuade African Americans and other minorities to participate in clinical trials, become organ donors, etc. Currently only 8% of people on the national list to donate bone marrow are black, but about 12% of the population is black. In bone marrow, even more so than for solid organs such as kidneys and livers, it is important to find a donor of the same ethnic group.[94] Barriers to adequate health care include lack of education, lack of empowerment, economic issues such as transportation, child care, time off from work, etc. To address these issues, some medical centers are using grant money from the National Cancer Institute to hire women from the community to do outreach, such as spreading the word about mammograms and helping distrustful or overwhelmed patients to navigate the health care system.[95] This grass-roots effort is one effective way to gain the trust needed in the minority communities.

Eighth, leaders in the minority communities have an ethical responsibility to address the many rumors and myths surrounding HIV/AIDS, vaccinations, etc. that are spreading within their communities. This is not to say that what has happened in the past should be ignored or forgotten. The minority communities cannot close their eyes to events like the Tuskegee Syphilis Study. Instead, civic and church leaders within these communities should begin an honest dialogue with the community about HIV/AIDS, clinical trials, and other health-related issues. It is time for leaders in the minority communities to work with the medical establishment for the health and safety of their constituents.

Ninth, underrepresentation in clinical trials can lead to results that do not account for a variety of factors—genetic, cultural, racial, religious, linguistic, as well as variables related to age and gender—that could have a significant impact on how well new drugs perform in the real world. To address these shortcomings, the following policy solutions have been proposed: government regulatory changes; increased collaboration between government and private industry on clinical trial design; increased community involvement in patient participation; scientific journal oversight of patient breakdowns; new, specialized training for review boards; reallocation of research funding to avoid duplication and address disparities; increased public education; increased focus on easing the patient participation process; and guaranteed insurance coverage for all related costs.[96] Instituting these policy solutions would not only increase minority representation in clinical trials but would also go a long way toward gaining the trust of the minority populations in the United States.

Racial and ethnic disparities in health care constitute a complex issue that pertains to individuals, institutions, and society as a whole. Unless we address these disparities and begin to eradicate them, we will never attain the goal of providing high-quality health care in the United States. If we do not make this a priority now, everyone will pay the price in the future.

Notes

1. Committee on Understanding and Eliminating Racial and Ethnic Disparities in Health Care, Institute of Medicine, *Unequal Treatment: What Healthcare Providers Need to Know About Racial and Ethnic Disparities in Health Care* (Washington, D.C.: National Academy Press, 2002).

2. A. Gifford, W. Cunningham, and K. Heslin et al., "Participation in Research and Access to Experimental Treatments by HIV-Infected Patients," *New England Journal of Medicine* 346, no. 18 (May 2, 2002): 1373–1382.

3. G. Corbie-Smith, S. Thomas, and D. St. George, "Distrust, Race, and Research," *Archives of Internal Medicine* 162, no. 21 (November 25, 2002): 2458–2463.

4. The term "medical profession" is a social construct and in this chapter is being used in a broad sense. The medical profession is composed of millions of individuals in which many may be racist and insensitive, but there are many of whom are not racist. For lack of a better term, the term "medical profession" will be used to designate medical professionals in the United States knowing full well not all are being deemed racist.

5. See Committee on Understanding and Eliminating Racial and Ethnic Disparities in Health Care, *supra* note 1, at 4.

6. United States Department of Health and Human Services, Agency for Healthcare Research and Quality (AHRQ), *2007 National Healthcare Disparities Report,* Washington, D.C., February 2008.

7. The Tuskegee Syphilis Study will be discussed in more depth later in this article. For a more detailed analysis of the Tuskegee Syphilis Study see, J. H. Jones, *Bad Blood: The Tuskegee Syphilis Experiment—A Tragedy of Race and Medicine* (New York: The Free Press, 1981).

8. G. W. Allport and L. Postman, *The Psychology of Rumor* (New York: Henry Holt, 1947): at ix.

9. P. Turner, I *Heard It Through the Grapevine: Rumor in African American Culture* (Berkeley: University of California Press, 1993): at 4.

10. *Id.,* at 5.

11. Allport and Postman make a case that legends are often little more than solidified rumors. See Allport and Postman, *supra* note 8, at 167.

12. *Id.,* at xv and 108.

13. See Turner, *supra* note 9, at 138.

14. V. Gamble, "A Legacy of Distrust: African Americans and Medical Research," *American Journal of Preventative Medicine* 9, no. 6, Supplement (1993): 35–38.

15. *Id.,* at 35. See also, T. D. Weld, *American Slavery as It Is: Testimony of a Thousand Witnesses* (New York: 1939); F. N. Boone, *Dr. Thomas Hamilton: Two Views of a Gentleman of the Old South* (New York: Phylon, 1967); and J. M. Sims, *The Story of My Life* (New York: Appleton, 1998).

16. *Id.,* at 35–36.

17. For a more detailed analysis of the influence of the Paris school on American medicine, see E. Ackerknecht, *Medicine at the Paris Hospital, 1794–1848* (Baltimore: Johns Hopkins Press, 1967); R. Shryock, *The Development of Modern Medicine: An Interpretation of the Social and Scientific Factors Involved* (New York: Elsevier, 1947); M. Foucault, *The Birth of the Clinic: An Archeology of Medical*

Perception (New York: Routledge Classics, 1973); and G. Gerald, *Edward Garvis and the Medical World of Nineteenth Century America* (Knoxville: Turner, 1978).

18. T. Savitt, "The Use of Blacks for Medical Experimentation and Demonstration in the Old South," *Journal of Southern History* 48, no. 3 (1972): 332–333.

19. *Id.*, at 333.

20. G.-M. Fry, *Night Riders in Black Folk History* (Athens: University of Georgia Press, 1991): at 174–176.

21. *Id.*, at 174–178.

22. *Id.*, at 176. See also Guttmacher, "Bootlegging Bodies," *Society of Medical History of Chicago* 4, no. 2 (January 1935): 353–402.

23. *Id.* (Fry), at 171.

24. For a more detailed analysis of the black migration to industrial centers, see D. Henderson, "The Negro Migration of 1916–1918," *Journal of Negro History* 6, no. 2 (January 1921): 383–498.

25. See Fry, *supra* note 20, at 171.

26. *Id.*, at 172.

27. D. C. Humphrey, "Dissection and Discrimination: The Social Origins of Cadavers in America, 1760–1915," *Bulletin of the New York Academy of Medicine* 44, no. 9 (1970): 819–827, at 822. Humphrey also cites T. S. Sozinsky, "Grave-Robbing and Dissection," *Penn Monthly* 19 (1879): 216.

28. *Id.* (Humphrey), at 824.

29. *Id.*, at 824–825.

30. See Gamble, *supra* note 14, at 36.

31. *Id.*, at 36. See also, T. W. Murrell, "Syphilis and the American Negro," *Journal of the American Medical Association* 54, no. 11 (1910): 846–849 at 847; and H. H. Hazen, "Syphilis in the American Negro," *Journal of the American Medical Association* 63, no. 6 (1914): 463–468 at 463.

32. J. G. Caldwell and E. V. Price et al., "Aortic Regurgitation in the Tuskegee Study of Untreated Syphilis," *Journal of Chronic Diseases* 26, no. 3 (1973): 187–194; S. Hiltner, "The Tuskegee Syphilis Study Under Review," *Christ Century* 90, no. 43 (1973): 1174–1176; R. H. Kampmeier, "The Tuskegee Study of Untreated Syphilis," *South Medical Journal* 65, no. 10 (1972): 1247–1251; R. H. Kampmeier, "Final Report on the 'Tuskegee Syphilis Study,'" *South Medical Journal* 67, no. 11 (1974): 1349–1353; S. Olansky and L. Simpson et al., "Environmental Factors in the Tuskegee Study of Untreated Syphilis," *Public Health Report* 69, no. 7 (1954): 691–698; D. H. Rockwell and A. R. Yobs et al., "The Tuskegee Study of Untreated Syphilis: The 30th Year of Observation," *Archives of Internal Medicine* 114 (1964): 792–798; S. H. Schuman and S. Olansky et al., "Untreated Syphilis in the Male Negro: Background and Current Status of Patients in the Tuskegee Study," *Journal of Chronic Diseases* 2, no. 5 (1955): 543–558.

33. In August, 1972, HEW appointed an investigatory panel which issued a report the following year. The panel found the study to have been "ethically unjustified" and

argued that penicillin should have been provided. See A. Brandt, "Racism and Research: The Case of the Tuskegee Syphilis Study," *Hastings Center Report* 8, no. 6 (December 1978): 21–29 at 21; and Ad Hoc Advisory Panel, Department of Health, Education and Welfare, *Final Report of the Tuskegee Syphilis Study* (Washington, D.C.: Government Printing Office, 1973). For a more detailed analysis of the Tuskegee Syphilis Study see, A. Caplan, "When Evil Intrudes," *Hastings Center Report* 22, no. 6 (November–December 1992): 29–32; H. Edgar, "Outside the Community," *Hastings Center Report* 22, no. 6 (November–December 1992): 32–35; P. A. King, "The Dangers of Difference," *Hastings Center Report* 22, no. 6 (November–December 1992): 35–38; and J. H. Jones, "The Tuskegee Legacy: AIDS and the Black Community," *Hastings Center Report* 22, no. 6 (November–December 1992): 38–40.

34. For a more detailed analysis of the impact of birth control on the African American community, see R. G. Weisbord, "Birth Control and the Black American: A Matter of Genocide?" *Demography* 10, no. 3 (1973): 571–590.

35. Norplant is the trade name for a birth control product consisting of six thin capsules that, upon being implanted in the woman's arm, releases an ovulation-inhibiting hormone. See Turner, *supra* note 9, at 221.

36. *Id.,* at 222. See also, Editor, "One Well-Read Editorial," *Newsweek* 31, December 1990, at 65–66; and D. Kimelman, "Poverty and Norplant," *Philadelphia Inquirer* 12, December 1990, at A-18.

37. T. Abate, "Brave New World of Genetics Explored at Academy of Science Meeting," *San Francisco Chronicle,* February 25, 2002, E-1.

38. *Id.,* at E-1.

39. For a more detailed analysis of the effects of race on medical care see, J. H. Geiger, "Race and Health Care: An American Dilemma," *New England Journal of Medicine* 335, no. 12 (1996): 815–816; M. E. Gornick, P. W. Eggers, and T. W. Reilly et al., "Effects of Race and Income on Mortality and Use of Services Among Medicare Beneficiaries," *New England Journal of Medicine* 335, no. 11 (1996): 791–799.

40. D. Y. Wilkenson, "For Whose Benefit? Politics and Sickle Cell Anemia," *The Black Scholar* 5, no. 8 (1974): 26–31. See also King, *supra* note 33, at 37.

41. *Id.*

42. *Id.* (Wilkenson), at 30.

43. See C. Curtis, *Vaccines Are Dangerous: A Warning to the Black Community* (Brooklyn: A&B Books, 1991).

44. B. O'Connor, "Foundations of African-American Mistrust of the Medical Establishment," unpublished manuscript, Hahnemann University Medical School, Philadelphia, Pennsylvania, at 10–11.

45. A national survey, conducted by the Roper Starch Worldwide polling company, found that out of 500 blacks, 18% said they believed AIDS was a man-made virus; 9% in the general population agreed. When asked more specifically whether HIV and AIDS were part of a plot to kill blacks, 9% of the all-black group said it was definitely true compared to 1% in the general group. See L. Richardson, "An Old

Experiment's Legacy: Distrust of AIDS Treatment," *New York Times*, April 21, 1997, at A-9.

46. See Gamble, *supra* note 14, at 37. See also, S. B. Thomas and S. C. Quinn, "The Tuskegee Syphilis Study, 1932 to 1972: Implications for HIV Education and AIDS Risk Education Programs in the Black Community," *New York Times*, April 21, 1997, at A-9.

47. See Turner, *supra* note 9, at 158. See also E. A. Kloniff and H. Landrine, "Do Blacks Believe That HIV/AIDS Is a Government Conspiracy Against Them?" *Preventative Medicine* 28, no. 4 (1998): 451–457; G. Corbie-Smith, S. B. Thomas, M. V. Williams, and S. Moody-Ayers, "Attitudes and Beliefs of African Americans Toward Participation in Medical Research," *Journal of General Internal Medicine* 14, no. 9 (1999): 537–546.

48. Centers for Disease Control, "HIV/AIDS in the United States-Fact Sheet," March 2008, at 1–5, available at http://www.cdc.gov/hiv/resources/factsheets/print /us.htm (last visited January 9, 2009).

49. It should be noted that "age, sex, diet, underlying disease, and the concomitant use of other medications, race and genetic factors may play pivotal parts in the variability of subjects' responses to a medication." See T. King, "Racial Disparities in Clinical Trials," *New England Journal of Medicine* 346, no. 18 (May 2, 2002): 1400–1402.

50. See Gifford et al., *supra* 2, at 1373–1382.

51. *Id.*, at 1376–1379. The NIH and the FDA both established guidelines encouraging inclusion of more women and minority groups in clinical trials. See National Institutes of Health, "Guidelines on the Inclusion of Women and Minorities as Subjects in Clinical Trials," *Federal Register 59* (1994): 14508–14513; and Food and Drug Administration, *Modernization Act of 1997* (FDAMA or the Act), Public Law No. 105–115 (November 21, 1997). It should be noted that experts at the NIH challenged the findings of Gifford et al. saying that because the study was based on patient interviews in 1996–1998, it was therefore out of date.

52. See Gifford et al., *supra* note 2, at 1379.

53. See Corbie-Smith et al., *supra* note 3, at 2458–2463.

54. See King, *supra* note 49, at 1402.

55. *Id.*, at 1402. See also L. Fogarty, D. Roter, and S. Larson et al., "Patient Adherence to HIV Medication Regimens: A Review of Published and Abstract Reports," *Patient Education Council* 46, no. 2 (2002): 93–108.

56. See King, *supra* note 49, at 1401.

57. J. Merz, "Report Claims Clinical Trials Miss Many Populations," *Washington Post*, April 3, 2008, available at http://www.irbforum.org/forum/read/2/167/167Vt? PHPSESSID=656c640dfe552e73efb2e3877c277473 (last visited December 11, 2008).

58. See Committee on Understanding and Eliminating Racial and Ethnic Disparities in Health Care, *supra* note 1, at 2.

59. *Id.*, at 3–4.

60. United States Department of Health and Human Services, Agency for Healthcare Research and Quality (AHRQ), *supra* note 6, at 5–6.

61. *Id.*, at 6.

62. *Id.*, at 7.

63. D. Williams, H. Gonzalez, and H. Neighbors et al., "Prevalence and Distribution of Major Depressive Disorder in African Americans, Caribbean Blacks, and Non-Hispanic Whites," *Archives of General Psychiatry* 64, no. 3 (March 2007): 305–315.

64. M. Halpern, E. Ward, and A. Pavluck et al., "Association of Insurance Status and Ethnicity with Cancer Stage at Diagnosis for 12 Cancer Sites: A Retrospective Analysis," *Lancet Oncology* 9, no. 3 (March 2008): 222–231.

65. N. Powe et al., "Black Americans Still Wary of Clinical Trials," *Medicine Online* (January 14, 2008), available at http://www.medicineonline.com/news/12/10849 /Black-Americans-Still-Wary-Of-clinical (last visited December 11, 2008).

66. Editor, "Did Tuskegee Damage Trust on Clinical Trials?" CNN.com, March 19, 2008, archived from original: http://en.wikipedia.org/wiki/Tuskegee_syphilis_experiment - see ref 22 at this link: http://www.cnn.com/2008/HEALTH/03/17/clinical.trials.ap/index.html (last visited December 11, 2008).

67. T. Sequist, G. M. Fitzmaurice, and R. Marshall et al., "Physician Performance and Racial Disparities in Diabetes Mellitus Care," *Archives of Internal Medicine* 168, no. 11 (June 9, 2008): 1145–1151; and L. Minnema "Race May Limit Care," *Washington Post*, June 17, 2008, available at <<http://www.washingtonpost.com/wp-dyn/content/article/2008/06/13/AR2008061303263 (last visited December 22, 2008).

68. *Id.* (Sequist et al.), at 1145. See also K. A. Schulman, J. A. Berlin, and W. Halrell et al., "The Effect of Race and Sex on Physicians' Recommendations for Cardiac Catheterization," *New England Journal of Medicine* 340, no. 8 (1999): 618–626; J. M. Abreu, "Conscious and Nonconscious African American Stereotypes: Impact on First Impression and Diagnostic Ratings by Therapists," *Journal of Consulting and Clinical Psychology* 67, no. 3 (1999): 387–393; and M. Van Ryn and J. Burke, "The Effect of Patient Race and Socio-Economic Status on Physician's Perceptions of Patients," *Social Science and Medicine* 50, no. 6 (2000): 813–828.

69. D. Satcher, "Our Commitment to Eliminate Racial and Ethnic Health Disparities," *Yale Journal of Health Policy, Law, and Ethics* 1, no. 1 (2001): 1–14.

70. *Id.*, at 1.

71. National Commission for the Protection of Human Subjects of Biomedical and Behavioral Research, *The Belmont Report: Ethical Principles and Guidelines for the Protection of Human Subjects of Research* (Washington, D.C.: US Government Printing Office, 1979): at B-1.

72. E. D. Pellegrino and D. C. Thomasma, A *Philosophical Basis of Medical Practice* (New York: Oxford University Press, 1981): at 213.

73. See Committee on Understanding and Eliminating Racial and Ethnic Disparities in Health Care, *supra* note 1, at 2.

74. See Corbie-Smith et al., *supra* note 3, at 2460.

75. See Powe et al., *supra* note 65, at 2.

76. See Gifford et al., *supra* 2, at 1373–1375.

77. *Id.*, at 1373.

78. See King, supra note 28, at 1402. See also, C. K. Svensson, "Representation of American Blacks in Clinical Trials of New Drugs," *Journal of the American Medical Association* 261, no. 2 (1989): 263–265.

79. Centers for Disease Control and Prevention, "United States HIV/AIDS Statistics," *HIV/AIDS Surveillance Report* 13, no. 2 (June 2001): 1–4.

80. See Powe et al., *supra* note 65. A. Gardner, "Black Americans Still Wary of Clinical Trials," *US News and World Report* (January 20, 2008), available at http://health .usnews.com/usnews/health/healthday/080114/black-americans-still-wary-of-clinical-trials.htm (last visited December 22, 2008).

81. G. Barrett, "Deadly Delay," *Newsweek Web Exclusive* (February 17, 2008), available at http://www.newsweek.com/id/112952/output/print (last visited December 11, 2008).

82. See United States Department of Health and Human Services, Agency for Healthcare Research and Quality (AHRQ), *supra* note 6, at Chapter 4, "Priority Populations," at 1–10.

83. M. Gilliam, "Health Care Inequality Is Key in Abortion Rates," *Philadelphia Inquirer,* August 10, 2008, available at http://www.philly.com/inquirer/currents /20080811_health-care_inequality_is_key_in_abortion_rates.html?adString=ing .currents/currents;!category=currents;&randomOrd=081308104817 (last visited December 22, 2008).

84. *Id.*, at 2.

85. US Department of Health and Human Services, "Key Themes and Highlights from the National Healthcare Disparities Report," 2007, at 1–11, available at http:// www.ahrq.gov/qual/nhdr07/Key.htm (last visited December 11, 2008).

86. See Committee on Understanding and Eliminating Racial and Ethnic Disparities in Health Care, *supra* note 1, at 5–6.

87. Council on Ethical and Judicial Affairs, Code of Medical Ethics: Current Opinions with Annotations, *American Medical Association,* Chicago, 1998, at 9.121.

88. See Corbie-Smith et al., *supra* note 3, at 2462.

89. *Id.*, at 2462.

90. See US Department of Health and Human Services, *supra* note 74, at 10.

91. M. Angell, "The Forgotten Domestic Crisis," *New York Times,* October 13, 2002, at Wk-13.

92. S. G. Stolberg, "Race Gap Seen in Health Care of Equally Insured Patients," *New York Times,* March 21, 2002, at A-1, A-34.

93. See Gardner, *supra* note 80, at 3.

94. E. Cohen, "Tuskegee's Ghosts: Fear Hinders Black Marrow Donation," CNN.com, February 7, 2007, at 1–2, available at http://www.cnn.com/2007/HEALTH/02/07 /bone.marrow/index.html (last visited January 9, 2009).

95. See Barrett, *supra* note 81, at 2–3.

96. A. Mozes, "Report Claims Clinical Trials Miss Many Populations," *US News & World Report*, April 1, 2008, available at http://health.usnews.com/usnews /health/healthday/080401/report-claims-clinical-trials-miss-many -populations.htm (last visited April 3, 2008).

Chapter 10

Sexual and Gender Minority Health

What We Know and What Needs to Be Done

Kenneth H. Mayer   Judith B. Bradford   Harvey J. Makadon
          Ron Stall   Hilary Goldhammer   Stewart Landers

Over the past few decades, clinicians, public health researchers, and officials have become increasingly aware that lesbian, gay, bisexual, and transgender (LGBT) persons constitute sexual and gender minorities who have unique health care needs.[1,2] This recognition was enormously heightened by the emergence of the AIDS epidemic, which demonstrated that sexual behavior could have major public health consequences. But the realization that sexual minorities have specific health care needs could arguably have begun with Alfred Kinsey, whose work illuminated the important roles that sexual expression plays in people's lives.[3,4] Certainly, by the early 1970s, debates in the American Psychiatric Association about whether homosexual behavior was pathological suggested that clinicians were aware that their gay and lesbian patients had specific needs that could best be addressed by knowledgeable practitioners. The American Psychiatric Association ultimately recognized that homosexuality was not a psychiatric illness[5] but that societal and internalized homophobia may affect access to appropriate care and cause mental distress, which in turn might compromise optimal mental health.

Changing social norms, led by the women's liberation movement, challenged societal assumptions on gender roles and identities and helped to empower the gay liberation movement to demand civil liberties for sexual minorities. As part of the ethos of community-based activism, sexual minorities developed autonomous health facilities designed to provide culturally sensitive care.

By 1980, there were dozens of loosely networked clinics, mental health programs, and provider groups that focused on sexual minority health. These institutions were among the first to recognize an increase in sexually transmitted infections among men who have sex with men and to identify the need for safer-sex interventions. Because of their emerging expertise, public health officials increasingly looked to sexual minority clinical programs to assist in understanding the spread of new infections among men who have sex with men and to test promising solutions. Notable examples of these collaborations were the first hepatitis B vaccine trials in the late 1970s, which were often conducted in centers like the Howard Brown Clinic in Chicago, Illinois, which a cooperative of gay medical students and other health professionals founded in 1974.[6] The relationships that emerged from these collaborations enabled sexual-minority community programs and public health investigators to rapidly mobilize and collaborate when the AIDS epidemic was first recognized.

To respond to the spread of AIDS, many of the early sexual-minority clinical programs rapidly developed sustained partnerships with local academic centers and federal public health agencies. Clinics such as Fenway Community Health in Boston, Massachusetts, developed not only some of the first programs for the counseling and care of people living with HIV/AIDS in the United States, but also the infrastructure needed to administer competitively reviewed grants from the National Institutes of Health and the Centers for Disease Control and Prevention. This unprecedented development of freestanding health centers in sexual-minority communities, as well as the enhanced attention that clinicians and researchers needed to devote to understanding sexual-minority patients' lifestyles, created a new paradigm that demonstrated the feasibility of conducting large-scale surveys and clinical trials in these communities.

Many of the first people to respond to the HIV/AIDS epidemic were lesbians, bisexuals, and transgender persons who helped their HIV-infected peers. Many of these clinicians, public health professionals, and activists learned firsthand that HIV transmission was abetted by other clinical concerns, including other sexually transmitted infections, substance use, depression, and stress related to societal stigmatization of sexual minorities. They also became aware that other clinical problems appeared to be more prevalent among sexual minorities than among heterosexuals, such as excessive tobacco use, human papillomavirus–associated anal neoplasia, and body image concerns.

The recognition that most LGBT health issues were insufficiently understood led the Institute of Medicine to commission a report in 1999 on the status of lesbians' health,[7] which highlighted the need for new population-based research on the true prevalence and incidence of clinical problems in lesbians. National LGBT organizations such as the Gay and Lesbian Medical Association, the National Gay and Lesbian Task Force, and the Human Rights Campaign recognized the importance of advocacy for further research and resources focused on sexual minority health and health care delivery. By the mid-1990s, almost 100 organizations joined together to form the National Coalition for LGBT Health to concentrate on advocating for these goals. The importance of these issues was duly recognized by the Department of Health and Human Services when it included lesbians and gay men as a population group experiencing health disparities in *Healthy People 2010: Understanding and Improving Health*[8] and subsequently provided support to the Gay and Lesbian Medical Association and the National Coalition for LGBT Health to convene an expert panel to draft a companion document to *Healthy People 2010*. This companion document[2] (which, unfortunately, the new administration in 2001 ignored) is still available online.

As with any minority population, the optimal provision of health care and prevention services to sexual and gender minorities requires providers to be sensitive to historical stigmatization, to be informed about continued barriers to care and the differential prevalence of specific risk factors and health conditions in these populations, and to become aware of the cultural aspects of their interactions with LGBT patients. We present current evidence on the issues most relevant to sexual and gender minority health. Although additional research is needed, since Kinsey's time other research pioneers have made important strides in conducting well-designed, population-based studies on LGBT health, and practitioners have developed useful guidelines and programs that should inform best practices in today's society.

Defining and Measuring Sexual and Gender Minorities

Groups and individuals must be counted to receive attention, and enumeration requires reasonably precise definitions to label groups and sort individuals. Although the science of counting population groups is imperfect, enough consensus has developed to create acceptable projections on the basis of race/ethnicity and gender. However, increasing diversity within the US population has necessitated the development of a more nuanced understanding of minority group membership, including identification, behavior, and cultural beliefs. The LGBT population comprises many diverse groups, increasingly referred to as *sexual and gender minorities*. The classification of lesbians, gays, and bisexuals within research studies is generally made on the basis of sexual orientation. The term *sexual orientation* encompasses more than sexual behavior, because individuals may identify with a specific sexual minority group without expressing those behaviors. Women primarily oriented to other women are referred to as *lesbians*, men primarily oriented to other men as *gay*, and individuals oriented to both men and women as *bisexual*.[9]

Gender is a construct of biological, psychosocial, and cultural factors generally used to classify individuals as male or female. *Transgender* is an inclusive term to describe people who have gender identities, expressions, or behaviors not traditionally associated with their birth sex. Transgender people may identify more strongly with another gender (e.g., natal females who identify as men, natal males who identify as women) or with a variance that falls outside dichotomous gender constructions prevalent in Western cultures (e.g., individuals who feel they possess both or neither gender). In other cultures, ranging from American Indian to several in Asia, transgender persons are recognized as part of traditional society. *Intersex* refers to persons born with atypical genital or reproductive anatomy who usually identify as male or female, although some may change their gender identity in the course of their development.[10]

Sexual and gender identity are characterized by fluidity and change, as many individuals who report same-sex behavior identify as heterosexual and others consider themselves to be alternately heterosexual, bisexual, and homosexual (or some other variation in pattern), and as self-perception changes over time.

Some racial/ethnic minorities who engage in same-sex relations may be less likely to identify as gay or bisexual,[11,12] possibly because they identify gay culture with white society or because they fear an LGBT identity would alienate them from family and community.[13] For some in the LGBT population, *gay* and *lesbian* are conventional terms, applicable to middle-aged and older individuals. Sexual-minority youths may prefer terms such as *queer* or *questioning*. Individuals within transgender communities report more than 100 terms to convey what "outsiders" combine into the generalized term *transgender*.[14]

Awareness of sexual minority orientation appears to be occurring at younger ages; on average, initial same-sex experience occurs around ages 14 to 16 years.[15,16] On the opposite end of the age spectrum, it is important to note that sexual and gender minorities do age. For the first time in US history, there is an identifiable cohort of LGBT elders, many of whom lack access to culturally competent health care and social services.[17]

From the perspective of population- and practice-based research, progress has been made to include sexual orientation as a demographic variable in several government surveys;[18] however, these surveys typically have just one question about sexual orientation and none for transgender identity.[19] Because of the paucity of measures, these data can be misleading and limited in usefulness. In the first national probability sample survey to specifically examine the sexual behaviors of US adults, 3 constructs—behavior, attraction, and identity—measured sexual orientation.[20] Individual and subgroup percentages varied substantially across these 3 measures. Men were twice as likely as women to identify as homosexual and more than twice as likely to report same-sex behavior since puberty. Respondents who lived in or near major urban areas or had advanced education were more likely to report same-sex behavior and were more likely to identify as homosexual or bisexual than those in nonurban areas. Latino and Asian men were less likely to report same-sex behavior but approximately twice as likely to report same-sex desire, attraction, or appeal compared with black or white men. Thus, the use of a single measure may mask subgroup differences, contributing to the general perception that sexual and gender minorities are far less numerous and diverse than is actually the case.

Despite their limitations, government surveys with sexual orientation measures have helped increase awareness for policy makers and the general public that LGBT people are distributed throughout the United States and, to some extent, may help distinguish how sexual minorities are alike and different from the general population. The most prominent government survey with a sexual orientation measure was the 2000 US Census, which counted about 1.2 million individuals who identified as living with a same-sex partner.[21] (See Figure 10.1 for a depiction of the distribution of same-sex households across the nation.)

Sexual identity, behavior, and attraction were more recently measured in the 2002 National Survey of Family Growth, leading to the finding that 4.1% of the US population aged 18 to 44 years (more than 4.5 million individuals) identified as homosexual or bisexual.[22] Among women aged 18 to 44 years in the National Survey of Family Growth, 1.3% thought of themselves as homosexual and 2.8% as bisexual; among men aged 18 to 44 years, 2.3% thought of themselves as homosexual and 1.8% as bisexual.

To increase understanding of LGBT population groups and their health-related needs, it is critical that population-based surveys and social behavioral

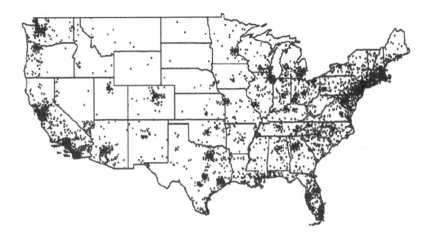

Figure 10.1. Same-Sex Households in the Continental United States, by County: 2000

Source: Data were from the US Census Bureau.[66]

Note: 1 dot = 100 same-sex households. Total = 594391 same-sex households.

research studies continue to expand and improve the measurement of sexual and gender minority identity and behavior. To this end, the National Institute of Child Health and Human Development has recently awarded funding to Fenway Community Health to develop the first federally funded population research center focused on LGBT health. This initiative will be developed in conjunction with the Inter-University Consortium for Political and Social Research of the University of Michigan in Ann Arbor; the Boston University School of Public Health; and a national consortium of academic investigators, university centers, and community-based organizations.

Unique Clinical Concerns of Sexual and Gender Minority Populations

In light of previous societal and professional misconceptions of sexual and gender minorities, it is not surprising that clinicians and public health researchers are only now learning about the range of health disparities and unique clinical issues affecting LGBT people. Existing research, although limited, points to a higher prevalence of certain conditions among LGBT patients that merit attention.[1,2,23,24] Many of the issues that disproportionately affect sexual and gender minorities, such as substance abuse, overweight and obesity, and tobacco use,[1,2,24] are among the leading health indicators designated by *Healthy People 2010*[8] (Table 10.1). Clinicians and public health professionals need to understand the dynamics and expression of these health issues in

Table 10.1. Leading Health Indicators and Sexual and Gender Minorities

Leading Health Indicators in the General US Population[a]	Areas of Increased Concern for Sexual and Gender Minorities[b]
Physical activity	
Overweight and obesity	√
Tobacco use	√
Substance abuse	√
Responsible sexual behavior	√
Mental health	√
Injury and violence	√
Environmental quality	
Immunization	
Access to care	√

[a] According to Healthy People 2010.[8]

[b] According to Makadon et al.[24]

LGBT people to fill the voids left by previous biases. To educate a new generation of clinicians, the American College of Physicians has published the first comprehensive text on the care of sexual and gender minority patients, *The Fenway Guide to Lesbian, Gay, Bisexual, and Transgender Health.*[24]

Among the most significant areas of clinical concern for LGBT patients are mental health disorders, particularly diagnoses of depression and anxiety.[25] Some studies have also found a higher prevalence of eating and body image disorders among gay and bisexual men compared with their heterosexual peers.[26] Mental health disorders are not inherent to being a sexual minority person but can manifest as a result of leading marginalized lives, enduring the stress of hiding one's sexuality, or facing verbal, emotional, or physical abuse from intolerant family members and communities.[27-29]

Although adolescents and young adults today have an easier time coming out because of greater general acceptance and more visible role models, recent studies suggest that LGBT youths are still at greater risk for suicide attempts than non-LGBT youths.[30] Clinicians and service providers need to be sensitive to the potential stressors of coming out and the process of forming a positive identity as an LGBT person, and should be prepared to answer questions and make referrals. Clinical and public health professionals can work to develop programs that specialize in the care of LGBT populations and can advocate for policies that diminish the stigma LGBT people encounter.

Some studies have found higher rates of substance use in sexual and gender minorities compared with heterosexual cohorts, although some of the earliest research recruited participants from bars, resulting in selection bias.[31] Recreational drug use, particularly stimulant use, among gay men has been associated with higher rates of unsafe sexual practices and HIV and other sexually transmitted infections.[32,33] Male-to-female transgender individuals may also be at higher risk for drug use and sexual risk behaviors.[34] Researchers have also found higher rates of heavy alcohol use and related problems among lesbians and bisexual women, and possibly gay and bisexual men, compared with heterosexuals.[35,36] There is strong evidence to suggest a higher prevalence of tobacco use in sexual minorities as well.[37-39] Several promising LGBT-specific tobacco cessation interventions have been developed; more information on these programs can be found through the National LGBT Tobacco Control Network website.[40]

Lesbians are more likely than women of other sexual orientations to be overweight and obese,[41] putting them at increased risk for cardiovascular disease, lipid abnormalities, glucose intolerance, and morbidity related to inactivity. Transgender patients may have enhanced cardiovascular risks because of exogenous hormone use.[42] Individuals who are HIV infected can be at higher risk for lipid abnormalities, depending on their regimen.[43]

Clinicians and epidemiologists have expressed concern that some LGBT populations are at increased risk for some cancers. Because of discomfort with the medical community, lesbians may seek routine breast and cervical cancer screening less often than heterosexual women.[44,45] In addition, lesbians and their providers may underestimate their risk of cervical cancer.[46] Many lesbians may have multiple risk factors for cervical cancer, including a history of sex with men at an early age.[47] Lesbians and bisexual women, independent of their current sexual practices, require the same schedule of Papanicolaou tests and human papillomavirus vaccination as other women.

Anal cancer is an important health concern for men who have sex with men. Because of the high prevalence of anal human papilloma virus in men who engage in receptive anal intercourse, trials are under way to evaluate the use of the human papillomavirus vaccine in men who have anal intercourse. There is growing evidence that routine anal Papanicolaou tests for men who are HIV infected is cost-effective in preventing anal cancer.[48] Although the data are less clear on the benefit of routine anal Papanicolaou tests for at-risk HIV-uninfected men who have sex with men, some experts recommend routine screening for this population, though perhaps less frequently than they do for HIV-infected men who have sex with men.[48]

Transgender individuals who have undergone sex reassignment surgery but retain pretransition organs or tissue remnants need careful follow-up for potential oncological problems commonly associated with their natal sex, including prostate,[49] breast, cervical, and ovarian cancer. Transgender health in general has not been a focus of specialized clinical care because of an even greater lack of data and resources than with gay and lesbian health. Transgender individuals have had to struggle to have their clinical issues taken seriously and to find appropriate resources for care. Guidelines for the care of transgender people are available online[50] but are not yet widely disseminated or taught. Transgender people also face financial barriers to care, given that transitional therapies with either medication or surgery are expensive and rarely covered by insurers in the United States.[51]

Intersex individuals, sometimes referred to as people who have a variation or disorder of sex development, are not traditionally included as an LGBT population, but they have some of the same health care and stigmatization problems. Intersex children and adults require specialized approaches to medical, surgical, and emotional care. A consortium of clinicians, parents, patients, and advocates recently developed guidelines on the care of children with intersex conditions.[52] In the past few years, the medical community has recognized that genital variations should not automatically be surgically altered in infancy and that gender identity formation is the result of complex biological and social factors and may not be fully evolved until adulthood.[53]

Clinical care issues are not the only concerns unique to LGBT patients. LGBT individuals' family lives can affect their engagement and satisfaction with care. Increasingly, LGBT individuals are developing socially sanctioned long-term relationships and are raising families. Many of these people seek support in finding appropriate services, such as LGBT-friendly adoption agencies and legal resources. Individuals are also coming out at earlier ages[15] and turning to their clinicians for support—hence the need for primary providers sensitized to sexual and gender minority health concerns. In addition, many LGBT elders have fewer family connections than non-LGBT elders and are less protected when a partner dies or while hospitalized with a life-threatening illness than people who have legally sanctioned marriages by traditional family law.[17] Public health advocacy for policy changes and supportive programs will make a difference in ensuring equity for sexual and gender minority patients at these later stages of life.

Barriers to Optimal Health Care for Sexual and Gender Minority Patients

Optimal health care for LGBT populations requires access to both competent medical personnel and sensitive prevention services. However, sexual and gender minorities continue to encounter numerous barriers to accessing care, clustering around 4 main issues: (1) reluctance by some LGBT patients to disclose sexual or gender identity when receiving medical care, (2) insufficient numbers of providers competent in dealing with LGBT issues as part of the provision of medical care, (3) structural barriers that impede access to health insurance and limit visiting and medical decision-making rights for LGBT people and their partners, and (4) a lack of culturally appropriate prevention services. Each of these barriers is important individually and together they form a challenging gauntlet of barriers to the receipt of medical care for many LGBT citizens (see Ramchand and Fox[54] for an overview of these barriers in the case of American gay and bisexual men).

LGBT patients have multiple reasons for not disclosing their sexual or gender identity to providers, including fears of homophobic reactions, confidentiality concerns, past negative experiences with providers, and fear of being stigmatized. To the extent that these concerns cause LGBT patients to delay receipt of care or withhold information that may be important to treatment, effective medical care can be compromised. But disclosure of sexual or gender minority identity is likely to improve care only if providers offer culturally competent and well-informed services in return—for example, the provider is aware of the unique health concerns of LGBT populations and is able to assess partnership status and sexual behavior without assumptions or judgment. Although attitudes are changing,[55] societal misperceptions and discomfort about homosexual behavior and identity persist, even among health care personnel.[56,57] Unfortunately, neither professional schools nor continuing education programs provide the training needed to improve the attitudes, knowledge, and skills of physicians and other health care professionals in caring for LGBT people.[58,59] Consequently, there are not enough clinicians who can provide optimal care to LGBT patients.

The structure of health insurance in the United States, which is largely financed through employers, can also inhibit LGBT people's access to clinical care. For example, only some organizations and legal jurisdictions extend insurance coverage to domestic partners, in effect denying coverage to unmarried partners of employed LGBT individuals. Furthermore, when antidiscrimination laws are not in place to prevent the loss of employment as a result of being identified as a sexual or gender minority, the danger of losing health insurance coverage is amplified. In addition to structural barriers to obtaining health insurance, lack of marriage rights for most LGBT long-term relationships means that even partners in decades-old relationships may be denied medical decision-making rights and prevented from providing crucial support during a partner's medical crisis.

Many of the variables associated with health risks among LGBT populations may be unique to these populations and thus require tailored prevention services.[40,60] Unfortunately, there are few LGBT-specific prevention services to deal with violence victimization, substance abuse, mental health concerns, and other health care needs, except in large metropolitan areas.[2] Even then, most of these services have not been as thoroughly evaluated as HIV-prevention services focusing on gay men. That said, the evidence base for efficacy trials of HIV-prevention models among gay men[61] suggests that innovative prevention models to address the most important epidemics LGBT populations face might improve health outcomes, thereby lowering the demand for expensive health care services. Improvements in access to medical care and effective prevention services for LGBT patients could concomitantly improve the health care delivery for other vulnerable populations.

Creating a Healthier Environment for Sexual and Gender Minority Patients

The provision of optimal care to sexual and gender minority patients requires welcoming clinical and program environments that promote good communication and allow individuals to feel comfortable discussing matters of their sexual identity, behavior, attractions, and any conflicts they may be experiencing.[62] It is critical to train providers and other staff to speak with patients and clients in a nonjudgmental, gender-appropriate, and professional way. These techniques should be taught during professional education[58] and staff training in health care and service facilities and should be reinforced with nondiscrimination policies in clinical and program settings, intake forms that ask about gender identities and same-sex partners, and visual cues in waiting and examination rooms that signal acceptance, such as brochures that discuss LGBT health risks and promotion.[63] Clinicians' efforts should be synergistic with those of public health departments, which could do more to ensure that their programs are culturally competent for this group. A handful of large city health departments (Boston, Chicago, Los Angeles, New York, and San Francisco) now have specific staff members dedicated to working with LGBT populations. However, acknowledgment of the public health issues affecting LGBT persons and plans and resources to address those issues at the state and federal level are still lacking.

To the extent public health has acknowledged the public health issues affecting LGBT persons, efforts have primarily occurred in the "traditional" realms of HIV/AIDS, sexually transmitted infections, and hepatitis. Activities to tailor public health prevention messages to the LGBT community in the areas of tobacco cessation, cancer, alcohol use, healthy weight, asthma, and cardiovascular health have been scant. Further, there has been a substantial dearth of data collection and analysis on the risk behaviors of and protective health factors for LGBT persons. However, Colorado, Massachusetts, North Dakota, and Vermont currently collect information about sexual orientation through their Behavioral Risk Factor Surveillance System.[64] The first transgender question to appear on a statewide Behavioral Risk Factor Surveillance System survey was in Massachusetts in 2007 (K. Cranston, MDiv, director, Massachusetts HIV/AIDS Bureau, written communication, August 18, 2007).

With the increasing weight of evidence-based data indicating that LGBT people experience substantial health disparities, it is incumbent upon federal and state public health officials to develop programs to remedy these disparities. Although LGBT patients make up approximately 2% to 5% of the US adult population, the proportion of resources allocated for their public health needs is substantially lower, particularly when looked at on a program-by-program basis. Schools of public health have been slow to incorporate teaching and research into LGBT health issues.[65] Advocacy for improving public health policy and the quality and number of public health programs for LGBT populations has been hampered by a lack of resources as well as by limited population-based data and the need to focus advocacy efforts on basic civil rights issues (employment, recognition of relationships, etc.).

The Road Ahead

More work is needed to improve data, resources, and public policy on sexual and gender minority health. Advocacy for better prevention, care and treatment, and the elimination of health disparities among LGBT populations needs to be supported by well-designed studies. Accordingly, it is essential that large national data sets that measure the health status of Americans include measures of sexual attraction, identity, and behavior and that more information is gathered on how to ask questions that best measure these constructs. Furthermore, it is important to learn how to collect this information confidentially to ensure the safety and privacy of respondents. As larger data sets become available, new resources to support innovative ways to study sexual and gender minority populations will be essential. It will be particularly important to understand the issues for people who may have multiple identities, such as LGBT people who are from racial or ethnic minority groups or who have disabilities.

Culturally appropriate programs need to be developed and refined to improve disparities in smoking, alcohol use, mental health, healthy weight, cancer prevention activities, and sexually transmitted infections. Federal agencies and public health organizations must disseminate the best practices of successful programs. Future national public health planning documents, such as *Healthy People 2020*, should incorporate new findings gathered on the health care needs of sexual and gender minority populations. As we learn more about health disparities and effective programs to address them, medical care providers, public health workers, and other human services workers who interact on a daily basis with LGBT persons will need training. Without such training, sexual and gender minorities will continue to interact with a health care system that is unaware, insensitive, and unprepared to meet their needs.

Acknowledgments

This work was supported in part by the National Institute of Child Health and Human Development (grant 1R21HD051178–01A2).

We give special thanks to Julie Honnold and Lauretta Safford of the Community Health Research Initiative Group, Virginia Commonwealth University, and to Kirsten Barrett for the census map figure.

Note: The content is solely the responsibility of the authors and does not necessarily represent the official views of the National Institute of Child Health and Human Development or the National Institutes of Health.

Human Participant Protection

No protocol approval was needed for this study.

Notes

1. Dean L, Meyer IH, Robinson K, et al. Lesbian, gay, bisexual, and transgender health: Findings and concerns. J *Gay Lesbian Med Assoc.* 2000;4:102–151.

2. *Healthy People 2010: Companion Document for Lesbian, Gay, Bisexual, and Transgender (LGBT) Health.* San Francisco: Gay and Lesbian Medical Association;

2001. Available at http://www.glma.org/_data/n_0001/resources/live/Healthy CompanionDoc3.pdf. Accessed September 14, 2007.

3. Kinsey AC, Pomeroy WB, Martin CE. *Sexual Behavior in the Human Male.* Philadelphia: W.B. Saunders; 1948.

4. Kinsey AC, Pomeroy WB, Martin CE, Gebhard PH. *Sexual Behavior in the Human Female.* Philadelphia: W.B. Saunders; 1953.

5. *Diagnostic and Statistical Manual of Mental Disorders, Fourth Edition.* Washington, DC: American Psychiatric Association; 2000.

6. Howard Brown Health Center. *Mission and overview.* Available at http://www .howardbrown.org/hb_aboutus.asp?id=21. Accessed October 1, 2007.

7. Solarz AL, ed. *Lesbian Health: Current Assessment and Directions for the Future.* Washington, DC: National Academy Press; 1999.

8. *Healthy People 2010: Understanding and Improving Health.* Washington, DC: US Department of Health and Human Services; 2000. Available at http://www.healthy people.gov/document. Accessed October 1, 2007.

9. Johnson C, Mimiaga M, Bradford J. Health care issues among lesbian, gay, bisexual, transgender, and intersex (LGBTI) populations in the United States: Introduction. *J Homosex* 2008;54(3):213-24. Available at http://www.tandfonline.com/doi/pdf /10.1080/00918360801982025.

10. Leidolf E, Curran M, Scout, Bradford J. Intersex mental health and social support options in pediatric endocrinology training programs. *J Homosex* 2008;54(3):233-42. Available at http://www.ncbi.nlm.nih.gov/pubmed/18825861.

11. Pathela P, Hajat A, Schillinger J, Blank S, Sell R, Mostashari F. Discordance between sexual behavior and self-reported sexual identity: A population-based survey of New York City men [published correction appears in *Ann Intern Med.* 2006;145(12): 936]. *Ann Intern Med.* 2006;145(6):416–425.

12. Ross MW, Essien EJ, Williams ML, Fernandez-Esquer ME. Concordance between sexual behavior and sexual identity in street outreach samples of four racial/ethnic groups. *Sex Transm Dis.* 2003;30:110–113.

13. US Department of Health and Human Services. Men of color who have sex with men and HIV/AIDS in the United States. *HRSA CAREAction,* 2003. Available at http:// www.taadas.org/publications/prodimages/HRSA%20CAREAction.%20Reaching %20Men%20of%20Color%20Who%20Have%20Sex%20With%20Men.pdf. Updated 2008 version here: ftp://ftp.hrsa.gov/hab/MSMofcolor.pdf . Accessed January 23, 2008.

14. Xavier J, Honnold J, Bradford J. *The Health, Health-Related Needs, and Lifecourse Experiences of Transgender Virginians.* Richmond: Virginia Department of Health; 2007. Available at http://www.vdh.virginia.gov/epidemiology/DiseasePrevention /documents/pdf/THISFINALREPORTVol1.pdf. Accessed January 23, 2008.

15. D'Augelli A, Hershberger S. Lesbian, gay, and bisexual youth in community settings: Personal challenges and mental health problems. *Am J Community Psychol.* 1993;21:421–448.

16. Bradford J. *Lesbian Health in the US: Our Foundation and Our Future.* Paper presented at Annual Conference of the Gay and Lesbian Medical Association, September 22–24, 2005, Montreal, Quebec.

17. Cahill S, South K, Spade J. *Outing Age: Public Policy Issues Affecting Gay, Lesbian, Bisexual and Transgender Elders.* New York: The Policy Institute of the National Gay and Lesbian Task Force Foundation; 2000.

18. Sell R. Gaydata.org: Data sources index. Available at http://gaydata.org/ds001 _Index.html. Accessed January 28, 2008.

19. Bradford J, Mayer K. Demography and the LGBT population: What we know, don't know, and how the information helps to inform clinical practice. In: Makadon H, Mayer K, Potter J, Goldhammer H, eds. *The Fenway Guide to Lesbian, Gay, Bisexual, and Transgender Health.* Philadelphia: American College of Physicians; 2007:28.

20. Laumann E, Gagnon J, Michael R, Michaels S. *The Social Organization of Sexuality: Sexual Practices in the United States.* Chicago: University of Chicago Press; 1994.

21. Simmons T, O'Connell M. Married-couple and unmarried-partner households: 2000. *Census 2000 Special Reports.* Washington, DC: US Census Bureau; 2003.

22. Mosher WD, Chandra A, Jones J. Sexual behavior and selected health measures: Men and women 15–44 years of age, United States, 2002. *Advance Data from Vital and Health Statistics* no. 362. Hyattsville, MD: National Center for Health Statistics; 2005.

23. Wolitski RJ, Stall R, Valdiserri RO, eds. *Unequal Opportunity: Health Disparities Affecting Gay and Bisexual Men in the United States.* New York: Oxford University Press; 2007.

24. Makadon H, Mayer K, Potter J, Goldhammer H, eds. *The Fenway Guide to Lesbian, Gay, Bisexual, and Transgender Health.* Philadelphia: American College of Physicians; 2007.

25. Cochran SD, Mays VM, Sullivan JG. Prevalence of mental disorders, psychological distress, and mental health services use among lesbian, gay, and bisexual adults in the United States. *J Consult Clin Psychol.* 2003;71:53–61.

26. Kaminski PL, Chapman BP, Haynes SD, Own L. Body image, eating behaviors, and attitudes toward exercise among gay and straight men. *Eat Behav.* 2005;6:179–187.

27. Meyer IH. Prejudice, social stress, and mental health in lesbian, gay and bisexual populations: Conceptual issues and research evidence. *Psychol Bull.* 2003;129: 674–697.

28. Safren SA, Heimberg RG. Depression, hopelessness, suicidality, and related factors in sexual minority and heterosexual adolescents. *J Consult Clin Psychol.* 1999;67: 859–866.

29. Mills TC, Paul J, Stall R, et al. Distress and depression in men who have sex with men: The urban men's health study [published correction appears in *Am J Psychiatry.* 2004;161(4):776]. *Am J Psychiatry* 2004;161:278–285.

30. Silenzio VMB, Pena JB, Duberstein PR, Cerel J, Knox KL. Sexual orientation and risk factors for suicidal ideation and suicide attempts among adolescents and young adults. *Am J Public Health* 2007;97:2017–2019.

31. Song Y, Sevelius J, Guzman R, Colfax G. Substance use and abuse. In: Makadon H, Mayer K, Potter J, Goldhammer H, eds. *The Fenway Guide to Lesbian, Gay, Bisexual, and Transgender Health.* Philadelphia: American College of Physicians; 2007: 209–212.

32. Colfax G, Vittinghoff E, Husnik MJ, et al. Substance use and sexual risk: a participant- and episode-level analysis among a cohort of men who have sex with men. *Am J Epidemiol.* 2004;159:1002–1012.

33. Colfax G, Coates TJ, Husnik MJ, et al. Longitudinal patterns of methamphetamine, popper (amyl nitrite), and cocaine use and high-risk sexual behavior among a cohort of San Francisco men who have sex with men. *J Urban Health* 2005;82: i62–i70.

34. Clements K, Wilkinson W, Kitano K, Marx R. HIV prevention and health service needs of the transgender community in San Francisco. *Int J Transgenderism* 1999;3:1–2.

35. Drabble L, Midanik LT, Trocki K. Reports of alcohol consumption and alcohol-related problems among homosexual, bisexual and heterosexual respondents: Results from the 2000 National Alcohol Survey. *J Stud Alcohol* 2005;66:111–120.

36. Burgard SA, Cochran SD, Mays VM. Alcohol and tobacco use patterns among heterosexually and homosexually experienced California women. *Drug Alcohol Depend.* 2005;77:61–70.

37. Tang H, Greenwood GL, Cowling DW, Lloyd JC, Roeseler AG, Bal DG. Cigarette smoking among lesbians, gays, and bisexuals: How serious a problem? (United States). *Cancer Causes Control* 2004;15:797–803.

38. Gruskin EP, Greenwood GL, Matevia M, Pollack LM, Bye LL. Disparities in smoking between the lesbian, gay, bisexual population and the general population in California. *Am J Public Health* 2007;97:1496–1502.

39. Stall R, Greenwood G, Acree M, et al. Prevalence and correlates of tobacco smoking among gay and bisexual men. *Am J Public Health* 1999;89:1875–1878.

40. National LGBT Tobacco Control Network website. *Resources.* Available at http://www.lgbttobacco.org/resources.php?ID=18. Accessed February 26, 2008.

41. Boehmer U, Bowen DJ, Bauer GR. Overweight and obesity in sexual minority women: Evidence from population-based data. *Am J Public Health* 2007;97: 1134–1140.

42. Futterweit W. Endocrine therapy of transsexualism and potential complications of long-term treatment. *Arch Sex Behav.* 1998;27:209–226.

43. Brown TT, Cofrancesco J. Metabolic abnormalities in HIV-infected patients: An update. *Curr Infect Dis Rep.* 2006;8:497–504.

44. Powers D, Bowen DJ, White J. The influence of sexual orientation on health behaviors in women. *J Prev Interv Community* 2001;22:43–60.

45. Matthews AK, Brandenburg D, Johnson T, Hughes TL. Correlates of under-utilization of gynecological cancer screening among lesbian and heterosexual women. *Prev Med.* 2004;38:105–113.

46. Marrazzo JM. Barriers to infectious disease care among lesbians. *Emerg Infect Dis.* 2004;10:1974–1978.

47. Diamant AL, Schuster M, McGuigan K, Lever J. Lesbians' sexual history with men: Implications for taking a sexual history. *Arch Intern Med.* 1999;159:2730–2736.

48. Palefsky JM, Cranston RD. Anal squamous intraepithelial lesions (ASIL): Diagnosis, screening and treatment. *UpToDate* website. Available at http://patients.uptodate.com/topic.asp?file=tumorhiv/2317 (subscription required). Accessed January 23, 2008.

49. van Haarst EP, Newling DW, Gooren LJ, Asscheman H, Prenger DM. Metastatic prostatic carcinoma in a male-to-female transsexual. *Br J Urol.* 1998;81:776.

50. World Professional Association for Transgender Health, Inc., website. Available at http://www.wpath.org/publications_standards.cfm. Accessed February 26, 2008.

51. Kaufman R. Introduction to transgender identity and health. In: Makadon H, Mayer K, Potter J, Goldhammer H, eds. *The Fenway Guide to Lesbian, Gay, Bisexual, and Transgender Health.* Philadelphia: American College of Physicians; 2007:336.

52. Consortium on the Management of Disorders of Sex Development. *Clinical Guidelines for the Management of Disorders of Sex Development in Childhood.* Rohnert Park, CA: Intersex Society of North America; 2006. Available at http://www.dsdguidelines.org/files/clinical.pdf. Accessed January 23, 2008.

53. Lee PA, Houk CP, Ahmed SF, Hughes IA, and the International Consensus Conference on Intersex Working Group. Consensus statement on management of intersex disorders. *Pediatrics* 2006;118:e488–e500.

54. Ramchand R, Fox C. Access to optimal care among gay and bisexual men: Identifying barriers and promoting culturally competent care. In: Wolitski RJ, Stall R, Valdiserri RO, eds. *Unequal Opportunity: Health Disparities Affecting Gay and Bisexual Men in the United States.* New York: Oxford University Press; 2007.

55. Smith DM, Mathews WMC. Physicians' attitudes toward homosexuality and HIV: Survey of a California medical society-revisited (PATHH-II). *J Homosex.* 2007;52:1–9.

56. Schatz B, O'Hanlan K. *Anti-Gay Discrimination in Medicine: Results of a National Survey of Lesbian, Gay, and Bisexual Physicians.* San Francisco: American Association of Physicians for Human Rights; 1994.

57. O'Hanlan KA, Cabaj RP, Schatz B, et al. A review of the medical consequences of homophobia with suggestions for resolution. *J Gay Lesbian Med Assoc.* 1997;1: 25–35.

58. Makadon HJ. Improving health care for the lesbian and gay communities. *N Engl J Med.* 2006;354:895–897.

59. Tesar CM, Rovi SL. Survey of curriculum on homosexuality/bisexuality in departments of family medicine. *Fam Med* 1998;30:283–287.

60. Stall R, Paul J, Greenwood G, et al. Alcohol use, drug use and alcohol-related problems among men who have sex with men: The Urban Men's Health Study. *Addiction.* 2001;96:1589–1601.

61. Herbst J, Sherba RT, Crepaz N, et al. A metaanalytic review of HIV behavioral interventions for reducing sexual risk behavior of men who have sex with men. J *Acquir Immune Defic Syndr.* 2005;39:228–241.

62. Makadon HJ, Mayer KH, Garofalo R. Optimizing primary care for men who have sex with men. *JAMA.* 2006;296:895–897.

63. Gay and Lesbian Medical Association. *Provider Guidelines for Creating a Welcoming Environment.* San Francisco: Gay and Lesbian Medical Association; 2006. Available at http://www.qahc.org.au/files/shared/docs/GLMA_guide.pdf. Accessed September 27, 2007.

64. Sell R. *Behavioral Risk Factor Surveys.* Available at http://gaydata.org/02_Data _Sources/ds002_BRFS/ds002_BRFS.html. Accessed January 28, 2008.

65. Corliss HL, Shankle MD, Moyer MB. Research, curricula, and resources related to lesbian, gay, bisexual, and transgender health in US Schools of Public Health. *Am J Public Health* 2007;97:1023–1027.

66. US Census Bureau. *Census 2000, Summary File 1, Table PCT014.* Available at http://www.socialexplorer.com/pub/reportdata/metabrowser.aspx?survey=C2000&ds=SF1&var=PCT014004&header=Truefactfinder2.census.gov. Accessed December 14, 2007.

Chapter 11

Mental Disorders, Health Inequalities, and Ethics

A Global Perspective

Emmanuel M. Ngui   Lincoln Khasakhala   David Nndetei
Laura Weiss Roberts

Introduction

The burden and inequalities in mental healthcare throughout the world are critically important health issues, and taken together present immense ethical challenges. In this chapter we examine mental health issues globally, with special emphasis given to the developing nations, because of the limited research and increased burden of mental disorders in these nations. We also provide an overview of the ethical considerations in international mental health and renewed interest in approaches that integrate mental health into primary care services (Table 11.1).

Mental disorders account for an enormous global burden of disease that is largely underestimated and underappreciated. In a given year, about 30% of the population worldwide is affected by a mental disorder and over two thirds of those affected do not receive the care they need (Chisholm et al., 2007; Kessler et al., 2005b; Wittchen, Jonsson, & Olesen, 2005). About 14% of the global disease burden is attributed to neuropsychiatric disorders, mostly depression, alcohol-substance abuse and psychoses (Murray & Lopez, 1996; Prince et al., 2007). In the USA, about 57.7 million adults experience a mental disorder annually, and 1 in 17 people have a serious mental health condition (Kessler, Chiu, Demler, & Walters, 2005a). These figures translate into hundreds of millions

Table 11.1. Summary of Key Issues in Global Mental Health

Issue	Key points
Burden of mental disorders	• The global burden of mental disorders is enormous, under-appreciated, and largely unmet.
	• Annually, about 30% of the population worldwide is affected by a mental disorder and over two thirds of those affected do not receive the care they need. Depression, alcohol and substance abuse and psychoses are among the most prevalent conditions.
	• Mental health problems have major economic and social cost.
	• Many nations have limited capacity (e.g., infrastructure, workforce, resources) needed to assess, identify and treat mental health disorders.
Ethics, human rights and social justice	• Human rights and social justice frameworks are critical in understanding and addressing mental health inequalities.
	• In many nations, limited or no policies exist to address basic needs and human rights of people with mental illness and standards of ethical conduct of research and treatment of mental disorders are inadequate or lacking.
	• Ethical principles of beneficence, autonomy, respect for persons and non-malfeasance for people living with mental disorders foster human dignity and promote human rights and social justice.
Mental health inequalities and unmet needs	• Mental disorders are associated and embedded within the broader social and economic context.
	• Poverty increases the risk of developing mental disorders, which in turn increase the risk of living in poverty due to disability or loss of gainful employment.
	• Mental disorders are determined by multiple and interacting social, psychological and biological factors. The underlying social determinants of mental disorders (e.g., low levels of education, unemployment) also are key determinants of living in poverty.

Table 11.1. Continued

Issue	Key points
	• Unmet mental health needs contribute to profound suffering and deaths largely because people cannot access needed treatment.
	• Shortages of mental health providers and resources result in unnecessary institutionalization of people with mental illness even though these conditions can be managed effectively in the community if services were available.
	• In most developing nations, the burden of caring for people with mental illness disproportionately falls on women and children.
Stigma and discrimination	• Mental health stigma and discrimination are major barriers to effective management of mental disorders.
	• Stigma, myths and misconceptions of mental illness contribute to much of the discrimination and human rights violation experienced by people with mental disorders.
	• Stigma and discrimination increase social isolation and unmet needs for mental health services, negatively influence choice of mental health careers, and limit development of policies and human rights protections for people living with mental disorders and their families.
	• Limited access to modern psychiatric services increases beliefs that mental disorders are untreatable which further increases stigma and discrimination and patient's reliance on traditional healers who may not have adequate skills and training to help people with serious mental disorders.
Integration of mental health into primary health care services	• In many developing nations, mental health services are provided at the tertiary level with limited or no integration to primary care interventions.
	• The majority of individuals with mental disorders and their families live in overt poverty and cannot access or afford appropriate and available specialized mental health services provided at tertiary-level health facilities serviced by psychiatrists.

(continued)

Table 11.1. Continued

Issue	Key points
	• Extreme and growing shortages of mental health workers further compounds the problem of access to mental health services resulting in limited access to services and reliance on traditional healers in some nations.
	• In the absence of integrated proper-functioning health systems it is impossible to provide mental health services for most individuals with mental disorders and their families in developing nations.
	• Integrating mental health into primary care services is a critical, affordable and cost-effective approach to delivering services for people living with mental disorders.
	• Such integrated systems of primary care can reduce unmet needs and social stigma and discrimination by decreasing social isolation, neglect and institutionalization of people with mental disorders.
Impact on economic development	• The economic burden of mental disorders is great. Mental disorders significantly impair economic growth through their effects on labor supply, earnings, participation and productivity.
	• Unmet mental health care needs are associated with increased risk of social problems (e.g., school dropout, alcohol and drug use, disability, unemployment, unsafe sexual behaviors, crime and poverty) that may influence economic growth.
	• In many developing nations, limited efforts have been made to address or modify the social determinants of health, including actions that allow people to adopt and maintain healthy lifestyles and those that create living conditions and environments that support health.
	• Mental health promotion is an integral part of health promotion theory and practice where persons with mental illness need affordable, available, accessible and appropriate sustainable mental health services for them to continue education (children and youth) or remain in economic-sustaining livelihoods (employment).

Table 11.1. Continued

Issue	Key points
	• These associations play a major role in risk behaviors, such as unsafe sexual behavior, road trauma and physical inactivity resulting in lack of meaningful, or dismissal from, employment, and in turn become an associated cause for depression and alcohol and drug use among people with mental disorders and their families.
Mental health data	• Lack of reliable mental health data within and across nations is pervasive and a critical barrier in addressing unmet mental health needs.
	• Limited data hinder better understanding of mental health needs and limit policy, interventions and resources needed to address mental disorders.
	• Data limitations put mental health needs on the back burner of policy development and resource allocation.
	• Better collection of mental health data are needed in the developing nations and among rural and racial groups in developed nations.

of people suffering from mental disorders globally including depression (154 million), schizophrenia (25 million) and alcohol use disorders (91 million) (Schmidt, Norman, & Boshuizen, 1990; WHO/WONCA, 2008). Suicides account for about 1 million deaths annually (WHO, 2002).

The projected burden of mental health disorders is expected to reach 15% by the year 2020, when common mental disorders (depression, anxiety and substance-related disorders including alcohol) will disable more people than complications arising from AIDS, heart disease, traffic accidents and wars combined. Almost one third (28%) of disability-adjusted life-years in 2005 were attributed to neuropsychiatric disorders (e.g., unipolar affective disorder[(10%]) (Murray & Lopez, 1996).

The burden of unmet mental health needs is especially high among children and youths (Flisher et al., 1997; Kataoka, Zhang, & Wells, 2002; Ngui & Flores, 2007). About 10% to 20% of all children are affected by one or more mental or behavioral problems (WHO, 2001b). In the USA, 1 in 5 children suffer from a mental disorder, with 1 in 10 affected by a serious mental or emotional disorder (US Department of Health and Human Services, 1999). Only 15% to 30% of these children, however, receive the treatment they need (WHO/WONCA, 2008). Kataoka found that 79% of children 6 to 7 years of age with mental disorders do not receive the care they need (Kataoka et al., 2002). Data from the developing nations is less reliable, but estimates from the Western Cape region of South Africa suggest that 17% of children and adolescents suffer from mental disorders (Kleintjes et al., 2006), whereas in conflict areas such as Mosul, Iraq, it is as high as 35% of children and youths (Al-Jawadi & Abdul-Rhman, 2007).

In light of this evidence, the ethical concerns associated with international mental health disparities are profound. Human rights and social justice frameworks are arguably central ethical tenets of public health (Beauchamp, 1999). According to the International Covenant of Economic, Social and Cultural Rights, "everyone has a right to the highest attainable standard of physical and mental health" (Earle, 2006, p. 327). As such, addressing global mental health inequalities and the underlying determinants of mental disorders promotes human rights and social justice in any society. These frameworks call for the ethical care of people living with mental illness and global advocacy of beneficence, autonomy, respect for individuals, non-malfeasance and empowerment of all people, and particularly those who are marginalized, stigmatized and discriminated against (Roberts & Dyer, 2004; Sheppard, 2002). Paul Farmer observes that the needs of the world's poor are often not recognized and the underlying structural inequalities that contribute to these conditions are frequently neglected or ignored by the international public health and foreign policy communities (Farmer, 2003). He calls for the inclusion and integration of human rights agenda, including resource equity and social justice in health diplomacy and international health assistance (Mann, 1996).

Initiatives and strategies to address health must systematically incorporate mental health as a key part of overall health. Application of the human rights and social justice frameworks in mental health require concerted effort and commitment to address the underlying determinants of mental health problems including fair, equitable, and ethical distribution of resource distribution (e.g., treatment), inclusive mental health and primary care policies and strengthened legal and human rights protection for people living with mental disorders and their families.

In many developing nations, standards for ethical conduct of research and treatment are inadequate or lacking. Addressing inequalities and unmet mental health needs, especially in the developing nations, will require establishment and strengthened ethical standards in research and treatment of people with mental health problems. Goodman (2008) observes that "ethics is essential for building trust in developing world ... ethics and trust are required for a successful research programme ... health of communities depends on more and better research; and that such research is necessary for reducing disparities" (Goodman, 2008, p. 89). Indeed, repeated demonstrations of integrity by economically established countries towards all people affected by mental illness and its burden throughout the world is a precondition for ethically sound and humane healthcare. Moreover, intensive and more appropriately attuned ethics education is critically important in understanding and addressing mental health inequalities and in the preparation of clinicians caring for people living with mental illness (Chipp et al., in press; Hoop, DiPasquale, Hernandez, & Roberts, 2008; Jain, Dunn, & Roberts, in press; Lehrmann, Hoop, Hammond, & Roberts, 2009; Roberts, Johnson, Brems, & Warner, 2008) in rural and underserved areas.

Inequalities in Mental Health

Inequalities in mental health exist, are pervasive and often ignored as illustrated by the neglect of a mental health focus in the Millennium Development Goals (United Nations, 2000). According to the World Health Organization (WHO), health inequalities can be defined as "differences in health status or in the distribution of health determinants between different population groups" (WHO, 2007). Health inequity is those inequalities in health considered unfair and unjust (Kawachi, Subramanian, & Almeida-Filho, 2002). Inequity in mental health exists in access to care, use and outcomes of care (e.g., morbidity and mortality) and can occur by geographical region (rural/urban), gender, socioeconomic status, racial or ethnic background and sexual orientation among other things.

Mental health inequalities are strongly associated and embedded within the broader social and economic context. An inverse relationship between socio-economic status and mental disorders has been documented (Dalgard, 2008; Hunt, McEwen, & McKenna, 1979; Kessler et al., 1994). In almost all nations the poor are at a higher risk of developing mental disorders compared to the non-poor. Poverty is both a "determinant and a consequence of poor mental health" (Murali & Oyebode, 2004, p. 217). Mental disorders increase the likelihood of living in poverty, perhaps because of their influence on functionality and ability to get or sustain employment. Conversely, poverty increases the likelihood of developing mental disorders (Bostock, 2004; Das et al., 2007; Murali & Oyebode, 2004).

The consequences of mental health inequalities include continued unnecessary suffering and premature deaths, increased stigma and marginalization, lack of investment in mental health workforce and infrastructure and limited or lack of treatment for people suffering from these conditions. In many developing nations with mental health policies, scarce resources and infrastructure, ineffective advocacy and the lack of political will limits effective mental health legislations and interventions (WHO, 2005b). These nations often lack effective mental health champions who can galvanize communities and policy makers to address mental health needs. Families of people with mental health problems are often marginalized and are limited in their ability to champion for mental health issues due to the stigma associated with these disorders. Some progress, however, is being made to redress the challenges posed by mental health problems (Eaton, 2009), but these efforts are few and need to be scaled up to adequately meet mental health needs.

Unmet Mental Health Needs

Mental health inequalities have contributed to profound suffering and death worldwide largely because people cannot access the treatment they need. Estimates for untreated serious mental disorders in developing countries range from 75% to 85% (WHO, World Mental Health Consortium, 2004). Over 80% of people suffering from mental disorders (e.g., epilepsy, schizophrenia, depression, intellectual disability, alcohol use disorders and those committing suicide) live in developing countries (Bertolote, Fleischmann, De Leo, & Wasserman, 2004). Untreated cases range from 32.2% for schizophrenia (including other non-affective psychosis) to 56.3% for depression, to 78.1% for alcohol and drug use disorders (Kohn, Saxena, & Levav, 2004). In Kenya, for example, the number of unidentified cases of mental illness attending a national hospital was 40% (Makanyengo, Othieno, & Okech, 2005), with unidentified cases of depression between 53% and 66.2% at the sub-district and district hospitals, respectively. Almost a quarter of patients attending general health facilities in Kenya have undiagnosed alcohol abuse problems (Ndetei et al., 2009). Rural areas in developing nations, as in economically established countries (Roberts et al., 2007), are especially affected by mental health disparities.

Many developing nations have no policies to address the basic needs and rights of individuals with mental illness, which contributes to limited prioritization of mental health in health planning, resource allocation, and workforce development, further increasing unmet mental health needs. Research shows that in developing nations patients often leave hospitals without knowing their diagnosis or what medications they are taking (Gerteis, Edgman-Levitan, Daley, & Delbanco, 1993; Ndetei, Mutiso, Khasakhala, & Kokonya, 2007b), wait too long for referrals, appointments and treatment (Murray & Tantau, 1998) and are not respected or given adequate emotional support (Botelho, Lue, & Fiscella, 1996; Sobel, 1995). In many communities, the burden of caring for the sick is placed on women and increasingly children because of the high adult morbidity and mortality due to HIV/AIDS and other infectious diseases. This has resulted in age and gender inequities in primary caregiver's responsibilities for people living with mental illness. Moreover, increased international migration of health workers from developing to the developed nations (Connell, Zurn, Stilwell, Awases, & Braichet, 2007; Kirigia, Gbary, Muthuri, Nyoni, & Seddoh, 2006; Stilwell et al., 2003, 2004) and internal migration from rural poorer communities to more wealthier urban communities in the developing nations has further worsened the shortage of mental healthcare workers (Mwaniki & Dulo, 2008; Ndetei, Khasakhala, & Omolo, 2008; Ndetei et al., 2007b). As a result, the majority of people with mental illness in developing nations go untreated despite the availability of effective treatment. These large treatment gaps are not surprising given that in many developing countries there is no budget for mental health services. Not only are mental health services scarce, but individuals who have mental disorders attending public medical services are required to meet the cost of their treatment (psycho-active drugs), while treatment for physical health problems is freely provided (Ndetei, Khasakhala, Kingori, Oginga, & Raja, 2007a; WHO, 2005b). This disproportionately affects poorer people who are at greater risk of having mental disorders.

Stigma and Discrimination

The burden of mental disorders in developing countries is compounded by high rates of stigma and discrimination, which are major obstacles in the provision and utilization of mental health services (Horwitz, Roberts, & Warner, 2008; Okasha, 2002; Onyut et al., 2009; Ssebunnya, Kigozi, Lund, Kizza, & Okello, 2009). Research documents increasing social distance and stigmatization of people living with mental disorders in sub-Saharan Africa (Adewuya & Makan- juola, 2005, 2008) even among mental health providers (Ndetei et al., 2009). The stigma, myths and misconceptions surrounding mental illness contribute too much of the discrimination and human rights violations experienced by people with mental disorders (Ndetei et al., 2007a). The laws, practices and social norms in many nations give extensive powers to guardians of people with mental disorders to decide where they live, their movements, their per- sonal and financial affairs and their care, including their commitment to mental hospitals (Ndetei et al., 2007a). Research, however, shows that clinicians and others, including family members, inaccurately judge what patients value (Gerhart, Koziao-McLain, Lowenstein, & Whiteneck, 1994; Laine et al., 1996; Roberts et al., 2003; Roberts, Warner, Anderson, Smithpeter, & Rogers, 2004a; Roberts, Green Hammond, Warner, & Lewis, 2004b), resulting in unnecessary restrictions in the rights to work, education, marriage and participation in community or family functions.

Stigma associated with mental disorders can also influence career choices resulting in fewer people choosing to work in the mental healthcare field. Studies involving medical students in Colombia ($n = 375$) (Pailhez, Bulbena, López, & Balon, 2010), Saudi Arabia ($n = 54$) (El-Gilany, Amr, & Iqbal, 2010) and Spain ($n = 207$) (Pailhez et al., 2010), and medical residents in Romania ($n = 112$) (Voinescu, Szentagotai, & Coogan, 2010), published in a special collection, recently demonstrated the negative attitudes that exist towards the medical specialism of psychiatry. For example, 82% of the Saudi Arabian students and 52% of the Romanian students in these survey projects endorsed the statement that "if a student expresses interest in psychiatry, he or she risks being ... seen by others as odd, peculiar, or neurotic." Large proportions of students had been actively discouraged by their medical school teachers, family members, friends, and fellow students from going into psychiatry (El-Gilany, Amr, & Iqbal, 2010; Voinescu, Szentagotai, & Coogan, 2010).

Limited knowledge of the causes, symptoms and treatment of mental illness often leads to common but erroneous beliefs that these conditions are caused by individuals themselves or by supernatural forces, possession by evil spirits, curse or punishment following the individual's family or is part of family lineage (Mohit, 2001). Disturbingly, physicians in training in some developing or economically disadvantaged countries hold these same beliefs, even after undergoing psychiatric training (Roberts, 2010). For example, 23–40% of Nigerian medical students in one study endorsed supernatural causes of mental illness, such as charms, evil spirits and witchcraft (Aghukwa, 2010). These beliefs increase stigma, discrimination and social isolation of individuals living with mental illness and limits resources for their care. Without effective diagnosis and treatment options, mental disorders are seen as untreatable, resulting in patients being undervalued and perceived as not able to contribute to society. In developing nations and in some communities in developed nations, the limited availability of modern mental health services and providers is offset by reliance on traditional and faith healers (Beals et al., 2005; Hewson, 1998; Ngoma, Prince, & Mann, 2003; Ovuga, Boardman, & Oluka, 1999; Sorsdahl et al., 2009). Although these alternative healers play a critical role, they often lack the necessary training and skills to provide effective care for people with serious mental illness.

Mental Disorders and Economic Development

The economic burden of mental disorder is great. In the USA the indirect costs associated with these disorders is estimated to be over $79 billion, with about $63 billion reflecting the loss of productivity because of illnesses (Manderscheid, Druss, & Freeman, 2007). In Canada, the economic burden of mental illness in 2003 was about $34 billion ($1,056 per capita), with depression and schizophrenia accounting for about $5 billion and $2.7 billion annually, respectively (Patra et al., 2007). Mental health conditions cost between 3% and 4% of the gross national product in the European Union member countries (Gabriel & Liimatainen, 2000; WHO, 2005c).

The effect of mental disorders extends beyond individual and family suffering to national economic development. Mental health well-being is strongly related to many economic development sectors (e.g., education, employment, law enforcement and incarceration) (Gureje & Jenkins, 2007) and several Millennium Development Goals (United Nations, 2000) (e.g., eradicating extreme poverty and hunger, reduce child mortality and improve maternal health) (Gureje & Jenkins, 2007; Miranda & Patel, 2005; WHO, 2002). These conditions can influence economic growth through their effects on labor supply, earnings, participation and productivity (Dewa & Lin, 2000; WHO, 2002). Depression, for instance, can negatively affect education, employment and productivity (Berndt et al., 1998; Kessler & Frank, 1997), but productivity gains after effective treatment exceed direct treatment costs (Simon et al., 2001).

Economic loss associated with decreased labor force participation and institutionalization of people with mental disorders is great. In the USA, about 3% of men and 4.5% of women cannot work or engage in regular activities because of mental or emotional problems. Men with mental disorders earn 21% less than men without mental disorders (Robins & Regier, 1991). In Kenya, the economic loss associated with institutionalization of mental and behavioral disorders is about $13 million (Kirigia & Sambo, 2003), a large amount in a country where over half of the population live on less than a dollar per day and have no safe drinking water (UNDP, 2000). Unmet mental health needs can create social problems (e.g., unemployment, substance abuse, poverty) that may increase crime and political instability. Sen observes, "there is plenty of evidence that unemployment has many far-reaching effects other than loss of income, including psychological harm, loss of work motivation, skill and self-confidence, increase in ailments and morbidity (and even mortality rates), disruption of family relations and social life, hardening of social exclusion and accentuation of racial tensions and gender asymmetries" (Sen, 1999, p. 94). In many developing nations these social problems are further compounded by poor governance, corruption and social morbidity due to natural and manmade disasters (e.g., wars), which increase mental health problems, erode social cohesion and capital and limit economic growth (Dewa & Lin, 2000; Njenga, 2002; WHO, 2002).

Integrating Mental Health into Primary Health Care Services

The mismatch between the global burden of mental disorders and availability of mental health resources is alarming. According to WHO, there is less than one psychiatrist for every 100,000 people in much of south-east Asia, and less than one psychiatrist for every 1 million people in sub-Saharan Africa (Jacob et al., 2007; WHO, 2005b). Nigeria, for example, has 100 psychiatrists for its population of 114 million (Gureje & Lasebikan, 2006). Globally, only 2% of national budgets are devoted to mental health (WHO, 2005b). About 70% of African and 50% of south-east Asian countries devoted less than 1% of their health budget on mental health (Jacob et al., 2007).

Given the scarcity of mental health providers in developing nations, the few psychiatric hospitals that exist are often understaffed, crowded and may not provide the quality of care needed. Most psychiatric hospitals are located in urban settings and away from family members, which further increases the social isolation and cost for families. In some countries, these hospitals are simply "warehouses" where patients are kept from the rest of the society because of limited resources and capacity to manage effectively their conditions. In developed nations (e.g., USA), deinstitutionalization of people with mental illness results in many patients, mostly racial/ethnic minorities, being incarcerated because of limited access and availability of basic mental health services in the community.

One key strategy for addressing inequalities in mental health care is to ensure the integration of mental health with other primary care services. Ongoing efforts to implement and enhance primary care in developing countries (Rohde et al., 2008; Tejada de Rivero, 2003; Walley et al., 2008) must include mental health care as a critical component of overall population health and well-being. Chan and Van Weel observe that

> for too long, mental disorders have been largely overlooked as part of strengthening primary care. This is despite the fact that mental disorders are found in all countries, in women and men, at all stages of life, among the rich and poor, and in both rural and urban settings. It is also despite the fact that integrating mental health into primary care facilitates person-centred and holistic services, and as such, is central to the values and principles of the Alma Ata Declaration. (WHO/WONCA, 2008, p. vii)

Reasons for integrating mental health into primary care include the enormous social and economic burden, the interwoven nature of physical and mental problems, and the significant treatment gaps of mental health problems (WHO/WONCA, 2008). Moreover, since primary care for mental health problems is affordable and cost-effective, such integration would generate good outcomes, promote access to care and respect for human rights (WHO/WONCA, 2008).

Community mental health services can help reduce social stigma and discrimination by reducing the social isolation, neglect and institutionalization of people living with mental health problems. Effective community management of mental disorders also helps people realize that people with mental illness can live productive lives, contribute to society and be integrated with society.

Data and the Global Burden of Mental Health Problems

Efforts to address mental health problems must also address the pervasive lack of reliable data within and across nations (WHO, 2005a). Health systems in many developing nations do not routinely collect mental health data (Ndetei et al., 2007b), which can limit the ability of nations to accurately determine the burden of these conditions and develop plans to address them. Data limitations put mental health needs on the backburner for most policy makers and make it difficult for governments and international agencies to devote more resources to address mental disorders. Strategies such as adding reliable mental health measures to ongoing population surveys (e.g., The Demographic Health Survey) can significantly improve availability of data for advocacy, program planning and policy formation in many countries.

In conclusion, health reform agendas in the developed and developing nations need to provide legal protection, services and human rights to people living with mental disorders. These policies must protect people with mental disorders from abuse, neglect and discrimination, and afford them the care they need. Justice requires that people with mental illness receive the same societal and legal protection given to other people with physical health conditions. Ethical and human rights challenges in caring for people living with mental illness and their families exist. These include (1) justification to provide mental health services to communities when primary healthcare services are inaccessible, unavailable and unaffordable and therefore unsustainable in rural and hard-to-reach areas; (2) lack of public awareness on mental health and limited knowledge about the causes of mental illness, which have resulted in mental health being given low priority by the policy makers and health providers; (3) the vicious circle between mental ill-health and poverty; (4) the role played by stigma towards individuals who have mental illness and their families; and (5) inadequate developed mental health policies, resulting in limitations to bring about major reforms in the implementation of mental health policies and service delivery needed by mental health systems.

Although the idea of health without mental health sounds absurd, mental health is perhaps the most neglected aspect of health in developed and developing nations. Addressing mental disorders often appears to be an afterthought in health and social policy development, added to existing "more important health issues" rather than a part of individual and population overall health and well-being. In defining health, the WHO clearly articulated the importance of mental health by including it with overall physical and social well-being. By putting it in between the state of "physical" and "social" well-being, this definition symbolically shows how mental health ties physical health and social well-being together. Neglect of mental health needs in health policies often translates to neglect in research, funding, services and infrastructure (e.g., the development of competent mental health workforce) especially in poor and underserved communities (WHO, 2001a, 2001b). Mental health is vital to our understanding of health and economic development and must be prioritized in health planning, resource allocation and fully integrated with other primary care services.

References

Adewuya AO, Makanjuola RO. Social distance towards people with mental illness amongst Nigerian university students. *Social Psychiatry & Psychiatric Epidemiology* 2005;40(11):865–868. [PubMed: 16234984]

Adewuya AO, Makanjuola RO. Social distance towards people with mental illness in southwestern Nigeria. *Australian & New Zealand Journal of Psychiatry* 2008;42(5):389–395. [PubMed: 18473257]

Aghukwa C. Medical students' beliefs and attitudes toward mental illness: Effects of a psychiatric education. *Academic Psychiatry* 2010;34:67–70. [PubMed: 20071734]

Al-Jawadi AA, Abdul-Rhman S. Prevalence of childhood and early adolescence mental disorders among children attending primary health care centers in Mosul, Iraq: A cross-sectional study. *BMC Public Health* 2007;7:274. [PubMed: 17910748]

Beals J, Novins DK, Whitesell NR, Spicer P, Mitchell CM, Manson SM. Prevalence of mental disorders and utilization of mental health services in two American Indian reservation populations: Mental health disparities in a national context. *American Journal of Psychiatry* 2005;162(9):1723–1732. [PubMed: 16135633]

Beauchamp DE. Public health as social justice. In: Beauchamp DE, Steinbock B., eds. *New ethics for the public's health.* New York: Oxford University Press; 1999, pp. 105–114.

Berndt ER, Finkelstein SN, Greenberg PE, Howland RH, Keith A, Rush AJ, et al. Workplace performance effects from chronic depression and its treatment. *Journal of Health Economics* 1998;17(5):511–535. [PubMed: 10185510]

Bertolote JM, Fleischmann A, De Leo D, Wasserman D. Psychiatric diagnoses and suicide: Revisiting the evidence. *Crisis: Journal of Crisis Intervention & Suicide* 2004;25(4):147–155.

Bostock J. The high price of poverty. Poverty and debt are major risk factors for mental ill health in deprived communities and groups. *Mental Health Today* 2004 November:27–29. [PubMed: 15575585]

Botelho R, Lue B, Fiscella K. Family involvement in routine health care: A survey of patients' behaviors and preferences. *Journal of Family Practice* 1996;42:572–576. [PubMed: 8656167]

Chipp C, Dewane S, Brems C, Johnson ME, Warner TD, Roberts LW. "If only someone had told me ...": Lessons from rural providers. *Journal of Rural Health,* 2011 Winter; 27(1):122-30/ DOJ 10. 1111/j.1748-0361.2010.00314.x. See http://www.ncbi.nlm.nih.gov/pubmed/21204979.

Chisholm D, Flisher AJ, Lund C, Patel V, Saxena S, Thornicroft G, et al. Scale up services for mental disorders: A call for action. *Lancet* 2007;370(9594):1241–1252. [PubMed: 17804059]

Connell J, Zurn P, Stilwell B, Awases M, Braichet J-M. Sub-Saharan Africa: Beyond the health worker migration crisis. *Social Science and Medicine* 2007;64:1876–1891. [PubMed: 17316943]

Dalgard OS. Social inequalities in mental health in Norway: Possible explanatory factors. *International Journal of Equity in Health* 2008;7(27)10. 10.1186/1475-9276-7-27. See http://www.equityhealthj.com/content/pdf/1475-9276-7-27.pdf.

Das J, Do QT, Friedman J, McKenzie D, Scott K. Mental health and poverty in developing countries: Revisiting the relationship. *Social Science and Medicine* 2007;65(3):467–480. [PubMed: 17462803]

Dewa C, Lin E. Chronic physical illness, psychiatric disorder and disability in the workplace. *Social Science and Medicine* 2000;51:41–50. [PubMed: 10817467]

Earle S. Promoting public health: Part 1. *Nursing Management* 2006;13(7):32–35. [PubMed: 17111966]

Eaton J. A new movement for global mental health and its possible impact in Nigeria. *Nigerian Journal of Psychiatry* 2009;7(1):14–15.

El-Gilany A, Amr M, Iqbal R. Students' attitudes toward psychiatry at Al-Hassa Medical College, Saudi Arabia. *Academic Psychiatry* 2010;34:71–74. [PubMed: 20071736]

Farmer, P. *Pathologies of power: Health, human rights, and the new war on the poor.* Berkeley: University of California Press; 2003.

Flisher AJ, Kramer RA, Grosser RC, Alegria M, Bird HR, Bourdon KH, et al. Correlates of unmet need for mental health services by children and adolescents. *Psychologic Medicine* 1997;27(5):1145–1154.

Gabriel P, Liimataine M. *Mental health in the workplace.* Geneva: International Labour Office; 2000 [accessed February 17, 2010]. Available at http://www.who .int/mental_health/policy/services/13_policies%20programs%20in%20work place_WEB_07.pdf.

Gerhart K, Koziao-McLain J, Lowenstein S, Whiteneck G. Quality of life following spinal cord injury: Knowledge and attitudes of emergency care providers. *Annals of Emergency Medicine* 1994;23(4):807–812. [PubMed: 8161051]

Gerteis M, Edgman-Levitan S, Daley J, Delbanco T. *Through the patient's eyes: Understanding and promoting patient-centered care.* San Francisco: Jossey-Bass; 1993.

Goodman, K. Ethics, evidence and innovation. Global forum update on research for health. In: Gehner M, Jupp S, Matlin SA, editors. *Fostering innovation for global health.* Vol. 5. Woodbridge: Pro-Brook; 2008, pp. 88–90.

Gureje O, Jenkins R. Mental health in development: Re-emphasising the link. *Lancet* 2007;369(9560):447–449.

Gureje O, Lasebikan VO. Use of mental health services in a developing country. Results from the Nigerian survey of mental health and well-being. *Social Psychiatry & Psychiatric Epidemiology* 2006;41(1):44–49. [PubMed: 16341828]

Hewson MG. Traditional healers in Southern Africa. *Annals of Internal Medicine* 1998;128(12/1):1029–1034. [PubMed: 9625666]

Hoop J, DiPasquale T, Hernandez J, Roberts LW. Ethics and culture in mental health care. *Ethics and Behavior* 2008;18:353–372.

Horwitz R, Roberts LW, Warner TD. Mexican immigrant women's perceptions of health care access for stigmatizing illnesses: A focus group study in Albuquerque, New Mexico. *Journal of Health Care for the Poor and Underserved* 2008;19(3): 857–873. [PubMed: 18677075]

Hunt S, McEwen J, McKenna S. Social inequalities and perceived health. *Effective Health Care* 1979;2(4):151–160. [PubMed: 10270615]

Jacob KS, Sharan P, Mirza I, Garrido-Cumbrera M, Seedat S, Mari JJ, et al. Mental health systems in countries: Where are we now? *Lancet* 2007;370(9592): 1061–1077. [PubMed: 17804052]

Jain S, Dunn L, Roberts L. Psychiatric residents' needs for education about informed consent, principles of ethics and professionalism, and caring for vulnerable populations: Results of a multisite survey. *Academic Psychiatry* 2011;35: 184-190. 10.1176/appi.ap.35.3.184 Available at http://ap.psychiatryonline.org /article.aspx?Volume=35&page=184&journalID=17.

Kataoka SH, Zhang L, Wells KB. Unmet need for mental health care among US children: Variation by ethnicity and insurance status. *American Journal of Psychiatry* 2002;159(9):1548–1555. [PubMed: 12202276]

Kawachi I, Subramanian SV, Almeida-Filho N. A glossary for health inequalities. *Journal of Epidemiology and Community Health* 2002;56(9):647–652. [PubMed: 12177079]

Kessler R, Chiu W, Demler O, Walters E. Prevalence, severity, and comorbidity of 12-month DSM-IV disorders in the National Comorbidity Survey Replication (NCS-R). *Archives of General Psychiatry* 2005a;62(6):617–627. [PubMed: 15939839]

Kessler R, Demler O, Frank R, Olfson M, Pincus H, Walters E, et al. Prevalence and treatment of mental disorders, 1990 to 2003. *New England Journal of Medicine* 2005b;352(24):2515–2523. [PubMed: 15958807]

Kessler RC, Frank RG. The impact of psychiatric disorders on work loss days. *Psychological Medicine* 1997;27(4):861–873. [PubMed: 9234464]

Kessler RC, McGonagle KA, Zhao S, Nelson CB, Hughes M, Eshleman S, et al. Lifetime and 12-month prevalence of DSM-III-R psychiatric disorders in the United States. Results from the National Comorbidity Survey. *Archives of General Psychiatry* 1994;51(1):8–19.

Kirigia J, Gbary A, Muthuri L, Nyoni J, Seddoh A. The cost of health professionals' brain drain in Kenya. *BMC Health Services Research* 2006;6:89. [PubMed: 16846492]

Kirigia J, Sambo L. Cost of mental and behavioural disorders in Kenya. *Annals of General Hospital Psychiatry* 2003;2(1):7. [PubMed: 12892565]

Kleintjes S, Flisher A, Fick M, Railoun A, Lund C, Molteno C, et al. The prevalence of mental disorders among children, adolescents and adults in the Western Cape, South Africa. *South African Psychiatry Review* 2006;9:157–160.

Kohn R, Saxena S, Levav I. The treatment gap in mental health care. *Bulletin of the World Health Organization* 2004;82:858–866. [PubMed: 15640922]

Laine C, Davidoff F, Lewis C, Nelson E, Kessler R, Delbanco T. Important elements of outpatient care: A comparison of patients' and physicians' opinions. *Annals of Internal Medicine* 1996;125:640–645. [PubMed: 8849148]

Lehrmann J, Hoop JG, Hammond K, Roberts L. Medical students' affirmation of ethics education. *Academic Psychiatry* 2009;33:470–477. [PubMed: 19933891]

Makanyengo MA, Othieno CJ, Okech ML. Consultation liaison psychiatry at Kenyatta National Hospital, Nairobi. *East Africa Medical Journal* 2005;82(2):79–84.

Manderscheid R, Druss B, Freeman E. *Data to manage the mortality crisis: Recommendations to the substance abuse and mental health services administration.* Washington, DC: SAMHSA; 2007 [Accessed March 3, 2010]. Available at http://www.promoteacceptance.samhsa.gov/10by10/summit_presentations.aspx.

Mann J. Health and human rights. *British Medical Journal* 1996;312(7036): 924–925. [PubMed: 8616294]

Miranda JJ, Patel V. Achieving the Millennium Development Goals: Does mental health play a role? *Public Library of Science (PLoS) Medicine* 2005;2(10):e291.

Mohit A. Mental health and psychiatry in the Middle East: Historical development. *Eastern Mediterranean Health Journal* 2001;7:336–347. [PubMed: 12690751]

Murali V, Oyebode F. Poverty, social inequality and mental health. *Advances in Psychiatric Treatment* 2004;10:216–224.

Murray C, Lopez A. editors. The global burden of disease: A comprehensive assessment of mortality and disability from diseases, injuries and risk factors in 1990 and projected to 2020. *Global Burden of Disease and Injury Series.* Cambridge, MA: Harvard School of Public Health on behalf of the World Health Organization and the World Bank; 1996.

Murray M, Tantau C. Must patients wait? *Journal of Quality Improvement* 1998;24:423–425.

Mwaniki D, Dulo C. *Migration of health workers in Kenya: The impact on health service delivery.* EQUINET discussion paper 55. Harare: EQUINET, ECSA HC, and IOM; 2008 [accessed January 22, 2010]. Available at http://www.aspeninstitute .org/sites/default/files/content/images/migration%20of%20health%20workers %20in%20kenya.pdf.

Ndetei D, Khasakhala L, Kingori J, Oginga A, Raja S. *Baseline study: The mental health situation in Kangemi informal settlement Nairobi, Kenya.* 2007a [accessed February 7, 2010]. Available at http://www.basicneeds.org.uk.

Ndetei D, Khasakhala L, Kuria M, Mutiso V, Ongecha F, Kokonya D. The prevalence of mental disorders in adults in different level general medical facilities in Kenya: A cross-sectional study. *Annals of General Psychiatry* 2009 [accessed January 22, 2010]. Available at http://www.annals-general-psychiatry.com/content/2018/2011 /2011.

Ndetei D, Khasakhala L, Omolo J. *Incentives for health worker retention in Kenya: An assessment of current practice.* EQUINET discussion paper 62. Harare: AMHF, EQUINET, ECSA-HC; 2008 [accessed 22 January 2010]. Available at http://www.equinetafrica.org/bibl/docs/DIS62HRndetei.pdf.

Ndetei D, Mutiso V, Khasakhala L, Kokonya D. The challenges of human resources in mental health in Kenya. *South African Psychiatric Review* 2007b;10:33–36.

Ngoma MC, Prince M, Mann A. Common mental disorders among those attending primary health clinics and traditional healers in urban Tanzania. *The British Journal of Psychiatry* 2003;183(4):349–355. [PubMed: 14519614]

Ngui EM, Flores G. Unmet needs for specialty, dental, mental, and allied health care among children with special health care needs: Are there racial/ethnic disparities? *Journal of Health Care for the Poor & Underserved* 2007;18(4):931–949. [PubMed: 17982216]

Njenga FG. Challenges of balanced care in Africa. *World Psychiatry* 2002;1(2): 96–98. [PubMed: 16946862]

Okasha A. Mental health in Africa: The role of the WPA. *World Psychiatry* 2002;1(1):32–35. [PubMed: 16946819]

Onyut LP, Neuner F, Ertl V, Schauer E, Odenwald M, Elbert T. Trauma, poverty and mental health among Somali and Rwandese refugees living in an African refugee settlement—An epidemiological study. *Conflict Health* 2009;3(6)10. 1186/1752-1505-1183-1186.

Ovuga E, Boardman J, Oluka EGAO. Traditional healers and mental illness in Uganda. *Psychiatric Bulletin* 1999;23:276–279.

Pailhez G, Bulbena A, López C, Balon R. Views of psychiatry: A comparison between medical students from Barcelona and Medellín. *Academic Psychiatry* 2010;34:61–66. [PubMed: 20071732]

Patra J, Popova S, Rehm J, Bondy S, Flint R, Giesbrecht N. *Economic cost of chronic disease in Canada 1995–2003.* Ontario: Ontario Chronic Disease Prevention Alliance and the Ontario Public Health Association; 2007.

Prince M, Patel V, Saxena S, Maj M, Maselko J, Phillips MR, et al. No health without mental health. *Lancet* 2007;370(9590):859–877. [PubMed: 17804063]

Roberts L, Warner T, Anderson C, Smithpeter M, Rogers M. Schizophrenia research participants' responses to protocol safeguards: Recruitment, consent, and debriefing. *Schizophrenia Research* 2004a;67:283–291. [PubMed: 14984889]

Roberts L, Warner T, Nguyen K, Geppert C, Rogers M, Roberts B. Schizophrenia patients' and psychiatrists' perspectives on ethical aspects of symptom re-emergence during psychopharmacological research participation. *Psychopharmacology* 2003;171:58–67. [PubMed: 12756518]

Roberts LW. Stigma, hope, and challenge in psychiatry: Trainee perspectives from five countries on four continents. *Academic Psychiatry* 2010;34:1–4. [PubMed: 20071716]

Roberts LW, Dyer AR. *Concise guide to ethics in mental health care.* Washington, DC: American Psychiatric Publishing; 2004.

Roberts LW, Green Hammond K, Warner T, Lewis R. Influence of ethical safeguards on research participation: Comparison of perspectives of people with schizophrenia and psychiatrists. *American Journal of Psychiatry* 2004b;161: 2309–2311. [PubMed: 15569905]

Roberts LW, Johnson ME, Brems C, Warner TD. Ethical disparities: Challenges encountered by multidisciplinary providers in fulfilling ethical standards in the care of rural and minority people. *Journal of Rural Health* 2007;23:89–97. [PubMed: 18237331]

Roberts LW, Johnson ME, Brems C, Warner TD. When providers and patients come from different backgrounds: Perceived value of additional training on ethical care practices. *Transcultural Psychiatry* 2008;45:553–565. [PubMed: 19091725]

Robins L, Regier D. *Psychatric disorders in America: The epidemiological catchment area study.* New York: Free Press; 1991.

Rohde J, Cousens S, Chopra M, Tangcharoensathien V, Black R, Bhutta ZA, et al. 30 years after Alma-Ata: Has primary health care worked in countries? *Lancet* 2008;372(9642):950–961. [PubMed: 18790318]

Schmidt HG, Norman GR, Boshuizen HP. A cognitive perspective on medical expertise: Theory and implication. *Academic Medicine* 1990;65(10):611–621. [PubMed: 2261032]

Sen, A. *Development as freedom.* New York: Anchor; 1999.

Sheppard M. Mental health and social justice: Gender, race and psychological consequences of unfairness. *British Journal of Social Work* 2002;32(6):779–797.

Simon GE, Barber C, Birnbaum HG, Frank RG, Greenberg PE, Rose RM, et al. Depression and work productivity: The comparative costs of treatment versus nontreatment. *Journal of Occupational & Environmental Medicine* 2001;43(1):2–9. [PubMed: 11201765]

Sobel DS. Rethinking medicine: Improving health outcomes with cost-effective psychosocial interventions. *Psychosomatic Medicine* 1995;57(3):234–244. [PubMed: 7652124]

Sorsdahl K, Stein DJ, Grimsrud A, Seedat S, Flisher AJ, Williams DR, et al. Traditional healers in the treatment of common mental disorders in South Africa. *Journal of Nervous & Mental Disease* 2009;197(6):434–441. [PubMed: 19525744]

Ssebunnya J, Kigozi F, Lund C, Kizza D, Okello E. Stakeholder perceptions of mental health stigma and poverty in Uganda. *BMC International Health and Human Rights* 2009;9:5. [PubMed: 19335889]

Stilwell B, Diallo K, Zurn P, Dal Poz M, Adams O, Buchan J. Developing evidence-based ethical policies on the migration of health workers: Conceptual and practical challenges. *Human Resources for Health* 2003;1:8. [PubMed: 14613524]

Stilwell B, Diallo K, Zurn P, Vujicic M, Orvill A, Dal Poz M. Migration of health-care workers from developing countries: Strategic approaches to its management. *Bulletin of the World Health Organization* 2004;82(8):595–600. [PubMed: 15375449]

Tejada de Rivero DA. Alma-Ata revisited. *Perspectives in Health* 2003;18(2):1–6.

UNDP. *Human development report 2000.* Oxford, UK: Oxford University Press; 2000.

United Nations. *United Nations millennium declaration: Resolution adopted by the general assembly* (No. A/RES/55/2; 8th plenary meeting). New York: United Nations General Assembly; 2000 [accessed February 20, 2010].

US Department of Health and Human Services. *Mental health: A report of the surgeon general.* Washington, DC: Department of Health and Human Services; 1999 [accessed January 29, 2010]. Available at http://www.surgeongeneral.gov/library/mentalhealth/home.html.

Voinescu B, Szentagotai A, Coogan A. Attitudes towards psychiatry—A survey of Romanian medical residents. *Academic Psychiatry* 2010;34:75–78. [PubMed: 20071737]

Walley J, Lawn JE, Tinker A, de Francisco A, Chopra M, Rudan I, et al. Primary health care: Making Alma-Ata a reality. *Lancet* 2008;372(9642):1001–1007. [PubMed: 18790322]

WHO. *Atlas: Mental health resources in the world.* Geneva: World Health Organization; 2001a.

WHO. *The world health report 2001: Mental health: New understanding, new hope.* Geneva: World Health Organization; 2001b.

WHO. *Health, economic growth, and poverty reduction: The report of working group 1 of the Commission on Macroeconomics and Health.* Geneva: World Health Organization, Commission on Macroeconomics and Health; 2002.

WHO. *Atlas of child and adolescent mental health resources, global concerns, implications for the future.* Geneva: World Health Organization; 2005a.

WHO. *Atlas: Mental health resources in the world.* Geneva: World Health Organization; 2005b.

WHO. *The economics of mental health in Europe.* Helsinki: WHO European Ministerial Conference on Mental Health; 2005c [accessed January 12, 2010]. Available at http://www.euro.who.int/_data/assets/pdf_file/0008/88595/E85445.pdf.

WHO. World Mental Health Survey Consortium. Prevalence, severity, and unmet need for treatment of mental disorders in the World Health Organization World Mental Health Surveys. *Journal of the American Medical Association* 2004;291: 2581–2590. [PubMed: 15173149]

WHO. *Ten statistical highlights in global public health (Part1): World health statistics.* Geneva: World Health Organization; 2007.

WHO/WONCA. *Integrating mental health into primary care: A global perspective.* Geneva: World Health Organization and World Organization of Family Doctors (WONCA); 2008.

Wittchen HU, Jonsson B, Olesen J. Towards a better understanding of the size and burden and cost of brain disorders in Europe. *European Neuropsychopharmacology* 2005;15(4):355–356. [PubMed: 15916884]

Chapter 12

Incarceration Nation

Health and Welfare in the Prison System in the United States

Martin Donohoe

The mood and temper of the public in regard to the treatment of crime and criminals is one of the most unfailing tests of any country. A calm, dispassionate recognition of the rights of the accused and even of the convicted criminal, ... [and] the treatment of crime and the criminal mark and measure the stored-up strength of a nation, and are the sign and proof of the living virtue within it.

—Winston Churchill[1]

Introduction

This chapter discusses various aspects of the United States' criminal justice system, with particular attention to women when applicable. Topics include the epidemiology of incarceration, juvenile detention, racism, the so-called War on Drugs, the prison-industrial complex, healthcare of prisoners, rehabilitation, and the death penalty. Suggestions for improving the criminal justice system are offered.

Lockdown: Who Are the People Behind Bars in the United States?

More than 2 million people are currently behind bars in the United States, a country that incarcerates almost three quarters of a million individuals and spends $41 billion per year on corrections.[2-4] The number of people under correctional supervision—behind bars, on parole, or on probation—is now 6.5 million, or 1 in every 32 adults.

Jails are correctional facilities housing accused persons awaiting trial or, in some jurisdictions, convicted criminals serving sentences up to 1 year. Most inmates stay for less than 1 month.[5] Prisons are facilities housing convicted inmates for longer sentences. It costs more than $30,000 per year to house a prisoner and up to $70,000 to fund 1 jail spot.[6]

Between 1972 and 2000, the number of people behind bars increased 6-fold.[4] No other Western democratic country has ever imprisoned more of its citizens. The US rate of incarceration is 699/100,000, with Russia's a close second at 644/100,000. Our rate is 6 times higher than those of Britain, Canada, or France.[5] California's prison system is larger than that of France and Germany combined.[7]

Women Behind Bars

US prisons and jails now hold more than 180,000 women—up 750% since 1980.[8,9] The yearly growth rate of women in prison is from 1.5 to 2 times higher than that of men.[6,10] One out of every 109 women in the United States is on parole, probation, or in jail or prison.[11]

Almost 80% of women in state prisons lack a high school degree; 15% were homeless at least once in the year before their arrest; and 65% are mothers of minor children and expect to resume their parenting role upon release from prison.[11]

Women have traditionally suffered disproportionately from biased justice systems throughout the world.[12] In addition to facing economic, social, legal, and political marginalization, as well as various forms of abuse,[13-15] women have been incarcerated and put to death for a variety of dubious reasons. Examples include the witch hunts of Medieval Europe, the Salem Witch Trials of colonial America, and the double standards of Victorian era morality, which supported the criminalization of certain behaviors for women but not for men.[12]

Kids on the (Cell) Block

Juvenile detention facility populations are also burgeoning. Females younger than 18 years represent 26% of juvenile arrests and 14% of those detained in residential facilities.[16]

Overcrowding is rampant in juvenile detention centers. Violence in such facilities injures 2,000 youths each month, and the use of isolation and restraints is not uncommon.[17] Nearly 1,000 incarcerated youths per month commit suicidal acts.[17] Youth crime recidivism rates are as high as 40%.[16]

Recent years have seen a trend toward trying youths in adult courts. Physicians for Human Rights, through its Health and Justice for Youth Campaign, is calling for an end to the transfer of youth to adult court, on the basis of recent neurologic research relevant to moral development and culpability, studies on recidivism in adolescent behavior, and the desirability of rehabilitation in juvenile justice.[18]

Schools or Prisons: Misplaced Priorities

There was a proposition in a township there to discontinue public schools because they were too expensive. An old farmer spoke up and said if they stopped the schools they would not save anything, because every time a school was closed a jail had to be built. It's like feeding a dog on his own tail. He'll never get fat. I believe it is better to support schools than jails.

—Mark Twain[19]

More money is put into prison construction than into schools. That, in itself, is the description of a nation bent on suicide. I mean, what's more precious to us than our children? We're going to build a lot more prisons if we don't deal with the schools and their inequalities.

—Jonathan Kozol[19]

Between 1985 and 2000, state spending on corrections grew at 6 times the rate of state spending on higher education.[20] Declining state support for colleges and universities, combined with rising tuition and fees, puts higher education increasingly out of reach for the middle class and poor, which in turn fuels the cycles of poverty and crime.

Race and Detention

The incarceration rate for African-Americans is 1,815/100,000, compared with 609/100,000 for Latino Americans, 235/100,000 for Caucasian Americans, and 99/100,000 for Asian Americans.[4] From arrest to sentencing, racism pervades the US criminal justice system. A person of color is more likely than a white person to be stopped by the police, to be abused by the police during that stop, to be arrested, to be denied bail, to be charged with a serious crime, to be convicted, and to receive a harsher sentence.[21,22] African American youth are 6 times more likely than whites to be both sentenced and incarcerated, 9 times more likely if charged with a violent crime.[23] The average length of stay for a Latino youth admitted for a drug offense to juvenile facilities is double the length of stay for a white youth.[23] Minority youths are significantly more likely to be sent to adult courts than their white counterparts.[24] In 2002, there were more black men behind bars than in college or university.[4]

"The War on Drugs"

The majority of US detainees are nonviolent offenders, incarcerated as part of the so-called War on Drugs, a multibillion-dollar initiative focused on law enforcement, interdiction, supply reduction, and prohibition,[25] which has been as effective in reducing drug use as the Iraq War has been in reducing terrorism.

The "War on Drugs" has a racist 20th century history, beginning with the "Chinese Opium Act," largely a response to widespread immigration, poverty, and disease among Asian Americans in San Francisco in the early 1900s.[26] The criminalization of marijuana, while arguably successful or necessary, has its origins in fears of Mexican immigrants "going loco."[26]

Although nearly three quarters of illicit drug users are of European American ancestry and only 15% are African American, African Americans make up 37% of those arrested and a disproportionate number of those imprisoned on drug charges.[27] Inequitable sentencing laws exacerbate the disparity between black and white inmates. For example, African American cocaine users tend to use less expensive crack cocaine, whereas whites prefer the powdered form.[4,27] Penalties for crack possession significantly exceed those for powder. Such bias has led critic Mark Crispin Miller to characterize the "War on Drugs" as "a race war waged by legal means."[4]

Between 1986 and 2000, there was a 400% increase in the number of women imprisoned for drug crimes.[28] Women are almost twice as likely as men to be imprisoned for drug-related offenses.[29]

Most Americans favor rehabilitation and alternative sentencing (restitution, community service) over the costly and counterproductive strategy of mass incarceration for drug use and possession. In Arizona, taxpayers saved $2.6 million in the first year after legislation passed mandating drug treatment instead of prison for nonviolent drug offenders.[28] Other alternatives to incarceration of drug abusers include the following:

- Shifting money away from interdiction and military intervention (such as the billions of dollars spent trying to end Columbian cocaine production, which has only fueled civil war and decimated peasants' incomes without offering them assistance producing alternative crops)
- Education and social marketing against substance abuse
- Vaccinations against illegal substances, currently in the theoretical and experimental stages
- Methadone and buprenorphine for opiate detoxification
- Research into other agents to facilitate detoxification and abstinence
- Treating substance abuse as a chronic illness[28]

The interventions available are dollar for dollar much more effective than interdiction and punishment.[28] Furthermore, one must note the irony that, currently, legal, harmful substances such as tobacco and alcohol kill orders of magnitude more individuals than heroin, cocaine, and marijuana combined.

Finally, while we lose $4 billion to burglary and robbery each year, we lose much more than that—an estimated $200 billion—to corporate fraud.[30] Fines for corporate environmental and social abuses are often miniscule and are considered a "cost of doing business" that does not severely impact companies' overall balance sheet.[31,32] Some corporations have been linked directly to human rights abuses, and many heavily lobby Congress to weaken environmental and occupational safety and health standards and to dismantle social legislation designed to protect the public's health.[31]

Prison Life

Prisons: De Facto Mental Institutions

One in 6 US prisoners is mentally ill.[24] Rates are higher among female inmates than among male inmates. Up to 5% of prisoners are actively psychotic at any given time. Ten percent of state inmates receive psychotropic medications.[33] Mental illness is much more common in juvenile than in adult facilities: Between 50% and 75% of incarcerated youth suffer from a mental health disorder.[34]

Prisons, now the primary supplier of mental health services in the United States, house 3 times as many men and women with mental illness as mental hospitals do.[24] The mentally ill are frequently victimized by other prisoners; punished by guards, whose custodial training does not qualify them to recognize and treat symptoms of mental illness; and sometimes housed in solitary confinement, which can exacerbate or cause acute psychosis. In a survey of female jail detainees in a large midwestern city, only one quarter of those who needed mental health services received them while in jail.[35]

The so-called Prison Litigation Reform Act bars lawsuits by inmates seeking damages for mental or emotional injury suffered while in custody when there is no proof of significant injury.[24] Under a federal circuit court ruling which upheld this legislation, inmates cannot sue guards for humiliation, mental torture, or nonphysical sadistic treatment unless, in effect, they have broken bones or blood to show for it. This is one of many ways in which US laws fail to meet standards mandated by the United Nations Convention Against Torture.[24] Recent widespread and credible reports of torture of prisoners by the Central Intelligence Agency and armed forces in the "War on Terror" cannot help but undermine the confidence of those incarcerated within the United States that they will not be subject to similar abuses.[36]

Overcrowding and the Prison-Industrial Complex

> Corporations [have] no moral conscience. [They] are designed by law to be concerned only for their stockholders, and not, say, what are sometimes called their stakeholders, like the community or the work force ...
>
> —Noam Chomsky[37]

As of 2000, 22 states and the federal prison system operated at 100% or more of capacity.[24] Along with the "War on Drugs," other contributors to prison overcrowding include the increasing use of mandatory minimums, repeat offender ("Three Strikes You're Out") laws, truth-in-sentencing regulations, and decreased judicial independence. One in 11 prisoners is now serving a life sentence; one quarter of them have no option of parole.[38]

As a result of overcrowding, and prompted by the often-illusory promises of free-market effectiveness, a private prison boom has occurred over the past 15 years. This development has benefitted from the prevailing political philosophy, which disparages the effectiveness of (and even need for) governmental social programs and touts the efficiencies of private industry, despite evidence to the contrary (for example, overhead for the Medicaid and Medicare programs is dramatically lower than that for private health insurance).

The American Correctional Association is the leading trade group pushing prison privatization. Corrections Corporation of America (CCA), the GEO Group (formerly Wackenhut), Correctional Medical Services, and other for-profit companies (e.g., Westinghouse, AT&T, Sprint, MCI, Smith Barney, American Express, and General Electric)[39] have aggressively marketed themselves to state and local governments, primarily in rural areas, promising jobs and new income for impoverished communities.[39] As they do for other industries, these governments offer tax breaks, subsidies, and infrastructure assistance.

Rural communities, eager for outside investment in the face of declines in logging, farming, mining, and manufacturing, are enticed by the promise of new jobs and profits to be re-invested in the community. Such promises often prove ephemeral, even misleading. A 2001 study by the Bureau of Justice Assistance found that rather than the projected 20% savings, the average savings from prison privatization was only 1%.[8,40,41] This estimate did not take into account the hidden monetary subsidies provided by communities, nor the fact that often so-called savings result from private prisons selecting the least costly inmates.[8,40,41] Private prison guards are paid significantly less than those in public prisons, and job turnover exceeds 50% (vs. 16% per year in public prisons).[8,40,41] Newly built prisons tend to attract large-scale national chain stores such as Walmart, which prompts the demise of locally controlled enterprises and shifts locally generated tax revenues to distant corporate coffers.[4]

The private prison industry is well connected in Washington, DC, having donated $1.12 million to 830 candidates in the 2000 elections.[8] The recently indicted former House speaker Tom Delay's (R–TX) Foundation for Kids accepted a $100,000 donation from CCA last year.[40] His brother Randy has lobbied the Texas Bureau of Prisons to send its prisoners to GEO's new Reeves County Detention Facility (a Reeves county judge is facing a lawsuit over his role in allowing the joint venture between GEO and Reeves County to go forward).[40]

Jails and Faith-Based Initiatives

A parallel development in the privatization of prison services has been the increasing presence of politically powerful faith-based prisoner management companies.[2] Supported by corrections budgets under President George W. Bush's Faith-Based Initiatives Program, these predominantly evangelical Christian groups include Prison Fellowship Ministries, founded in 1976 by Charles Colson, who served time for his role in the Watergate affair.[42] These programs offer perks ranging from better cell location to job training and post-release placement in exchange for participation in prayer groups, courses in "creationism," and even "conversion therapy" for homosexuals. It is unclear how many prisoners signing up for these programs are sincere in their desire to "find Christ," as opposed to merely seeking improved living conditions, fellowship, and enhanced options for housing and job placement after discharge.[42]

Some programs promise to "cure" sex offenders through prayer and Bible study and substitute for evidence-based programs that employ aversion therapy and normative counseling. Highly recidivist and dangerous criminals may be released back into society armed with little more than polemics about sin.[42]

Prison Labor

Prison labor can provide inmates with the means to accrue money, albeit at a very low salary, to support them after release. As of late 2001, almost 4,000 inmates in 36 states were working in private sector companies, and an additional 23,000 federal prisoners were working for Federal Prison Industries in various production and service capacities.[41] Federal wages average 92 cents per hour; state wages range from 23 cents to 7 dollars per hour. Prisoners keep 20%, with the rest going to restitution, to offset incarceration, and to support their families.[41] The 80% spent on such deserving sources is laudable, yet prisoners' low pay means that upon release most have few financial resources, making crime an attractive or desperate option. Objections to prison labor include the undercutting of unions and the shift of manufacturing and service jobs from the law-abiding poor to the incarcerated. Such a shift has also occurred with the exodus of jobs with US companies to prisons in Mexico or China (and other countries known for human rights abuses), despite laws that ban the importation of goods made by prison laborers.[43]

Health Issues of Prisoners

According to 1997 Bureau of Justice statistics, almost one third of state and one quarter of federal inmates surveyed had a physical impairment or mental condition.[33] These percentages likely represent underestimates. Fifty-two percent of state and 34% of federal inmates were under the influence of alcohol or other drugs at the time of their offenses.[33] Although rates of alcohol and opiate dependency among arrestees are approximately 12% and 4%, only 28% of jail administrators report that their institutions had ever detoxified arrestees.[44]

Health problems commonly encountered in adults of both sexes include dental caries and periodontal disease, tuberculosis (including multidrug-resistant tuberculosis), hepatitis B and C, human T lymphotropic virus types I and II, and sexually transmitted diseases such as gonorrhea, chlamydia, syphilis, and human papillomavirus infection (which can lead to cervical cancer).[45]

Women and men in correctional facilities face 5-fold higher rates of HIV infection than those in the general population.[46] In a reverse of what is seen outside prison walls, infection rates for women exceed those of men, 3.5% to 2.2%.[47] Rates of hepatitis C are 9 to 10 times higher in inmates than among the general population.[48]

Imprisoned women are a high-risk obstetric population. They are more likely than nonincarcerated women to smoke, abuse alcohol and illegal drugs, and have medical comorbidities, yet less likely to have received antenatal care.[49] Incarceration is associated with increased odds of low birth weight and preterm birth for women younger than 40.[50] Adolescents are particularly vulnerable: only one third of juvenile correctional facilities provide prenatal services; a mere 30% provide parenting classes.[16] Given their age, education, income prospects, and inexperience in parenting, those who gain custody of their children post-discharge are at risk for abuse and neglect.

Unfortunately, prison gynecologic care is often treated as a specialty service, leaving it more vulnerable than other primary care services to budget cuts.[8] And while post-discharge maternity case management can offset obstetric risks for women released before their due dates, such programs, when they exist, are underfunded.[50]

Healthcare

A society should be judged not by how it treats its outstanding citizens but by how it treats its criminals.

—Fyodor Dostoevsky[19]

In the early 1970s, fewer than 30% of US jails had medical facilities and only about 1 in 5 had a formal arrangement with any medical provider.[51] In *Estelle* v. *Gamble* (1976), the Supreme Court affirmed an inmate's constitutional right to medical care, citing the Constitution's Eighth Amendment prohibition of cruel and unusual punishment.[45] Nevertheless, in 1999, Amnesty International found that prison healthcare was woefully substandard, reporting that women inmates suffered from neglect manifested by a failure to refer seriously ill inmates for treatment and by a lack of qualified personnel, healthcare resources, and appropriate mental healthcare.[52] Today, many institutions remain noncompliant with the American Medical Association's standards for healthcare of the incarcerated, which include regularly scheduled sick calls, an initial medical screening, and ongoing medical, dental, and psychiatric care.[53]

Today, 40% of inmate care (in 34 states) is provided by private corporations, the remaining 60% by government entities.[8,51] The quality of healthcare provided by private corporations is often substandard and shoddy. Correctional Medical Services, the nation's largest (and cheapest) provider of prison medicine, has been the subject of investigations and lawsuits for negligent and incompetent care and for trying to cut costs by transferring its sickest patients to state facilities (commonly referred to as "patient dumping").[8,51] Despite receiving more than half a billion dollars in taxpayer money per year, the company has refused to account for how that money is spent and how much is gleaned off the top for profit.[51] A recent evaluation by the New York State Commission on Corrections found a pattern of medical negligence in the "care" provided by for-profit Prison Health Services, which resulted in several deaths.[51] As of late 2004, Prison Health Services was defending itself against more than 1,000 lawsuits.[8]

Although on the whole, privatized prison healthcare is worse than government-sponsored care, some states' systems reach appalling nadirs. A federal judge recently placed California's prison healthcare system into receivership, citing an "unconscionable degree of suffering and death" in the state's 33 lockups, which resulted in almost 1 needless death per day.[53] These deaths, as well as much unnecessary suffering, have no doubt been facilitated by California's requirement that inmates must make co-payments of $5 per visit, a deterrent to all but the most critically ill.[8]

Some states have developed formal relationships with academic medical centers, resulting in the development of specialized treatment programs and improved health outcomes.[54,55,56] Many institutions have also begun to incorporate hospice and palliative medicine programs[57] in response to the aging prison population, which in turn is a consequence of an aging population and longer sentences.

Abuse of Female Prisoners

Ninety-two percent of girls entering the juvenile justice system have been subjected to prior emotional, physical, or sexual abuse, and 40% have been raped.[58] At least 1 in 5 women on death row has been assaulted or sexually harassed while in prison, and a third of them report that corrections officers observed them when they used the toilet, showered, or dressed.[59] Despite laws prohibiting sexual abuse against women by correctional officers, rape and abuse of women prisoners is rampant and often occurs with impunity.[3,8] Perpetrators seldom face charges. Correctional authorities tend to deny the seriousness of the problem. It has become more difficult for prisoners subjected to sexual harassment to seek redress since the 1996 passage of the so-called Prison Litigation Reform Act.[59]

Rehabilitation and Release

Each year, more than 600,000 prisoners are released from prison, 4 times as many as were released in 1980.[60] Unfortunately, in the 1990s, funding for rehabilitation was dramatically cut, reducing inmates' access to drug treatment, education, and job training programs. Meanwhile, newly released and paroled convicts face restrictions on their ability to get federally subsidized housing, welfare, and healthcare. Many lack job prospects, a function of limited resumés and the enhanced feasibility of background searches facilitated by improved technology. More than 60% of employers would not knowingly hire an ex-offender,[4] which is understandable given the lack of funding for education and job-skills training behind bars and high rates of criminal recidivism.

Although many children may be better off not reuniting with their now-released mothers, numerous barriers to family reunification exist for those willing women capable of resuming their maternal roles. These include reunification timelines that enable states to begin proceedings to terminate parental rights if a child has been in foster care for 15 out of the last 22 months; lack of contact with children, who often live many miles away; lack of affordable child care; and restrictions on public assistance after release for certain offenders.[11]

Only Maine, Massachusetts, Utah, and Vermont allow prisoners to vote.[61] Eleven states have lifetime bans on ex-felons voting, despite recommendations from the National Commission on Federal Election Reform, led by former presidents Gerald Ford and Jimmy Carter, that all states let former felons vote.[59,60] Thirteen percent of black men do not possess the right to vote.[62] Some have argued that the disenfranchisement of black ex-felons in Florida, accompanied by overly aggressive purging of voter rolls by election officials (e.g., the elimination of all voters with names that matched those of ex-felons, with an over-representation of "typical African-American names"), led to the slim victory of George W. Bush over Al Gore in the 2000 election.[63]

The Death Penalty

> When in *Gregg* v. *Georgia* the Supreme Court gave its seal of approval to capital punishment, this endorsement was premised on the promise that capital punishment would be administered with fairness and justice. Instead, the promise has become a cruel and empty mockery. If not remedied, the scandalous state of our present system of capital punishment will cast a pall of shame over our society for years to come. We cannot let it continue.
>
> —Justice Thurgood Marshall, 1990[64]

> As one whose husband and mother-in-law have died the victims of murder assassination, I stand firmly and unequivocally opposed to the death penalty for those convicted of capital offenses. An evil deed is not redeemed by an evil deed of retaliation. Justice is never advanced in the taking of a human life. Morality is never upheld by a legalized murder.
>
> —Coretta Scott King[64]

The Death Penalty: Methods of Execution

Throughout history, convicted (and often suspected) criminals have been executed. Hanging, shooting by firing squad, and the guillotine were predominant modes of execution until the early 1880s, when the electric chair was developed by dentist Alfred Southwick.[65] New York became the first state to adopt the electric chair, thanks in part to the aggressive lobbying of Thomas Edison, who tried to use features of the device to secure a bigger share of the electricity market from his competitor, George Westinghouse.[66] Over the next half century, other states followed New York and began to use the electric chair.

After its first use by the state of Texas in 1982, lethal injection increased rapidly in popularity. Developed by University of Oklahoma anesthesiologist Stanley Deutsch as an ideal (and inexpensive) way to bring about a speedy and "extremely humane" demise,[67] it is now the predominant mode of execution.[65] Most states use a "death cocktail" of the anesthetic sodium thiopental, followed by the paralytic agent pancuronium bromide, followed by potassium chloride to stop the heart.[68] Ironically, the American Veterinary Medical Association and 19 states, including Texas, prohibit the use of neuromuscular blocking agents such as pancuronium to kill animals, since the drug does not inhibit awareness (although phenobarbital does).[68] The National Coalition to Abolish the Death Penalty has called upon every manufacturer and distributor of the drugs used in lethal injection to publicly condemn and prohibit the use of their products in executions and to allow independent monitoring of compliance.[70]

Although a popular misconception, to the contrary, execution by electrocution or lethal injection is not humane. For instance, the Georgia Supreme

Court declared in 2001 that the electric chair, "with its specter of excruciating pain and its certainty of cooked brains and blistered bodies," violated the prohibition against cruel and unusual punishment.[71] In one study of 49 inmates executed by lethal injection in 4 states, 43 showed levels of anesthetic lower than that required for surgery, and 21 had concentrations consistent with awareness.[69]

The Death Penalty: Law and Epidemiology

In 1972, the US Supreme Court (*Furman* v. *Georgia*) temporarily halted executions. States rewrote their death penalty laws, and 4 years later the Supreme Court ruled that these new laws were constitutional (*Gregg* v. *Georgia*).[72] As of November 29, 2005, 38 states had laws allowing capital punishment.[73]

Since 1976, 32 states have carried out 1,000 executions. Texas leads all other states by a wide margin. Former governor (now President) George W. Bush presided over a record 152 executions. Despite the fact that a third of the inmates executed under him were represented by lawyers who were sanctioned at some time for misconduct, Bush has claimed repeatedly that the death penalty is infallible.[21,74,75]

There are currently approximately 50 women (out of 3,500 people) on death row.[59] Ten out of approximately 150 women sentenced to death since 1976 have been executed.[59] Women on death row tend to have strong histories of physical and sexual victimization and substance abuse. Because of their small numbers, they are often effectively kept in isolation. Many are denied access to religious and other prison services, despite the purported safeguards of the Religious Land Use and Institutionalized Persons Act of 2000.[59]

Only a small fraction of death row inmates are ever actually executed. Life expectancy on death row is 13 years.[76] Since 1976, an estimated collective extra $1 billion has been spent to implement the death penalty in the 38 states that have it.[77] As with other aspects of the criminal justice system, racism plays a significant role in capital punishment, with those killing a white person much more likely to be sentenced to death than those killing an individual of a racial minority.[21] Furthermore, extensive criminological data agree that the death penalty is not a deterrent to violent crime and that in fact, in some cases, it may even be an incitement.[78]

The Death Penalty: Errors, Exonerations, and Public Opinion

Serious constitutional errors mar about two thirds of state and federal capital cases, such as ineffective assistance of defense counsel (including unqualified, underqualified, and even sleeping attorneys), prosecutorial misconduct, and improper jury instructions.[79,80]

Since 1973, more than 120 people have been released from death row with evidence of their innocence.[73] Due to the work of The Innocence Project[81] and others, DNA evidence has increasingly been used to exonerate the unjustly accused.[2] The Justice for All Act of 2004 grants any inmate convicted of a federal crime the right to petition a federal court for DNA testing to support a claim of innocence and increases the financial compensation due wrongfully convicted federal prisoners.[2] However, some states not only lack such a safeguard, but in fact are trying to remove convicted defendants' rights to petition for post-conviction DNA testing.[82,83] Provisions of recent "anti-terrorism" legislation also limit the rights of those accused and/or convicted of capital crimes, including rights of appeal.

False confessions of men and women sentenced to death are surprisingly common. They can occur as a result of coercion, exhaustion, or mental impairment.[84] Almost one quarter of those eventually cleared by DNA testing confessed to police.[84,85] False confessions can be discouraged by more open interrogation procedures, which could also save money by decreasing the costs of appeals. Currently only Alaska, Illinois, Maine, and Minnesota require the videotaping of every interrogation and confession.[84,86]

Public opinion in favor of the death penalty has been waning, down from 80% in 1994 to 64% in 2005 (50% when the choice of life without parole is presented as an alternate sentencing option).[73] Despite such majority support, 80% of Americans feel that innocent people have been executed in the past 5 years.[87]

Illinois and Maryland have called for a halt to executions, and 3 major cities (Philadelphia, Pittsburgh, and San Francisco) have called for a moratorium on capital punishment.[88] In 1997, the American Bar Association called for an immediate halt to executions. Every year since 1997, the United Nations Commission on Human Rights has passed a resolution calling on countries that have not abolished the death penalty to establish a moratorium on executions.[89] Amnesty International and Human Rights Watch have also called for an end to the death penalty.

The Death Penalty: Special Populations

Between 2002 and March 1, 2005, when the US Supreme Court (*Roper* v. *Simmons*) struck down the constitutionality of the death penalty for youths younger than 18 at the time of the crime, the United States was the only country to legally and openly execute a juvenile defendant.[90,91] *Roper* v. *Simmons* brings the United States into line with 7 international treaties that prohibit the execution of juveniles, including the Convention on the Rights of the Child (which the United States has not signed).[90]

There are currently 2,225 people in the United States sentenced to life in prison without parole for crimes they committed as children, in violation of the

Convention on the Rights of the Child.[92] Blacks are 10 times more likely than whites to receive this sentence.[92] At least 132 nations outlaw life sentences without parole for juvenile defendants.[92]

From 1976 to 2002, when the Supreme Court ruled unconstitutional their execution (*Atkins* v. *Virginia*), the United States executed at least 34 mentally retarded individuals.[93] The Court, in *Ford* v. *Wainwright* (1986), has also barred the execution of prisoners who are too mentally ill to understand that they are going to die, although only Louisiana prevents the state from forcing antipsychotic drugs on a prisoner to make him or her sane enough to execute.[72]

The Death Penalty and Health Professionals

Despite the opposition of the American Medical Association, the American Public Health Association, and the American Nurses Association to the participation of health professionals in executions, in 2001 a disappointing 3% of randomly selected physicians were aware of AMA guidelines prohibiting their participation in executions, and 41% indicated that they would perform at least 1 action in the process of lethal injection for capital punishment disallowed by the AMA.[94]

Conclusions

It is troubling that the United States, the world's wealthiest nation, incarcerates a greater percentage of its citizens than any other country; has a criminal justice system marred by racism and substandard healthcare; until recently executed juveniles and the mentally retarded; and continues to execute adults, placing it in the company of states known for human rights abuses, such as China, Iran, and Saudi Arabia.[95]

We have locked up drug users with more hardened criminals in overcrowded institutions, creating ideal conditions for the nurturing and mentoring of more dangerous criminals. We have prioritized punishment over rehabilitation, releasing ex-cons without the necessary skills to maintain abstinence from drugs, with financial and employment prospects that make returning to a life of crime an attractive or desperate survival option. It is shameful that as the richest country on earth, which loudly proclaims to be the planet's greatest democracy, we have failed to develop a criminal justice system that is fair and just and one that would actually lower crime and make us all more safe. Instead, like so many other social services, we have turned over significant portions of the criminal justice system to enterprises that value profit over human dignity and development and community improvement.

Nicholas Freudenberg[10] has recommended a series of public policy goals that would reduce the adverse health effects of incarceration and facilitate the re-entry of prisoners into society. They are the following: improved quality of health, mental health, and substance abuse services in correctional facilities, and the development of gender-specific programs; improved discharge planning and linkages with community service providers; expanded and improved vocational and employment programs for inmates and ex-offenders; and reduced stigmatization of ex-offenders. Along with increased alternatives to incarceration, achievement of these aims would reduce drug use and criminal recidivism, improve the healthcare of ex-offenders and of the general public (e.g., through decreased transmission of infectious diseases and fewer acts of violence by the intoxicated or untreated mentally ill), improve family and societal cohesion, and save money.

To Freudenberg's suggestions, I would add that health professionals need to pay greater attention to the social ills that foster substance abuse and other crimes, particularly the growing chasm between the rich and poor, the haves and the have-nots. We all share the responsibility to hold our government accountable for creating a fair system of justice that combines reasonable punishment with restitution and the smooth re-entry of rehabilitated criminals into society.

Notes

1. Southern Center for Human Rights homepage. Available at http://www.schr.org/. Accessed January 11, 2006.

2. Rothstein MA. Genetic justice. *N Engl J Med.* 2005;352:2667–2668. Abstract.

3. US: Number of Aging Prisoners Soaring—Corrections Officials Ill-Prepared to Run Geriatric Facilities. *Human Rights Watch,* 2012. http://www.hrw.org/news/2012/01/26/us-number-aging-prisoners-soaring.

4. Street P. Race, place, and the perils of prisonomics. *Z Magazine* 2005;July/August:80–85.

5. Beck A J, Karberg, J C (2001). *Prison and jail inmates at midyear 2000.* 2001. Washington, DC: US Department of Justice. http://www.ojp.usdoj.gov/bjs/pubalp2.htm. Accessed January 11, 2006.

6. Women's Prison Association (WPA). *WPA focus on women and justice.* 2003; August. Available at http://www.wpaonline.org/pdf/Focus_August2003.pdf. Accessed January 11, 2006.

7. Roosevelt M. Bizarre, draconian and disproportionate? *Time* 2002;November 11:65–66.

8. Thayer L. Hidden hell: Women in prison. *Amnesty Now* (Amnesty International). 2004;Fall:10–13.

9. DeGroot AS. HIV infection among incarcerated women: Epidemic behind bars. *AIDS Reader* 2000;10:287–295. Abstract.

10. Freudenberg N. Adverse effects of US jail and prison policies on the health and well-being of women of color. *Am J Public Health* 2002;92:1895–1899. Abstract.

11. Women's Prison Association. *WPA focus on women and justice: Barriers to reentry.* 2003;October. Available at http://www.wpaonline.org/pdf/Focus_October2003 .pdf. Accessed January 11, 2006.

12. Kurshan N. *Women and imprisonment in the US: History and current reality.* Available at http://prisonactivist.org/women/women-and-imprisonment.html. Accessed January 11, 2006.

13. Donohoe MT. Individual and societal forms of violence against women in the United States and the developing world: An overview. *Curr Womens Health Rep.* 2002;2:313–319. Abstract.

14. Donohoe MT. Violence against women: Partner abuse and sexual assault. *Hospital Physician* 2004;40:24–31.

15. Donohoe MT. Violence and human rights abuses against women in the developing world. *Medscape Ob/Gyn and Women's Health* 2003;8(2). Posted November 26, 2003. Available at http://www.medscape.com/viewarticle/464255.

16. Committee on Adolescence, American Academy of Pediatrics. Health care for children and adolescents in the juvenile correctional care system. *Pediatrics* 2001;107:799–803. Abstract.

17. Physicians for Human Rights. *Health and justice for youth campaign: Unhealthy and inappropriate facilities.* Available at http://www.phrusa.org/campaigns/juv _justice/conditions.html. Accessed January 11, 2006.

18. Physicians for Human Rights. *Health and justice for youth campaign: Juveniles in adult prisons.* Available at http://www.phrusa.org/campaigns/juv_justice /adult.html. Accessed January 11, 2006.

19. WriteAPrisoner.com homepage. Available at http://writeaprisoner.com/prison-quotes.htm. Accessed January 11, 2006.

20. Ambrosio TJ, Schiraldi V (Justice Policy Institute). *From classrooms to cell blocks: A national perspective.* Available at http://www.justicepolicy.org/article.php?id=40. Accessed January 11, 2006.

21. Bright SB. Will the death penalty remain alive in the twenty-first century? International norms, discrimination, arbitrariness and the risk of executing the innocent. *Wisconsin Law Rev.* 2001;1:1–33.

22. Sikora AG, Mulvihill M. Trends in mortality due to legal intervention in the United States, 1979–1997. *Am J Public Health* 2002;92:841–843. Abstract.

23. Physicians for Human Rights. *Health and justice for youth campaign: Juveniles in Adult prisons.* Available at http://www.phrusa.org//campaigns/juv _justice/race.html. Accessed January 11, 2006.

24. Human Rights Watch. *Ill-equipped: US prisons and offenders with mental illness.* Available at http://www .hrw.org/reports/2003/usa1003/. Accessed January 11, 2006.

25. Davies R. Prison's second death row. *Lancet* 2004;364:317–318. Abstract.

26. Kraut A. *Silent travelers: Germs, genes and the immigrant menace.* Baltimore: Johns Hopkins Press; 1994.

27. Human Rights Watch. *Incarcerated America.* 2003; April. Available at http://www .hrw.org/backgrounder/usa/incarceration/us042903.pdf. Accessed January 11, 2006.

28. Women's Prison Association. *Focus on women and justice: Trends in sentencing.* Available at http://www.wpaonline.org/pdf/Focus_Trends_May2004.pdf. Accessed January 11, 2006.

29. Marshall MF. Health care for incarcerated women. Letter from the president column. ASBH (American Society of Bioethics and Humanities) *Exchange* 1999;Winter:2,8.

30. Bartlett DL, Steele JB. Corporate welfare. *Time* 1998;November 9:36–79.

31. Chernoff PA. Sentencing environmental offenders. *PSR Quarterly* 1993;3:183–186.

32. Donohoe MT. Causes and health consequences of environmental degradation and social injustice. *Soc Sci Med.* 2003;56:573–587. Abstract.

33. Kendig NE. Correctional health care systems and collaboration with academic medicine. *JAMA.* 2004;292:501–503. Abstract.

34. Physicians for Human Rights, Health and Justice for Youth Campaign. The "criminalization" of mental health problems. Available at http://www .phrusa.org/campaigns/juv_justice/mental.html. Accessed January 11, 2006.

35. Teplin A, Abram K, McClelland GM. Mentally disordered women in jail: Who receives services? *Am J Public Health* 1997;87:604–609.

36. Priest D. CIA holds terror suspects in secret prisons. *Washington Post* 2005; November 2. Available at http://www.washingtonpost.com/wp-dyn/content /article/2005/11/01/AR2005110101644_pf.html. Accessed January 11, 2006.

37. The Internet Movie Database. *Memorable quotes from* The Corporation. Available at http://www.imdb.com/title/tt0379225/quotes. Accessed January 11, 2006.

38. Mauer M, King RS, Young MC. *The meaning of life: Long-term prison sentences in context.* The Sentencing Project. 2004;May. Available at http://www.sentencingproject.org/pubs_06.cfm. Accessed January 11, 2006.

39. Cottin H. US substitutes jails for schools. *Workers World.* Available at http:// www.workers.org/ww/2002/prisons0912.php. Accessed January 11, 2006. Talvi SJA. Cashing in on the cons: Undercover at the American Correctional Association's 2005 Winter Conference. *In These Times* 2005;February 4. Available at http:// www.inthesetimes.com/site/main/article/1924/. Accessed January 11, 2006.

40. Singleton L. Felons: The American worker's newest competitor. *The ultimate field guide to the US economy.* Available at http://www.fguide.org/Bulletin/prislabr.htm. Accessed January 11, 2006.

41. Shapiro SM. Jails for Jesus. *Mother Jones* 2003;November/December:55–59, 98–99.

42. Watson J. Prison products sold in the US *The Oregonian* 2002;December 4:A8.

43. Fiscella K, Pless N, Meldrum S, Fircella P. Alcohol and opiate withdrawal in US jails. *Am J Public Health* 2004;94:1522–1524. Abstract.

44. Glaser JB, Greifinger RB. Correctional health care: A public health opportunity. *Ann Intern Med.* 1993;118:139–145. Abstract.

45. McClelland GM, Teplin LA, Abram KM, Jacobs N. HIV and AIDS risk behaviors among female jail detainees: Implications for public health policy. *Am J Public Health* 2002;92:818–825. Abstract.

46. Spaulding A, Stephenson B, Macalino G, Ruby W, Clarke JG, Flanigan TP. Human immunodeficiency virus in correctional facilities: A review. *Clin Infect Dis.* 2002;35:305–312. Abstract.

47. Voelker R. New initiatives target inmates' health. *JAMA.* 2004;291(13):1549–1551.

48. Knight M, Plugge E. Risk factors for adverse perinatal outcomes in imprisoned pregnant women: A systematic review. *BMC Public Health* 2005;5:111.

49. Bell JF, Zimmerman FJ, Cawthon ML, et al. Jail incarceration and birth outcomes. *J Urban Health: Bull NY Acad Med.* 2004;81:630–644.

50. Hylan WS. Sick on the inside: Correctional HMOs and the coming prison plague. *Harper's Magazine* 2003;August:44–54.

51. Amnesty International. *"Not my sentence": Violations of the human rights of women in custody.* 1999. Available at http://web.amnesty.org/library/Index/ENGAMR510191999?open&of=ENG-USA. Accessed January 11, 2006. As cited in Reviere R, Young VD. Aging behind bars: Health care for older female inmates. *J Women Aging* 2004;16:55–69.

52. Council on Scientific Affairs, American Medical Association. Health status of detained and incarcerated youths. *JAMA.* 1990;263:987–991. Abstract.

53. von Zielbauer P. Private health care in jails can be a death sentence. *New York Times* 2005; February 27. Reprinted at Common Dreams News Center. Available at http://www.commondreams.org/headlines05/0227-02.htm. Accessed January 11, 2006.

54. Raimer BG, Stobo JD. Health care delivery in the Texas prison system: The role of academic medicine. *JAMA.* 2004;(292):485–489. Abstract.

55. Applebaum KL, Manning TD, Noonan JD. A university-state-corporation partnership for providing correctional mental health services. *Psychiatric Services* 2002;53:185–189. Abstract.

56. Craig EL, Craig RE. Prison hospice: An unlikely success. *Am J Hosp Palliat Care* 1999;16:725–729. Abstract.

57. Physicians for Human Rights, Health and Justice for Youth Campaign. *Girls in the system.* Available at http://www.phrusa.org/campaigns/juv_justice/girls.html. Accessed January 11, 2006.

58. American Civil Liberties Union and American Friends Service Committee. *The forgotten population: A look at death row in the United States through the experiences of women.* 2004; December. Available at http://www.afsc.org/forgotten-population/forgotten-population.pdf. Accessed January 11, 2006.

59. Ripley A. Outside the gates. *Time* 2002;January 21:56–63.

60. The Sentencing Project. *Felony disenfranchisement in the United States.* 2005. Available at http://www.sentencingproject.org/losing_03.cfm. Accessed January 11, 2006.

61. Street P. Dark connections: Empire abroad, prisons at home. *Z Magazine* 2003;January:41–45.

62. Palast G. *The best democracy money can buy.* London: Penguin Books; 2003.

63. Death penalty quotes. Available at http://www.geocities.com/aboaev/quotes /dp.html. Accessed January 11, 2006.

64. Staff. Pulling the plug on the electric chair. *Mother Jones* 2000;May/June:27.

65. Aaron C. Death is different. *In These Times* 2002;September 13.

66. Groner JI. Lethal injection: A stain on the face of medicine. *BMJ.* 2002;325:1026–1028. Abstract.

67. Brauchli C. Inhumane drug used in many executions. Common Dreams News Center. October 18, 2003. Available at http://www.commondreams.org/views03 /1018-05.htm. Accessed January 11, 2006.

68. Staff. Medical collusion in the death penalty: An American atrocity. *Lancet* 2005;356:1361.

69. Staff. *Drug companies and their role in aiding executions.* National Coalition to Abolish the Death Penalty, 2002. Available at http://www.ncadp.org/assets /applets/report.pdf. Accessed January 11, 2006.

70. *Dawson* v. *The State of Georgia and Moore* v. *The State of Georgia.* Available at http://www.soundportraits.org/data/on-air/ga_decision.pdf. Accessed January 11, 2006.

71. Silverstein K. By reason of insanity. *Mother Jones* 2001;September/October:26–31.

72. Death Penalty Information Center. *Facts about the death penalty.* November 29, 2005. Available at http://www.deathpenaltyinfo.org/FactSheet.pdf. Accessed January 11, 2006.

73. Hightower J. George W Bush's deadly absolutism. *Hightower Lowdown* 2000;2:4.

74. Carlson M. Why this test helps Bush. *Time* 2000;June 11:34.

75. Appel JM. Wanted dead or alive? Kidney transplantation in inmates awaiting execution. *J Clin Ethics* 2005;Spring:58–60.

76. Warshaw A. *Gulf War veteran explains his opposition to the death penalty.* The Moratorium Campaign. 2003;Winter/Spring:15.

77. American Civil Liberties Union. *The case against the death penalty.* Available at http://sun.soci.niu.edu/~critcrim/dp/dppapers/aclu.antidp. Accessed January 11, 2006.

78. Liebman JS, Fagan J. *A broken system: Error rates in capital cases, 1973–1995.* Available at http://www2.law.columbia.edu/instructionalservices/liebman/. Accessed January 11, 2006.

79. Liebman JS, Fagan J, Gelman, et al. *A broken system, Part II: Why there is so much error in capital cases, and what can be done about it.* Available at

http://www2.law.columbia.edu/brokensystem2/index2.html. Accessed January 11, 2006.

80. The Innocence Project. Available at http://www.innocenceproject.org/. Accessed January 11, 2006.

81. Ripley A. After the exoneration. *Time* 2000;December 11:96.

82. Neuman C. Why DNA exonerations may get rarer. *Time* 2005;Oct 2:22.

83. Bennett B. True confessions? *Time* 2005;December 12:45–46.

84. Tyre P. Reversing the verdict. *Newsweek* 2002;December 10:56–58.

85. Dobb E. False confessions: Scaring suspects. *Amnesty Now* 2002;Winter:6–9,28.

86. Novak V. A change in the weather on the way? *Time* 2001;May 21:40.

87. Staff, Equal Justice USA. Four major cities urge moratorium. *Moratorium News* 2000;Spring:1.

88. Amnesty International Staff. *The death penalty.* Available at http://web.amnesty.org/pages/deathpenalty-index-eng. Accessed January 11, 2006.

89. Zissis C. Spare the child. *Amnesty International* 2004;Winter:5.

90. Physicians for Human Rights. Health and Justice for Youth Campaign. *The juvenile death penalty.* Available at http://www.phrusa.org/campaigns/juv_justice/death_pen.html. Accessed January 11, 2006.

91. Staff. End juvenile life without parole. *Amnesty International* 2005;Winter:21.

92. Execution Database, Death Penalty Information Center. Available at http://www.deathpenaltyinfo.org/getexecdata.php. Accessed January 11, 2006.

93. Farber NJ, Aboff BM, Weiner J, et al. Physicians' willingness to participate in the process of lethal injection for capital punishment. *Ann Intern Med.* 2001;135:884–888. Abstract.

94. Amnesty International. *Executions around the world, 2004.* Available at http://www.deathpenaltyinfo.org/article.php?did=127&scid=30#interexec. Accessed January 11, 2006.

95. The death penalty: An international perspective, 2004. Available at interexechttp://www.deathpenaltyinfo.org/article.php?did=127&scid=30#interexec. Accessed 12/9/05.

Part Three

Women's Health

Throughout most of recorded history, women have been subjugated by men, confined to home and hearth, where despite limited opportunities for public advancement, they have provided child care and promoted community cohesiveness, essential functions for public health.

The United States' Declaration of Independence of 1776 states that "all men are created equal, that they are endowed by their creator with certain unalienable rights, that these are life, liberty, and the pursuit of happiness." This nation's founding document excluded women from such rights. A few years after this document's signing, the French Revolution culminated in the French Assembly's Declaration of the Rights of Man and Citizen (of 1789), calling similar rights "self-evident and unalienable." Two years later French playwright, feminist, and anti-slavery activist Olympe de Gouges wrote, in the Declaration of the Rights of Women and the Female Citizen, "Woman is born free and lives equal to Man in her rights." For her brazen proclamation, she was executed.

The 1848 Declaration of Sentiments from the Seneca Falls Convention, which marked the beginning of the women's rights movement in the United States, was a plea for the end of discrimination against women in all spheres of society, including allowing full suffrage. Susan B. Anthony and Elizabeth Cady Stanton, mothers of this movement, were followed by Margaret Sanger, who introduced birth control in 1916. Four years later, the ratification of the Nineteenth Amendment to the US Constitution gave women the right to vote. In 1923, the National Woman's Party proposed an equal rights amendment to the Constitution, an updated version of which passed Congress in 1972 but which failed to achieve ratification by two-thirds of the states by the 1982 deadline.

Despite this setback, women struggled to achieve significant gains in the twentieth century, including the passage of Title VII of the Civil Rights Act of 1964, which prohibited employment discrimination on the basis of race, color, religion, national origin, or sex; and Title IX of the Education Amendments, which prohibits sex discrimination in all aspects of education programs that receive federal support (expanded by the Supreme Court in 1997 to include athletic programs). In 1975 the Supreme Court denied states the right to exclude women from juries and two years later opened the draft to women. Today, more than 210,000 women are actively serving in the US military, and one out of every seven soldiers serving in the wars in Iraq and Afghanistan is a woman.

In 1960, the first oral contraceptive was approved by the Food and Drug Administration, giving women control over their reproductive capacities, and as a result increasing their educational and career opportunities. In the 1973 landmark *Roe* v. *Wade* case, the Supreme Court declared that the US Constitution protects a woman's right to terminate an early pregnancy, enhancing women's reproductive freedom. Women's freedom has also been advanced through court decisions enforcing sexual harassment statutes, opening previously all-male clubs to their membership, and through laws such as the Violence Against Women Act and the Family and Medical Leave Act.

Women have made tremendous strides in education. Today, over one-half of students receiving bachelor's degrees and almost one-half of entering medical students are female.[1] Nevertheless, women are still paid about 77 cents on the dollar compared with men working similar jobs,[2] they provide the bulk of child care and do the majority of cooking and cleaning, and their hard-won reproductive freedoms are under assault by well-funded conservative and religious groups.

Worldwide, women suffer even greater hardships, including impaired access to reproductive health care and political, legal, educational, economic, and social marginalization. Lack of access to quality education, when combined with inadequate contraception, leads to higher rates of pregnancy and childbirth and fewer opportunities for economic advancement. Many women suffer painfully destructive genital-cutting procedures and some are put to death for crimes such as adultery. Men continue to dominate politics in the United States and abroad, creating and enforcing laws that prevent women from enjoying the rights granted them in the United Nations' Universal Declaration of Human Rights.

Women's marginalization has important effects on public health, some of which are discussed in the selections included in this section.

Chapter Thirteen (by Martin Donohoe) provides an overview of various forms of individual and societal violence against women. Societal violence against women is defined as structural forms of discrimination or depravation that affect women as a class, such as excess poverty, impaired access to employment and education, divorce restrictions, salary inequalities, political marginalization, and limited availability of reproductive health services.[3]

Chapter Fourteen (by Martin Donohoe) considers myriad barriers to abortion in the United States as well as the effects of US policy on reproductive health care worldwide. Since the article was written, anti-abortion zealots have increased their campaigns, and the current conservative majority on the Supreme Court makes possible the overturning of *Roe* v. *Wade*.

The autobiographical narrative by Eleanor Cooney in Chapter Fifteen describes the author's harrowing ordeal of rape and robbery during an illegal abortion, the type of demeaning scenario largely unfamiliar to young women in America today, who may not appreciate the reproductive rights won by their mothers' generation.

Former secretary-general of the United Nations Kofi Annan said that "gender equality is critical to the development and peace of every nation"[4] and "there is no tool for development more effective than the empowerment of women"[5] (http://www.un.org/News/Press/docs/2005/sgsm9738.doc.htm). Readers are encouraged to visit the women's health page of the Public Health and Social Justice website at http://phsj.org/womens-health/, where they will find other articles, regularly updated open-access slide shows, and links to many organizations working for equality and justice for women worldwide. There are also links to articles that deal specifically with domestic violence and female genital cutting.

Notes

1. Association of American Medical Colleges. *Medical school enrollment shows diversity gains: Number of first-time applicants also up, demonstrating interest in medicine as a career.* Retrieved from https://www.aamc.org/newsroom/newsreleases/2010/152932/101013.html.

2. Institute for Women's Policy Research. *The gender-wage gap, 2009.* Retrieved from http://www.iwpr.org/publications/pubs/the-gender-wage-gap-2009.

3. Heise, L. L., Raikes, A., Watts, C., & Zwi, A. Violence against women: A neglected public health issue in less developed countries. *Social Science & Medicine,* 1994, *39*(9), 1165–1179.

4. Annan, K. *Empowerment of women the most effective development tool, Secretary-General tells Commission on Status of Women.* Press Release SG/SM/9738, WOM/1489. Retrieved from http://www.un.org/News/Press/docs/2005/sgsm9738.doc.htm.

5. Ibid.

Chapter 13

Individual and Societal Forms of Violence Against Women in the United States and the Developing World

An Overview

Martin Donohoe

Introduction

This chapter reviews individual and societal forms of violence against women that occur in the United States and throughout the world. Its purpose is to assist readers in recognizing and managing these phenomena, and to encourage them to advocate locally and nationally for solutions to public health and human rights issues facing women worldwide. The incorporation of societal and structural forms of violence against women into the medical curriculum, to complement current curricular offerings on domestic violence/partner abuse, would likely enhance the willingness and abilities of health professionals to become more active in clinical work, research, and public policy in women's health.

Heise et al.[1] have divided violence against women into individual and societal forms. Individual violence against women is defined as any act of verbal or physical force, coercion, or life-threatening depravation that causes physical or psychological harm, humiliation, or arbitrary depravation of liberty, or that perpetuates female subordination.[1] Examples of this include partner abuse, sexual assault (including marital rape), forced prostitution, forced non-compliance with contraception, female genital mutilation, and sex slavery. Societal violence against women is defined as structural forms of discrimination or depravation that affect women as a class.[1] Examples of this include excess poverty, impaired access to employment or education, divorce restrictions, salary inequalities, political marginalization, and impaired access to reproductive health services.

Individual Violence Against Women

Partner Abuse and Sexual Assault in the United States

The following briefly discusses the epidemiology and management of partner abuse and sexual assault in the United States as a prelude to a discussion of the broader scope of the problem of violence against women worldwide. More detailed discussions of domestic violence and rape can be found elsewhere.

Domestic violence is seen in all age, race, and socioeconomic brackets.[2] Estimates of the lifetime prevalence of assault and sexual abuse range from 15 to 25%.[3-5] Each year, two to four million women are assaulted, and every fifteen seconds a woman is beaten.[4] Annual incidence of one or more episodes of intimate partner violence is 17%.[6] The estimated incidence of abuse in pregnancy ranges from 8 to 20%.[7-10] Fifty to 70% of mothers of abused children have been abused themselves.[11] Over one-half of women murdered in the United States are killed by a current or former partner, and one-half to three-quarters of the 1,000 to 1,500 murder-suicides per year involve domestic violence.[5,12] Child abuse is seen in one-third to one-half of families where partner abuse occurs.[13]

Rape, defined as unwanted, forced penetration—orally, vaginally, or anally—is reported by 33 to 46% of women who are physically abused.[5] Annual incidence is greater than 80 per 100,000 women and lifetime prevalence may reach as high as 25% since rape is a very under-reported crime. Spousal rape occurs in up to 10 to 15% of all marriages and tends to be more violent and less frequently reported than non-spousal rape.[5] It is not illegal in many US states and other countries. Rape results in a 25% chance of pregnancy, up to a one in four chance of acquiring a sexually transmitted disease (rates of gonorrhea are 6–12%, chlamydia 4–17%, and syphilis 0.5–3%), and a one to two per thousand odds of acquiring HIV (depending on the nature of the forced sex, infectivity of the perpetrator, and presence of erosions or sores on the victim or rapist).[14]

Physical sequelae of partner abuse include trauma, chronic pain, eating and sleeping disorders, sexually transmitted diseases, irritable bowel syndrome,[15] and a delayed risk of hypertension, arthritis, and heart disease.[5] Victims of domestic violence have a five-fold increased risk of developing a psychiatric disorder; 10% of domestic violence victims attempt suicide.[5] Rape victims show a much higher prevalence of alcoholism and drug abuse than the general population, with the substance abuse beginning after the rape. Early psychological sequelae of rape include withdrawal, confusion, psychological numbing, a sense of vulnerability/hopelessness/loss/betrayal, shock, denial, and distrust of others. Long-term psychological outcomes include depression, anxiety disorders, phobias, anorexia/bulimia, substance abuse, and post-traumatic stress disorder.[14]

Health care providers should make routine, repeated assessments of women for domestic violence in all clinical settings; maintain a supportive, non-judgmental attitude; avoid victim-blaming; validate the woman's experiences, building on her strengths, and transferring power and control to her; be available, providing frequent follow-up; and involve social services. They should discover the nature and duration of the abuse; assess for child abuse and ensure children's safety by following mandated reporting laws; keep detailed records, including photographs; testify in court as needed; and not recommend marriage counseling.[5,16] Practitioners should ensure the victim's safety, assist her in obtaining a restraining order, provide her with phone numbers of shelters and hot lines, and help her develop a plan for a quick exit, including a safe place to go. Patients should have important items (such as driver's license, birth certificate, credit cards, and documents related to their children's health) handy in case a rapid exit is required.

In caring for victims of sexual assault, providers should obtain a full medical history, evaluate and treat physical injuries, obtain cultures, treat pre-existing infections, offer post-exposure human immunodeficiency virus prophylaxis and post-coital contraception (versus in utero paternity testing followed by selective abortion for those who might already be pregnant),[17] arrange medical follow-up, and provide counseling.[14]

Screening practices of primary care providers vary, but on the whole physicians frequently fail to recognize violence against women.[18] This results from fears of offending, feelings of powerlessness, time constraints, a low confidence in their ability to affect change, a sense of their own vulnerability, and deficits in education and training. Doctors frequently underestimate the prevalence of domestic violence in their patients and communities. Compassionate asking and trust building are useful in getting patients to discuss abuse.[19]

Regrettably, the availability of domestic violence shelters in the United States is poor, with up to 70% to 80% of women and 80% of children turned away on any given night in major cities.[13] Shelters are woefully under-funded. Average length of stay at a US shelter is fourteen days; most allow a thirty-day maximum stay. Over 50% of all homeless women and children become homeless as a direct result of fleeing domestic violence.

Individual Violence Against Women in the Developing World

As in the US, women in the developing world suffer verbal, emotional, physical, and sexual abuse. Worldwide at least one woman in three has been beaten, forced into sex, or otherwise abused in her lifetime.[1] In countries such as Bangladesh, Cambodia, Mexico, and Zimbabwe, many see wife-beating as justified. In rural Egypt, up to 81% of women say that wife-beating is justified under certain circumstances.[1] In the developing world, resources for victims are often extremely limited. For example, Mexico City, the most heavily populated city in the world, has only one shelter for battered women.[20]

Other types of individual violence against women noted more frequently in the developing world than in the United States include dowry-related murder, bride-burning, forced abortion and sterilization, divorce restrictions, forced prostitution, and child prostitution. Even so, an estimated 300,000 children under age 18 work in the sex trade in North America; their exploitation fuels a $7 billion-a-year industry.[21] One to two million women and girls are being trafficked annually around the world for the purposes of forced labor, forced prostitution, servile domestic labor, or involuntary marriage.[21] Selective abortion, malnutrition, and killing of female children is not uncommon, and may account for the ratio of male to female births in China being 1.1:1.0, and for higher infant mortality rates among girls in numerous poorer nations.[22] Some women use suicide as "vengeance" against an abusive spouse. Others commit post-rape suicide or are killed by friends or relatives to "cleanse the family honor" after a rape. These types of killings constitute 47% of homicides in Alexandria, Egypt.[1]

South Africa has recently suffered a "rape epidemic."[23] Their official rape rate is 104 per 100,000 people (versus 34 per 100,000 in the US), the highest rate in the world. An estimated 50,000 rapes occur annually, but only 1 in 35 are reported. Victims are at high risk of acquiring HIV infection, due to rates of infection of up to 40% in young adult males and because of the poor availability of post-rape antiretroviral drugs in government hospitals.[23]

Other disturbing phenomena include sex slavery at animist shrines in Ghana, Benin, and Togo;[24] the widespread belief in some parts of sub-Saharan Africa that having sex with a virgin cures HIV infection; and physicians' performance of virginity exams to certify women as pure and "marry-able," which occurs in Turkey and elsewhere.[25]

Female Genital Mutilation

Female genital mutilation ranges from simple clitoridectomy to infibulation (removal of the clitoris and labia minora, stitching the labia major together, and leaving a small opening posteriorly for urine and menstrual blood); the most extreme forms constitute a surgical "chastity belt."[26] This practice should not be called "female circumcision," as the male equivalent of clitoridectomy would be penectomy. Female genital mutilation represents the cultural control of women's sexual pleasure and reproductive capabilities. Mutilation procedures were formerly used in the US and the United Kingdom as treatments for hysteria ("floating womb"), epilepsy, melancholy, lesbianism, and excessive masturbation.

Worldwide, one hundred million women, most in sub-Saharan Africa, have been affected by female genital mutilation.[26] These women are found across all socioeconomic strata and in all major religions. Two million girls are mutilated per year. Operations are most commonly carried out on young girls between ages four and ten; physicians perform about 12% of procedures.[27] Cutting is often done under non-sterile conditions and without anesthesia. Complications and sequelae include bleeding, infection, dyspareunia, painful neuromas, keloids, dysmenorrhea, infertility, decreased sexual responsiveness, shame, fear, and depression.[27] Physicians managing those who have suffered genital mutilation need to be sensitive to cultural identity issues and aware of the availability of deinfibulation procedures.[26]

The United Nations, World Health Organization, and Federation International Gynecology and Obstetrics (FIGO) have all condemned female genital mutilation.[26] It is illegal to perform it in the US under child abuse statutes. Some have called this prohibition "cultural imperialism"; others note that we have outlawed other coercive and abusive "cultural practices," including slavery, polygamy, child labor, and the denial of appropriate, life-saving medical care to sick children.[28] Immigrant women who fear that they are likely to face a forced operation upon return to their countries of origin have successfully petitioned for political asylum.

Societal/Structural Violence Against Women

Societal violence against women involves economic, legal, political, and educational structures; repressive, entrenched belief systems; and social phenomena that deny women basic human rights and/or impede women's abilities to achieve their full potentials.[1] After a brief review of the historical subjugation of women and ideals of beauty, I will focus on teen pregnancy and single motherhood, impaired access to abortion services, economic marginalization, and gender-based harassment.

The Historical Subjugation of Women and Ideals of Beauty

Most of human history has been marked by the subjugation and marginalization of women. Examples include witch trials and burnings at the stake in the Middle

Ages (and later in Salem, Massachusetts); the Chamberlin family's hoarding of its invention of the obstetrical forceps, motivated by profit and the desire for fame; and J. Marion Sims's early operative gynecologic surgeries on slaves, performed without anesthesia.[29] These examples can be contrasted with the relatively rapid acceptance of chloroform for obstetrical anesthesia, after its introduction for other surgical procedures, mostly due to its use by Queen Victoria and its promotion by Charles Darwin and Charles Dickens.[30]

Many historical ideals of beauty have been dangerous and/or have involved the subjugation of women.[31] These include the ancient Greek practice of wrapping newborn baby girls' heads; Roman and Persian women's applying antimony to make their conjunctivae sparkle; the use of belladonna eye drops by sixteenth and seventeenth century women to dilate their pupils and make their eyes appear doe-like; the Elizabethan era practice of hair plucking and the use of lead-based ceruce makeup; Chinese foot binding, which causes pain and puts women at high risk of osteoporosis, falls, and balance problems;[32] and the longstanding practice of corseting. More recent examples include breast implants, available since 1903; tapeworms to cause malabsorption and promote weight loss, employed by opera singer Maria Callas; 11th and 12th rib removals; botulinum toxin injections; and liposuction.[31,33] Today plastic surgeons perform more than one million cosmetic procedures annually, a 153% increase over last decade's rates.[34]

Certainly today most women freely opt for these appearance-altering interventions, yet they are motivated by societal norms promoted by a media which values appearance over character, style over substance.[34] Women who have been sexually abused report more body dissatisfaction and self-consciousness, and may opt for cosmetic procedures more often than those without a sexual abuse history.[35] Regrettably, today only 29% of teens state that they are "happy with the way I am."[36] Sixty percent of girls in grades 9 through 12 are trying to lose weight (compared to 24% of boys), and 5% to 10% of females over age 18 have an eating disorder.[37] Girls who diet are at increased risk of smoking initiation;[38] many see smoking as a helpful weight loss aid.

Teen Pregnancy

Greater than 50% of high school-age adolescents are sexually active; average age at first intercourse is 17 for girls and 16 for boys.[39,40] Current birth rates to girls age 15 to 19 are 55 per 1,000 per year; these have gradually decreased since 1960.[39,40] Up to two-thirds of adolescents use condoms, three times as many as did so in the 1970s. Nevertheless, the US has rates of teen pregnancy which are three to ten times higher than those among the industrialized nations of Western Europe.[41] US teen poverty rates are higher by a similar magnitude.[42] Six out of seven US teen births are to the 40% of girls living at or below the poverty level. Two-thirds of teen mothers were raped or abused as children.[42]

The role of adult males in teen pregnancy is under-recognized. In California in 1993, 71% of teen pregnancies (for whom a father was reported) were fathered by adult men with an average age of 22.6 years, or five years older than the mothers.[42] More births were fathered by men over 25 than by boys under 18. Sexually transmitted disease and acquired immunodeficiency syndrome rates among teenage girls were two to four times higher than among age-matched teenage boys; instead, teenage girls' rates were closer to adult male rates.[42] Statutory rape, in which adult perpetrators or boyfriends have sexual intercourse with underage girls, is infrequently reported by providers, who cite as reasons the appearance of consensual "adult relationships," a lack of confidence in the criminal justice system, confidentiality, fear of deterring patients from seeking health care and social services follow-up, and the risk of physical retaliation.[11] States are evenly split on whether or not mandated reporting is required.[43]

Only 8% of US high schools provide condoms, despite the fact that promotion and distribution of condoms does not increase teen sexual activity.[44,45] Many health plans fail to cover all contraceptive methods, even though all methods are more effective and less costly than no method.[46] Many fewer plans cover abortion than cover sterilization, leaving poor women in the unenviable position of having to choose sterilization if they lack the resources for adequate contraception or for an abortion (which may become necessary even when accepted contraceptive methods are used as directed).[47] On a positive note, the US House of Representatives recently voted to reinstate the contraceptive coverage for federal employees that President Bush has omitted in his 2002 budget proposal.[48]

The availability of emergency contraception should help further decrease teen pregnancy rates. However, some Catholic hospitals prohibit discussion of emergency contraception, even with rape victims.[49] Unfortunately, recent so-called Welfare Reform legislation allocated to states fifty million dollars over five years to teach abstinence, rather than to provide contraceptives.[50]

The vast majority of sex education programs in the US do not affect teenage behavior in any substantial way.[51] They neither promote more sexual activity, nor do they significantly reduce unprotected sex. The few programs that do work give teenagers a clear and narrow message—delay having sex, but if you have sex, always use a condom. Good programs also teach teens how to resist peer pressure.[51]

Single Motherhood

Twenty-one percent of US children currently live in solo-mother families. Of white children born since 1980, 50% will spend some part of their childhood in a single parent family, compared with 80% of African-American children. The current US divorce rate is just under 50%.[52] Over 50% of children in solo-mother families live below the poverty line.[53] On average, children from single-parent families show poorer school performance, a higher risk of teen pregnancy, increased rates of delinquency, and decreased overall mental health.[53]

Fifty percent of mothers of preschoolers and 70% of mothers of school-age children work outside the home. One-half of working mothers' children are cared for by relatives, three-eighths are in family day care, and one-eighth are in day care centers, many of which are poorly regulated and experience high worker turnover. The US is one of the only industrialized countries without paid maternity leave and health benefits guaranteed by law. The Family and Medical Leave Act of 1993 guarantees only unpaid leave, and only to individuals from establishments employing at least fifty workers.[54] Forty-four percent of working women are ineligible, and low-wage workers are disproportionately excluded.

Access to Pregnancy Care

Many women lack access to comprehensive prenatal and obstetrical care. Almost 600,000 women die each year from complications related to pregnancy and childbirth, nearly 99% of them in developing nations.[55] About one-quarter of pregnant women experience a serious complication during labor or at delivery, including excessive bleeding, infection, and pre-eclampsia.[55] The US lags behind most of the industrial world in infant mortality, due in large part to lack of universal access to health insurance.[56]

Access to Abortion Services

Since abortion was legalized in 1973, more than 30 million US women have had this procedure.[57] Between 1.2 and 1.4 million abortions are performed in the US, a rate of 20 abortions per 1,000 fertile women per year.[57] There are 314 induced abortions for every 1,000 recognized pregnancies.[58] Forty-eight percent of those obtaining abortions are over age 25, 59% white, 20% married, and 56% have children. By age 45, the average female will have had 1.4 unintended pregnancies; 43% will have had an induced abortion.[59] Fifty-eight percent of women with unintended pregnancies get pregnant while using birth control.[57] This is not surprising, given one-year contraceptive failure rates ranging from 2 to 3% for IUDs, to 7% for contraceptive pills, to 21% for periodic abstinence.[57]

Since the 1973 *Roe* v. *Wade* decision legalizing abortion, various barriers have been erected in the path of those seeking to obtain one. The Hyde Amendment of 1977 cut off Medicaid funding for nearly all abortions. Before former president William Clinton took office, discussion of abortion in federally funded health clinics was prohibited. Upon taking office, current president George W. Bush reinstated the Mexico City Policy, a Reagan-era rule that bans US family planning aid to overseas groups[60] that provide abortions or abortion referrals, even if they do so with private, non-US funds.[59] Thirty-nine states have parental notification laws,[61] which have led to a rise in late trimester abortions and to increased numbers of abortions in neighboring states without such laws. Recently, the Bush Administration drafted a policy that would let states define unborn children as persons eligible for medical coverage.[62]

In 1994, only 12% of ob/gyn residency programs required training in abortion methods, down from 25% in 1985, even though only 10–15% of ob/gyn residents are morally opposed to abortion.[63–65] Today approximately one-third of medical schools teach something about abortion, through mandatory coursework, elective classes, lectures, or Planned Parenthood rotations, although no hard data exist on the percentage of students exposed and exactly what they learn.[66] In the US, 86% of counties and 30% of metropolitan areas have no abortion provider.[59] Abortions cost approximately $350; most patients pay out of pocket.[57] Only one out of three patients has insurance coverage, and only one out of three insurance companies cover the procedure after the deductible is met.[57] Often patients are reluctant to file claims due to confidentiality concerns.

Other obstacles to abortion include bans on specific methods, mandated waiting periods, spousal notification laws, regulation of abortion facility locations, and zoning ordinances designed to keep abortion clinics from being built in certain areas.[67] Both patients and providers face harassment by individuals and organized groups. Between 55% and 86% of providers report harassment.[57] There were 166 violent incidents reported in 1997, including 7 arsons, 11 death threats, 6 assaults, 62 stalkings, 65 cases of vandalism, and 1 attempted murder.[68] The availability of mifepristone (RU-486) for medical pregnancy termination has the potential to improve women's access to safe abortion.[69]

Worldwide there are 36 to 53 million abortions performed per year. Abortion on request is permitted in only 22% of countries (6% of developing countries).[70] Although international abortion laws are being slowly liberalized, one-third of the developing world lives where abortion is prohibited, or allowed only in cases of rape or incest or to save the mother's life. Many procedures are performed illegally, outside the traditional health care system, which explains in part why 70,000 women (8 per hour) die annually from abortions; these fatalities constitute 13% of all maternal deaths.[57] One-quarter to one-half of maternal deaths in Latin America are due to unsafe abortions. For every one abortion death, there are 30 infections or injuries. In some countries, lack of access to contraception has been a bigger issue than lack of access to abortion services.[57] The average number of lifetime abortions for a woman in Russia is nine; it was 18 in Romania, prior to the fall of Communism.

Despite abortion foes' arguments that having an abortion leads to irrevocable psychological harm, most data suggest only a self-limited sense of loss and guilt and minimal to no long-term emotional or psychological sequelae.[71] Indeed, women denied abortions often experience resentment and distrust, and their children may face social and occupational deficiencies.[72]

Education, Work, and Income Inequalities

In the developing world, there exists a large gender gap in access to primary and secondary education.[73] Fertility rates vary in inverse proportion to literacy rates. Women do two-thirds of the world's work, receive 10% of global income, and own only 1% of global property.[74] Each year, an estimated 50,000 women are brought to the US to work under conditions of forced servitude; even so, the Justice Department has prosecuted only 250 cases in the last two years involving such victims.[75] Women working full-time in the US make $0.75 for each $1.00 made by males; this ratio has remained essentially stagnant over the last two decades.[76] Today 53% of mothers return to work within one year of giving birth, two-thirds of these full-time, up from 17% returning to work in 1976.[77] While women make up 46% of the US work force, they hold less than 2% of senior-level management positions in Fortune 500 companies.[76]

Nevertheless, from 1987 to 1999, the number of female-owned firms doubled to 9.1 million; the number of workers employed by these firms quadrupled, to 27.5 million, and sales of these firms quadrupled, to 3.6 trillion dollars. The fastest growing fields of employment for women are construction, wholesale trade, transportation, communications, agriculture, and manufacturing.[78]

Gender-Based Sexual Harassment

Sexual harassment occurs when there exists a quid pro quo, i.e., the threat or expectation of inappropriate behavior in response to a woman's actions, or if there exists a hostile work environment.[79] Gender discrimination, psychological abuse, and sexual harassment are reported by high percentages of medical students and residents.[80] In a recent study of US women physicians,[81] 48% of respondents had experienced gender-based harassment, and 37% sexual harassment. Harassment was more common in medical school than in internships and residency, and more common in training than in practice. Higher rates were reported by physicians who were younger, divorced, or in historically male specialties. Lower rates were reported by Asians, those satisfied with their careers, those in government jobs, and the politically very conservative. Perceived gender bias by female academic physicians is associated with lower career satisfaction.[82] After adjustment for work hours, practice type, and specialty, female internists in one study still made 14% less than their male colleagues.[83] On the other hand, Baker[84] found no difference in earnings among young male and female physicians with similar practice characteristics, although older men and certain specialists did earn more than their female colleagues. The Physician Work Life Study,[85] however, found lower rates of pay and higher burnout rates among female physicians.

It should be noted that while the Civil Rights Act of 1964 prohibits discrimination based on race and sex, it does not prohibit discrimination based on sexual orientation, and hence this still occurs, often overtly, in many settings.

Other International Forms of Structural Violence Against Women

Outside the United States, widespread violations of women's rights occur through social, legal, and political marginalization.[1] In Afghanistan, after the Taliban militia took over in 1996, human rights abuses were perpetrated primarily against women.[86] These included gender-based violence, denial of access to education and health care, and limited opportunities for employment. Female employment rates decreased from 62 % to 12%. Afghanistan's maternal mortality rate is among the world's highest, and is likely to increase, at least in the short term, as a consequence of the current war. Afghanistan ranks lowest on the United Nation's (U.N.'s) Development and Gender-Disparity Indices. The current interim government plans to continue many Islamic law statutes which make it difficult for female victims of violence to achieve justice and safety. In Pakistan, four witnesses are required for a rape conviction.[87] Worldwide, including recently in the former Yugoslavia and in Chechnya, rape continues to be used in war, for domination, humiliation, control, "soldierly bonding," and ethnic cleansing; it is often carried out in front of family members. It has been recognized as a war crime since the Nuremberg Trials.

Conclusions

Individual and societal violence against women remains common, both in the US and internationally. Societal violence often begets, or at least facilitates, individual violence. Societal forms of violence are being increasingly seen as violations of basic human rights.[88] Even so, the US has still not signed the U.N.'s Convention on the Elimination of All Forms of Discrimination Against Women[89] nor the U.N.'s Convention on the Political Rights of Women.[90]

Hopefully this brief overview will encourage educators to broaden the scope of health professions education beyond domestic violence to include other national and international forms of individual and structural violence against women. Curricular offerings should include a historical perspective and cover the medical profession's obligations and roles in combating violence against women with their patients, in their institutions and communities, and in the world-at-large. Ideally this chapter will prompt practitioners and policy makers to become more aware of inequities and injustices; to discuss these issues with their patients, colleagues, and students; and to lobby at the local, national, and even global level for changes in law and policy to protect victims and to improve the status of women.

Acknowledgments

The author gratefully acknowledges the excellent technical assistance of Linda Ward, Betty Ward, Peggy Miner, Cari Gandrud, and Lynn San Juan.

Notes

1. Heise, L.L., et al., Violence against women: A neglected public health issue in less developed countries. *Social Science Medicine*, 1994. 39(9): pp. 1165–1179.

2. Bauer, H.M., M.A. Rodriguez, and E. Perez-Stable, Prevalence and determinants of intimate partner abuse among public hospital primary care patients. *Journal of General Internal Medicine*, 2000. 15: pp. 811–817.

3. Coker, A.L., et al., Frequency and correlates of intimate partner violence by type: Physical, sexual, and psychological battering. *American Journal of Public Health*, 2000. 90(4): pp. 553–559.

4. McCauley, J., et al., The "Battering Syndrome": Prevalence and clinical characteristics of domestic violence in primary care internal medicine practices. *Annals of Internal Medicine*, 1995. 123(10): pp. 737–746.

5. Council on Scientific Affairs Report: Violence against women. *Journal of American Medical Association*, 1992. 267(23): pp. 3184–3189.

6. Schafer, J., R. Caetano, and C.L. Clark, Rates of intimate partner violence in the United States. *American Journal of Public Health*, 1998. 88(11): pp. 1702–1704.

7. Gazmararian, J.A., et al., Prevalence of violence against pregnant women. *Journal of American Medical Association*, 1996. 275(24): pp. 1915–1920.

8. Newberger, E.H., S.E. Barham, and E.S. Liberman, Abuse of pregnant women and adverse birth outcome. *Journal of American Medical Association*, 1992. 267(17): pp. 2370–2372.

9. Eisenstat, S.A. and L. Bancroft, Domestic violence. *New England Journal of Medicine*, 1999. 341(12): pp. 886–892.

10. Martin, S.L., et al., Physical abuse of women before, during and after pregnancy. *Journal of American Medical Association*, 2001. 285(12): pp. 1581–1584.

11. Elders, M.J. and A.E. Albert, Adolescent pregnancy and sexual abuse. *Journal of American Medical Association*, 1998. 280(7): pp. 648–649.

12. Marzuk, P.M., K. Tardiff, and C.S. Hirsch, The epidemiology of murder-suicide. *Journal of the American Medical Association,* 1992. 267(23): pp. 3179–3183.

13. Jensen, R.H., Domestic violence facts. *Ms.,* 1994. V(2): pp. 44–51.

14. Hampton, H.L., Care of the woman who has been raped. *New England Journal of Medicine,* 1995. 332(4): pp. 234–237.

15. Drossman, D., et al., Sexual and physical abuse and gastrointestinal illness. *Annals of Internal Medicine,* 1995. 123(10): pp. 782–794.

16. Randall, T., Domestic violence intervention calls for more than treating injuries. *Journal of American Medical Association,* 1990. 264: pp. 939–940.

17. Hammond, H.A., J.B. Redman, and C.T. Caskey, In utero paternity testing following alleged sexual assault: A comparison of DNA-based methods. *Journal of the American Medical Association,* 1995. 273(22): pp. 1774–1777.

18. Rodriguez, M.A., et al., Screening and intervention for intimate partner abuse. *Journal of American Medical Association,* 1999. 282(5): pp. 468–474.

19. Gerbert, B., et al., A qualitative analysis of how physicians with expertise in domestic violence approach the identification of victims. *Annals of Internal Medicine,* 1999. 131: pp. 578–584.

20. Olavarrieta, C.D. and J. Sotelo, Domestic violence in Mexico. *Journal of American Medical Association,* 1996. 275(24): pp. 1937–1941.

21. Documentary, *Stolen lives: Children in the sex trade.* Fanlight Productions, 1997.

22. Reuss, A., Missing women. *Dollars and Sense,* 2001(May/June): pp. 40–43.

23. Hawthorne, P., An epidemic of rapes. *Time,* 1999(November): p. 59.

24. Simmons, A.M., "Wife of the Gods" stirs up Ghana, *Los Angeles Times,* 1999. p. 24.

25. Frank, M.W., et al., Virginity examinations in Turkey. *Journal of American Medical Association,* 1999. 282(5): pp. 485–490.

26. Toubia, N., Female circumcision as a public health issue. *New England Journal of Medicine,* 1994. 331(11): pp. 712–716.

27. Council of Scientific Affairs: Female genital mutilation. *Journal of American Medical Association,* 1995. 274(21): pp. 1714–1716.

28. Schroeder, P., Female genital mutilation — a form of child abuse. *New England Journal of Medicine,* 1994. 331(11): pp. 739–740.

29. Ojanuga, D., The medical ethics of the "father of gynaecology" Dr. J. Marion Sims. *Journal of Medical Ethics,* 1993. 19: pp. 28–31.

30. Rose, P., *Parallel lives: Five Victorian marriages.* New York: Random House, 1984.

31. Henig, R.M., The price of perfection. *Civilization,* 1996. May/June: pp. 54–61.

32. Cummings, S.R., X.U. Ling, and K. Stone, Consequences of foot binding among older women in Beijing China. *American Journal of Public Health,* 1997. 87(10): p. 1680.

33. Kalb, C., Our quest to be perfect. *Newsweek,* 1999(August): pp. 52–59.

34. Newman, C., The enigma of beauty. *National Geographic*, 2000(January): pp. 94–121.

35. Kerney-Cooke, A. and D.M. Ackard, The effects of sexual abuse on body image, self-image, and sexual activity of women. *Journal of Gender-Specific Medicine*, 2000. 3(6): pp. 54–60.

36. Phillips, K., How *Seventeen* undermines young women. *Extra!*, 1993.

37. Carlson, M., J. McDowell, and A. Park, Girl power. *Time*, 1998(June): pp. 60–62.

38. Austin, S.B. and S.L. Gortmaker, Dieting and smoking initiation in early adolescent girls and boys: A prospective study. *American Journal of Public Health*, 2001. 91(3): pp. 446–450.

39. Dickinson, A., Teenage sex. *Time*, 1999(November): p. 160.

40. Stodghill, R., Where'd you learn that? *Time*, 2000.

41. Population action report: Study ranks global reproductive health. *The Nation's Health*, 2001: p. 7.

42. Males, M.A., Adult involvement in teenage childbearing and STD. *Lancet*, 1995. 346: pp. 64–65.

43. Elstein, S.G and N. Davis, *Sexual relationships between adult males and young teen girls: Exploring the legal and social responses*. Washington, DC: American Bar Association Center on Children and the Law, 1997.

44. Kirby, D., et al., The impact of condom distribution in Seattle schools in sexual behavior and condom use. *American Journal of Public Health*, 1999. 89(2): pp. 182–188.

45. Schuster, M.A., et al., Providing high school students with access to condoms does not increase teen sex. *Family Planning Perspectives*, 1998. 222: p. 12.

46. Trussell, J., et al., The economic value of contraception: A comparison of 15 methods. *American Journal of Public Health*, 1995. 85: pp. 494–503.

47. Donohoe, M.T., Adolescent pregnancy. *Journal of American Medical Association*, 1996. 276(4): p. 282.

48. Staff, Contraceptive coverage for federal employees upheld. *The Nation's Health*, 2001: p. 5.

49. Human Rights Watch: *World report: Women and human rights*. 2001.

50. Morse, J., Preaching chastity in the classroom. More sex-education classes are teaching kids only abstinence. Will they listen? *Time*, 1999(Oct): pp. 79–80.

51. Kirby, D., *Sex education in the schools*. Menlo Park, CA: Henry J. Kaiser Family Foundation, 1994.

52. Dickinson, A., I do's and don'ts. There are no rules for making a happy marriage. Two books offer up some advice anyway. *Time*, 2001: p. 81.

53. UNICEF, *Half of solo mothers in poverty in Australia, Canada and US*. UNICEF, 1996.

54. Chavkin, W., What's a mother to do? Welfare, work and family. *American Journal of Public Health,* 1999. 89(4): pp. 477–479.

55. Safe motherhood. *Journal of the American Medical Association,* 1998. 279(14): p. 1058.

56. Himmelstein, D., S. Woolhandler, and I. Hellander, *Bleeding the patient: The consequences of corporate health care.* Monroe, ME: Common Courage Press, 2001.

57. Grimes, D.A., A 26-year-old woman seeking an abortion. *Journal of American Medical Association,* 1999. 282(12): pp. 1169–1175.

58. Abortion Surveillance: Preliminary analysis-United States. *Morbidity and Mortality Weekly Report,* 1998. 47: pp. 1025–1028.

59. Henshaw, S.K. Unintended pregnancy in the United States. *Family Planning Perspectives,* 1998. 30: pp. 24–29.

60. Pozner, J.L., Self-gagged on gag rule. *Extra!,* 2001(May/June): pp. 7–8.

61. Lacayo, R., What can a kid decide? *Time,* 2000: p. 32.

62. Hodge, R.D., Weekly review. *Harper's Magazine Online.* 2001.

63. Talley, P.P. and G.R. Bergus, Abortion training in family practice residency programs. *Family Medicine,* 1996. 28: pp. 245–248.

64. MacKay, H.T. and A.P. MacKay, Abortion training in obstetrics and gynecology residency programs in the United States. *Family Planning Perspectives,* 1995. 27: pp. 112–115.

65. Lazarus, E.S., Politicizing abortion: Personal morality and professional responsibility of residents training in the United States. *Social Science Medicine,* 1997. 44(9): pp. 1417–1425.

66. Edwards, T.M., How med students put abortion back in the classroom. *Time,* 2001: pp. 59–60.

67. NARAL report: Access to safe abortions increasingly difficult. *The Nation's Health,* 2001(Apr): p. 11.

68. Moore, M. and K. Glynn, *Adventures in a TV nation.* New York: HarperCollins, 1998.

69. Gibbs, N., The pill arrives. *Time,* 2000(October): pp. 40–49.

70. Indriso, C. and A. Mundigo, Abortion in the developing world. *American Journal of Public Health,* 1999. 89(12): pp. 1890–1892.

71. Adler, N.E., et al., Psychological responses after abortion. *Science,* 1990. 248: pp. 41–4.

72. Hogue, C., et al., Answering questions about long-term outcomes, in *A clinician's guide to medical and surgical abortion,* M. Paul et al., Editors. Churchill Livingstone: New York, 1999.

73. UNICEF, *Education gender gap.* 1997, UNICEF.

74. Caldicott, H., *If you love this planet: A plan to heal the earth.* New York: W.W. Norton & Company, 1992.

75. Numbers. *Time*, 2000(April): p. 23.

76. Jones, B., Giving women the business. *Harper's Magazine*, 1997(December): pp. 47–58.

77. McLaughlin, L., Working moms. *Time*, 2000(November): p. 13.

78. Rutherford, M., Women run the world. *Time*, 1999(June).

79. Cloud, J., Sex and the law. *Time*, 1998. 23: pp. 48–54.

80. VanIneveld, C.H.M., et al., Discrimination and abuse in internal medicine residency. *Journal of General Internal Medicine*, 1996. 11: pp. 401–405.

81. Frank, E., D. Brogan, and M. Schiffman, Prevalence and correlates of harassment among US women physicians. *Archives of Internal Medicine*, 1998. 158(4): pp. 352–358.

82. Carr, P.L., A.S. Ash, and R.H. Friedman, Faculty perceptions of gender discrimination and sexual harassment in academic medicine. *Annals of Internal Medicine*, 2000. 132: pp. 889–896.

83. Ness, R.B., F. Ukoli, and S. Hunt, Salary equity among male and female internists in Pennsylvania. *Annals of Internal Medicine*, 2000. 133: pp. 104–110.

84. Baker, L.C., Differences in earnings between male and female physicians. *New England Journal of Medicine*, 1996. 334(15): pp. 959–964.

85. McMurray, J.E., et al., The work lives of women physicians. *Journal of General Internal Medicine*, 2000. 15: pp. 372–380.

86. Rasekh, Z., et al., Women's health and human rights in Afghanistan. *Journal of American Medical Association*, 1998. 280(5): pp. 449–451.

87. *Harper's index*. 1999(May 17).

88. Miller, A.M., Uneasy promises: Sexuality, health, and human rights. *American Journal of Public Health*, 2001. 91(6): pp. 861–864.

89. Convention of the Elimination of All Forms of Discrimination Against Women. The General Assembly of the United Nations, 1952.

90. Convention of the Political Rights of Women. 1952.

Chapter 14

Obstacles to Abortion in the United States

Martin Donohoe

Introduction

Despite being a legal (and commonly used) medical procedure, numerous barriers have been placed in the way of women attempting to exercise their right to abortion and in the way of healthcare providers and educators attempting to assist women in exercising this right. This issue of "Women's Health in Context" considers obstacles, particularly those erected by the current United States administration, and calls for reform, education, and activism by those concerned about women's reproductive healthcare.

Epidemiology of Abortion

More than 42 million American women have had an abortion since its legalization by the United States Supreme Court in 1973.[1,2] In 2002, 1.29 million abortions took place, down by 5% (about 1.36 million) in 1996 and by nearly 27% since 1980.[2,3] More than half of abortions occur in women younger than 25, with a third of all abortions occurring in women aged 20–24.[2] Nearly half (49%) of all pregnancies are unintended.[4] More than 30% of these occur in married women. Fifty-four percent of women with unintended pregnancies become pregnant while using birth control.[5] By age 45, the average female will have had 1.4 unintended pregnancies, and 43% will have had an induced abortion.[4]

Note: An earlier version of this article was published in the *Journal of the American Medical Women's Association.* Donohoe MT. Increase in obstacles to abortion: The American perspective in 2004. *J Am Med Women's Assn.* 2005;60(1):16–25. Available at http://www.ncbi.nlm.nih.gov/pubmed/16845763. Accessed June 21, 2005.

Abortion remains one of the safest medical procedures available.[6-10] It is more dangerous to carry a fetus to term than to undergo an abortion before 21 weeks; the risk of death with childbirth is 11 times higher.[2] More important, a delay in having abortion until after 15 weeks of pregnancy, when medical risks associated with abortion increase significantly, is more common among adolescents than among older women.[2] Most data suggest that only a self-limited sense of loss and guilt occurs after a woman has an abortion, and there seem to be minimal to no long-term emotional and psychological sequelae.[11] Anxiety symptoms have been identified as the most common adverse response in the short term.[11] Women denied abortions often experience resentment and distrust, and their children may face social and occupational deficiencies.[12]

Barriers to Abortion

Barriers to abortion are manifold and include legal point of viability; cost and coverage; the availability of mifepristone, an oral abortifacient; provider availability; harassment of patients and providers; laws designed to limit the provision of abortion services; and a culture of pseudoscience which promotes the dissemination of misinformation regarding human reproduction through a wasteful diversion of the public's tax revenues.

Legal Point of Viability

Roe v. *Wade*[13] protects the privacy and availability of abortion procedures at less than 24 weeks, the point of legal viability.[14] After viability, states can ban abortion, except when necessary to protect the woman's life or health.

Costs and Coverage

An average self-paying patient was charged $372 for a surgical abortion at 10 weeks and between $438 and $490 for a medical abortion in 2001.[15] Second-trimester surgical abortions are 2 to 3 times more expensive than first-trimester surgical abortions. Most patients pay out of pocket.[15,16] Only 26% of abortions are billed directly to public or private insurance.[15] Most insured patients are reluctant to file claims because of concerns about confidentiality. Some health plans cover sterilization but not abortion, leaving poor women in the unenviable position of having to choose sterilization if they lack the resources for adequate contraception.[17-19]

The 1978 Hyde Amendment prohibits federal Medicaid dollars from being spent on abortion, except to preserve a woman's life or in cases of rape or incest.[20] Twenty-two states allocate a portion of their share of Medicaid funding to cover abortion. The Hyde Amendment was applied to Medicare, which covers disabled women, in 1998. Women of color are more likely than white women to be poor, to lack health insurance, and to rely on government healthcare programs. Thus, they are disproportionately harmed by prohibitions on public funding for abortions.[21,22] In addition, black women and Hispanic women are more likely than white women to have an abortion.[23] Higher rates of abortion are explained, in part, by higher rates of unintended pregnancy, a greater proportion of conceptions that end in abortion, and greater poverty.

The Defense Department, through TRICARE, provides health coverage to military personnel and their families. TRICARE has instituted a permanent ban on abortion coverage, except when the life of the woman is endangered.[20,24] American Indians and Alaskan natives covered by the Indian Health Service are subject to the Hyde Amendment.[20] The Federal Employees Health Benefits Program pays for abortions only in cases of life endangerment, rape, or incest. Women in federal prisons are allowed to obtain an abortion only when their lives are endangered or when the pregnancy is the result of rape,[20] which may be difficult to prove.

Legal Barriers

Between 1995 and 2003, approximately 350 anti-choice measures were enacted, including statutes that protect pharmacists who refuse to fill birth control prescriptions on moral or religious grounds.[25,26] In 2003, 10 states introduced 15 measures that would ban all or most abortions.[27,28] In 2004, Michigan enacted a ban on abortion.[29] The ban prevents physicians from performing most abortions, even in cases when a woman's life or health is in danger (e.g., a woman with diabetes or a heart condition). However, on June 14, 2005, the American Civil Liberties Union, the Center for Reproductive Rights, and the Planned Parenthood Federation of America sought to block the ban in federal court. The law has been enjoined pending the court's decision.

In the month of January 2005 alone, 15 states introduced 19 bills that would require counseling and waiting periods for abortion; and 12 states introduced 17 bills that would mandate parental involvement in minors' abortions. Twenty-three states already have mandated waiting periods for women wishing to obtain an abortion,[30] augmenting patients' exposure to anti-choice harassment and increasing the gestational age at which pregnancy termination occurs, thereby also enhancing the risk associated with the procedure.[31,32]

On April 27, 2005, the House of Representatives passed the "Teen Endangerment Act."[33] The first section of the law (which is also known as the "Child Custody Protection Act") would make it a federal crime for anyone other than a parent to accompany a young woman across state lines for an abortion without complying with the home state's parental involvement statutes.[32,34,35] Although 33 states enforce parental consent or notification laws for minors seeking an abortion,[2] 24 of these have parental involvement requirements that meet the Teen Endangerment Act's restrictive definition of a "parental involvement law."[32] This barrier would delay an abortion for a teenager determined to have one but unable to draw on her parents' assistance, increasing its economic cost and placing additional physical and emotional burdens on her.

The second section of the Teen Endangerment Act (Child Interstate Abortion Notification Act) would make it a federal crime to provide an abortion to a teenager outside of her home state unless the physician has notified a parent at least 24 hours in advance. There is no exception made for when an abortion may be necessary to protect a young woman's health. It further requires a 24-hour waiting period and written notification even if a parent accompanies his or her daughter to an out-of-state abortion provider.[32] The Senate is currently considering a bill similar to the Teen Endangerment Act but without interstate abortion notifications.

Parental notification laws can be dangerous if a pregnancy results from incest or if the adolescent's home environment is abusive or otherwise unstable. A national survey of female adolescents found that mandated parental notification laws would likely increase risky or unsafe sexual behavior and, in turn, the incidence of sexually transmitted disease (STDs) and adolescent pregnancy.[36] Others have found that parental consent and notification laws could prevent up to half of teens from using Planned Parenthood services, including contraception, while only stopping 1% from having sex.[37] Based on the projected number of additional pregnancies, births, abortions, and untreated STDs and resulting pelvic inflammatory disease, the potential annual costs of parental consent and law enforcement reporting requirements in 1 state (Texas) have been estimated at $43.6 million for girls younger than 18 years currently using publicly funded services.[38] In May 2005, the US Supreme Court agreed to hear a case involving New Hampshire's parental notification law, which had been ruled unconstitutional by the First US Circuit Court of Appeals because it contained no health exception in the event of a medical emergency.[39]

Targeted regulation of abortion provider (TRAP) laws are designed to add excessive regulations and extra costs to abortion clinics.[40,41] TRAP regulations far exceed the usual recommendations and requirements of respected scientific organizations. Increased retrofitting, design, and training costs, combined with increased licensing fees and burdensome documentation requirements, have put some clinics out of business and forced others to close temporarily or reduce services. Zoning ordinances have also been passed to force clinics to move. Some facilities shut down and do not reopen. The overall effects of TRAP laws and unfair zoning ordinances are to decrease access and increase costs of abortion.[42] As of 2004, 19 states and Puerto Rico enforce TRAP laws that apply to abortions performed at any stage of pregnancy, and 14 states enforce TRAP laws that apply only to abortions performed after the first trimester.

Forty-six states have enacted "refusal clauses," which allow employers to refuse to provide contraceptive coverage in their health plans; pharmacists to refuse to dispense, or provide referrals for, oral contraceptive pills; and certain medical personnel, health facilities, and/or institutions to refuse to provide abortion services.[28] Healthcare professionals can deny patients' requests for information on, or referral for, family planning services, regardless of patients' healthcare needs.[17,27,28,43,44] The Weldon Federal Refusal clause, signed by President George W. Bush in December 2004, allows federally funded health-care entities to deny women information on abortion services, even if state laws mandate that such information be given upon request.[45] The National Family Planning and Reproductive Health Association filed suit soon afterward, on the basis that the Weldon clause is in conflict with the requirements of Title X, the nation's only federal program solely dedicated to providing family planning and reproductive healthcare to low-income and uninsured women.

The current administration has aggressively attempted to grant rights usually available only to living US citizens to the unborn, creating a movement for "fetal rights." It has extended coverage under the State Children's Health Insurance Program (SCHIP) to fetuses, while failing to extend full prenatal care to all women.[17,43,46] The mission of the federal Advisory Committee on Human Research Protection, which oversees the safety of human research volunteers, has been expanded to include embryos.[47-49] The "unborn victims of violence law" criminalizes harming fetuses and was signed into law by President Bush on April 1, 2004.[50] The National Abortion Rights Action League (NARAL) argues that this legislation is an attempt to undermine *Roe* v. *Wade*.[51] In February 2005, a Cook County, Illinois, judge ruled that parents of a frozen embryo accidentally destroyed by a Chicago fertility clinic could file a wrongful death lawsuit.[52] By contrast, the European Court of Human Rights declined to extend full human rights to fetuses.[53]

The so-called Partial Birth Abortion Ban criminalizes the seldom performed and often lifesaving (for the mother) procedure known as intact dilatation and extraction.[14,54] The ban makes no exceptions for the health of the woman. A federal appeals court judge in San Francisco blocked the administration from enforcing the ban against Planned Parenthood of America clinics and their doctors, who perform roughly half the nation's abortions.[55] Two other courts have also struck down the ban.[56] Courts have also blocked the United States Justice Department's attempts to access confidential medical records as part of their case against opponents of the law.[57] The present US Supreme Court previously ruled that a similar 2000 Nebraska State Law was unconstitutional.[3]

In 2001, more than 20 states had biased counseling laws,[58] often (mis)labeled "mandated informed consent" or "women's right to know" laws, which employ scare tactics and unbalanced data to convince women that abortion is especially dangerous. Similar biased (dis)information is promulgated at up to

4,000 "crisis pregnancy centers" nationwide, some of which receive federal and state funding.[59,60] Staffs try to dissuade clients from having abortions through exaggeration of risks, myths, and fetal photographs.

Limited Availability of Mifepristone

Oral mifepristone allows medical termination of pregnancies up to 49 days from the last menstrual period.[61-64] Many women are unable to obtain this drug because of lack of awareness of its existence, providers' lack of knowledge and fears of prescribing it, and cost. Medicaid restricts funding for mifepristone to cases of rape, incest, or to preserve the pregnant woman's life. The current administration has asked the United States Food and Drug Administration (FDA) to reconsider its approval of mifepristone. Currently proposed state and federal legislation aims to curtail the availability of mifepristone and to limit the number of prescribing doctors.[65,66]

Provider Availability

Over one third of US women live in the 87% of counties in the United States, including 30% of metropolitan areas, that have no abortion provider.[7] The situation is worst in rural areas.[15,67] Only 1,800 physicians provided abortion services in 2000, down 11% from 2,400 in 1996.[3,7] Only 12% of obstetrics and gynecology residency programs required abortion training in the mid-1990s, down from 25% in 1985.[68-72] More recently, Espey and colleagues[73] conducted a survey on abortion education throughout the 4 years of medical school. The results show that abortion education remains limited in US medical schools. Most states bar nonphysicians from performing abortions.[74]

Harassment of Patients and Providers

Since 1977, there have been 80,000 reported acts of violence and/or disruption at abortion clinics in the United States and Canada, including 7 murders, 17 attempted murders, 41 bombings, 166 arsons, 125 assaults, and 654 anthrax threats (480 of them since September 11, 2001).[15,75,76] Patients are often harangued, belittled, defamed, and taunted with verbal and physical threats, despite the federal Freedom of Access to Clinic Entrances Act.[46,77] Between 55% and 86% of providers report that they have been harassed.[16]

The environment in which this harassment occurs has been perpetuated by the federal administration's philosophy and anti-choice rhetoric. For example, when President Bush declared January 20, 2002, 2 days before the 29th anniversary of *Roe* v. *Wade*, "National Sanctity of Life Day," he likened abortion to terrorism: "On September 11, 2001, we saw clearly that evil exists in this world, and that it does not value life.... Now we are engaged in a fight against evil and tyranny to preserve and protect life. In so doing, we are standing again for those core principles upon which our nation was founded."[78] Such rhetoric is permissive of extremism, in that it likens the "battle" against prochoice advocates and abortion providers to that against malevolent suicide bombers.[14]

Effects of United States' Policy on Access to Abortion Worldwide

US policy has affected access to abortion and other reproductive health services worldwide. Lack of access to reproductive education, condoms, and contraceptives in the developing world has led to a large need for abortion, which has not been matched by appropriate numbers of providers and facilities.[79,80] One third of the developing world lives where abortion is prohibited or allowed only in cases of rape or incest or to save the mother's life.[81] At least 80,000 women die annually from unsafe abortions (8 per hour).[82] Unsafe abortion deaths account for 13% of all maternal deaths.[82] For every 1 abortion death, 30 women suffer injuries, severe blood loss, or infection.[82] In 2001, President Bush reinstated the global gag rule first adopted by President Ronald Reagan in 1984 and later rescinded by President Bill Clinton in 1993.[83-85] This edict prevents US government aid from being used by any organization operating outside the country that discusses, advocates for, or performs abortions. Since the resumption of the global gag rule, at least 430 organizations in 50 countries have stopped performing abortions or speaking about abortion laws in order to qualify for US funds.[86] In 2005, the Bush administration has blocked the release of $34 million for the United Nations Population Fund, which provides women's healthcare, promotes women's rights, and prevents violence against women in 140 countries.[87] Furthermore, despite the recommendation of a World Health Organization (WHO) expert committee that mifepristone and misoprostol should be added to its essential medicines list, the WHO, possibly in response to US Department of Health and Human Services pressure, has still failed to act.[88]

Pseudoscience and Ideology Trump Science

The Bush administration has displayed a consistent pattern of disregarding sound science and making appointments to key scientific posts based on ideology rather than scientific expertise and experience.[89] This has had wide-ranging, detrimental effects on women's reproductive health and rights.

For instance, limiting unwanted pregnancies through comprehensive sex education programs and increased availability of contraception would seem to be one approach to decreasing the number of abortions that would please most Americans. As opposed to abstinence-only sex education, comprehensive sex education programs delay initiation of sexual intercourse by teens, reduce the frequency of intercourse, decrease numbers of sexual partners, increase condom and contraception use, lower rates of STDs, and reduce the number of unwanted pregnancies.[90,91] They are supported by the scientific community[92] and by many Americans.[91,93,94]

In 1988, only 2% of US schools relied solely on abstinence-only sex education; by 1999, 23% did.[90] The federal government will spend approximately $170 million on abstinence-only education programs in fiscal year 2005, more than twice the amount spent in fiscal year 2001.[95] Over 80% of the abstinence-only curricula, used by over two-thirds of grantees in 2003, contain false, misleading, or distorted information about reproductive health, including false information about the effectiveness of contraceptives; false information about the risks of abortion; and scientific errors, including mistaken information regarding HIV transmission.[96] The curricula blur science and religion and treat stereotypes about boys and girls as scientific fact.[96] These stereotypes undermine girls' achievement, claim that girls are weak and need protection, and reinforce male sexual aggressiveness.[96] In late 2001, the administration redefined "success" for these programs as "completion of a course" or "a commitment to abstain from sexual activity," rather than by actual outcomes such as delayed onset of sexual activity or decreased teen pregnancy rates.[96,97] The diversion of government funds to abstinence-only programs represents a shift of financial resources away from effective measures to reduce the need and demand for abortions.[97] Combined with Bush administration cuts to family planning programs and the diversion of funds away from other social programs into the administration's so-called Healthy Families Initiative, this will likely increase the number of unwanted pregnancies and thus the number of women seeking pregnancy termination.[90,97,98]

Although the FDA approval of prescription emergency contraception (EC) has increased women's options for the prevention of unwanted pregnancy, only one quarter of reproductive age women in the United States have heard about EC, and some pharmacists refuse to fill prescriptions for EC.[17,42,44,99] Arkansas, Mississippi, and South Dakota explicitly protect pharmacists who refuse to dispense EC; other states are considering similar legislation.[100] The American College of Obstetricians and Gynecologists, the American Academy of Family Physicians, and the American Academy of Pediatrics support over-the-counter (OTC) availability of EC.[101] Even so, the FDA, influenced by the opinions of political appointees, ignored its own advisory panel's 23–4 vote to approve Barr Pharmaceuticals' petition to sell levonorgestrel EC (Plan B) OTC.[102] In June 2005, however, New Hampshire became the seventh state to allow pharmacists to dispense EC without a prescription, and New York is considering following suit.[103] The other 6 states are Alaska, California, Hawaii, Maine, New Mexico, and Washington. And, on June 23, 2005, the New York State Senate approved a bill that would allow pharmacists to dispense EC to women who do not have a prescription. It is unclear whether Governor George Pataki will sign the bill.[104]

Conclusions

Although some barriers to abortion in the United States are long-standing, many new ones have been erected since the current president took office. The Bush administration has limited public access both to scientifically sound sex education and to effective methods of STD prevention and contraception. It has attempted to prevent (or at least delay) availability of EC. The administration's policies opposing women's right to choose have been backed by pseudoscience and by inflammatory rhetoric. These policies have helped to create an environment in which women inclined toward abortion may be delayed in undergoing, or even have to forgo, the procedure. President Bush has nominated a number of anti-choice judges for the federal bench, and may have the opportunity to select 1 or even 2 new Supreme Court justices. This would shift the current balance in favor of abortion rights to one in which *Roe* v. *Wade* could be overturned, making abortion illegal in many states and/or circumstances.

Preserving women's access to abortion services will require vigilance, legislative efforts at the federal and state levels, and court challenges to unjust laws. Advocates should continue to lobby at the state and federal level for access for women to a full range of reproductive health options. Acts of harassment and violence against abortion providers and clinics should be treated by law enforcement officials as acts of domestic terrorism. Efforts to prevent the government from inserting itself into the doctor-patient relationship through legislation should be countered aggressively.[105] Finally, healthcare providers and educational institutions should enhance their professional and public education programs to ensure the promulgation of scientifically sound information regarding contraception and abortion and the availability of trained providers for women who choose to exercise their legal right to terminate an unwanted pregnancy.

Notes

1. Finer LB, Henshaw SK, *Estimates of US abortion incidence in 2001 and 2002*, The Alan Guttmacher Institute, 2005. Available at http://www.guttmacher.org/pubs/2005/05/18/ab_incidence.pdf. Accessed June 21, 2005.

2. The Alan Guttmacher Institute, *Facts in brief: Induced abortion*, May 18, 2005. Available at http://www.agi-usa.org/pubs/fb_induced_abortion.html. Accessed June 21, 2005.

3. Tumulty K, Novak V. Under the radar: Thirty years after *Roe* v. *Wade,* the White House is pressing its case against abortion delicately. An inside look at the strategy. *Time* 2003 (January 27):38–41.

4. Henshaw SK. Unintended pregnancy in the United States. *Fam Plann Perspect.* 1998;30:24–29, 46.

5. Jones RK, Darroch JE, Henshaw SK, Contraceptive use among US women having abortions in 2000–2001, *Perspect Sex Reprod Health* 2002;34:294–303.

6. Elam-Evans LD, Strauss LT, Herndon J, et al. Abortion surveillance—United States, 1999. *MMWR Surveill Summ.* 2002;51(SS-9):1–9,11–28.

7. Finer LB, Henshaw SK. Abortion incidence and services in the United States, 2000. *Perspect Sex Reprod Health* 2003;35:6–15.

8. Lawson HW, Frye A, Atrash HK, Smith JC, Shulman HB, Ramick M. Abortion mortality, United States, 1972 through 1987. *Am J Obstet Gynecol.* 1994;171:1366–1372.

9. Maureen P. Office management of early induced abortion. *Clin Obstet Gynecol.* 1999;42:290–305.

10. Bartlett LA, Berg CJ, Shulman HB, et al. Risk factors for legal induced abortion-related mortality in the United States, *Obstet Gynecol.* 2004;103:729–737.

11. Bradshaw Z, Slade P. The effects of induced abortion on emotional experiences and relationships: A critical review of the literature. *Clin Psychol Rev.* 2003;23:929–958.

12. Hogue C, Lichtenberg ES, Borgatta L, et al., Answering questions about long-term outcomes, in *A Clinician's Guide to Medical and Surgical Abortion,* M. Paul et al., eds. New York: Churchill Livingstone; 1999.

13. *Roe* v. *Wade* (1973). 410 US 438.

14. Greene MF, Ecker JL. Abortion, health and the law. *N Engl J Med.* 2004;350:184–186.

15. Henshaw SK, Finer LB. The accessibility of abortion services in the United States, 2001. *Perspect Sex Reprod Health* 2003;35:16–24.

16. Grimes DA. A 26-year-old woman seeking an abortion. *JAMA.* 1999;282:1169–1175.

17. Westhoff C. Emergency contraception. *N Engl J Med.* 2003;349:1830–1835.

18. Sonfield A, Gold RB, Frost JJ, Darroch JE. US insurance coverage of contraceptives and the impact of contraceptive coverage mandates, 2002. *Perspect Sex Reprod Health* 2004;36:72–79.

19. *Uneven and unequal: Insurance coverage and reproductive health.* New York: The Alan Guttmacher Institute; 1994.

20. Staff. *The appropriations process and discriminatory abortion funding restrictions.* NARAL Pro-Choice America 2003. Available at http://www.naral.org/facts /loader.cfm?url=/commonspot/security/getfile.cfm&PageID=7832. Accessed June 21, 2005.

21. Donovan P. *The politics of blame: Family planning, abortion and the poor.* New York: The Alan Guttmacher Institute; 1995.

22. NARAL Foundation. *The reproductive health and rights of women of color.* 2000. Available at http://www.naral.org/publications/loader.cfm?url=/commonspot /security/getfile.cfm&PageID=2435. Accessed June 21, 2005.

23. Jones RK, Darroch JE, Henshaw SK, Patterns in the socioeconomic characteristics of women obtaining abortions in 2000–2001. *Perspect Sex Reprod Health* 2002;34:226–235.

24. Staff. *The Bush administration's reproductive rights record.* National Organization for Women. November 2002. Available at http://www.now.org/issues/abortion /roe30/record.html. Accessed June 21, 2005.

25. NARAL Pro-Choice America. *Memorandum re anti-choice state legislative trends.* October 9, 2003. Available at http://www.naral.org/facts/loader.cfm?url= /commonspot/security/getfile.cfm&PageID=5586. Accessed June 21, 2005.

26. Davis SS. Can a pharmacist refuse to dispense birth control? *Time* 2004(June 7):22.

27. Yeoman B. The quiet war on abortion. *Mother Jones* 2001(September /October):46–51.

28. NARAL Pro-Choice America. *Refusal clauses: Dangerous for women's health.* January 1, 2005. Available at http://www.naral.org/facts/loader.cfm?url= /commonspot/security/getfile.cfm&PageID=16140. Accessed June 22, 2005.

29. Michigan Center for Reproductive Rights groups ask court to block abortion ban. http://www.crlp.org/pr_05_0614michigan.html. Accessed June 20, 2005.

30. NARAL *Foundation. Mandatory waiting periods and the freedom to choose.* Available at http://www.naral.org/facts/loader.cfm?url=/commonspot/security /getfile.cfm&PageID=1792. Accessed June 22, 2005.

31. Staff, American Medical Association. Induced termination of pregnancy before and after *Roe* v. *Wade*: Trends in the mortality and morbidity of women. *JAMA.* 1992;268:3238.

32. Center for Reproductive Rights. *The Teen Endangerment Act: Harming young women who seek abortions.* April 2005. Available at http://www.crlp.org/pub _fac_ccpa.html. Accessed June 22, 2005.

33. American Civil Liberties Union. *House approves Teen Endangerment Act; ACLU denounces measure, says it puts politics before young women's health.* Press release. April 27, 2005. Available at http://www.aclu.org/ReproductiveRights /ReproductiveRights.cfm?ID=18134&c=223. Accessed June 22, 2005.

34. NARAL Pro-Choice America. *The "Child Custody Protection Act" and the inadequacy of judicial bypass procedures.* July 19, 2004. Available at http://www .naral.org/facts/loader.cfm?url=/commonspot/security/getfile.cfm&PageID= 13289. Accessed June 22, 2005.

35. Planned Parenthood Federation of America. *Teenagers, abortion, and government intrusion laws.* 2004. Available at http://www.plannedparenthood.org/library /ABORTION/laws.html. Accessed June 21, 2005.

36. Jones RK, Purcell A, Singh S, Finer LB. Adolescents' reports of parental knowledge of adolescents' use of sexual health services and their reactions to mandated parental notification for prescription contraception. *JAMA*. 2005;293:340–348.

37. Reddy DM, Fleming R, Swain C. Effect of mandatory parental notification on adolescent girls' use of sexual health care services. *JAMA*. 2002;288:710–714.

38. Franzini L, Marks E, Cromwell PF, et al. Projected economic costs due to health consequences of teenagers' loss of confidentiality in obtaining reproductive health care services in Texas. *Arch Pediatr Adolesc Med*. 2004;158:1140–1146.

39. Staff. *US Supreme Court agrees to review state's abortion law*. CNN online. May 23, 2005. Available at http://www.cnn.com/2005/LAW/05/23/scotus.abortions .ap/. Accessed June 22, 2005.

40. Bader EJ. Abortion decline. *Z Magazine* 2003(Apr);16(4). Available at http: //www.zmag.org/ZMagSite/Apr2003/baderprint0403.html. Accessed June 22, 2005.

41. Center for Reproductive Rights. *Targeted Regulation of Abortion Providers (TRAP): Avoiding the TRAP*. Available at http://www.reproductiverights.org/pub_fac _trap.html. Accessed June 28, 2005.

42. Chavkin W. Sex, lies and silence: Reproductive health in a hostile environment. *Am J Public Health* 2001;91:1739–1741.

43. Snyder U. Thirty years after *The Joy of Sex*—Unintended pregnancy in the United States. *Medscape Ob/Gyn and Women's Health*. Available at http://www .medscape.com/viewarticle/442319. Accessed June 22, 2005.

44. Adams KE, Donohoe MT. Reproductive rights—commentary: Provider willingness to prescribe emergency contraception. *American Medical Association Virtual Mentor* 2004 (September);6(9). Available at http://www.ama-assn.org /ama/pub/category/12783.html. Accessed June 22, 2005.

45. Krisberg K. Refusal clause seen as threat to reproductive health, gag on information. *The Nation's Health* 2005(February):1, 10. Available at http://www .medscape.com/viewarticle/498617. Accessed June 22, 2005.

46. NARAL Pro-Choice America Foundation. *Proactive trends update* (Memorandum, October 8, 2003). Available at http://www.naral.org/facts/loader.cfm?url= /commonspot/security/getfile.cfm&PageID=4021. Accessed June 22, 2005.

47. Weiss R. New status for embryos in research. *Washington Post* October 30, 2002. Available at http://www.uams.edu/orsp/articles/11_1_02.htm. Accessed June 22, 2005.

48. US Department of Health & Human Services. *HHS names 11 to secretary's advisory committee on human research protection*. Press release. January 3, 2003. Available at http://www.hhs.gov/news/press/2003pres/20030103.html. Accessed June 22, 2005.

49. Society for Women's Health Research. *Issue: Human research protection*. July 22, 2004. Available at http://www.womenshealthresearch.org/policy/issues_hsp .htm. Accessed June 22, 2005.

50. The White House. Office of the Press Secretary. *President Bush signs Unborn Victims of Violence Act of 2004.* April 1, 2004. Available at http://www .whitehouse.gov/news/releases/2004/04/20040401-3.html. Accessed June 22, 2005.

51. NARAL Pro-Choice America. *The "Unborn Victims of Violence Act" is not the solution to domestic violence.* January 1, 2004. Available at http://www.naral.org /facts/loader.cfm?url=/commonspot/security/getfile.cfm&PageID=7970. Accessed June 22, 2005.

52. Paulson A. Lawsuit over an embryo fuels debate on when life begins. *Christian Science Monitor* March 23, 2005. Available at http://www.csmonitor.com/2005 /0323/p02s02-ussc.html. Accessed June 22, 2005.

53. Center for Reproductive Rights. *Court rejects use of European human rights law to establish fetal rights.* July 8, 2004. Available at http://www.crlp.org/pr_04 _0708france.html. Accessed June 22, 2005.

54. Associated Press Staff. *Bush signs ban on late-term abortion.* Available at http://www.cnn.com/2003/ALLPOLITICS/11/05/abortion.ap/index.html. Accessed June 22, 2005.

55. Liptak A. US judge in San Francisco strikes down federal law banning form of abortion. *New York Times* June 2, 2004.

56. Center for Reproductive Rights. *Federal abortion ban struck down in Nebraska case: Third court finds ban unconstitutional.* September 8, 2004. Available at http://www.reproductiverights.org/pr_04_0908pba.html. Accessed June 22, 2005.

57. Office of the City Attorney, City and County of San Francisco. *Herrera blocks Ashcroft bid for medical records.* Available at http://www.ci.sf.ca.us/site /cityattorney_page.asp?id=23313. Accessed June 22, 2005.

58. American Civil Liberties Union Reproductive Freedom Project. *Biased counseling against abortion.* April 11, 2001. Available at http://www.aclu.org/Reproductive Rights/ReproductiveRights.cfm?ID=9046&c=143. Accessed June 22, 2005.

59. Staff. Crisis pregnancy centers pose threat to women's health, choices. *The Nation's Health* 2002(August):16.

60. NARAL Pro-Choice America. *Congress should not legitimize deceptive "crisis pregnancy centers" or fund campaign to mislead women.* January 1, 2005. Available at http://www.prochoiceamerica.org/facts/loader.cfm?url= /commonspot/security/getfile.cfm&PageID=16473. Accessed June 22, 2005.

61. Blumenthal P, Johnson J, Stewart F. *The approval of mifepristone (RU486) in the United States: What's wrong with this picture?* MedGenMed. July 26, 2000. Available at http://www.medscape.com/viewarticle/408923. Accessed June 22, 2005.

62. Trupin SR, Moreno C. *Medical abortion: Overview and management.* MedGenMed. March 8, 2002. Available at http://www.medscape.com/viewarticle/429755. Accessed June 22, 2005.

63. Barclay L. Lower-dose mifepristone abortion regimen effective with high satisfaction. *Medscape Medical News* February 15, 2005. Available at http://www.medscape.com/viewarticle/499420. Accessed June 22, 2005.

64. Prine L, Lesnewski R, Berley N, Gold M. Medical abortion in family practice: A case series. *J Am Board Fam Pract.* 2003;16:290–295. Available at http://www.medscape.com/viewarticle/461866. Accessed June 22, 2005.

65. NARAL Pro-Choice America. *RU-486/mifepristone.* Available at http://www.naral.org/Issues/ru486/index.cfm. Accessed June 22, 2005.

66. Bill H.R.1079. RU-486 Suspension and Review Act of 2005. Available at http://www.theorator.com/bills109/hr1079.html. Accessed June 22, 2005.

67. Bennett T. Reproductive health care in the rural United States. *JAMA.* 2002; 287:112.

68. Talley PP, Bergus GR. Abortion training in family practice residency programs. *Fam Med.* 1996;28:245–248.

69. MacKay HT, MacKay AP. Abortion training in obstetrics and gynecology residency programs in the United States. *Fam Planning Perspect.* 1995;27:112–115.

70. Lazarus ES. Politicizing abortion: Personal morality and professional responsibility of residents training in the United States. *Soc Sci Med.* 1997;44:1417–1425.

71. Shanahan MA, Metheny WP, Star J, Peipert JF. Induced abortion: Physician training and practice patterns. *J Reprod Med.* 1999;44:428–432.

72. Almeling R, Tews L, Dudley S. Abortion training in US obstetrics and gynecology residency programs, 1998. *Fam Plann Perspect.* 2000;32:268–271, 320.

73. Espey E, Ogburn T, Chavez A, Qualls C, Leyba M. Abortion education in medical schools: A national survey. *Am J Obstet Gynecol.* 2005;192:640–643.

74. American Civil Liberties Union. *State restrictions that may apply to early medical abortion. Physician only laws.* February 1, 2000. Available at http://www.aclu.org/ReproductiveRights/ReproductiveRights.cfm?ID=9025&c=143. Accessed June 22, 2005.

75. Clarkson F. Terror in the name of the Lord. *Ms Magazine.* 2002/2003 (December/January):77–81.

76. NARAL Pro-Choice America. *Clinic violence.* Available at http://www.naral.org/Issues/violence/index.cfm. Accessed June 22, 2005.

77. Diamond S. Abortion politics. *Z Magazine* 1995. Available at http://www.zmag.org/ZMag/articles/may95diamond.htm. Accessed June 22, 2005.

78. Bush GW. *National Sanctity of Human Life Day proclamation,* January 18, 2002. Available at http://www.whitehouse.gov/news/releases/2002/01/20020118-10.html. Accessed June 22, 2005.

79. Donohoe MT. Individual and societal forms of violence against women in the United States and the developing world: An overview. *Curr Women's Hlth Rep.* 2002;2:313–319.

80. DaVanzo J, Adamson DM. *Family planning in developing countries: An unfinished success story* (Population Matters Issue Paper). Santa Monica, CA: RAND; 1998.

81. Indriso C, Mundigo A. Abortion in the developing world. *Am J Public Health* 1999;89:1890–1892.

82. World Health Organization. *Abortion: A tabulation of available data on the frequency and mortality of unsafe abortion,* Third Edition. Geneva: World Health Organization; 1997.

83. Center for Reproductive Rights. *The Bush global gag rule: Endangering women's health, free speech and democracy.* Available at http://www.crlp.org/pub_fac _ggrbush.html. Accessed June 22, 2005.

84. The White House. Office of the Press Secretary. *Memorandum for the administrator of the United States Agency for International Development.* January 22, 2001. Available at http://www.planetwire.org/wrap/files.fcgi/1177_bush _mexico_city_memorandum.htm. Accessed June 22, 2005.

85. Planned Parenthood Federation of America (PPFA). *Bush Administration expands the global gag rule.* Available at http://www.planetwire.org/details/4270. Accessed June 22, 2005.

86. National Organization for Women. *Reproductive rights historical highlights.* Available at http://www.now.org/issues/abortion/roe30/timeline.html. Accessed June 22, 2005.

87. 34 Million Friends of UNFPA. *Bush Administration to withhold UNFPA funding.* Available at http://www.34millionfriends.org/index.htm. Accessed June 22, 2005.

88. Editors. Abortion drugs must become WHO essential medicines. *Lancet* 2005;365:1826.

89. Union of Concerned Scientists. *Specific examples of the abuse of science.* Available at http://www.ucsusa.org/global_environment/rsi/page.cfm?pageID=1398. Accessed June 22, 2005.

90. Donohoe MT. Teen pregnancy: A call for sound science and public policy. *Z Magazine* 2003;16(4):14–16.

91. Kirby DJ. Sex education in the schools. In: Garrison JA, Smith MD, Besharov DJ, eds. *Sexuality and American social policy.* Menlo Park, CA: Henry J. Kaiser Family Foundation; 1994.

92. NIH Consensus Statement: Interventions to prevent HIV risk behaviors. *National Institutes of Health* 1997;15:15–16.

93. Kaiser Family Foundation. *Sex education in America: A view from inside the nation's classrooms.* Menlo Park, CA: The Kaiser Family Foundation; 2000.

94. Kirby D. Sexuality and sex education at home and school. *Adolesc Med.* 1999;10:195–209.

95. Waxman HA. *Abstinence-only education.* Government Reform Minority Office. Available at http://www.democrats.reform.house.gov/investigations.asp? Issue=Abstinence-Only+Education. Accessed June 22, 2005.

96. Waxman HA. *The content of federally funded abstinence-only education programs.* United States House of Representatives Committee on Government Reform—Minority Staff, Special Investigations Division, December 2004. Available at http://reform.democrats.house.gov/Documents/20041201102153-50247 .pdf. Accessed June 22, 2005.

97. Planned Parenthood. *The assault on birth control and family planning programs, October 2003.* A Planned Parenthood report on the Bush Administration and its allies. Available at http://www.plannedparenthood.org/pp2/portal/files /portal/medicalinfo/birthcontrol/report-031030-birth-control.pdf. Accessed June 22, 2005.

98. Olson S. Marriage promotion, reproductive injustice, and the war against poor women of color. *Dollars and Sense: The Magazine of Economic Justice* 2005 (January/February). Available at http://www.dollarsandsense.org/archives /2005/0105olson.html. Accessed June 22, 2005.

99. Donohoe MT. Violence against women: Partner abuse and sexual assault. *Hospital Physician* 2004;40:24–31.

100. Cantor J, Baum K. The limits of conscientious objection: May pharmacists refuse to fill prescriptions for emergency contraception? *N Engl J Med.* 2004;351:2008–2012.

101. Kolata G. Debate on selling morning-after pill over the counter. *New York Times* December 12, 2003.

102. Grimes DA. *Politics, power and procreation.* MedGenMed. June 15, 2005. Available at http://www.medscape.com/viewarticle/505887. Accessed June 22, 2005.

103. Heavey S. *Seventh state eases "morning-after" pill access.* Reuters Health Information. June 17, 2005.

104. A Victory for Women [editorial]. *New York Times* June 23, 2005.

105. Drazen JM. Inserting government between patient and physician. *N Engl J Med.* 2004;350:178–179.

Chapter 15

The Way It Was

Eleanor Cooney

The Beatles ruled. The mini was in. I was seventeen, and pregnant. What happened next is what could happen again.

In 1959, when I was a precocious smarty-pants still in grade school, I wrote a fake letter to Doris Blake, the *New York Daily News* advice columnist. I pretended to be a teenage girl "in trouble." I spun a tale of a liquor-soaked prom night and passing out in the back of a car. I included a cast of entirely fictional characters—a worthless boyfriend, a mentally unstable mother, a strict, brutal father. I ended my letter with: "Now I think I am pregnant. Please help me. I am desperate."

I'm not sure what I expected, but my letter was not printed, and no advice was forthcoming. The silence was utter. Possibly Miss Blake, like Nathanael West's Miss Lonelyhearts, had a drawer where such letters were tossed. If so, the other letters in that drawer were no doubt a lot like mine—except that they were not written by wise-ass children. They were real. And for the writers of those letters, the silence was real. And I remember thinking: *Gee, what if I really were that girl I made up? What would I do?*

One summer night some years later, when I was not quite 18, I got knocked up. There was nothing exciting or memorable or even interestingly sordid about the sex. I wasn't raped or coerced, nor was I madly in love or drunk or high. The guy was another kid, actually younger than I, just a friend, and it pretty much happened by default. We were horny teenagers with nothing else to do.

Nature, the ultimate unsentimental pragmatist, has its own notions about what constitutes a quality liaison. What nature wants is for sperm and egg to meet, as often as possible, whenever and wherever possible. Whatever it takes to expedite that meeting is fine with nature. If it's two people with a bassinet and a nursery all decorated and waiting and a shelf full of baby books, fine. If it's a 12-year-old girl who's been married off to a 70-year-old Afghan chieftain, fine. And if it's a couple of healthy young oafs like my friend and me, who knew perfectly well where babies come from but just got stupid for about 15 minutes, that's fine, too.

In the movies, newly pregnant women trip, fall down the stairs, and "lose the baby." Ah. If only it were that easy. In real life, once that egg is fertilized and has glided on down the fallopian tube, selected its nesting place, and settled in, it's notoriously secure, behaves like visiting royalty. Nature doesn't give a fig about the hostess's feelings of hospitality or lack of them. If the zygote's not defective, and the woman is in good health, almost nothing will shake it loose. Anyone who's been pregnant and didn't want to be knows this is so.

On November 5, 2003, three decades after *Roe* v. *Wade* established a woman's constitutional right to terminate a pregnancy, President George W. Bush signed the Partial Birth Abortion Ban [PBAB] bill into law. We've all seen the photograph: The president sits at a table with a modest little smile on his lips. Nine guys—senators and congressmen—stand behind him, watching that signature go onto the paper, giddy grins on their faces. They look almost goofy with joy.

Two of these happy fellows are actually Democrats: Jim Oberstar and Bart Stupak. The rest are Republicans to their marrow: the bill's sponsor, Rick Santorum, as well as Steve Chabot, Orrin Hatch, Henry Hyde, Tom DeLay, Mike DeWine, and Dennis Hastert.

Be assured that it's not just "partial-birth" abortion they're so happy about passing a law against. It's all the law heralds. Like some ugly old wall-to-wall carpeting they've been yearning to get rid of, they finally, *finally* loosened a little corner of *Roe*. Now they can start to rip the whole thing up, roll it back completely, and toss it in the dumpster.

For with the PBAB, Bush and Co. have achieved the first federal legal erosion of *Roe v. Wade* since its adoption in 1973. *Roe* states that a woman may terminate a pregnancy up to the point of "viability," approximately 24 weeks. After that, states may prohibit or restrict abortion, but exceptions must be made to preserve "the life or health of the woman." The PBAB has been around the block before—in 1995, 1997, 1999, and 2000. What stopped it before was always the debate over allowances for women's health. President Clinton vetoed it three times because it disallowed exceptions to prevent serious disabling injury to the woman. But when the bill came up again in 2002, allowances for prevention of disabling injury to the mother were left out, as were those for rape and incest. A "partial-birth" abortion would be permitted only as a last resort to save the mother's life, or if the fetus was already dead. In other words, the risk of permanent injury to the woman if she proceeds with the pregnancy is not a good enough reason to perform one—not in Santorum's book. She has to be literally on death's doorstep. A couple of Democrats tried to offer an amendment that brought up that pesky women's health issue again. The bill's authors objected. Women and their doctors will just use the amendment as a loophole! Chabot worried it would create "a phony ban" and Santorum predicted it would be defeated. It was.

One Democratic senator proposed a nonbinding resolution, expressing " . . . the sense of the Senate that . . . *Roe* v. *Wade* was appropriate and secures an important constitutional right and should not be overturned." This amendment passed in the Senate by a 52–46 vote. The House version of the PBAB lacked any such amendment.

In conference, the Republicans quickly took care of that feeble bleat on behalf of *Roe:* They simply deleted it. When the bill landed on Bush's desk, the resolution to reaffirm *Roe* was gone.

What, you might ask, is "partial-birth" abortion? Most of us know that the term is not a medical one. Invented by the pro-life folks in the last decade or so, it's a vague reference to "intact dilation and extraction," or D&X. Introduced in 1992, D&X is a variation on a similar, well-established second- (and sometimes third-) term procedure—"dilation and evacuation," or D&E—used after the fetus has grown too large to be vacuumed or scraped out in a simple D&C, or "dilation and curettage."

In a D&E, the fetus is usually dismembered inside the uterus and extracted in pieces. Old obstetrics books from as far back as the 1700s have disquieting illustrations of the various tools of yore used for fetal dismemberment. Nowadays, powerful gripping forceps are used, making the procedure much less dangerous for the woman.

The D&X was developed with the same objective. An inherent hazard of D&E—aside from potential damage by the instruments themselves and the risk of leaving tissue behind, increasing the chances of infection—is that fetal bones begin to calcify at about 13 weeks. As they are broken up, the sharp bone ends can puncture, scrape, and perforate. Hence the "intact" dilation and extraction. The fetus is brought out whole instead of being pulled apart bit by bit. The head is punctured and then collapsed by suction or compression so that it will fit through the partially dilated cervix. The fetus is dead, but in one piece. This, specifically, is the procedure the PBAB has sought to criminalize—when the fetus is killed while its body is outside the uterus, therefore "partially born."

Under the PBAB of 2003, a D&X would be permitted only to save the woman's life or if the fetus is dead. It would require a girl who'd been impregnated by her uncle, father, or brother, and who, out of shame, ignorance, and fear had hidden her condition until it was obvious to the world, to carry the fetus to term and give birth. If a woman discovers, late in her pregnancy, that the fetus has, say, anencephaly—a brain stem but no actual brain—then she must carry it to term, give birth, and let it die on its own.

Since lurid descriptions of partial-birth abortion have been so effective in rallying support for the bill, perhaps some balance is needed. I've read and heard hundreds of accounts of pre-*Roe* abortion, and there was a wide range of danger, squalor, sanitary conditions, provider skill, follow-up care. The well-heeled and well-connected often flew to Puerto Rico or Sweden and checked into clinics. Of the ones who couldn't do that, some were lucky enough to find competent, compassionate doctors. Some were treated kindly and recovered without incident. The other extreme was pain, terror, and death worthy of the Inquisition. A typical picture emerges, though, and it matches up just about perfectly with a story told to me by a woman I know.

After a date rape (by a "poet") during a trip to Paris in 1967 when she was 23, she found herself pregnant. She tried the usual "remedies"—scalding hot baths, violent jumping, having someone walk on her belly. When she got home to Minnesota, she was two months along. A doctor friend there said he couldn't help her himself, but sent her to a local prostitute who did abortions.

The prostitute had her own speculum. The procedure was done on the prostitute's bed: The catheter was inserted through the cervix and left there. After four days of high fever, chills, bleeding, and passing big chunks of tissue, she landed in the hospital. They said her uterus was perforated, that she had acute peritonitis and an "incomplete" abortion. She was given a huge dose of penicillin and treated as if she were some sort of contemptible lower life form. The emergency-room doctor snarled, "What have you done to yourself?" Later, she realized that the first doctor—her friend—had known all along that she'd probably get desperately ill. Only then could a hospital legally give her a D&C.

She recovered—sterile, violently allergic to penicillin, and so "paralyzed and ashamed" by the experience that she stayed away from men for four years. Who says deterrence doesn't work?

Then there's the famous 1964 police photograph of a woman's corpse on a motel-room floor in Connecticut. She's kneeling naked, face down as if to Mecca, legs bent to her chest, bloody towels bunched under her. The case had made local headlines, but the picture wasn't seen by the general public until *Ms. Magazine* ran it in a 1973 article lauding the ruling of *Roe* v. *Wade*. Details emerged about the woman's life and death: She was 27, married with two young daughters, but estranged from her violent husband. Her lover had performed the abortion, using borrowed instruments and a textbook. When she started hemorrhaging, he panicked, fled the motel, and left her there.

Compared to those two women, I got off easy. By the middle of September, I'd missed two periods and my cigarettes were tasting peculiar. I was bound for freshman year at college in Boston, though, so I just ignored the facts and went off to school. It took a third missed period and almost throwing up in the backseat of a car packed with kids to penetrate my adolescent thick headedness.

I had a savvy friend in New York, Kat, who only dated rich older men. I figured she'd be the one to call. Soon a long ride on buses and trains took me out to a house in a Boston suburb. The doctor's wife answered the door.

There was no waiting room, no magazines, no other patients. The house was completely ordinary, perhaps a touch run-down. She showed me into a room off the front hall and vanished.

Except for a small sink, the office was just a regular room, a parlor, with green walls and venetian blinds and a worn rug on the floor. A tall, battered, glass-doored porcelain cabinet stood in a corner. Through the glass, I could see on the shelves a dusty disorderly jumble of stethoscopes, hypodermics, bottles, little rubber hammers, basins, forceps, clamps, speculums, wads of cotton. There were rust stains in the sink and a tired old examining table.

The doctor, a little nervous man with glasses and a bald head, came in. I explained my problem. I have to examine you, he said. And he said: Everything has to be clean, very clean. He went to the sink and washed and washed his hands.

He finished and stood there without saying anything. His eyes were sort of glittering behind his glasses, and he acted as if I was supposed to know what to do next. I glanced around for a gown, but he was looking impatient, so I just took off my underwear and climbed onto the table.

He didn't bother with a glove. He poked around a while, then told me that I'd waited too long, I was too far gone, it would be too risky for him, and that would be $25.

And I was back out on the suburban street, the door shut firmly behind me.

Kat told me to come to New York and bring $500. I slept on the couch in her apartment. Kat's roommate, Elaine, gave me the address of a doctor over in Jersey City. I took a train and walked 10 blocks to a street of old brownstones, some of them with their windows boarded up. There had been no calling ahead for an "appointment"; you were supposed to just show up.

This doctor had a waiting room, with dark walls and a very high ceiling, the front room of the brownstone. It was full of people, facing each other along opposite walls, sitting in old, cracked, brown leather parlor chairs with stand-up ashtrays here and there, like in a bus station. A set of tall sliding wooden doors stood closed between that room and the next. Everyone was smoking, including me. The air was blue.

Several Puerto Rican–looking women chattered away in Spanish and seemed perfectly cheerful. There were a few men, who looked as if they might be accompanying somebody, and some more women who sat silent and staring.

And there was a couple who stood out like a pair of borzoi among street mutts: a man and woman, tall, slim, expensively dressed WASPs, faces grim, looking like people who'd taken a seriously wrong turn off the highway. I remember feeling sorry for them.

The tall wooden doors separated. A potbellied man in shirtsleeves who resembled Harpo Marx minus the fun stood there. His eyes moved around the room. He looked at the Puerto Rican women, the tall WASP woman, then at me, then the WASP woman again, considered for a moment, turned back to me, and pointed.

You, he said.

I got up and went in. He slid the doors shut. We were alone.

The windows in here had been nailed over with plywood, and the floor was ancient linoleum. There was a smell of insecticide. Boxes and bundles of paper were piled high in the dim corners and on a rolltop desk, and along the walls were shelves crammed messily with stethoscopes, hypodermics, speculums. The examining table was the centerpiece of the room, antique and massive, from the last century, dark green leather, steel and ceramic, designed so that the patient did not lie flat but in a semi-reclining position. Instead of stirrups, there were obstetrical leg supports. A tall old-fashioned floor lamp with a rose silk shade and a fringe, the only light in the room, stood next to the table alongside a cylinder of gas. An unlit crystal chandelier dangled in the overhead shadows.

The doctor had a trace of some sort of European accent. German, I guessed. He was about a foot shorter than I was, and behaved with obsequious deference, as if I had dropped in for an afternoon sherry. He gestured toward the examining table with a courtly flourish. I sat between the leg supports while he stood close and asked questions: Last period, how many times had I had sex, was I married, how many men had I had sex with, did they have large or small penises, were they circumcised, what positions, did I like it?

He moved the floor lamp closer. I put my legs in the apparatus and looked up at the chandelier.

He didn't bother with a glove, either. He thrust several fingers in, hard, so I could feel the scrape of his nails.

Ouch! I said politely.

Ouch, he mocked. Never mind your ouch. He pushed his fingers in harder and pressed down on my belly with his other hand.

You are very far along, he said. It will be a very difficult procedure. Come back tomorrow. Be here at seven o'clock in the evening. Give me one hundred dollars now because this will be difficult. You can pay the rest when you come back. Bring cash. Five hundred more.

I borrowed the extra hundred from Kat, and enlisted someone I knew to ride out to Jersey City with me on the train, a guy who was something of an ex-boyfriend. Even though I was enigmatic about why we were going to Jersey City at night, he guessed what was up, and seemed fairly entertained at the prospect.

This time, there was no one in the waiting room. The doctor looked very annoyed when he saw that I wasn't alone. My friend stayed out there while I went into the office. The doctor locked the door behind us.

When I was on the table, he stood between my legs and pressed and ground his pelvis against me and then put his fingers in for a while.

Then he said: You are too far gone. I cannot do it.

I put my legs down and sat up. He stood next to me, leaned on me heavily, and rubbed his two hands up my thigh, all the way up, so that his fingertips collided with my crotch. I understood then that he'd known perfectly well on my last visit that he wasn't going to go through with it.

You are a beautiful girl, a beautiful girl, he breathed moistly onto my face as his hands slid up and down, up and down. It is too late. Take my advice. Have the baby. Have the baby.

He unlocked the sliding doors and beckoned my friend in.

Get married, he said. Have the baby.

Hey, I'm not the guy, said my friend.

What about my hundred dollars? I asked.

Get out of here, the doctor said, and turned his back.

When we got to my friend's train stop, he walked off whistling a jaunty tune. Good luck, he said, and was gone.

Today, chat rooms and message boards related to abortion show a disturbing trend among some young people: Not only is disinformation rife ("The only reason abortion is still legal," writes one correspondent, "is becuz the babies organs are prossed and some of that money is forwarded to the libral party."), but many young people haven't the remotest notion of pre-*Roe* reality. Abortion's been legal since before they were born. Some even believe that abortion was invented with *Roe* v. *Wade*.

Abortion was not always illegal before *Roe*. Into the 19th century, what a woman did with her early pregnancy was considered a purely domestic matter. Until "quickening," when the fetus was perceived to be alive and kicking, it wasn't even considered a pregnancy, but a "blocking" or an "imbalance," and women regularly "restored the menses," if they so chose, through plants and potions. Abortifacients became commercially available by the mid-1700s.

Quality control was not great, and the earliest abortion legislation, in the 1820s and '30s, appears to have been an effort to curtail poisoning rather than abortion itself. According to several historians of the issue, as abortion—both through drugs and direct procedures—became a bigger and bigger commercial venture, "orthodox" physicians, who were competing with midwives, homeopaths, and self-styled practitioners of all stripes, pushed to make abortion illegal. The nascent American Medical Association established its dominance over lay practitioners through abortion laws, and women were kept in their place. Eugenics played a role, too: With "undesirables" breeding prolifically, motherhood was hailed as a white woman's patriotic duty, abortion a form of treason. By the mid-1800s, most of the "folk" knowledge had been lost and abortion became "infanticide." Between 1860 and 1880, antiabortion laws spread city by city, state by state. Now there was a ruthlessly pragmatic aspect: In the aftermath of the slaughter of half a million men during the Civil War, the births were needed. First the men were conscripted, then the women.

Demand for abortion continued to grow in spite of the laws. Periods of relative tolerance gave way to periods of stricter enforcement, which inevitably corresponded to periods of women's activism. In the late 19th century, it was when they demanded a voice in politics. After World War II and through the 1960s, it was when they demanded sexual freedom. All kinds of change, rebellion, and upheaval were busting out then, and the reflexive reaction of the authorities was to crack down. For women getting illegal abortions, this era was particularly marked by fear, secrecy, ignorance, shame, and danger. This was the era that put the rusty coat hanger into the collective consciousness.

The day after I returned from Jersey City, there was another doctor in a seedy little basement office in New York, who didn't even touch me. He said the only way to do it at this point would be to perform a miniature caesarean, not something he could do in his office.

Kat and Elaine were plainly getting tired of having me and my problem on their couch. They came up with a phone number in Florida. I called. A male voice said I should fly to Miami. They'd meet me and take me to one of the islands, to a clinic. Give us the telephone number of where you're staying now in New York. We'll call you back and confirm the arrangements.

He called back within an hour. It was set: Fly to Miami next Thursday, between the hours of noon and five. Wear something bright red so we'll know you when you get off the plane. And bring eight hundred dollars, in cash.

One last thing, he said. You must not tell anyone where you're going.

They understand that I'm over three months, right? I said.

Yeah, yeah. They know. It's all set.

I hung up. This didn't feel good at all. Florida, the islands, wads of cash, distant voices.

I thought about doing what I should have done in the first place: calling my mother.

Not calling her in the beginning wasn't because my mother was a prude or religious or anything like that. Hardly. It was because I was naturally secretive, had wanted to take care of things on my own. I just wanted it to go away. But there was a limit to even my pigheadedness. I thought about how sad it would make my mother if I just disappeared. My mother, who was right there in the city, swung into action instantly. She made arrangements with a doctor she knew, and borrowed the $1,500 it would cost because of the added risk.

This doctor had a clean, modern office in Midtown. He drew a diagram showing the difference between a first-trimester D&C and what I'd be having. After three months, he said, the placenta and the blood vessels that feed it grow too complex to simply be scraped out. To do so would be to just about guarantee a hemorrhage. In a normal birth or miscarriage, he said, the uterus contracts, shearing off the placenta and pinching off the connecting blood vessels. We induce a miscarriage, he said, by injecting a saline solution into the amniotic sac. The fetus dies. The uterus rejects it by contracting. That way, no hemorrhage. Then we go in and take it out. If it were done any other way, it could easily kill you.

A date was made for the following week. I was off of Kat and Elaine's couch and on my mother's.

One evening, my mother's phone rang. It was the man in Florida. He'd tracked me down through Kat, and he was angry. What the hell had happened? Where was I? They'd waited all day at the airport in Miami, met every plane. I apologized, told him I'd made other arrangements here at home. He said I was a fucking bitch who owed money to him and a lot of other people, told me to go fuck myself, and hung up.

Maybe everything would have been peachy if I'd gone to the islands. Maybe I'd have come back with a tan and heartwarming stories of kindness and caring that I'd remember fondly through the years. A rather different picture always comes to mind, though, and it involves a morgue in a run-down little hospital with heat and flies, and then a dinghy with an outboard, or maybe a fishing boat with a rumbling, smoky diesel engine, heading out into the Caribbean at night bearing a largish canvas bag weighted with cinder blocks....

That year in the 1960s, several thousand American women were treated in emergency rooms for botched abortions, and there were at least 200 known deaths. Comparing my story with others from the pre-*Roe* era, what impresses me is how close I veered to mortal danger in spite of not living under most of the usual terrible strictures. Unlike so many of the women I've read about and talked to, especially the teenagers, I was quite unburdened by shame and guilt. I'd never, ever had the "nice girls don't do it" trip laid on me. I came from a religion-free background. I wasn't worried in the least about "sin," was not at all ambivalent about whether abortion was right or wrong. I wasn't sheltered or ignorant. I didn't face parental disapproval or stigmatization of any kind. I had no angry husband. My mother would have leapt in and helped me at any point. There was no need at all to keep my condition secret and to procrastinate, but I did it anyway. What does this say about how it was for other young girls and women who didn't have my incredible luck? I was luckier than most in another department, too—being raped by the abortionist was a major hazard of the era. I merely got diddled by a couple of disgusting old men. It was nasty and squalid, but it certainly didn't kill me. As I said, I got off easy.

Ironically, it was the medical profession, which had made abortion illegal in the first place, that started to speak out. Doctors treating the desperately sick women who landed in hospitals with raging peritonitis, hemorrhages, perforated uteruses, and septic shock often had to futilely watch them die, because the women had waited too long to get help—because they were confused and terrified, because what they had done was "illegal" and "immoral."

One doctor's "awakening" is vividly described in *The Worst of Times*, a collection of interviews with women, cops, coroners, and practitioners from the illegal abortion era. In 1948, when this doctor was an intern in a Pittsburgh hospital, a woman was admitted with severe pelvic sepsis after a bad abortion. She was beautiful, married to someone important and wealthy, and already in renal failure. Over the next couple of days, despite heroic efforts to save her, a cascade of systemic catastrophes due to the overwhelming infection culminated with the small blood vessels bursting under her skin, bruises breaking out everywhere as if some invisible fist were punching her over and over, and she died. Being well-to-do didn't always save you.

Her death was so horrible that it made him, he recalls, physically ill. He describes his anger, but says he didn't quite know with whom to be angry. It took him another 20 years to understand that it was not the abortionist who killed her—it was the legal system, the lawmakers who had forced her away from the medical community, who "... killed her just as surely as if they had held the catheter or the coat hanger or whatever. I'm still angry. It was all so unnecessary."

All so unnecessary.

In the same book, a man who assisted in autopsies in a big urban hospital, starting in the mid-1950s, describes the many deaths from botched abortions that he saw. "The deaths stopped overnight in 1973." He never saw another in the 18 years before he retired. "That," he says, "ought to tell people something about keeping abortion legal."

In February 2004, seven abortion doctors in four states sued Attorney General John Ashcroft, claiming that D&X was indeed a medically necessary procedure. Ashcroft retaliated by subpoenaing their hospitals for the records of all patients who'd had late-term abortions in the past five years—most long before the PBAB—to determine, ostensibly, if any D&Xs had actually been prompted by health risks. In June, a federal judge in San Francisco declared the PBAB to be unconstitutional—saying it was vague, placed an "undue burden" on abortion rights, and contained no exception for a woman's health—but she did not, in deference to other cases wending their way through the legal system, completely lift the ban.

One doctor, writing about D&X, said something that particularly struck me—that the actual practice of medicine, the stuff that goes on behind closed doors, is often gruesome, gory, and messy. Saws whine, bones crack, blood spatters. We outside of the profession are mostly shielded from this reality. Our model is white sheets, gleaming linoleum, and Dr. Kildare. Face-lift, hip replacement, bypass, liver transplant—many people would faint dead away at a detailed description of any of these. Doctors roll up their sleeves, plunge in, and do tough, nervy, drastic, and risky things with our very meat-bone-and-gristle bodies, under occasionally harrowing circumstances.

The gruesome aspect of D&X has been detailed and emphasized, but as a procedure, it's in line with the purpose of medicine: to get a hard flesh-and-blood job done. What makes it different from other procedures is that it can involve a live fetus. This puts it in a class by itself. But the woman undergoing a D&X knows this. If she's doing it, there will be powerfully compelling reasons, and it's not for anyone else to decide if those reasons are compelling enough.

Women of all kinds seek and have always sought abortion: married, single, in their twenties, thirties, and forties, teenagers. Some have no children, some have several already. Some never want children, some want children later. They are churchgoers, atheists, agnostics. They are morally upright pillars of the community, they are prostitutes. They're promiscuous, they're monogamous, they're recent virgins. They get pregnant under all kinds of circumstances: consensual sex, nonconsensual sex, sex that falls somewhere between consensual and nonconsensual. Some are drunk or using drugs, some never even touch an aspirin. Some use no birth control, some use birth control that fails.

The desperate teenager I invented in my letter to Doris Blake in 1959 surely had hundreds, maybe thousands, of real-life counterparts at the very moment I put the envelope in the mail. All kinds of women are vulnerable and are affected by the particulars of abortion law, but the ones most profoundly affected are the very young, and it's a one-two punch from both nature and society. First, nature itself conspires to make teenagers defenseless—they're lushly fertile, their brains are flooded with sex hormones, and their judgment, practical knowledge, and common sense have been known to be less than perfect.

Teenagers—especially those who are poor and uneducated—are by far the group having the most elective late-term abortions. If we truly wish to protect the young and vulnerable, promote a "culture of life," as President Bush said so grandly in his signing speech, then we must make teenage girls a top priority. Make sure they don't get pregnant in the first place, and not just by preaching "abstinence only." If they do get pregnant, don't throw a net of fear, confusion, and complication over them that will only cause them to hide their conditions for as long as they can. Because that's exactly what they'll do. You could argue that "partial-birth" abortion is the price a society pays when it calculatedly keeps teenage girls ignorant instead of aggressively arming them with the facts of life and, if necessary, the equipment to protect themselves from pregnancy.

I was hardly one of those tragically vulnerable teenagers. I suppose I was the kind of wanton female the lawmakers and wrath-of-God types look down on. There's no doubt that I was stupid and irresponsible, and I certainly knew better than what you might have surmised from my actions. By some standards, I suppose you could say I was a slut. Those sleazy doctors left no doubt that that's how they saw me. Some would say I got what I deserved, or that I deserved to die.

The arguments would be endless, but they would be irrelevant to the facts: From the moment I started looking for an abortion, not once did I even consider going through with the pregnancy. Not for one second. It simply was not going to happen. Nothing, and I mean nothing, was going to stop me, and it could have cost me my life. And this is what I had in common with millions and millions of women throughout time and history. When a woman does not want to be pregnant, the drive to become unpregnant can turn into a force equal to the nature that wants her to stay pregnant. And then she will look for an abortion, whether it's legal or illegal, clean or filthy, safe or riddled with danger. This is simply a fact, whatever our opinion of it. And whether we like it or not, humans, married and unmarried, will continue to have sex—wisely, foolishly, violently, nicely, hostilely, pleasantly, dangerously, responsibly, carelessly, sordidly, exaltedly—and there will be pregnancies: wanted, unwanted, partly wanted, partly unwanted.

A society that does not accept the facts is a childish society, and a society that makes abortion illegal—and I believe that the PBAB is a calculated step in exactly that direction—is a cruel and backward society that makes being female a crime. It works in partnership with the illegal abortionist. It puts him in business, sends him his customers, and employs him to dispense crude, dirty, barbaric, savage punishment to those who break the law. And the ones who are punished by the illegal abortionist are always women: mothers, sisters, daughters, wives.

It's no way to treat a lady.

Part Four

Obesity, Tobacco, and Suicide by Firearms: The Modern Epidemics

In the nineteenth and early twentieth centuries, the focus of public health was on sanitation, clean water, and epidemics of infectious diseases, such as cholera, yellow fever, and influenza. Major progress in hygiene occurred, including measures promulgated by Florence Nightingale, whose attention to cleanliness and wound management in Crimean War theater hospitals led to changes in nursing care that have had an arguably greater effect on hospital-associated mortality than any scientific advance since. With the discovery of new vaccines for diseases such as polio and smallpox (eradicated from the planet except for caches at the CDC and the State Research Center of Virology and Biotechnology [VECTOR] in Koltsovo, Russia[1]), antibiotics, and ongoing advances in surgical technique, infectious disease epidemics became less significant contributors to morbidity and mortality in the United States. Shamefully, millions in the developing world still die each year from vaccine-preventable and antibiotic-treatable diseases, an issue noted in other chapters' readings.

Despite recent scares involving severe acute respiratory syndrome (SARS) and bird flu, the major modern epidemics facing the developed world are now diseases resulting from obesity and tobacco abuse.

Chapter Sixteen (by Martin Donohoe) explores the causes and health and economic consequences of obesity; the "obesity economy"; nutrition, exercise, and television; the role of the food and beverage industry in promoting consumption of unhealthy foodstuffs; the flipside of obesity, pathological underweight; and gluttony. Medical and surgical treatments for obesity are reviewed along with public health approaches to combating obesity. As life expectancy increases in the developing world, obesity is becoming a major problem there as well, with enormous anticipated health care costs expected over coming decades consequent to multiple associated chronic conditions.

Chapter Seventeen (by Martin Donohoe) provides an overview of the tobacco epidemic, then examines one specific public health response, the WHO Framework Convention on Tobacco Control (World Tobacco Treaty). The chapter describes the tremendous power of the tobacco industry, achieved through lobbying and the efforts of those passing through the revolving door between industry and government, over US government regulation and the government's ultimately unsuccessful attempt to scuttle the convention. US objections to this convention mirror the unwillingness of our country to enter into a number of other international agreements designed to protect human and environmental health and human rights (discussed in other chapters).

Chapter Eighteen (by Matthew Miller and David Hemenway) reviews data showing how the easy availability of firearms increases the rate of suicide in the United States. Despite increasing recognition of psychiatric illness and greater availability of antidepressant medications, each year 35,000 Americans commit suicide.[2] Almost twice as many individuals take their own lives each year than are murdered. The widespread availability of firearms in the United States plays a major role because a majority of completed suicides involve guns. The authors argue that restricting access to firearms prevents attempted and completed suicides.

This section emphasizes the importance of a public health approach to major health care issues, a method frequently overlooked by clinicians more attentive to learning and implementing therapies for obesity- and tobacco-related diseases and learning surgical techniques to treat firearm injuries than to decreasing population-wide levels of obesity, smoking, and gun violence. Further information regarding these topics can be found on the obesity and tobacco industry pages of the Public Health and Social Justice website at http://phsj.org/obesity/ and http://phsj.org/tobacco-industry/ respectively.

Notes

1. Centers for Disease Control and Prevention. *Emergency preparedness and response—Smallpox.* December 29, 2004. Retrieved from http://www.bt.cdc.gov/agent/smallpox/basics/outbreak.asp.

2. Crosby, A. E, Ortego, L., & Stevens, M. R. Suicides—United States, 1999–2007. *Centers for Disease Control and Prevention Morbidity and Mortality Weekly Supplement,* January 14, 2001, *60*(01), 56–59. Retrieved from http://www.cdc.gov/mmwr/preview/mmwrhtml/su6001a11.htm?s_cid=su6001a11_e&source=govdelivery.

Chapter 16

Weighty Matters

Public Health Aspects of the Obesity Epidemic

Martin Donohoe

PART I

Causes and Health and Economic Consequences of Obesity

This chapter is derived from a 5-part series that describes public health aspects of the obesity epidemic. The prevalence of overweight and obesity has been rising in the United States for decades and has now reached epidemic proportions.[1] Part I describes the epidemiology and health consequences of obesity; part II discusses economic consequences of obesity, the obesity economy, and the roles of exercise, nutrition, and television; part III covers sodas, pouring contracts, and the food industry; part IV deals with obesity worldwide as well as pathologic underweight and gluttony; and part V discusses treatments and public health measures to combat obesity. Obesity affects men and women, but certain aspects of this medical and public health problem are unique to women, and these will be noted when relevant.

Epidemiology of Obesity in the United States

The average height/weight for American men and women today are, respectively, 5′9″/191 lbs. and 5′4″/164 lbs.[2] Overweight is classified as a body mass index (BMI) (weight [kg] /height [m^2]) = 25.0 and obesity as a BMI = 30.0. In 2005, 60.5% of US adults were overweight and 23.9% were obese.[1] The prevalence of obesity is nearly identical in men and women and ranges from 18%

among adults aged 18 to 29 years to 30% among adults aged 50 to 59 years.[1] Obesity is more common among lower-income individuals, rural Americans, non-Hispanic blacks, and those with less education.[1,3] Low socioeconomic status is more closely linked to obesity for women than for men.[4]

Some anthropologists have attached cultural explanations to the obesity epidemic among African Americans. During the lean centuries of slavery, when food was intermittently scarce and dietary choices limited, being overweight was both a protective mechanism and a sign of good health. Persistence of some of these factors may partially explain obesity among African Americans. However, poverty also plays a role because poor individuals tend to eat more calorie-laden fast food, and poverty is more common among African Americans than among Caucasians.[5] Others have cited an association between food insecurity and obesity. Since African Americans have higher levels of poverty and food insecurity and live in neighborhoods with fewer supermarkets and more fast-food restaurants, consumption of nutritious foodstuffs becomes impractical and is indeed more expensive, leading to overconsumption of low-cost, energy-dense (i.e., high in added sugars and fat) foods.[4,6]

Causes of obesity include poor diet and inadequate exercise. Genetic, hormonal, and environmental factors play a significant role, as can 1 type of adenovirus.[7] A child with 1 overweight parent has a 40% chance of being overweight; with 2 overweight parents, it's 80%.[8] A number of medications (from birth control pills to antidepressants and antipsychotic drugs) can also contribute to weight gain. Interestingly, 25% of pets in the United States are obese and obese pets are more likely to have obese owners, implying that such owners overfeed or underexercise their animals.[9]

Health Consequences of Overweight and Obesity

Morbidity and Mortality

Obesity contributes to almost 300,000 deaths per year in the United States alone and is the second largest behavioral contributor to death after tobacco smoking.[10,11] Overweight and obesity in adulthood are associated with large decreases in life expectancy and increases in early mortality, similar in magnitude to those seen with smoking.[12]

Obesity is associated with increased risk for hypertension, diabetes, dyslipidemia, coronary heart disease, obstructive sleep apnea, gastroesophageal reflux disease, gallstones, asthma, pseudotumor cerebri, certain cancers (such as breast, colon, cervical, and uterine), major depression and suicidality, and possibly early onset of puberty in girls.[13,14] The prevalence of type 2 ("adult-onset") diabetes—the type most commonly associated with obesity—increased 33% (to 6.5%) from 1992 to 2000, and continues to climb.[15] Current patterns of overweight and obesity could account for 14% of all deaths from cancer in men and 20% of those in women.[16]

Overweight and Obesity in Childhood and Adolescence

Overweight and obesity rates have doubled in children and tripled in adolescents since 1980, spurring an epidemic of hypertension, type 2 diabetes, and the metabolic syndrome in children—conditions rarely seen in this age group a few decades ago.[17-19] Obese children show decreases in physical and social functioning.[20] Severely obese children and adolescents have similar health-related quality of life as those diagnosed as having cancer.[21] Overweight and obesity in childhood are risk factors for obesity in young adulthood and middle age, so as the population ages, the contribution of obesity to US healthcare costs will increase.[22]

Obesity as a Barrier to Preventive Care

Obesity is a barrier to the receipt of preventive care, partially because obese individuals have more chronic health conditions. Addressing these conditions takes time during doctor visits, time that might otherwise be spent on provision of preventive services. It is also more time-consuming and difficult to perform certain procedures, particularly Pap smears, breast examinations, and colon cancer screening, on overweight persons.

The obese are less likely to be screened for colorectal cancer, which can be cured in its early stages.[23] Obese women receive fewer mammograms and Pap smears than their nonobese counterparts, despite having higher rates of breast and cervical cancer, both of which are curable when found early through screening.[24,25] To complicate matters, obese women are 20% more likely than their normal-weight counterparts to have false-positive mammograms, which leads to more unnecessary biopsies and associated anxiety.[26]

PART II

Treatments and Approaches to Combating the Problem

This section describes the economic consequences of obesity, the "obesity economy," and the roles played by nutrition, exercise, and television.

Economic Consequences of Obesity

In 2003, obesity-attributable national medical expenditures were $75 billion and ranged from $87 million in Wyoming to $7.7 billion in California.[19,27] Half of the healthcare costs associated with obesity are currently covered by

Medicare, which now classifies obesity as a disease.[19] Much of the increased costs of healthcare associated with the obese are due to prescription drugs, but complications from surgery are more common and hospital lengths of stay are longer for obese than for normal-weight individuals.[28,29]

The Obesity Economy

Today there is a growing "obesity economy."[5] The plus-size apparel market is worth $17 billion and accounts for 20% of women's clothing sales, up from 11% in 2001. Half of all US women wear size 14 or larger clothing, whereas in 1985 the average size was 8.[30] Companies have sprung up to cater to the morbidly obese, producing XXXL sizes, oversized autos, furniture, coffins, and specialized medical equipment such as lifts, special chairs, and toilets.

Nutrition, Fast Food, Supersizing, Sweeteners, and Soda

Major changes in the human diet have contributed to the rise in overweight and obesity. These include the beginning of agriculture more than 10,000 years ago and, more recently, changes in portion size, the spread of fast food franchises since the mid-20th century, the use of artificial sweeteners and trans-fatty acids in processed foods, and current high levels of consumption of sugar- and caffeine-containing sodas.

The Contributions of Agriculture to Nutrition and Society

The advent of agriculture, considered a watershed in human societal evolution, brought the benefits of community and local food production but also led to a class-based society with rulers, farmers, artisans, merchants, and soldiers, each with distinct duties and positions in the group hierarchy. It may have hastened, or even brought about, the advent of organized warfare. It also led to dramatic changes in diet and exercise.

Our Ancestors Expended Enormous Calories in Hunting and Gathering

They ingested up to 7,000 of the 75,000 different edible plant species on a predominantly vegetarian diet. The wild game they ate, when it was available, was high in protein but very low in fat, unlike today's grain-fed (and antibiotic- and hormone-treated) supermarket meat.[31] Today, humans eat a markedly decreased variety of foodstuffs, and most of the planet relies on just a few crops (wheat, corn, rice) for a large proportion of its calories.[32]

Fast Foods and Supersizing

In recent decades, portion sizes have grown, as has the size of restaurant dinner plates.[33,34] Americans now spend about one half of their food budgets and consume about one third of their calories outside the home.[18]

Fast food spending has increased 18-fold since 1970.[35] The US food industry produces 3,800 calories per person per day, although average caloric need is only 2,500 calories per person per day. Fast foods (super-sized, protein-poor, carbohydrate- and fat-rich meals) now comprise 10% of total caloric intake.[36] On any given day, 8% of Americans eat at McDonalds.[37] A typical American eats 30 pounds of French fries per year.[38]

Serving size and the caloric content of typical packaged and fast foods have ballooned over the last 50 years, as the following examples illustrate:[39]

- In 1954, a Burger King hamburger weighed 2.8 oz. and contained 202 calories. The same regular burger today weighs 4.3 oz. and contains 310 calories.

- A serving of McDonalds fries was 2.4 oz. and contained 210 calories when the restaurant chain began in 1955. Today, one serving is 7 oz. and contains 610 calories.

- In 1916, the typical size of a bottle of Coca-Cola was 6.5 fluid oz. and contained 79 calories. Today the typical bottle contains 16 fluid oz. and 194 calories.

- Some mega-sized fast food burgers on the market today contain well over 1,000 calories.

Fast food outlets tend to target poor inner city communities. Meals can be obtained inexpensively and conveniently, which helps consumers working 2 jobs, raising children solo, or lacking inadequate kitchen facilities. The fast food industry directly targets children, producing 20% of Saturday morning television and offering, often in collusion with the motion picture industry, prizes and inducements based on characters that appeal to youngsters.

Fast food restaurants tend to be clustered around schools.[40] Furthermore, some US hospitals have regional and national fast food franchises located on the grounds of their main medical centers, thus sending the wrong message to patients and their families about optimal nutrition.[41]

The consumption of fast and junk foods begins early in life. Each day, 3% and 10%, respectively, of US infants and toddlers eat candy; 4% and 23%, respectively, consume sweetened soda beverages.[42] Soft drinks, which account for 20% to 24% of calories for 2- to 19-year-olds, are associated with tooth decay and decreased consumption of healthier alternatives, such as fruits and vegetables.[43]

Americans of all ages are drinking more soda, and a majority of adults drink soda daily. Per capita soda consumption has more than doubled since 1970, from 24 gallons per year to 53 gallons per year.[18] One well-known convenience store chain offers sizes such as "Big Gulp" and "Super Big Gulp."[29]

Seventy percent of soft drinks consumed in the United States contain caffeine as an added ingredient. Evidence suggests that the mood-altering and physical dependence–producing effects of caffeine (a central nervous system stimulant) have contributed to high rates of consumption of caffeinated soft drinks.[44] Soda's addictive properties put imbibers at risk of caffeine-withdrawal symptoms such as headache.

The National School Lunch Program

The National School Lunch Program gives schools more than $6 billion per year to offer low-cost meals to more than 27 million schoolchildren at 99,000 schools and childcare centers.[45] Begun in 1946, the program, administered by the US Department of Agriculture, has the conflicting missions of providing healthy meals to children, regardless of income, and subsidizing agribusiness, shoring up demand for beef and milk.[35] As such, meals emphasize meat and dairy products at the expense of fruit and vegetables, contain high levels of fat, and fail to meet the government's own inadequate nutritional standards, which are out of date with current science and have not been updated since the 1970s.[19,45]

Eighty-one percent of schools serve lunches exceeding 30% fat content, less than 45% serve cooked vegetables other than potatoes (usually French-fried), and less than 10% serve legumes.[45] Overemphasis on milk products may increase long-term risk for breast cancer, particularly if the milk comes from cattle treated with recombinant bovine growth hormone (also known as recombinant bovine somatotropin).[46,47]

Such daily fare does not help to establish good nutritional habits in America's youth. Unfortunately, dramatic changes in the National School Lunch Program are unlikely to occur given the large amounts of political clout wielded (and campaign dollars donated) by the beef and dairy industries, which have former lobbyists in key positions in the Department of Agriculture.[19,45]

Exercise and Television

The Institute of Medicine has urged Americans to exercise 1 hour per day, double the 1996 recommendation by the Surgeon General.[48] However, 70% of American adults are not active in their leisure time; 40% are not active at all.[49] One third of children do not participate in the minimum recommended level of moderate or vigorous physical activity, and the number taking part in physical education courses has dropped significantly, in part due to school funding cuts.[19]

Neighborhoods with high levels of minorities and individuals of low socioeconomic status have a paucity of facilities that enable and promote physical activity, such as parks and gymnasia.[50] Perception of one's neighborhood as less safe is also associated with an increased risk of overweight in children, likely due to fear of exercising outdoors.[51] Lack of exercise has effects beyond obesity, as participating in daily physical education is associated with better school attendance, more positive attitudes about school, and better academic performance.[19]

Instead of exercising, many youth spend their time watching television and using other electronic media such as the Internet and video games. The average youth spends 67% more time watching TV per year than he/she spends in the classroom.[52] Thirty-two percent of children aged 2–7 years have televisions in their rooms, as do 65% of children aged 8–18 years, which diminishes parental control over viewing time and content.[53]

Increases in television viewing are associated with increased calorie intake among youth, especially of calorie-dense low-nutrient foods of the type promoted on TV.[54] Businesses spend an estimated $13 billion annually marketing food and drinks in the United States, much of it on television advertising.[55] American children are exposed to approximately 40,000 food advertisements per year, 72% of which promote candy, cereal, and fast food.[56] Convenience/fast foods and sweets comprise over 80% of foods advertised during children's programming.[57] African American–oriented television airs far more junk food ads targeted at kids than general-oriented networks.[58]

Neither the Federal Trade Commission nor the Federal Communications Commission has the authority to limit such advertising, despite the fact that children are vulnerable to exploitive advertising messages and unable to discern truth from fiction in ads.[59] The American Academy of Pediatrics, which argues that children are cognitively and psychologically defenseless against advertising, has called for severe restrictions on advertisements for junk food aimed at children.[60]

Intriguingly, overweight and obese characters on television represent less than half of their percentages in the general population.[61] Such characters are less likely to be considered attractive, to interact with romantic partners, or to display physical affection, no doubt perpetuating stereotypes and contributing to the poor self-image many overweight individuals face.[61] In the real world, the overweight and obese, especially women, suffer from various forms of stigmatization. For instance, overweight and obese women get fewer promotions and face more job discrimination, whereas heavyset men do not.[45]

PART III
A Look at Food and Beverage Industries

The last two parts of this chapter reviewed the health and economic consequences of obesity and described the contributing roles of nutrition, exercise, and television. This section will focus on the food and beverage industries and on their links to schools, healthcare organizations and facilities, and government.

Soda/Beverages

Besides the increase in food portion size, which has become commonplace in the United States in the past decade, another major contributor to increased caloric content is use of high fructose corn syrup, an artificial sweetener found in many processed products such as sodas and fruit drinks. In fact, one of the largest changes in the human diet over the last few decades has been the 1,000+% increase in consumption of this calorie-laden artificial sweetener.[62] A meta-analysis of 88 studies found a clear association between soft drink intake and increased energy intake and body weight; lower intakes of milk, calcium, and other nutrients; and increased risk for diabetes and other health problems.[63]

Pouring Contracts and Soda Consumption

Over the last decade, cash-strapped school districts attempting to gain additional income to compensate for cuts in educational and athletic programs have signed "pouring rights" contracts with soda manufacturers.[64] In 2002, 240 US school districts had exclusive "pouring rights" contracts with soft-drink companies. In return for the placement of soda machines on campus and exclusive marketing rights to district children, companies sponsor sports and other extracurricular activities. One school was required to print the soda's name on its rooftop so that it could be seen by planes arriving and leaving from a nearby airport. Schools, which should be promoting proper nutrition, have instead been offered incentives to sell sugar-laden beverages because the majority of revenue from such contracts is realized through student purchases.

Some school districts, such as Los Angeles and Pittsburgh, have bowed to parental and health professional pressure and banned the sale and marketing of soft drinks.[65,66] Additionally, federal law now requires school districts to have nutritional wellness policies in place; these will be strengthened over the coming few years and should help to curb pouring contracts.[66]

In early 2006, Coca-Cola, Pepsi, and other soft drink manufacturers announced new voluntary policies to remove soda and other sugary drinks from schools nationwide.[67] Nevertheless, soft drink advertising still reaches students through television and magazine advertisements and, in the classroom, via Channel One, a ubiquitous, free, corporate-sponsored, advertising-laden news summary watched daily by millions of school children.[68]

The Food Industry, Medical Groups, and Government

One would hope that organizations of medical professionals would take a strong stand against the purveyors of fast foods, sodas, and sweets. However, a number of such groups have taken money from these companies, presenting a troubling conflict of interest. For example, the American Dietetic Association published a fact sheet entitled "Straight Facts about Beverage Choices," supported by an unrestricted grant from the National Soft Drink Association.[69] The group has also accepted money from other corporate sponsors, such as Mars and Coca Cola, to support its professional meetings.[70] In exchange for getting to use the American Diabetes Association's (ADA's) label on its diet drinks, Cadbury Schweppes (makers of Dr. Pepper and chocolate candies) donated a few million dollars to the ADA.[71] The American Academy of Family Physician's magazine, *Family Doctor: Your Essential Guide to Health and Well-Being*, mailed to 50,000 US family physicians in 2004, contained advertisements from food companies that included McDonald's, Kraft (maker of Oreo cookies), and Dr. Pepper, among others.[71] And although children's hospitals should be providing healthy environments for patients, parents, and staff, many in the United States (more than in Canada) have fast food outlets and vending machines that sell suboptimal food choices.[72]

US sugar producers, the packaged food industry, and producers of high-fructose corn syrup sweeteners contribute generously to high-level politicians, and have exercised their influence on a number of occasions to weaken food standards and labeling laws in the United States. They have also successfully applied pressure, through their "representatives" at the Department of Health and Human Services, to the World Health Organization, causing it to revise and thereby weaken the organization's antiobesity guidelines.[73]

In 2005, the US Federal Trade Commission asked industry to self-regulate its food advertising. In response, companies accounting for an estimated two thirds of children's food and beverage television advertisements pledged to improve the mix of foods advertised to children under age 12 and to reduce their total number of food advertisements overall.[74,75] These companies included Burger King, Cadbury Adams, Campbell Soup, Coca-Cola, ConAgra, General Mills, Hershey, Kellogg, Kraft Foods, Mars, Masterfoods, McDonald's, PepsiCo, and Unilever.

Given historical examples of industry failing to self-regulate, more formal, government-mandated rules may become necessary. However, many of these companies have, and are continuing to develop, healthier food choices in response to consumer demand. Also, major political figures, such as former president Bill Clinton and former Arkansas governor and current Republican presidential candidate Mike Huckabee, have launched antiobesity initiatives.

PART IV
Obesity Worldwide, Pathological Underweight, and Gluttony

This section discusses obesity worldwide as well as the related topics of pathologic underweight and gluttony.

Obesity Worldwide

America's weight problem is occurring in the midst of a global epidemic of over-weight and obesity.[76] Although the world's underfed population has declined slightly to 1.1 billion, the number of overweight people has surged to match that figure.[77] Individuals who move from countries with lower rates of cancer and more healthy diets (such as many southeast Asian nations) within a generation adopt a less healthy American diet. As a result, they become more over-weight/obese and suffer higher rates of cancer and obesity-related illnesses.[78] Americanization of food choices and portion sizing, particularly through the cultural export of fast-food outlets, have made obesity a significant health problem in both developed and developing nations throughout the world.

Underweight and Pathological Behaviors: The Flip Side to the Obesity Epidemic

The flip side of the obesity epidemic in the United States is that many individuals suffer from abnormal self-image, particularly regarding their weight. The prevalence of eating disorders has risen in the United States and in developing countries, a possible consequence (in part) of the Western media's depiction of the "ideal," excessively thin woman.

As many as 66% of women and 52% of men have reported feelings of dissatisfaction or inadequacy regarding their body weight.[79] Sixty percent of girls in grades 9–12 are trying to lose weight, compared with 24% of boys.[79] The number-one wish of girls aged 11–17 is to lose weight.[80] Women are more likely to judge themselves as overweight when they are not, whereas men are the opposite.[81] Women who desire to lose weight are more likely to do so in the hopes of improving their appearance, whereas men who wish to lose weight are more likely to be concerned about their future health and fitness.[82]

Body-image distress is now classified as a psychological disorder. Five percent to 10% of females have an eating disorder such as anorexia nervosa or bulimia.[79] Male and female high school athletes are especially at risk for unhealthy weight-control behaviors, such as restricting food intake, vomiting, overexercising, using diet pills, inappropriately taking prescribed stimulants or insulin, and using nicotine.[83] Some adolescents dehydrate by restricting fluid intake, spitting, wearing rubber suits, taking daily steam baths and/or saunas, and using diuretics or laxatives.[83]

Consequences of abnormal weight-loss behaviors include delayed matura-tion, impaired growth, menstrual irregularities or loss of menses, increased rates of infection, eating disorders, and depression. Alternatively, such behav-iors can be a sign of depression or verbal, physical, or sexual abuse.[84,85]

Media images have contributed to a misguided perception of the "ideal" body. Today, models weigh 23% less than average women; in 1986 it was only 8%.[86] Modeling schools for teens create unrealistic expectations. Only a very "select" few models achieve financial success (of these select few, beginners earn $1,500 per day, those in the top tier $25,000 per day, and supermodels $100,000 or even more per day).

Food Insecurity and Hunger

Ironically, although the United States is the wealthiest nation, prone to over-consumption of natural resources and plagued by an epidemic of obesity, our country also faces an increasing maldistribution of wealth and significant levels of poverty and hunger.[32] The US Department of Agriculture estimates that 12% of US households suffer from food insecurity (limited or uncertain availability of nutritionally adequate and safe foods, or limited or uncertain ability to acquire acceptable food in socially acceptable ways), and that another 4% face outright hunger (the uneasy or painful sensation caused by the recurrent lack of access to food).[87] Twenty-five percent of children live in poverty, and 4 million go hungry each day.[88] At the same time, American households waste over $43 billion worth of food per year, 3 times as much as in 1985.[32] Worldwide, hunger-related causes kill as many people in 2 days as were killed in the atomic bombing of Hiroshima.[32]

Gluttony

A bizarre trend likely to be seen by the rest of the world as typical of American "affluenza" and overconsumption of resources is the recent dramatic increase in the number and popularity of eating contests. The most (in)famous of such events is Nathan's Annual Fourth of July Hot Dog Eating Contest—the World Cup of food bolting—in which past winners have consumed over 50 frankfurters and buns in just 12 minutes.[89] The International Federation of Competitive Eating sponsors more than 150 other annual gorgefests, involving such foods as chicken wings, oysters, and jalapenos, which it promotes through its official newsletter, *The Gurgitator*.[89]

PART V
Treatments and Public Health Approaches to Combating the Problem

This final section examines treatments as well as public health approaches to combating obesity.

Treatments for Obesity

Treatment for obesity involves decreasing caloric intake (especially simple carbohydrates, which can contribute to diabetes, and trans-fatty acids, which are highly atherogenic and increase risk of cardiovascular disease), exercising more, and possibly getting more sleep.[90] Adults should receive 45% to 65% of their calories from carbohydrates, 20% to 35% from fat, and 10% to 35% from protein.[48] However, with the exception of 1 trial conducted with individuals enrolled in Weight Watchers, the evidence to support the use of the major commercial and self-help weight loss programs is suboptimal.[91]

In some countries, insurance companies cover obesity treatment. Although most in the United States do not, they do cover myriad expensive health consequences of obesity.[92] Americans spend an estimated $30 billion each year on diet pills, diet foods, exercise videos, health club dues, and other weight loss tools.[7]

Weight loss drugs are a 1-billion-dollar per year business in the United States.[93] One study showed that nearly 5 million US adults used prescription weight loss pills between 1996 and 1998.[94] However, one fourth of users were not overweight, suggesting that such medication may be used inappropriately. Use was especially common among women.

Drug therapy may be appropriate for patients with a BMI greater than 30 or a BMI greater than 27 with additional risk factors, such as diabetes. Sibutramine and orlistat are approved for long-term use, but they have been found to reduce weight only by about 10% when combined with diet and exercise, and sibutramine can increase blood pressure.*,[95]

The anti-obesity drugs fenfluramine and dexfenfluramine were taken off the market in 1997, after numerous reports of cardiac valvulopathy.[94] Nonprescription supplements, essentially unregulated with respect to purity, composition, and effectiveness, can be dangerous, and should be avoided. In particular, compounds containing ephedra, which has been banned by the US Food and Drug Administration (FDA) but can still be found in a number of preparations sold in the United States and purchased abroad, should not be used. Future pharmaceutical treatments will likely be directed against hormones involved in the regulation of satiety, such as leptin and ghrelin, and may include vaccines.[93] Those with a BMI greater than 40 may be eligible for bariatric (weight loss) surgery. Procedures include the Roux-en-Y gastric bypass, stapled gastroplasty, and adjustable gastric banding, all designed to reduce stomach size and control caloric intake.[96] Although complication rates of almost 40% over a 180-day period have been reported, substantial health benefits are common, including excess weight loss of up to 70% and resolution of diabetes in 77% of patients.[97,98] In particular, recent data suggest a long-term mortality benefit from bariatric surgery for the severely obese.[99,100] More than 200,000 bariatric procedures are performed annually, and almost 1 billion dollars was spent on

---

*Note: Sibutramine was taken off the market by the Food and Drug Administration since it increased the risk of stroke and myocardial infaction. [Lowes R. Abbott withdraws sibutramine from market. Medscape Alerts 2010 (October 8). Available at http://www.medscape.com/viewarticle/730155. Accessed 1/15/11.]

such surgeries in 2002, even though only 0.6% of eligible adults underwent a procedure—suggesting a huge untapped market.[99,101]

Public Health Measures to Reduce Obesity

One objective of the Department of Health and Human Services' *Healthy People 2010* is reducing the prevalence of obesity to 15%.[102] Accomplishing this objective will require a multifarious approach involving providers, public health advocates, citizens, and legislators.

While less than half of obese US adults visiting a primary care physician for a well-care visit are counseled about weight loss, those counseled were more likely to attempt weight loss than those who do not receive counseling.[103] Improving healthcare provider education in nutrition might improve patient counseling, as would the increased use of nutritionists in primary care settings, a move which would likely be cost-saving. Providers need to counsel patients frequently regarding body weight, and be observant for signs and symptoms of body image problems and pathologic weight loss/gain behaviors. Healthcare professionals should promulgate guidelines regarding normal body weight, healthy dieting behaviors, and the value of regular exercise.

School- and community-based health education campaigns tailored to cultural background, gender, and age group, as well as health messages widely disseminated in the entertainment and news media, can help correct misperceptions regarding weight and promote healthy behaviors.[104] Public schools should enhance their health curricula at all levels, provide more healthful meal choices, and resist the invasion of fast foods, soda pop machines, and exclusivity contracts. Enhanced state funding for public education will relieve the financial pressures that lead administrators to even consider these contracts. Hospitals, too, should provide healthful selections in their cafeterias, and refuse to have fast food franchises on their premises.

The provision of healthier menu options in federally sponsored school lunch offerings has been shown to increase student participation in the National School Lunch Program.[105] Use of local produce from community-supported agriculture, especially organically grown produce, would decrease the adverse consequences of pesticides on the environment and the amount of harmful greenhouse gasses produced in the transportation of food over long distances.[32,47,106,107]

A school wellness policy provision included in the Child Nutrition and Women, Infants, and Children Reauthorization Act of 2004 mandated that schools that participate in federal nutrition programs create wellness policies on how to improve students' nutrition and health as well as set guidelines for all foods sold in school by 2006.[19] The Child Health Nutrition Promotion and School Lunch Protection Act, introduced in both the US Senate and

House of Representatives, called for updating decades-old federal nutrition standards for snack foods sold in cafeterias, stores, and vending machines on school grounds.[108] Furthermore, in 2005, 40 states introduced about 200 bills addressing nutrition in schools.[19]

Measures to optimize the amount of exercise undertaken by the obese include expanding the number of pedestrian malls in public places; increasing the availability of recreational centers, parks, and workplace gyms; encouraging people to walk or ride bicycles to work and school; requiring physical education at school; and providing insurance coverage for membership in athletic clubs and insurance discounts for participation in exercise programs.[104]

Health insurers should provide enhanced coverage for obesity prevention and treatment. Finally, governmental bodies should be purged of those with industry connections so that they can provide more aggressive, unbiased oversight of the weight loss industry. As noted in part III, a number of food and beverage companies have taken steps to restrict advertising to children.[109]

Because most consumers are unaware of the high levels of calories, fat, saturated fat, and sodium found in many menu items, provision of nutrition information on restaurant menus could potentially reduce the consumption of less healthful foods, and might spur restaurants to offer healthier choices.[110] As of January 1, 2006, all conventional foods were required to include information regarding the amount of trans-fatty acids (the most atherogenic type of lipids) they contain.[111] The FDA estimates that such labeling will prevent from 600 to 1,200 cases of coronary heart disease and 250 to 500 deaths each year.[112]

Public health authorities in New York, Chicago, and Los Angeles have proposed a ban on the use of artificial trans-fatty acids in these cities' restaurants.[112] Additionally, a bill was introduced in Congress to require food manufacturers to adjust the labeling of their products to better inform consumers of their trans-fat content.[113] Some claim that trans-fatty acids add flavor and texture to fried foods, but suitable, less dangerous cooking oil substitutes are available, yet underutilized.

Other measures that might decrease rates of obesity include prohibiting the distribution of toys and promotional games, the presence of play equipment, and the presence of video or other games at fast food outlets; requiring fast-food outlets to locate a minimum distance from youth-oriented facilities such as schools and playgrounds; limiting the total number or per-capita number of fast-food outlets in a community; limiting the proximity of all fast-food outlets to each other; charging a fee to fast food outlets and using the proceeds to mitigate the impact of poor nutritional content (e.g., construct parks, fund after-school programs, or provide nutrition education); and prohibiting drive-through service.[114]

A majority of Americans believe that the government should be involved in fighting obesity, particularly by regulating the marketing of "junk foods" to kids.[115] As of 2000, 19 states taxed non-nutritious foods, such as soft drinks and candy.

Finally, some have brought lawsuits against purveyors of junk foods to reclaim healthcare costs. Some states are considering class action suits of this nature, reminiscent of the partially successful lawsuits against the tobacco industry.

Conclusion

The obesity epidemic in the United States has multifactorial causes and is responsible for serious health consequences. Its contribution to suffering and death and its effect on national healthcare costs calls for urgent action. Confronting the obesity crisis will require the concerted efforts of healthcare providers, educators, legislators, and social advocates.

Notes

1. Centers for Disease Control and Prevention. State-specific prevalence of obesity among adults—United States, 2005. *MMWR.* 2006;55:985–988.

2. Staff. Notebook. *TIME* November 2, 2004:26.

3. US Department of Health and Human Services. *The Surgeon General's call to action to prevent and decrease overweight and obesity.* Rockville, MD: US Department of Health and Human Services; 2001.

4. Snyder U. Obesity and poverty. *Medscape Ob/Gyn and Women's Health* March 4, 2004. Available at http://www.medscape.com/viewarticle/469027. Accessed March 5, 2004.

5. Savitt TL. Black health on the plantation: Masters, slaves, and physicians. In: Leavitt JW, Numbers RL, eds. *Sickness and health in America: Readings in the history of medicine and public health.* Madison: University of Wisconsin Press; 1985.

6. Drewnowski A, Darmon N, Briend A. Replacing fats and sweets with vegetables and fruits: A question of cost. *Am J Publ Health* 2004;1555–1559.

7. Watson S. How fat vaccines will work. *Mental Floss* 2006 January/February: 30–32.

8. Wallis C. Word to parents. *TIME* June 7, 2004:103–104.

9. Staff. Notebook. *TIME* November 24, 2003:21.

10. Tumulty K. The politics of fat. *TIME* March 27, 2006:40–43.

11. Allison DB, Fontaine KR, Manson JE, Stevens J, VanItallie TB. Annual deaths attributable to obesity in the United States. *JAMA.* 1999;282:1530–1538. Abstract.

12. Peeters A, Barendregt JJ, Willekens F, et al. Obesity in adulthood and its consequences for life expectancy: A life-table analysis. *Ann Intern Med.* 2003;138:24–32. Abstract.

13. Carpenter KM, Hasin DS, Allison DB, Faith MS. Relationships between obesity and DSM-IV major depressive disorder, suicide ideation, and suicide attempts: Results from a general population survey. *Am J Publ Health* 2000;90:251–257.

14. Bailey-Shah S. Is obesity causing the early onset of puberty in girls? *KATU News.* Available at ://www.katu.com/printstory.asp?ID=85714. Accessed May 9, 2006.

15. Kluger J. The diabetes explosion. *TIME* September 4, 2000:58.

16. Calle EE, Rodriguez C, Walker-Thurmond K, Thun MJ. Overweight, obesity, and mortality from cancer in a prospectively studied cohort of US adults. *N Engl J Med.* 2003;348:1625–1638. Abstract.

17. Muntner P, He J, Cutler JA, Wildman RP, Whelton PK. Trends in blood pressure among children and adolescents. *JAMA.* 2004;291:2107–2113. Abstract.

18. Oregon Department of Human Services. *Bigger is not always better.* CD summary. 2002;51:1–2.

19. Krisberg K. Schools taking center stage in battle against childhood obesity. *The Nation's Health* 2005 September:1, 22–23.

20. Williams J, Wake M, Hesketh K, Maher E, Waters E. Health-related quality of life of overweight and obese children. *JAMA.* 2005;293:70–76. Abstract.

21. Schwimmer JB, Burwinkle TM, Varni JW. Health-related quality of life of severely obese children and adolescents. *JAMA.* 2003;289:1813–1819. Abstract.

22. Daviglus ML, Liu K, Yan LL, et al. Relation of body mass index in young adulthood and middle age to Medicare expenditures in older age. *JAMA.* 2004;292: 2743–2749. Abstract.

23. Rosen AB, Schneider EC. Colorectal cancer screening disparities related to obesity and gender. *J Gen Intern Med.* 2004;19:332–338. Abstract.

24. Wee CC, McCarthy EP, Davis RB, Phillips RS. Screening for cervical and breast cancer: Is obesity an unrecognized barrier to preventive care? *Ann Intern Med.* 2000;132:697–704.

25. Wee CC, McCarthy EP, Davis RB, Phillips RS. Obesity and breast cancer screening: The influence of race, illness burden, and other factors. *J Gen Intern Med.* 2004;19:324–331. Abstract.

26. Elmore JG, Carney PA, Abraham LA, et al. The association between obesity and screening mammography accuracy. *Arch Intern Med.* 2004;164:1140–1147. Abstract.

27. Ogden CL, Carroll MD, Curtin LR, McDowell MA, Tabak CJ, Flegal KM. Prevalence of overweight and obesity in the United States, 1999–2004. *JAMA.* 2006;295:1549–1555. Abstract.

28. Raebel MA, Malone DC, Connor DA, et al. Health services use and health care costs of obese and nonobese individuals. *Arch Intern Med.* 2004;164:2135–2140. Abstract.

29. Zizza C, Herring AH, Stevens J, Popkin BM. Length of hospital stays among obese individuals. *Am J Public Health* 2004;94:1587–1591. Abstract.

30. Kher U. How to sell XXXL. *TIME* 2003 (January 27):43–46.

31. Lemonick MD. How we grew so big. *TIME* 2004 (June 7): Special supplement on America's obesity crisis.

32. Donohoe MT. Causes and health consequences of environmental degradation and social injustice. *Soc Sci Med.* 2003;56:573–587. Abstract.

33. Young LR, Nestle M. The contribution of expanding portion sizes to the US obesity epidemic. *Am J Public Health* 2002;92:246–249. Abstract.

34. Nielsen SJ, Popkin BM. Patterns and trends in food portion sizes, 1977–1998. *JAMA.* 2003;289:450–453. Abstract.

35. Kadlec D. Chain reaction. *TIME* 2004 (June 7):99–100.

36. Ebbeling CB. *Marketing of fast food and sugar-sweetened beverages to children: Is it promoting obesity?* Stop Commercial Exploitation of Children. Available at http://www.commercialexploitation.com/articles/marketing_fast_food.htm. Accessed February 8, 2008.

37. Staff. Numbers. *TIME* 2003 (August 18):20.

38. Jeffery C. Want irrigation with that? *Mother Jones* 2003 (March/April):26.

39. Newman C. Why are we so fat? *National Geographic* 2004 (August):46–61.

40. Austin SB, Melly SJ, Sanchez BN, Patel A, Buka S, Gortmaker SL. Clustering of fast-food restaurants around schools: A novel application of spatial statistics to the study of food environments. *Am J Public Health* 2005;95:1575–1581. Abstract.

41. Cram P, Nallamothu BK, Fendrick AM, Saint S. Fast food franchises in hospitals. *JAMA.* 2002;287:2945–2946.

42. Staff. Junk food starts early. *TIME* 2003 (November 10):117.

43. Cullen KW, Ash DM, Warneke C, de Moor C. Intake of soft drinks, fruit-flavored beverages, and fruits and vegetables by children in grades 4 through 6. *Am J Public Health* 2002;92:1475–1478. Abstract.

44. Griffiths R, Vernotica EM. Is caffeine a flavoring agent in cola soft drinks? *Arch Fam Med.* 2000;9:727–734.

45. Yeoman B. Unhappy meals. *Mother Jones* 2003 (January/February):40–45, 81.

46. Michels KB, Willet WC. Breast cancer—early life matters. *N Engl J Med.* 2004;351:1679–1681. Abstract.

47. Donohoe MT. Genetically modified foods: Health and environmental risks and the corporate agribusiness agenda. *Z Magazine* 2006 (December):35–40.

48. Staff. Legislation, lawsuits aimed at obesity epidemic. *The Nation's Health* 2002 (October):31.

49. Staff. Most adults shun exercise during leisure time. *The Nation's Health* 2002 (June/July):29.

50. Powell LM, Slater S, Chaloupka FJ, Harper D. Availability of physical activity-related facilities and neighborhood demographic and socioeconomic characteristics: A national study. *Am J Public Health* 2006;96:1676–1680. Abstract.

51. Lumeng JC, Appugliese D, Cabral HJ. Neighborhood safety and overweight status in children. *Arch Pediatr Adolesc Med.* 2006;160:25–31. Abstract.

52. Worldwatch Institute. *Matters of scale: Brain drain.* July/August, 2004. Available at http://www.worldwatch.org/pubs/mag/2004/174/mos/. Accessed June 5, 2008.

53. Linn S. *Marketing to children: An overview.* Stop Commercial Exploitation of Children. Available at http://www.commercialexploitation.com/articles /marketing_to_children_an_overview.htm. Accessed June 5, 2008.

54. Wiecha JL, Peterson KE, Ludwig DS, Kim J, Sobol A, Gortmaker SL. When children eat what they watch: Impact of television viewing on dietary intake in youth. *Arch Pediatr Adolesc Med.* 2006;160:436–442. Abstract.

55. Consumers Union. *Consumers Union's opposition to HR 339, a bill shielding the fast food industry from the health effects of its food and beverages and failure to disclose those effects.* Available at http://www.consumersunion.org/pub/2004 /02/000877print.html. Accessed June 5, 2008.

56. Kunkel D. Children and television advertising. In: Singer DG, Singer JL, eds. *Handbook of children and the media.* Thousand Oaks, CA: Sage; 2001:375–393.

57. Harrison K, Marske AL. Nutritional content of foods advertised during the television programs children watch most. *Am J Public Health* 2005;95:1568–1574. Abstract.

58. Outley CW, Taddese A. A content analysis of health and physical activity messages marketed to African-American children during after school television programming. *Arch Pediatr Adolesc Med.* 2006;160:432–435. Abstract.

59. Staff. *Into the mouths of babes: Never too young to get hooked on junk food.* Stop Commercial Exploitation of Children. Available at http://www.commercialexploitation.com/articles/mouth_of_babes.htm. Accessed June 5, 2008.

60. Heller L. *Pediatricians call for more kids' ad restrictions.* Food Navigator USA. Available at http://www.foodnavigatorusa.com/news/printNewsBis.asp?id= 72531. Accessed June 5, 2008.

61. Greenberg BS, Eastin M, Hofschire L, Lachlan K, Brownell KD. Portrayals of overweight and obese individuals on commercial television. *Am J Public Health* 2003;93:1342–1348. Abstract.

62. Hill R. Nation's waist began to swell as corn-sugar intake surged. *Oregonian* March 31, 2004:D11.

63. Vartanian LR, Schwartz MB, Brownell KD. Effects of soft drink consumption on nutrition and health: A systematic review and meta-analysis. *Am J Publ Hlth.* 2007;97:667–675.

64. Pinson N. *School soda contracts: A sample review of contracts in Oregon public school districts.* 2004. Available at http://www.communityhealthpartnership .org/images/pages/soda_report/full_report.pdf. Accessed October 25, 2007.

65. Late M. LA schools ban sales of sodas. *The Nation's Health* November 9, 2002:9.

66. Smydo J. Back to school: Snacks, soft drinks banished as schools focus on nutrition. *Pittsburgh Post-Gazette* September 1, 2006. Available at http://www.post-gazette.com/pg/06244/718119-298.stm. Accessed November 27, 2007.

67. Hsuan A. Schools back off sweet soda deals. *Oregonian* November 15, 2006:A1, A3.7.

68. Hoynes W. News for a captive audience: An analysis of Channel One. *Extra!* May/June 1997. Available at http://www.fair.org/index.php?page=1383. Accessed October 28, 2007.

69. Levine J. *A conflict of interest: Unhealthy financial relationships between nutrition professionals and the food industry.* Available at http://www.commercial exploitation.com/articles/conflict_of_interest.htm. Accessed February 8, 2007.

70. McDonald CM, Karamlou T, Wengle JG, et al. Nutrition and exercise environment available to outpatients, visitors, and staff in children's hospitals in Canada and the United States. *Arch Pediatr Adolesc Med.* 2006;160:900–905. Abstract.

71. Mokhiber R, Weissman R. *Tuna meltdown.* Focus on the Corporation. May 2005. Available at http://lists.essential.org/pipermail/corp-focus/2004/000179.html. Accessed May 20, 2007.

72. Mokhiber R, Weissman R. *All fall down.* Focus on the Corporation. May 2004. Available at http://lists.essential.org/pipermail/corp-focus/2005/000204.html. Accessed May 16, 2007.

73. Mooney C. Eating away at science. *Mother Jones* May/June 2004:17–18.

74. Heller L. *Food firms restrict advertising to kids.* Food Navigator USA. July 19, 2007. Available at http://www.foodnavigator-usa.com/news/printNewsBis.asp?id=78342. Accessed July 19, 2007.

75. Heller L. *Marketing to kids: Nestle, Dannon non-committal could lead to regulations.* Food USA Navigator. October 12, 2007. Available at http://www.foodnavigator-usa.com/news/printNewsBis.asp?id=80537. Accessed October 14, 2007.

76. Caballero B. A nutrition paradox—underweight and obesity in developing countries. *N Engl J Med.* 2005;352:1514–1516. Abstract.

77. Staff. Global overweight, obesity expanding at rapid pace. *The Nation's Health* 2000;(May):14.

78. Goel MS, McCarthy EP, Phillips RS, Wee CC. Obesity among US immigrant subgroups by duration of residence. *JAMA.* 2004;292:2860–2867. Abstract.

79. Labi N. Girl power. *TIME* June 29, 1998. Available at http://www.time.com/time/magazine/printout/0,8816,988643,00.html. Accessed March 13, 2008.

80. Maine M. *Stop the madness, stop the body wars, stop the commercial exploitation of kids.* Stop Commercial Exploitation of Kids. Available at http://www.commercial exploitation.com/articles/stop_the_madness.htm. March 13, 2008.

81. Chang VW, Christakis NA. Self-perception of weight appropriateness in the United States. *Am J Prev Med.* 2003;24:332–339. Abstract.

82. Levy AS, Heaton AW. Weight control practices of US adults trying to lose weight. *Ann Intern Med.* 1993;119:661–666. Abstract.

83. Kuehn BM. Pediatricians warned about student athletes' risky weight-control tactics. *JAMA.* 2006;295:486–487. Abstract.

84. Donohoe MT. Violence against women: Partner abuse and sexual assault. *Hospital Physician* 2004;40:24–31.

85. Donohoe MT. Individual and societal forms of violence against women in the United States and the developing world: An overview. *Curr Womens Hlth Reports* 2002;2:313–319.

86. Jeffery C. Why women can't win for trying. *Mother Jones* 2006;(January/February):22–23.

87. Bickel G, Carlson S, Nord M. *Household food security in the United States: 1995–1998.* Washington, DC: Food and Nutrition Service, US Department of Agriculture;1999.

88. Ackerman S. The ever-present yet nonexistent poor. *Extra!* 1999;(January/February):9–10.

89. Kaufman F. Fat of the land. *Harper's Magazine* 2003;(October):65–71.

90. Lamberg L. Rx for obesity: Eat less, exercise more, and — maybe — get more sleep. *JAMA.* 2006;295:2341–2343. Abstract.

91. Tsai AG, Wadden TA. Systematic review: An evaluation of major commercial weight loss programs in the United States. *Ann Intern Med.* 2005;142:56–66. Abstract.

92. Bray GA. The epidemic of obesity. *West J Med.* 2000;172:78–79. Abstract.

93. Park A. Pills in the pipeline. *TIME* 2004 (June 7):90.

94. Khan LK, Serdula MK, Bowman BA, Williamson DF. Use of prescription weight loss pills among US adults in 1996–1998. *Ann Intern Med.* 2001;134:282–286. Abstract.

95. Staff. *Weight loss.* Prescriber's letter;2003(June):23.

96. Mitka M. Surgery for obesity: Demand soars amid scientific, ethical questions. *JAMA.* 2003;289:1761–1762. Abstract.

97. Encinosa WE, Bernard DM, Chen CC, Steiner CA. Healthcare utilization and outcomes after bariatric surgery. *Med Care* 2006;44:706–712. Abstract.

98. Encinosa WE, Bernard DM, Steiner CA, Chen CC. Use and costs of bariatric surgery and prescription weight loss medications. *Health Affairs* 2005;24:1039–1046. Abstract.

99. Sjostrom L, Narbro K, Sjostrom D, et al. Effects of bariatric surgery on mortality in Swedish obese subjects. *N Engl J Med.* 2007;357:741–752. Abstract.

100. Adams TD, Gress RE, Smith SC. Long-term mortality after gastric bypass surgery. *N Engl J Med.* 2007;357:753–761. Abstract.

101. Meguid MM. Review of Martin LF, *Obesity surgery.* New York: McGraw-Hill; 2004.

102. US Department of Health and Human Services. *Healthy people 2010* (conference ed., in 2 vols.). Washington, DC: US Department of Health and Human Services; 2000. Available at http://www.health.gov/healthypeople. Accessed March 28, 2008.

103. Galuska DA, Will JC, Serdula MK, Ford ES. Are health care professionals advising obese patients to lose weight? *JAMA.* 1999;282:1576–1578. Abstract.

104. Blumenthal SJ, Hendi JM, Marsillo L. A public health approach to decreasing obesity. *JAMA.* 2002;288:2178.

105. Wojcicki JM, Heyman MB. Healthier choices and increased participation in a middle school lunch program: Effects of nutrition policy changes in San Francisco. *Am J Public Health* 2006;96:1542–1547. Abstract.

106. Donohoe MT. Factory farms, antibiotics, and anthrax. *Z Magazine* 2003:28–30. Available at http://zmagsite.zmag.org/Jan2003/donohoe0103.shtml. Accessed March 28, 2008.

107. Donohoe MT. Roles and responsibilities of health professionals in confronting the health consequences of environmental degradation and social injustice: Education and activism. *Monash Bioethics Review,* 2008;27(Nos. 1 and 2):65-82.

108. Mitka M. Senate eyes school junk food. *JAMA.* 2006;295:2130.

109. Donohoe MT. Weighty matters: Public health aspects of the obesity epidemic. Part III—Sodas, pouring contracts, and the food industry. *Medscape* 2008.

110. Burton S, Creyer EH, Kees J, Huggins K. Attacking the obesity epidemic: The potential health benefits of providing nutrition information in restaurants. *Am J Publ Health* 2006;96:1669–1675.

111. Sheehan E. Food product labels to bear information on trans fats. *The Nation's Health* 2003 (September):1, 18.

112. Associated Press staff. *NYC health board bans trans fats at restaurants.* Available at http://www.cnn.com/2006/HEALTH/12/05/ny.trans.fat.ap/index.html. Accessed December 6, 2006.

113. Heller L. *New bill proposes stricter trans fat labeling.* Food USA navigator. Available at http://www.foodnavigatorusa.com/news/printNewsBis.asp?id=80513. Accessed October 14, 2007.

114. Ashe M, Jernigan D, Kline R, Galaz R. Land use planning and the control of alcohol, tobacco, firearms, and fast food restaurants. *Am J Public Health* 2003;93:1404–1408. Abstract.

115. Mello MM, Studdert DM, Brennan TA. Obesity—the new frontier of public health law. *N Engl J Med.* 2006;354:2601–2610. Abstract.

Chapter 17

Cigarettes

The Other Weapons of Mass Destruction

Martin Donohoe

Dirty Bombs

Although Americans have been concerned about possible "rogue states" or "evil empires" gaining access to weapons of mass destruction, we must not forget that there is an enemy that mass-produces and sells—with the complicity and financial support of both the US government and healthcare organizations—weapons of mass destruction. This enemy is none other than the tobacco industry, whose "dirty bombs" daily choke the breath from hundreds of millions worldwide, many of them women and children. One member of the highly profitable cabal producing these incendiary devices is Phillip Morris (now Altria), the world's largest multinational tobacco company, with $10 billion in sales in 2002 and a net worth almost double the prewar gross domestic product of Iraq.[1]

Worldwide Epidemic

Tobacco claims almost 450,000 lives per year in the United States* and 4.9 million worldwide.[2] The World Health Organization (WHO) predicts that, by 2030, smoking will become the leading cause of death globally, killing 10 million persons per year, most of them in developing countries.[2] Despite

---

*Each year, 400,000 people die from the direct effects of tobacco smoke and another 40,000 to 60,000 plus die from the indirect effects of tobacco smoke.

an overall decline in the numbers of smokers in the United States over the past few decades—including a decline in the number of women and high school students who smoke—the prevalence of cigarette smoking continues to increase in many developing countries.[3,4] Of the 1.3 billion smokers worldwide, 84% live in developing countries or in nations with transitional economies.[1] Furthermore, within countries, tobacco consumption is inversely related to socioeconomic level.[2] Higher smoking prevalence among the poor means that they bear more of the burden of the health and economic costs of tobacco.[5]

More than 250 million women worldwide smoke today, including 22% of women in developed countries and 9% of women in developing countries.[6] In addition, many women in Southeast Asia chew tobacco.

Health Consequences of Tobacco Use

Health consequences of tobacco use include cardiovascular disease (myocardial infarctions, abdominal aortic aneurysms, and peripheral vascular disease), stroke, chronic obstructive pulmonary disease, cancer at multiple sites (cancers of the mouth, tongue, throat, vocal cord, esophagus, stomach, lung, kidney, bladder, and cervix, along with some types of leukemia and multiple myeloma), peptic ulcer disease, osteoporosis, low birth weight and birth defects, tooth decay, skin wrinkling, and sexual dysfunction.[7]

Money Up in Smoke

In the United States, smoking is the leading cause of death and is responsible for more than $75 billion in direct medical costs.[8] Twenty-five million Americans alive today are expected to die of a smoking-related illness.[9] Medical care and lost productivity due to tobacco use costs each US citizen $550 per year.[6] By comparison, the war and reconstruction in Iraq will ultimately cost at least $200 billion, or $714 per US citizen.[10]

In my internal medicine practice in Oregon, I see many individuals who, hooked as teens, now cough and wheeze their way through each day; some are shackled to oxygen tanks, have become emaciated, and are dying painfully from emphysema, cancer, and heart disease. Many of my patients are uninsured (as are 43 million US citizens) and unable to afford the inhalers and other prescription drugs necessary to ease their suffering. Many will soon lose basic health services as a result of our state's budget crisis. Oregon, along with other states, has issued bonds backed by future tobacco settlement earnings to pay current bills rather than use the funds for smoking prevention and cessation programs or healthcare for smoking-related diseases. De-funding smoking prevention programs makes little long-term economic sense, as society saves $3 in medical costs for every $1 spent to prevent smoking.[6]

Death for Sale

Cigarettes are the most marketed products in the world—products that, when used as directed, cause enormous suffering and death. The United States is the world's leading exporter of cigarettes.[6] US tax money has been used to assist corporations in their marketing efforts to attract overseas smokers in the developing world, particularly women and children, to compensate for small declines in smoking prevalence at home.[11,12]

Smokescreen—PR, Advertising, Hollywood, and Women

In the early 20th century, smoking was largely a habit and pastime of men. The founder of the public relations industry, Edward Bernays, was hired by the American Tobacco Company to develop a campaign to encourage women to smoke.[13] Bernays tied smoking to the women's suffrage movement. Free cigarettes ("torches of liberty") were provided to suffragettes, who "brazenly" smoked them during public marches.

Today, one quarter of American women smoke. Women have been specifically targeted in tobacco advertising over the past few decades (e.g., "You've come a long way, baby"). The tobacco industry's marketing strategies have skillfully linked cigarette use to typical female values, such as independence, self-reliance, weight control, stress management, social progress and popularity, personal attractiveness, autonomy, self-fulfillment, youth, happiness, personal success, health, and lifestyles that are active, vigorous, and strenuous. Tobacco companies have also attracted positive publicity by sponsoring sporting events, such as the Virginia Slims Tennis Tournament.[14]

For decades, Hollywood has functioned as a conduit for the tobacco industry's marketing efforts. Many films feature characters who smoke. Smoking is often presented as edgy, sexy, and glamorous. The average number of "smoking incidents" per hour in major US films in 2002 was 10.9, essentially unchanged from 10.7 in 1950.[15]

The Framework Convention on Tobacco Control Treaty

WHO has spent the past 3 years crafting a Framework Convention on Tobacco Control Treaty.[1,2] One hundred ninety countries worked to finalize the treaty, which took effect on February 27, 2005, and was ratified by 49 nations (including Australia, Canada, Mexico, and the United Kingdom). Another 120 countries have signed but not yet ratified the treaty, which exempts tobacco control from free trade challenges, limits tobacco advertising, cracks down on tobacco smuggling, bans tobacco sales to and by minors, promotes agricultural diversification and alternative livelihoods for tobacco farmers, standardizes packaging (banning such deceptive terms as "light" and "mild"), and improves warning labels.[1,2]

United States Against the World—US Efforts to Undermine the WHO Treaty

US and international opinion surveys show overwhelming public support for the goals of the treaty.[1,16] Despite this, at the behest of William Steiger, Director of the US Office of Global Health Affairs, the US delegation to the treaty talks attempted to scuttle the agreement in the name of free speech and free trade.[17] The original US negotiator, Dr. Thomas Novotny, resigned after the Bush administration pressured him to lobby for the deletion of 10 of 11 provisions from the treaty, as outlined in a Phillip Morris memo.[18]

The current administration has strong ties to the tobacco industry.[18,19] President Bush's long-time chief political strategist and now assistant to the president, deputy chief of staff and senior advisor Karl Rove was a lobbyist and strategist for Phillip Morris (Altria); Kirk Blalock, a White House liaison to the business community, was a Phillip Morris public relations official; Charles Black, an informal advisor to Mr. Bush during the 2000 presidential campaign, was a Phillip Morris lobbyist in Washington; Daniel Troy, the Food and Drug Administration's (FDA) chief counsel, represented the tobacco industry when it sued the FDA over tobacco ad regulation; and Secretary of Health and Human Services Tommy Thompson received $72,000 in campaign contributions from Phillip Morris executives when he was governor of Wisconsin, and he has also served as an advisor for the primary tobacco lobbying firm in Washington, DC. In 2004, Thompson rejected his own advisory panel's recommendation to increase the federal tobacco tax.[18,19] Finally, both British American Tobacco PLC's Brown and Williamson unit and RJ Reynolds Tobacco Holdings, Inc. are represented by Barbour, Griffith and Rogers, a lobbying firm stocked with Republican operatives, including Haley Barbour, former GOP chairman, and Lanny Griffith, who was a White House aide to President George H. W. Bush.[18,19]

In the 2004 elections, tobacco companies contributed $3,480,901 through individual contributions and political action committees, 74% of which went to Republicans.[20] Tobacco companies have given more than $20 million to Republican candidates for federal office since 1997; Phillip Morris has been the leading overall campaign contributor to Republicans since 1989.

Only when its sole ally Germany dropped its opposition to the WHO treaty did Secretary Thompson announce that the United States would support the agreement. In May 2004, the United States became the 108th nation to sign on.[8] However, this does not guarantee that the US Senate will ratify the treaty (by the required two-thirds majority) or that President Bush will sign.

Bush apparently wants to have it "reviewed by lawyers" first. In either case, the United States, which should be leading the international community on important public health issues, instead has taken a generally obstructionist stance and only come around at the last minute.

In its efforts to scuttle another major public health treaty, as it did with the Kyoto Protocol on environmental pollution and global warming, the current administration has exhibited a callous disregard for human health. Furthermore, its laissez-faire attitude toward national tobacco regulation—in the face of the huge economic burden consequent to tobacco use and growing state and federal budget deficits—illustrates its contempt for the physical and economic well-being of our citizens.

Healthcare Organizations and Medical Schools—Whose Side Are They On?

It is not just the federal government but also the healthcare industry that has been complicit in its support of the tobacco industry. As of 1999, insurers (including some of the largest owners of health maintenance organizations) and mutual funds were invested heavily in tobacco stocks.[21] Cigna held $42.7 million worth of stock, MetLife $62.1 million, and Prudential $892 million. TIAA-CREF, whose mutual funds are owned by many academic health professionals, held $731.7 million worth of Phillip Morris stock alone.

From 1996 to 1998, Phillip Morris and Cigna collaborated to censor accurate information on the harms of smoking and environmental tobacco smoke so that it would not appear in Cigna health newsletters sent to employees of Phillip Morris and its affiliates.[22] Tobacco companies have also sponsored "research" claiming to disprove many of the health consequences of direct and environmental tobacco smoke. Some of Phillip Morris's "studies" were conducted at a shadowy facility located in Germany, with complex mechanisms in place that aimed to ensure the work done there could not be linked to Phillip Morris.[23]

The tobacco industry has "white-coated" itself since the 1940s, borrowing from medicine's prestige and public esteem in its ads featuring smoking doctors. As of late 2004, despite a decades-old plea from the American Medical Association for medical schools to divest their tobacco holdings, at least 5 of the nation's leading medical schools** had failed to do so, and those that had divested had done so with little publicity. These institutions have squandered critical opportunities for ethical and moral leadership in the anti-tobacco crusade. One possible reason: the continued funding of academic scientists and institutional programs.

**Cornell, Duke, Washington University, Yale, and possibly Penn, which refused to answer requests; Columbia is said to have divested but could not provide details to confirm divestment.

Clearing the Air: How to Disarm the Tobacco Industry

I ask readers to contact President Bush and their senators and representatives and urge them to support the WHO treaty; to back legislation to limit tobacco advertising (particularly that which influences children), provide for more pronounced warning labels, limit workplace smoking, and increase tobacco taxes; to crack down on international cigarette smuggling; to support legislation that would allow the FDA to regulate tobacco; and to stop using our tax dollars to promote smoking overseas. Instead, this money should be used to fund smoking education and cessation programs, as well as to provide medical care for victims of tobacco-related diseases, ideally both here in America and abroad. Concerned citizens should also lobby their state legislators to cease attempts to divert tobacco settlement dollars away from smoking education and cessation programs. Finally, patients and physicians should encourage medical schools to divest their tobacco stocks and publicize their decisions to do so.

It is time to put public health before political favoritism and the profits of corporations and academic institutions. It is time to clear the air and disarm the tobacco industry.

Notes

1. Lazarus D. *Bush tries to weaken tobacco treaty.* Common Dreams News Center. 2003 (April 30).

2. Who Health Organization Tobacco Free Initiative. *Frequently asked questions on the WHO FCTC and the context in which it was negotiated.* Available at http://www .who.int/tobacco/framework/faq/en/. Accessed March 6, 2005.

3. American Thoracic Society. *ATS guidelines: Cigarette smoking and health.* Available at http://www.utdol.com/application/topic.asp?file=ats_guid/19553 &type+A&slectedTitle=20~228. Accessed March 6, 2005.

4. Centers for Disease Control and Prevention. Cigarette use among high school students United States, 1991–2003. *MMWR.* 2004;53:499–502.

5. World Health Organization. *Tobacco free initiative: Economics.* Available at http://www.who.int/tobacco/research/economics/en/. Accessed March 6, 2005.

6. Mackay J, Eriksen M. *The tobacco atlas.* Geneva: World Health Organization; 2002.

7. Sackey JA, Rennard SI. *Patient information: Smoking cessation.* UpToDate online 12.2. Available at www.uptodate.com. Available to members at http://www.utdol .com/application/topic.asp?file=lung_dis/5094&type=A&selectedTitle=197~269. Accessed July 6, 2004.

8. Mokdad AH, Marks JS, Sroup DF, Gerberding JL. Actual causes of death in the United States, 2000. *JAMA.* 2004;291:1238–1245.

9. Late M. Health effects of smoking are more dangerous than thought. *The Nation's Health* 2004(August):1, 20.

10. Bennis P, Institute for Policy Analysis Iraq Task Force. *A failed "transition": The mounting costs of the Iraq war.* September 30, 2004. Available at http://www.ips-dc .org/iraq/failedtransition/A_Failed_Transition-webver.pdf. Accessed March 15, 2005.

11. Barry M. The influence of the US tobacco industry on the health, economy, and environment of developing countries. *N Engl J Med.* 1991;324:917–920.

12. Waxman H, Durbin RJ. *Administration promotes tobacco products abroad, letter to the president.* February 12, 2003. Available at http://www.democrats.reform.house .gov/story.asp?ID=600. Accessed March 5, 2005.

13. Stauber J, Rampton S. *Lies, damn lies and the public relations industry.* Monroe, ME: Common Courage Press; 1995.

14. Christen AG, Christen JA. The female smoker: From addiction to recovery. *Am J Med Sci.* 2003;326:231–234.

15. Staff. Harper's index. *Harper's Magazine* 2004(May):13.

16. Woodward T. Up in smoke. *San Francisco Bay Guardian* 2003(February 12). Available at http://www.takingontobacco.org/event/dhhsdemo/sfbg.html. Accessed March 6, 2005.

17. Yeoman B. Secondhand diplomacy. *Mother Jones* 2003(March/April). Available at http://www.motherjones.com/news/outfront/2003/03/ma_284_01.html. Accessed March 6, 2005.

18. Action on Smoking and Health. *Tobacco has strong ties to government.* 2001(March 7). Available at http://nosmoking.org/march01/03-07-01-1.html. Accessed March 6, 2005.

19. *Tobacco: Long-term contribution trends.* Available at http://www.opensecrets.org /industries/indus.asp?Ind=A02&Format=Print. Accessed March 7, 2005.

20. Himmelstein DU, Woolhandler S, Boyd JW. Investment of health insurers and mutual funds in tobacco stocks [letter]. *JAMA.* 2000;284:697.

21. Muggli ME, Hurt RD. A cigarette manufacturer and a managed care company collaborate to censor health information targeted at employees. *Am J Public Health* 2004;94:1307–1311.

22. Diethelm PA, Rielle JC, McKee M. The whole truth and nothing but the truth? The research that Phillip Morris did not want you to see. *Lancet* 2005;365;9461. Abstract. Available at http://www.thelancet.com/journal/vol365/iss9461/full /llan.365.9461.early_online_publication.32426.1. Accessed March 5, 2005.

23. Wander N, Malone R. Selling off or selling out? Medical schools and ethical leadership in tobacco stock divestment. *Acad Med.* 2004;79:1017–1026.

Chapter 18

Guns and Suicide in the United States

Matthew Miller
David Hemenway

This past June, in a 5-to-4 decision in *District of Columbia* v. *Heller*, the Supreme Court struck down a ban on handgun ownership in the nation's capital and ruled that the district's law requiring all firearms in the home to be locked violated the Second Amendment. But the Supreme Court's finding of a Second Amendment right to have a handgun in the home does not mean that it is a wise decision to own a gun or to keep it easily accessible. Deciding whether to own a gun entails balancing potential benefits and risks. One of the risks for which the empirical evidence is strongest,[1] and the risk whose death toll is greatest, is that of completed suicide.

In 2005, the most recent year for which mortality data are available, suicide was the second leading cause of death among Americans 40 years of age or younger. Among Americans of all ages, more than half of all suicides are gun suicides. In 2005, an average of 46 Americans per day committed suicide with a firearm, accounting for 53% of all completed suicides. Gun suicide during this period accounted for 40% more deaths than gun homicide.

Why might the availability of firearms increase the risk of suicide in the United States? First, many suicidal acts—one third to four fifths of all suicide attempts, according to studies—are impulsive. Among people who made near-lethal suicide attempts, for example, 24% took less than 5 minutes between the decision to kill themselves and the actual attempt, and 70% took less than 1 hour.[2]

Second, many suicidal crises are self-limiting. Such crises are often caused by an immediate stressor, such as the breakup of a romantic relationship, the loss of a job, or a run-in with police.

As the acute phase of the crisis passes, so does the urge to attempt suicide. The temporary nature and fleeting sway of many suicidal crises is evident in the fact that more than 90% of people who survive a suicide attempt, including attempts that were expected to be lethal (such as shooting oneself in the head or jumping in front of a train), do not go on to die by suicide. Indeed, recognizing the self-limiting nature of suicidal crises, penal and psychiatric institutions restrict access to lethal means for persons identified as potentially suicidal.

Third, guns are common in the United States (more than one third of US households contain a firearm) and are lethal. A suicide attempt with a firearm rarely affords a second chance. Attempts involving drugs or cutting, which account for more than 90% of all suicidal acts, prove fatal far less often.

The empirical evidence linking suicide risk in the United States to the presence of firearms in the home is compelling.[3] There are at least a dozen US case-control studies in the peer-reviewed literature, all of which have found that a gun in the home is associated with an increased risk of suicide. The increase in risk is large, typically 2 to 10 times that in homes without guns, depending on the sample population (e.g., adolescents vs. older adults) and on the way in which the firearms were stored. The association between guns in the home and the risk of suicide is due entirely to a large increase in the risk of suicide by firearm that is not counterbalanced by a reduced risk of nonfirearm suicide.

Moreover, the increased risk of suicide is not explained by increased psychopathologic characteristics, suicidal ideation, or suicide attempts among members of gun-owning households.

Three additional findings from the case-control studies are worth noting. The higher risk of suicide in homes with firearms applies not only to the gun owner but also to the gun owner's spouse and children. The presence of a gun in the home, no matter how the gun is stored, is a risk factor for completed suicide.

And there is a hierarchy of suicide risk consistent with a dose-response relationship. How household guns are stored matters especially for young people—for example, one study found that adolescent suicide was four times as likely in homes with a loaded, unlocked firearm as in homes where guns were stored unloaded and locked.

Many ecologic studies covering multiple regions, states, or cities in the United States have also shown a strong association between rates of household gun ownership and rates of completed suicide—attributable, as found in the case-control studies, to the strong association between gun prevalence and gun suicide, without a counterbalancing association between gun-ownership levels and rates of nongun suicide. We recently examined the relationship between rates of household gun ownership and suicide in each of the 50 states for the period between 2000 and 2002.[4] We used data on gun ownership from a large telephone

Table 18.1. Data on Suicides in States with the Highest and Lowest Rates of Gun Ownership, 2001-2005*

Variable	States with the Highest Rates of Gun Ownership	States with the Lowest Rates of Gun Ownership	Ratio of Mortality Rates
Person-years	195 million	200 million	
Percent of households with guns	47	15	
Male			
Number of firearm suicides	14,365	3,971	3.7
Number of nonfirearm suicides	6,573	6,781	1.0
Total number	20,938	10,752	2.0
Female			
Number of firearm suicides	2,212	286	7.9
Number of nonfirearm suicides	2,599	2,478	1.1
Total number	4,811	2,764	1.8

*Note: The states with the highest rates of gun ownership included here are Wyoming, South Dakota, Alaska, West Virginia, Montana, Arkansas, Mississippi, Idaho, North Dakota, Alabama, Kentucky, Wisconsin, Louisiana, Tennessee, and Utah. The states with the lowest rates of gun ownership included here are Hawaii, Massachusetts, Rhode Island, New Jersey, Connecticut, and New York. Data on gun ownership are from the 2001 Behavioral Risk Factor Surveillance System. Data on suicides are from the Centers for Disease Control and Prevention Web-Based Injury Statistics Query and Reporting System (WISQARS; www.cdc.gov/ncipc/wisqars).

survey (of more than 200,000 respondents) and controlled for rates of poverty, urbanization, unemployment, mental illness, and drug and alcohol dependence and abuse. Among men, among women, and in every age group (including children), states with higher rates of household gun ownership had higher rates of firearm suicide and overall suicides. There was no association between firearm-ownership rates and nonfirearm suicides. To illustrate the main findings, we presented data for the 15 states with the highest levels of household gun ownership matched with the six states with the lowest levels (using only six so that the populations in both groups of states would be approximately equal). In Table 18.1, the findings are updated for 2001 through 2005.

The recent Supreme Court decision may lead to higher rates of gun ownership. Such an outcome would increase the incidence of suicide. Two complementary approaches are available to physicians to help counter this possibility: to try to reduce the number of suicide attempts (e.g., by recognizing and treating mental illness) and to try to reduce the probability that suicide attempts will prove fatal (e.g., by reducing access to lethal means). Many US physicians, from primary care practitioners to psychiatrists, focus exclusively on the first approach. Yet international experts have concluded that restriction of access to lethal means is one of the few suicide prevention policies with proven effectiveness.[5]

In our experience, many clinicians who care deeply about preventing suicide are unfamiliar with the evidence linking guns to suicide. Too many seem to believe that anyone who is serious enough about suicide to use a gun would find an equally effective means if a gun were not available. This belief is invalid.

Physicians and other health care providers who care for suicidal patients should be able to assess whether people at risk for suicide have access to a firearm or other lethal means and to work with patients and their families to limit access to those means until suicidal feelings have passed. A website of the Harvard Injury Control Research Center can help physicians and others in this effort (www.hsph.harvard.edu/means-matter). Effective suicide prevention should focus not only on a patient's psychological condition but also on the availability of lethal means — which can make the difference between life and death.

Notes

1. Hemenway D. *Private guns, public health.* Ann Arbor: University of Michigan Press; 2004.

2. Simon OR, Swann AC, Powell KE, Potter LB, Kresnow MJ, O'Carroll PW. Characteristics of impulsive suicide attempts and attempters. *Suicide Life Threat Behav.* 2001;32:Suppl.:49–59.

3. Miller M, Hemenway D. The relationship between firearms and suicide: A review of the literature. *Aggress Violent Behav.* 1999;4:59–75.

4. Miller M, Lippmann SJ, Azrael D, Hemenway D. Household firearm ownership and rates of suicide across the 50 United States. *J Trauma* 2007;62:1029–1035.

5. Mann JJ, Apter A, Bertolote J, et al. Suicide prevention strategies: A systematic review. *JAMA.* 2005;294:2064–2074.

Food: Safety, Security, and Disease

Food is necessary for life. It supplies us with energy for thought and movement and helps us to grow, brings us together with family and friends, and is the focal point of many cultural rituals and religious traditions.

About ten thousand years ago we abandoned a hunter-gatherer lifestyle in favor of agriculture. This brought benefits such as economies of scale and food surpluses, allowing more people to live together, but it also was largely responsible for a division of labor into farmers, rulers, crafts people, and warriors, whose role it was to protect agricultural settlements and to battle for new areas to farm. This stratified society (the class system) is currently a contributor to many social injustices.

Developments in technology, including advanced irrigation systems, domestication of animals, the plow, and selective breeding, improved agricultural outputs and gave humans more leisure time to think and create. However, soil depletion due to failure to rotate crops, overgrazing, and slash-and-burn agriculture (the last a consequence of growing populations) led to wars and possibly the collapse of civilizations such as the Easter Islanders and the Anasazi Indians. Even so, many civilizations created sustainable food systems in which the environmental, social, and economic impacts of food production sustained the needs of the current generation and allowed for future generations to flourish.

In the nineteenth and twentieth centuries much changed. Society moved further away from the diverse diet of plants and animals, which had sustained us for millennia, toward monoculture and reliance on fewer and fewer crops. Populations reliant on monoculture became vulnerable to famine, as happened during the Irish potato famine, which led to widespread emigration. In the last century, pesticides, a byproduct of the development of poison gases used in World War I, were added to crops to increase yield. Despite some successes, many insects evolved resistance to these chemicals, which also had adverse health effects on those exposed to the chemicals, either through application or ingestion (see Chapter Seven). The largely plant-based diet supplemented with occasional meat from a hunting party's kill that supported humans for millennia has been increasingly supplanted by a diet rich in meat. This diet, along with exposure to pesticides, has contributed in part to certain cancers and other medical ills. Our growing population's demand for meat and poultry has led to the consolidation of small family farms into concentrated agricultural feeding operations. These factory farms confine animals in unhealthy (and often abusive) feedlots, contribute significant greenhouse gasses to the atmosphere (thus increasing global warming), and pollute our waterways with billions of tons of waste. Overuse of nontherapeutic, supposedly growth-promoting antibiotics by factory farms has become the dominant source of food-borne, antibiotic-resistant infections in humans. Outbreaks of such illnesses occur frequently, thanks to US government subsidies that have favored factory farms over smaller operations and because government agencies designed to protect the public from food-borne illnesses are underfunded. As with meat and poultry, our increasing demand for fish has led to overfishing, the collapse of many vital fisheries, and the creation of fish farms, with their attendant high concentrations of estuary-damaging waste.

Today just a handful of meat, dairy, and seed companies control food production. The technologies made possible by the discovery of DNA have been employed by large, profit-driven agribusiness corporations, whose manipulation of plant and animal genomes to create genetically modified plants and animals has gone largely unregulated. The dramatic rise in production of genetically modified foods over the last twenty years, including the use of plants and animals to produce pharmaceuticals and industrial chemicals (biopharming), constitutes perhaps the largest mass experiment conducted on humans without our consent (and in many cases even our knowledge). This experiment carries significant risks for our health, our environment, and the diversity and security of our food supply.

Other threats to our food supply include bovine spongiform encephalopathy ("mad cow disease"); irradiation of food (which carries uncertain health risks and for which the production of radioactive cobalt and cesium requires commercial reprocessing of high-level nuclear waste); and the carbon footprint of a global system of food production and distribution, such that the average meal travels over 1,500 miles to reach your plate. The shift from local to global food production and consumption has made it increasingly difficult for public health authorities to prevent and trace food-related health problems. Their jobs have been made more difficult by politicians beholden to corporate campaign donations and by industry scientists who hide data from the public (citing trade secrets) and advance a corporate-friendly agenda to ensure highly remunerative employment when they pass through the revolving door between government and industry.

Regrettably, at a time when 1.5 billion people do not consume enough calories to prevent stunted growth and other health risks, food commodities' speculation and trading and the diversion of food crops to biofuels has contributed significantly to a rise in global food prices. Some countries use food aid to advance political or corporate agendas, further contributing to the famines that kill millions worldwide each year. Rich governments and corporations are buying up rights to millions of hectares of agricultural land in developing countries in order to secure their own long-term food supplies. Worse, food is often employed as a weapon of war, with invading armies burning crops and planting land mines in the most fertile soil, often causing more deaths from starvation than from direct violence.

The chapters in this section address major threats to the food system. Chapter Nineteen (by Martin Donohoe) explains how the overuse of agricultural antibiotics has led to a rise in antibiotic, food-borne infections in humans. It reviews the checkered history of one of the world's largest agricultural biotechnology and pharmaceutical corporations, Bayer, which ignored calls from the FDA and numerous health care groups to remove its drug Baytril (enrofloxacin) from the market. Baytril was a major contributor to the increase in ciprofloxacin-resistant Campylobacter infections in humans. Interestingly, Bayer also manufactured ciprofloxacin (Cipro), an immensely profitable drug. The company negotiated a sweetheart deal with the US government to sell the drug at a significant profit (in time of national emergency with heightened fears of a biological weapons attack) to the government to stockpile it to be used in the case of a possible attack involving anthrax, a bacterium sensitive to the drug.

Chapter Twenty (by Martin Donohoe) reviews the health and environmental risks of genetically modified (GM) crops, including biopharmed crops (i.e., crops modified to produce pharmaceutical agents and industrial chemicals). It reviews international opposition to GM crops and describes efforts, unsuccessful thus far in the United States, to require labeling of foodstuffs produced from such crops. It criticizes efforts by corporations and their surrogates in government to market these crops to the developing world as a solution to world hunger. Textboxes provide brief overviews of golden rice–vitamin A deficiency and the precautionary principle.

Chapter Twenty-One (by Elanor Starmer, David Wallinga, Rick North, and Martin Donohoe) is a proposal calling for precautionary avoidance of nonmedicinal hormones, especially those intentionally added to the food system, which was adopted by the American Public Health Association in 2009. This chapter covers the adverse human, animal, and environmental consequences of the use of synthetic hormones such as steroid sex hormones and recombinant bovine growth hormone in, respectively, meat and dairy production.

The United Nation's Food and Agriculture Organization has stated that enough food is produced daily to provide every living person with over 2,700 calories per day, well over the 2,000 to 2,200 calories per day necessary for growth and daily activities. Sadly, half the world's food is wasted. Solving world hunger and improving the safety and long-term security of the world's food supply does not require dangerous technologies; many scientists argue that it could be accomplished through local, sustainable, organic agricultural practices tested over millennia. Most agree that it requires primarily political and social will. Further readings and regularly updated, open-access slide shows are available on the food safety/food justice issues page of the Public Health and Social Justice website at http://phsj.org/food-safety-issues/. It is hoped that the reader will explore the external links portion of this web page, make healthy food purchases, and advocate for a more safe, equitable, and sustainable system of food production and distribution.

Notes

1. Diamond, J. *Collapse: How societies choose to fail or succeed* (New York: Penguin), 2005.
2. Kent, G. *The right to adequate food*. Retrieved from http://www.fao.org/righttofood/kc/downloads/vl/docs/AH288.pdf.

Chapter 19

Factory Farms as Primary Polluter

Martin Donohoe

Over the past 15 years, factory farms have replaced small family farms as the primary producers of livestock for human consumption in the US These farms generate 1.4 billion tons of animal waste per year (130 times annual human waste production). One hog farm in North Carolina generates the same amount of waste as all of Manhattan. While Manhattan has a fairly effective sewage system, the hog farm's manure ferments in an open lake, seeps into the local water supply, creates an unbearable stench for nearby residents, and can be widely disseminated by floods and hurricanes. As sewage from factory farms permeates local rivers, fish die, ecosystems are disrupted, and the growth of bacteria, which can cause human infection, is promoted. Not surprisingly, factory farms have replaced industrial factories as the number one polluter of American waterways.

Almost all of the eight billion cattle, poultry, and swine raised for human consumption in the US each year receive antibiotics to "promote growth." The Union of Concerned Scientists estimates that non-therapeutic livestock use, primarily by large factory farms, accounts for 70 percent of antibiotic use in the US, an increase of 50 percent over the last 15 years. Agricultural antibiotic use facilitates the development of antibiotic-resistant bacteria. For instance, enterococcus bacteria resistant to the antibiotic vancomycin, and only partly responsive to recently developed antimicrobials, plague intensive care unit patients in increasing numbers; spread of this organism was likely promoted by the use of avoparcin, a vancomycin-like antibiotic fed to chickens. The Centers for Disease Control and Prevention have declared that antibiotic use in food animals is the dominant source of antibiotic resistance among food-borne pathogens affecting humans.

Campylobacter, the most common food-borne infection in the US, causes 2.5 million cases of diarrheal illness and 100 deaths annually. The incidence of food-borne Campylobacter resistant to fluoroquinolones, the class of antibiotic commonly used to treat this disease, rose from 13 percent in 1998 to 18 percent in 1999. Over the same period, fluoroquinolone use in animals rose 40 percent. Two fluoroquinolones, sarafloxacin (trade name Saraflox) and enrofloxacin (trade name Baytril), have been widely used on factory farms. Recently, the Food and Drug Administration declared that the only option to protect human health from antibiotic resistant Campylobacter is to cease the use of fluoroquinolones in poultry. In response to an FDA-proposed ban, Abbott Laboratories voluntarily withdrew sarafloxacin from the market. Despite calls from the American Public Health Association, Physicians for Social Responsibility, and others, Bayer Corporation has refused to pull Baytril off the market and is fighting the FDA-proposed ban.

Of note, outlawing the sub- and nontherapeutic use of antibiotics in factory farms and instead focusing on disease prevention and improved sanitation, diet, habitat, vaccination, and treatment of specific infections is not only more humane, but would minimally increase meat costs to consumers while helping to lower the estimated $4 billion spent each year on antibiotic-resistant infections in humans. Of course, increasing the proportion of vegetables and fruits in our diets would have direct health benefits to individuals, and also would cut down on agricultural antibiotic-associated human infections.

The Checkered History of Bayer

Based in Leverkusen, Germany, the Bayer Corporation employs 120,000 individuals worldwide and boasts annual sales of $28 billion. Its largest market is the US. It produces pharmaceuticals, genetically modified crops, is the third largest manufacturer of herbicides in the world, and dominates the insecticide market. Following its 2001 purchase of Aventis CropScience, it became the number one biotech company in Europe, where it controls over half of the genetically modified crop varieties up for approval for commercial use. In 2001, *Fortune Magazine* named Bayer "one of the most admired companies in the United States"; *Multinational Monitor*, on the other hand, labeled it one of the "ten worst corporations of the year."

The company has an ignominious history of unethical practices and violations of federal statutes. In World War I, Bayer helped to invent chemical warfare and developed the "school for chemical warfare" in Germany. In World War II it was part of the IG Farben conglomerate, which exploited slave labor at Auschwitz and conducted unethical human subject experiments. In the early 1990s, the company admitted knowingly selling HIV-tainted blood-clotting products, which infected up to 50 percent of hemophiliacs in some developed countries. US class action suits related to these sales were settled for $100,000 per claimant while European taxpayers were left to foot most of the bills for the care of these unfortunate patients. From 1995 on, Bayer has failed to follow its promise to withdraw its most toxic pesticides from the market, and failed to educate farmers in developing countries regarding health risks associated with exposure to its pesticides, undoubtedly thereby contributing to the 2 million to 10 million poisonings and 200,000 deaths per year that the World Health Organization attributes to pesticide exposure.

In 1998, Bayer paid Scottish adult volunteers $750 each to swallow doses of the insecticide Guthion to, according to the company, "prove the product's safety." In 2000, the FDA and the Federal Trade Commission cited Bayer for misleading claims regarding aspirin and heart attacks and strokes. That same year, it was fined by the Occupational Safety and Health Administration for workplace safety violations related to exposures to carcinogenic MDA, and by the Commerce Department for violations of export laws. In 2001, FDA-reported violations in Bayer's quality control contributed to a worldwide shortage in clotting factor for hemophiliacs.

Despite these egregious violations of common law and human rights, Bayer is seen by many as an established, caring company, known mainly for its aspirin, which many of us have used since youth. To maintain its public image, Bayer resorts to "greenwash," advertising designed to portray its products as ecofriendly (e.g., pesticides are called "crop protection"); "bluewash," identifying itself with the United Nations through its status as a signatory to the UN's global compact (despite its ongoing violations of this agreement); the promotion of a stealth anti-environmental health agenda, via sponsorship of the so-called wise use and responsible care movements and membership in corporate front groups such as the Global Crop Protection Federation (whose name belies its intent, which is not so much crop protection as the increased use of both genetically modified organisms and pesticides); and harassment/SLAPP suits (strategic lawsuits against private parties), designed to discredit (and deplete the financial resources of) watchdog groups such as the Coalition Against Bayer Dangers. Bayer is a member of numerous lobbying groups attacking "trade barriers" (i.e., environmental health and safety laws). The company has donated $600,000 to US politicians over the last five years, and gave $120,000 to President George W. Bush's 2000 election campaign.

Bayer produces a human fluoroquinolone, ciprofloxacin (trade name Cipro, similar chemically to the Baytril used agriculturally). Cipro is one of the two treatments of choice (along with the much cheaper and equally effective doxycycline) for anthrax. Bayer stands to make large profits off of Cipro through physician prescriptions ($4.50 per pill in the drugstore) and sales to the US government, for a proposed stockpile to treat a potential 10 million exposed patients (at $0.95 per pill, which is still twice what the government pays for Cipro under another program and over four times the price one generic manufacturer has proposed). Cipro's patent was set to expire in 2004, but it has been granted an additional 6 months patent protection under the FDA's pediatric extension bill, in exchange for conducting safety and efficacy tests on children. Cipro has been the bestselling antibiotic in the world for the last 8 years, and is currently the 11th most prescribed drug in the US (20th in sales). Gross sales in 1999 for Cipro were $1.04 billion; sales increased 20–25 percent one month after the 2001 anthrax mailings. Even at the reduced price, Bayer stands to make enormous profits by providing Cipro for the government stockpile, not to mention potential sales to all 280 million Americans.

The US government has the authority, under existing law, to license generic production of ciprofloxacin by other companies (which could cost as little as $0.20 per pill) in the event of a public health emergency. The government refused to deem the late 2001 spate of anthrax exposures, and the potential for a large scale anthrax attack, a public health emergency. Why? Because doing so would have weakened its case, presented to the World Trade Organization (WTO) meeting in Qatar, that the massive suffering consequent to 25 million AIDS cases in sub-Saharan African nations does not constitute enough of a public health emergency to permit these countries to obtain and produce cheaper generic versions of largely unavailable anti-AIDS drugs. The government's stance is likely related to the record $80 million dollars spent by drug companies on campaign donations in the most recent national elections. Fortunately, the WTO ministers voted in favor of the developing world.

Suggestions for Citizen Action

In the case of Bayer and its fluoroquinolone antibiotics, corporate profits and influence peddling are triumphing over public health and rational science. Stronger regulation over agricultural antibiotic use and pricing of human pharmaceuticals is urgently needed, as well as stiffer penalties for corporate malfeasance (fines and prison sentences). Concerned citizens should support locally produced, antibiotic-free meat from small farms (contact the Bayer Corporation, 100 Bayer Road, Pittsburgh, PA 15205–9741; 412-777-2000 to protest Bayer's failure to cease production of Baytril); and contact their legislators and the White House to demand increased availability of generic ciprofloxacin and anti-AIDS drugs, at home and abroad, under existing law and trade agreements.

Chapter 20

Genetically Modified Foods

Health and Environmental Risks and the Corporate Agribusiness Agenda

Martin Donohoe

In November 2003 Oregon voters defeated Measure 27, which would have required the labeling of genetically modified (GM) foods sold or distributed in the state. The ballot initiative, the first of its kind in the United States, would have covered wholesale and retail foods sold in supermarkets, but not in cafeterias, restaurants, prisons, or at bake sales and other public gatherings.

Measure 27's lopsided defeat (73 percent to 27 percent) was somewhat surprising, given that multiple polls conducted by the media, government, and industry showed that anywhere from 85 percent to 95 percent of citizens (both in Oregon and in the nation as a whole) favored labeling. However, the initiative's failure can be understood in light of its opponents outspending its proponents $5.3 million to $200,000. Small amounts of opposition funding came from grocers and farm groups, with only a miniscule portion from groups and individuals inside Oregon. Most came instead from large agribusiness corporations headquartered outside the state, such as Monsanto, DuPont, Syngenta, Dow AgroSciences, BASF, Aventis, Hoechst, and Bayer CropScience.

Many of these companies have manufactured chemical weapons (e.g., Hoechst: mustard gas; Monsanto: Agent Orange; Dow: napalm) and pesticides (Monsanto: DDT) throughout the 20th century. DuPont and Hoechst once produced most of the ozone-destroying chlorofluorocarbons known to have weakened the earth's atmospheric shield against carcinogenic ultraviolet radiation. Today, most of these corporations continue to make pesticides and agricultural antibiotics (overuse of which is the major contributor to food-borne, antibiotic-resistant infections in humans). Opposition groups were aided by an experienced team of public relations and political professionals, and hid behind scientific-sounding "advocacy groups," such as the Council for Biotechnology Information.

Opponents of Measure 27 funded advertisements describing increased, onerous, and complicated government oversight and frightened the public with unfounded fears of up to $1,500 in additional taxes per family. Realistic cost estimates for enactment of the initiative were actually between 79 cents per person per year and $4 per family per year—either way a small price to pay for information vital to consumer choice. The opposition accused the measure's supporters of being "against national policy and scientific consensus," "technophobic," and "anti-progress." They argued that labels would provide "unreliable, useless information that would unnecessarily confuse, mislead, and alarm consumers."

Within months of the measure's defeat, the anti-labeling lobby pushed a bill through the Oregon House of Representatives that would keep local governments from imposing any food labeling requirements and would prevent state agencies from adopting requirements stricter than porous federal regulations allow. Due to aggressive face-to-face and phone lobbying by safe food advocates, the bill was not brought up for a vote in the state senate prior to the legislature's adjournment for the year. However, to date eight states have enacted laws to prohibit counties and other local governments from banning or regulating GM seeds, and five other states are considering similar legislation.

GM foods come from plants and animals whose DNA has been altered through the addition of genes from other organisms. In development since 1982, GM crops became commercially available in 1994. Almost all GM foods are altered to resist herbicides (which are almost always manufactured by the same company) or agricultural pests. Today, according to industry estimates, GM crops are grown commercially by 8.25 million farmers on 222 million acres spread over 21 countries. Top producers are the United States (59 percent of world output), Argentina (20 percent), Canada (6 percent), Brazil (6 percent), and China (5 percent). Among crops today, 50 percent of corn, 75 percent of cotton, 83 percent of canola, and 85 percent of soybeans are genetically modified; 60 to 70 percent of processed foods available in the US today come from GM crops, yet interestingly, only 24 percent of Americans believe they have eaten GM foods.

Purported benefits of genetic modification include increasing growth rate and enhancing ripening, preventing spoilage, augmenting nutritional quality, changing appearance, and providing resistance to herbicides. Golden rice, the "poster child" of GM foods, is touted as the solution to the problem of Vitamin

A deficiency, a major cause of blindness in the developing world. However, golden rice is unlikely to live up to such a promise.

Health and Environmental Risks

Health and environmental risks of GM foods include allergies and toxicities from new proteins entering the food supply. This occurred when individuals who consumed GM L-tryptophan dietary supplements in the late 1980s developed deadly eosinophilia-myalgia syndrome. More recently, Bt (Bacillus thurigensis) corn (corn modified to resist the corn borer pest) has been shown to increase the sensitivity of mammals to other allergens; GM peas have caused lung inflammation in mice; and new, allergenic proteins have been identified in GM soy in South Korea. Bt cotton has reportedly caused dermatitis, respiratory illnesses, and allergic symptoms in Philippine and Indian farm workers. A once-secret Monsanto report found that rats fed a diet rich in GM corn had smaller kidneys and unusually high white blood cell counts, a sign of inflammation. A Russian Academy of Sciences report found an up to six-fold increase in death and severe underweight in infants of mothers fed GM soy.

The incidence of food allergies is increasing. Besides increased recognition and reporting, some scientists suggest that this may be due in part to GM foods. Currently the Food and Drug Administration (FDA) reports that 2 percent of adults and 5 percent of infants and young children in the US have food allergies.

Genes initially designed to protect crops from herbicides can also be transferred to native weeds, resulting in the creation of herbicide-resistant "superweeds." For instance, herbicide-resistant oilseed rape has transferred its resistance gene to charlock weeds and turnips in the United Kingdom and glyphosate (Roundup) resistance has been identified in pigweed in Missouri and Georgia, ryegrass in California, creeping bentgrass in Oregon, and maretail in multiple states.

GM plants and animals can interbreed with wild relatives, spreading novel genes into wild populations. They can out-compete or drive to extinction wild varieties or become bioinvaders in neighboring farms or other ecosystems. The end result is a further decrease in agricultural biodiversity, as well as economic harms to organic and other farmers relying on income from non-GM crops sold abroad. The United Nations Food and Agriculture Organization estimates that 75 percent of the genetic diversity in agriculture present at the beginning of the 20th century has been lost. GM crop production will hasten this seemingly irreversible change.

Multiple cases of GM contamination of non-GM crops have been reported. In a 2001 study, 7 percent of growers of organic corn, soybeans, and canola reported GM contamination. In Canada herbicide resistance has spread from

GM canola to wild relatives by pollination. In Japan GM canola has been found growing near some ports and roadsides. Since canola is not grown commercially in Japan, imported seeds likely escaped during transportation to canola oil–processing facilities. Heinz baby food sold in China was found to contain Bt toxin gene sequences.

In 2000 unapproved Aventis Starlink GM corn contaminated the food supply, resulting in $1 billion in food recalls and costing growers $110 million. Syngenta accidentally released hundreds of tons of GM corn, tagged with antibiotic resistance genes, to farmers between 2001 and 2004. In 2002 corn genetically modified by Prodigene to produce a pig vaccine contaminated soybeans in Nebraska and Iowa. The US Department of Agriculture (USDA) fined Prodigene $250,000 and reimbursed farmers over $3 million. Other farmers have not received such compensation, in particular those Mexican farmers whose native corn varieties, cultivated over centuries, have been contaminated with GM corn, despite their geographic isolation in mountain highlands.

In August 2006 contamination of wild creeping bentgrass with Roundup-resistant Miracle-Gro/Monsanto GM grass was discovered in Oregon, threatening the state's $374 million grass seed market. In a surprisingly candid moment, Scotts's Miracle-Gro spokesperson Jim King acknowledged, ''The fact that nature took its course was exactly what you would have expected to happen.'' Also in August 2006, Bayer CropScience announced that its herbicide-tolerant Liberty Link rice had contaminated the food supply between 1998 and 2001. Bayer delayed announcing the incident for 6 months and the US government delayed an additional 18 days. Economic consequences for the $1.5 billion US rice farm market could be huge: Japan has banned imports of US rice and the European Union is now testing all imported rice. Of the first 162 samples recently tested by the European Federation of Rice Millers, which represents about 90 percent of all EU trade in rice, 33 tested positive for Liberty Link contamination.

Other risks of GM foods include altered nutritional value of foodstuffs; transfer of antibiotic resistance genes into intestinal bacteria or other organisms, contributing to the growing multibillion-dollar public health problem of antibiotic resistance; and increased pesticide and herbicide use, when pests and weeds develop resistance to genetically engineered food toxins. Such increased pesticide and herbicide use has been documented in Bt cotton and Roundup-rReady crops (glyphosate is toxic to the placenta). GM plants also may adversely alter soil bacteria and consequently soil quality. Finally, non-target insects may be negatively affected by the excess pesticides used on pesticide-resistant crops, with ripple effects on other predator and prey organisms. (The US government has even used the war in Iraq as cover to introduce GM crops into the fertile crescent where agriculture began. For example, Order 81 of the

Coalition Provisional Authority sets regulations favoring the patented seeds of large multinationals over locally produced seeds.)

Farmers have faced intimidation and lawsuits from agribusiness. Percy Schmeiser was sued by Monsanto for theft of GM canola seeds. While he lost the case, the penalty was a one dollar fine. Scientists who have brought to light the adverse consequences of GM crops, such as Ignacio Chapela and Arpad Pusztai, have also faced harassment and academic marginalization, not surprising given the large amounts of money allocated to universities by agribusiness to support their agendas.

US regulatory agencies such as the Department of Agriculture, the Environmental Protection Agency, and the Food and Drug Administration rely on safety tests done by companies that make GM products, a case of the fox guarding the henhouse. The Department of Agriculture's Office of the Inspector General reported in January 2006 that the department has failed to regulate adequately field trials of GM crops.

A culture of intimidation currently threatens the US government's scientific enterprise, compromising the government's ability to base policy upon sound science in a number of different areas. For example, up to one-fifth of FDA scientists responding to a 2006 survey said that they "have been asked, for non-scientific reasons, to inappropriately exclude or alter technical information or their conclusions in an FDA scientific document." A NASA scientist was forced to alter a report on the dire consequences of global warming; important data regarding the utility of post-coital contraception were ignored by the FDA under pressure from the so-called "religious right"; and a government analysis on the true (higher) expected cost of the Medicare Part D drug bill was kept from Congress until it approved the plan, which places drug company profits before patient well-being.

Biopharming

Biopharming, the engineering of plants to produce pharmaceuticals such as enzymes, antibiotics, contraceptives, and vaccines, poses similar threats to environmental and human health. Purported rationales of biopharming include the ability to produce large amounts of drugs using farmers and farms, which are felt to be less expensive than technicians and manufacturing plants, respectively. Seeds and silos function as convenient, inexpensive storage systems. Major biopharm crops include corn, soybeans, tobacco, and rice. Tested agents include aprotinin (involved in blood clotting), trypsin (a pancreatic enzyme with research and industrial uses), and anti-sperm antibodies (for contraception) in corn. Insulin-producing safflower has been proposed.

Some 400 biopharm products are under development and over 300 open-air field trials have been conducted nationwide. Some corporate forecasts predict that biopharming will be a $200 million/year industry involving 10 percent of all US corn acreage within 10 years. However, the pharmaceutical industry's promise of cheaper medications and vaccines seems dubious, given its history of price gouging and excessive profits (which exceed those of any other industry). Furthermore, while savings might accrue to the drug companies, the potential health and environmental consequences of plants engineered to produce enzymes, antibiotics, abortifacients (agents which induce miscarriage), chemotherapy, vaccines, and industrial and research chemicals will be externalized, borne by food manufacturers, taxpayers, and local communities. Farmers are unlikely to be major beneficiaries of biopharming, as market forces, including foreign competition, will drive down compensation. Furthermore, the acreage required for biopharming is very small compared with commodity crop acreage, so only a very small number of growers will be involved.

Acceding to industry's desire for secrecy in product development, and not eager to frighten unsuspecting citizens, the US Department of Agriculture conceals the location of all biopharm crop sites from the public and even neighboring farmers, hides the identity of the drug or chemical being tested in most cases, and condones biopharm companies' practice of "anonymously" planting these crops without identifying security risks or notifying neighbors. Cases of contaminated food crops have already been reported, in the Prodigene case necessitating the destruction of hundreds of thousands of bushels of soybeans.

Ironically, a major site of testing is Hawaii, home to the country's most fragile ecosystem and greatest number of endangered species. The introduction of papayas genetically modified to resist ring-spot virus devastated Hawaii's $10 million papaya economy, as prices fell precipitately when traditional buyers Canada and Japan rejected the modified product. In August 2006 a federal district court judge ruled that the USDA violated the Endangered Species Act and the National Environmental Policy Act in granting biopharm crop permits in Hawaii.

Oregon Physicians for Social Responsibility's Campaign for Safe Foods last year introduced a bill to place a statewide four-year moratorium on biopharming. Despite strong opposition from corporate agribusiness front groups like Oregonians for Food and Shelter, the bill passed out of Senate committee. Nevertheless, the bill never came up for a vote before the full Republican-controlled legislature prior to the end of the legislative session. Five other states have considered similar bills, but none has ever made it out of committee.

Vertebrates and Trees

Plants and foodstuffs are not the only organisms undergoing genetic modification in the name of profit. Genetic modification of lower vertebrates suffered a setback in late 2002 when Washington state banned genetically engineered fish, which threatened to escape their "farms" and interbreed with wild stocks, possibly hastening the extinction of wild salmon and other fish. Nevertheless, fish farmed elsewhere continue to undergo genetic modifications to augment their size, color, or growth rate. California recently banned importation of GM Glofish, zebra fish with an inserted gene causing them to glow in the dark. The biopharming industry has now co-opted animals as drug production factories. Examples include transgenic sheep that produce alpha-1-antitrypsin (used to treat a human enzyme deficiency disease), cows whose udders produce lysostaphin (which promotes resistance to Staphylococcus aureus, the major cause of mastitis—or breast infection—in cattle), and rats that secrete an experimental human malaria vaccine in their milk. The potential health and environmental consequences of genetically modified animals are similar to those of GM crops.

On another note, although the Food and Drug Administration has asked the animal cloning industry to delay selling milk and meat products from its test-tube-replicated cows and pigs, companies are already selling such products, unlabeled, to unsuspecting consumers.

Approximately 230 experiments involving the genetic modification of 24 species of trees have transpired in at least 16 countries. Sites have generally been kept secret and the resulting trees are reportedly sterile. Genetically altered trees under development have included faster growing trees with stronger wood and greater wood and paper yields; hardier trees requiring less chemical bug and weed killers; disease-resistant trees; trees that would require fewer toxic chemicals for paper processing; and trees that change color when exposed to bioterror agents.

With the support of the Environmental Protection Agency (EPA), one company is testing trees altered to remove mercury ions from contaminated soil around Danbury, Connecticut. Danbury was historically the center of the US hat-making industry, which in past centuries used large amounts of mercury, a known developmental and neurotoxin that caused the "Danbury shakes" in exposed workers. Ironically, these trees will merely convert mercury ions into volatile elemental mercury, which will then be released into the atmosphere, converted by phytoplankton to organic mercury, dispersed over the world's oceans, and work its way from large fish to mammals to, eventually, nursing infants.

GM Foods and World Hunger

The food dictators who control intellectual property and patent monopolies over GM seeds and plants recently attempted, through the United Nations Food and Agriculture Organization and the World Health Organization, to use the famine in Zambia to market GM foods through aid programs, even as more than 45 African countries expressed a willingness to supply local, non-GM relief and voiced support for Zambia's desire to not pollute its crops with GM foods. Such pollution would have prevented Zambia from exporting its crops to many other countries that did not accept GM imports (further weakening its already fragile economy and in turn exacerbating the famine). Zimbabwe, Malawi, and Angola have also refused GM food aid.

GM foods are promoted as the solution to world hunger, yet increasing reliance on GM food furthers corporate control of agriculture, transmogrifying farmers into "bioserfs." This is accomplished via genetic use restriction technologies (GURTS). In v-GURTS, also known as "terminator technology," seeds are made sterile, via insertion of a gene that stops manufacture of a protein needed for germination, so that they cannot be cropped and resown. In t-GURTS, also known as "traitor technology," a regulatory gene is inserted, which in turn controls genes governing germination, growth, and other important characteristics of plant development. This regulatory gene can only be activated when the plant is sprayed with a proprietary chemical, which is sold separately. Terminator technology threatens to overturn traditional agricultural practices of farmers who, instead of saving seeds for next year's crop, are forced to buy seeds annually from biotech companies. Terminator seed threat goes far beyond such farmers' fields: terminator plants still produce pollen, which could spread and sterilize non-GM crops.

In 2000 the world's governments called for a moratorium, under the UN Convention on Biological Diversity, on developing and testing terminator technology. This ban was reconfirmed in March 2006. Nevertheless, the US, Canada, Australia, the United Kingdom, and New Zealand are all trying to overturn the ban. Of note, the World Council of Churches opposes terminator technology.

Because 60 to 70 percent of foods available today come from genetically modified crops, it may be impossible to outlaw GM foods altogether. However, labeling laws would allow consumer choice to drive the market, possibly putting the brakes on this rapidly expanding technology. In the US food substances are already labeled for vitamin, mineral, caloric, and fat content; wines containing sulfites warn those who are allergic and labels inform vegetarians of the source of various proteins so that they can avoid ingesting animal products.

Labeling of GM foods would help to prevent dangerous allergic attacks (studies suggest this could have occurred in unsuspecting consumers of soybeans modified with Brazil nut genes, which were never marketed); allow vegetarians to avoid, for instance, tomatoes modified with flounder genes; and help concerned individuals to avoid ingesting milk from cattle injected with recombinant bovine growth hormone (rBGH), which increases the level of potentially carcinogenic insulin-like growth factor I (IGF-1) in milk. Labeling will heighten public awareness of genetic engineering, grant people the freedom to choose what they eat based on their individual willingness to confront risk, and ensure a healthy public debate over the merits of genetic modification of foodstuffs.

The European Union (EU) has required labeling of GM foodstuffs since 1998; Japan, China, Australia, and other countries also mandate labeling. A few years ago, Vermont became the first state to require manufacturers of genetically modified seeds to label and register their products.

Mendocino, Marin, and Trinity Counties in California have voted to forbid planting of any genetically modified crops. A state bill to pre-empt local bans on GM crops passed the California House of Representatives, but failed to make it out of a Senate committee. The Cartagena Protocol on Biosafety of the UN's Convention on Biological Diversity allows countries to bar imports of GM seeds, microbes, animals, or crops that they deem a threat to their environments. It does not cover processed food made from GM crops. The US has not signed the protocol and actively opposes it. In March 2006 the UN Convention on Biological Diversity called for a precautionary approach to the genetic modification of trees.

Many countries ban the import of GM foods from the US; others have in place, or are actively considering, labeling laws and bans on GM food imports. The EU banned the planting and importation of GM foods from the US and elsewhere until recently, when it lifted the ban, in part due to a US lawsuit against the EU through the World Trade Organization. Even so, this year the Swiss banned GM crops and 164 local governments in the EU have banned or come out against such crops. There are over 3,000 GM-free zones in Europe, and others in Canada, Australia, and the Philippines. Danish law now compensates farmers whose fields have become contaminated with GM crops. The government then seeks recompense from the farmer whose field originated the genetic contamination, assuming the culprit can be pinpointed. Recently, some corporations producing GM foods have not been able to get insurance due to excessive liability risks.

Opponents of biopharming include the US National Academy of Sciences, the Union of Concerned Scientists, the British Medical Association (which favors a moratorium on GM foods), Consumers Union, the Grocery Manufacturers of America, the National Food Processors Association, the Organic Consumer's Association, and numerous environmental groups.

The Future

Public education, particularly in environmental and health science, should enhance citizens' ability to separate biased corporate pronouncements of safety from legitimate scientific concerns. Environmental education should be based on sound, independent, peer-reviewed science. Unfortunately, due to chronic under-funding of public schools, much environmental health is now taught via corporate-sponsored, biased curricula. Examples of such greenwashed curricula include Dow Chemical's "Chemipalooza," Exxon's "Energy Cube," and the American Nuclear Society's "Activities with the Atoms Family." The precautionary principle, a fundamental tenet of public health, should be the guiding concept behind agricultural science and policy. Campaign finance reform and publicly funded elections could lessen the grip of agribusiness on our legislative bodies.

US Representative Dennis Kucinich (D-OH) has introduced a bill to require labeling of GM foodstuffs, expand FDA oversight, increase regulations governing biopharming, and enhance research and policy initiatives to help developing nations feed themselves. Without tremendous public pressure, however, this bill is unlikely to come up for a vote before the full House.

Attempts by legislatures to pass laws prohibiting labeling should be exposed and vigorously opposed. Recently, the US House of Representatives passed a bill entitled the National Uniformity for Food Act. Vigorously supported by industry, which has donated millions to legislators, the bill would mandate uniform but weak national standards for food safety. The bill would render

---

The Precautionary Principle

Oregon Physicians for Social Responsibility's Campaign for Safe Foods and other food safety groups advocate the application of the precautionary principle in agricultural policy. The principle states that when evidence points toward the potential of an activity to cause significant, widespread or irreparable harm to public health or the environment, options for avoiding that harm should be examined and pursued, even though the harm is not yet fully understood or proven. The precautionary principle advises giving human and environmental health the benefit of doubt; including appropriate public participation in the discussion of policy choices; gathering unbiased scientific, technological and socioeconomic information; and considering less risky alternatives.

---

illegal over 200 state (and many more local) labeling laws. The US Senate will soon consider the bill.

Given the importance of food to human survival and environmental health, consumers should support local agriculture and patronize farmers' markets (which decreases transportation costs, pollution, and global warming); consider vegetarianism (which facilitates water conservation) or at least decrease their meat intake and avoid over-fished species; shun the highly processed, genetically manipulated comestibles available in large grocery chains and the fried, fat-flavored foodstuffs found in fast food franchises; and oppose International Monetary Fund, World Bank, and World Trade Organization structural adjustment programs, which exacerbate hunger in the developing world by forcing debtor nations to restructure their agricultural base toward GM export crops and away from nutritional foodstuffs for local consumption.

World hunger will not be solved through large-scale molecular manipulation of food crops whose cultivation has been carefully perfected over 10,000 years, but through individual actions and political and social will.

Golden Rice and Vitamin A Deficiency

Vitamin A deficiency, a major cause of blindness in the developing world, affects millions. Severe deficiencies blind 350,000 pre-school age children each year. Lesser deficiencies weaken the immune system, increasing the risk of measles, malaria, other infectious diseases, and death. Vitamin A deficiency is implicated in over one million deaths per year.

Golden rice, touted as the biotech solution to vitamin A deficiency, was developed in 1999 by Swiss and German scientists, who spliced two daffodil and one bacterial gene into japonica rice. The rice produces beta-carotene, which the body converts into vitamin A in the absence of other nutritional deficiencies (such as those for zinc, protein, and fats) and in individuals not suffering from diarrhea. Unfortunately, these nutritional deficiencies and diarrhea are common among those suffering from vitamin A deficiency. Furthermore, golden rice is not yet adapted to local climates in developing countries. The amounts of vitamin A it produces are minute: 3 servings of $1/2$ cup per day would provide only 10% of one's vitamin A requirement (6% for nursing mothers). To make matters worse, beta-carotene is a pro-oxidant and may be carcinogenic.

Vitamin A deficiency can be cured with small to moderate amounts of vegetables, However, cultivation of such vegetables has decreased in the face of increasing monoculture to produce export crops, in part a consequence of World Bank and International Monetary Fund policies. Vitamin A deficiency can also be cured with inexpensive supplements. As with most nutritional deficiencies, indeed world hunger in general, a lasting solution to vitamin A deficiency depends not on new forms of technology, but rather on political and social will and international cooperation.

Chapter 21

Opposition to the Use of Hormone Growth Promoters in Beef and Dairy Cattle Production (American Public Health Association Policy Statement, Adopted 2009)

Elanor Starmer   David Wallinga   Rick North
                                             Martin Donohoe

There is clear evidence that hormones originating outside the body can interfere with our own hormone function.[1] Estrogen is classified by IARC as a Group 1 human carcinogen, for example.[2] In 1971, the FDA stated that the use of DES (the first synthetic hormone) in pregnant women was contraindicated after science appeared showing higher cancer risks in their daughters.[3-5] These "DES daughters," we now know, are at least 40 times more likely than the general population to develop certain clear cell cancers of the vagina or cervix in in their teens or twenties.[6] Experience with DES constitutes some of the earliest and most compelling human evidence that disruption of the human endocrine system occurs from exogenous hormone exposure.

In its first scientific statement issued in June 2009, the Endocrine Society, citing the precautionary principle, determined that "results from animal models, human clinical observations, and epidemiological studies converge to implicate EDCs (endocrine disrupting chemicals) as a significant concern to public health."[7] The statement echoes the findings of a 1996 article in *American Academy of Pediatrics News*, which found that "scientific knowledge about [EDCs'] effects on humans ... appears sufficient to justify societal approaches to limiting population exposures."[8]

Fetuses and children are thought to be more vulnerable to the hormone-disrupting effects of exogenous hormones and hormone-like chemicals. A recent consensus conference reviewed the robust and growing body of science that exposure to environmental chemicals, especially in utero, can disrupt normal hormone function and alter child development, as well as alter fetal programming, adding to risks for hormone-related cancer and other chronic diseases later in life.[9] Today, many hormone-related chronic diseases are common and/or on the rise, including breast and prostate cancer,[9-12] thyroid disease[13-15] obesity and diabetes,[9,16-19] endometriosis,[20] uterine fibroids,[21] and infertility.[22,23] Early-stage breast development in young girls appears to be occurring at younger ages today as compared to 1991, as indicated by a recent study in *Pediatrics.*[24]

The relationship between these recent adverse trends in hormone-related development or chronic disease incidence and what likely are multiple social and/or environmental co-contributors is not completely understood. (Of course, population genetics do not shift over such a small time period.) On the other hand, biological plausibility and scientific findings now suggest that exogenous hormones such as those used in our food system may be one such contributor to these negative trends. In one 2007 study, for example, sperm concentration of male offspring was found to be inversely related to their mothers' self-reported beef consumption while pregnant, with possible links hypothesized to the six steroid hormones routinely used in American beef production.[25]

APHA Policy #200011, *The Precautionary Principle and Children's Health,* "encourages precautionary action to prevent potential harm to fetuses, infants, and children [from the continued manufacture and use of substances], even if some cause and effect relationships have not been established with scientific certainty."[26] APHA has reiterated its support for the precautionary principle in other policy, as well.[27] Because children cannot choose to avoid food, and because the use of exogenous hormone growth promoters in beef and dairy production is unnecessary, this policy resolution lays out a precautionary rationale and scientific evidence for public health action to remove these food production uses of exogenous hormones.

Synthetic Hormones in Beef Production

From FDA approval in 1954 until 1979, DES continued to be used as a growth-promoting synthetic estrogen in beef cattle production even after its human uses were halted.[28] Three natural steroid hormones—estradiol, testosterone, and progesterone, and three synthetic surrogates (zeranol, melengestrol, trenbolone) remain in widespread use by US and Canadian beef cattle producers to boost growth and production;[25,29] concurrent use of more than one steroid is approved.[30] One of them, trenbolone, is thought to have 8–10 times greater anabolic activity than testosterone.[31] It is widely acknowledged that the use of these hormone growth promoters results in residues in meat.[32,33] Residues of these hormone growth promoters also persist for weeks to months in manure and in feedlot runoff, raising concerns about the added exogenous hormone load to the environment.[34,35]

Since 1988, use of steroid hormones in cattle production has been illegal in Europe.[33] According to the European Commission's Scientific Committee on Veterinary Measures Related to Public Health, the decision to ban the use of such hormones was "based on the accumulating evidence on the fragility of the endocrine equilibrium in all stages of life as well as the potential genotoxicity of these compounds and their metabolites." The commission continues, "Exogenous hormone exposure may disrupt this delicate equilibrium as is evidenced by the pronounced effects of oestrogens and testosterone on functional imprinting. Thus even exposure to residual amounts of hormonally active compounds as present in meat and meat products needs to be evaluated in terms of potentially adverse effects to public health."[36] By contrast, the US government position is that hormone residues in beef from adult cattle pose no threat to human health. This assumption of safety, however, has remained untested by long-term epidemiologic studies and instead relies on dated research concerning the ability of estrogen (estradiol) to *mutate* genes. It fails to reflect more recent research that hormones and hormonally active chemicals may exert their toxicity instead via epigenetic changes.[23,37]

rBGH Use in Dairy Production

Since 1994, recombinant bovine growth hormone, also known as rBGH or rbST, has been injected into dairy cows to increase milk production, typically to increase production by an average of 11–15%.[38] rBGH was developed and marketed by Monsanto and sold to Elanco, a division of Eli Lilly, in October 2008. Though approved by the FDA in a controversial November 1993 decision, both Canada and the European Union in 1999 refused to approve the drug's use, officially citing harm to cows' health.[39,40] No significant scientific studies since then have led these bodies to reconsider their stance. Australia, New Zealand, and Japan have also prohibited its use.[41,42]

Although some studies (including a number funded by Monsanto) have failed to demonstrate that rBGH harms dairy cows,[43] virtually all independent analyses of the data reached a different conclusion.[44] In addition to the Canadian and European studies, the FDA's analysis of the data submitted by Monsanto demonstrated that use of rBGH increases the incidence of sixteen different harmful conditions in cows, including birth disorders, hoof problems, heat stress, diarrhea, increased somatic cell count, and mastitis, a painful udder infection.[45] Based on this evidence, the FDA requires these risks be listed on rBGH package inserts, but not on finished dairy products.[45] Virtually all animal-welfare organizations, including the Humane Society of the United States and the Humane Farming Association, oppose the use of rBGH.[46]

rBGH use presents an additional risk to human health in the form of antibiotic resistance. As more cows develop mastitis due to rBGH use, farmers necessarily increase their use of antibiotics to treat the udder infections.[47] There is now a consensus among scientists that antibiotic use in farm animals increases antibiotic resistance, which can then be transmitted back to humans through bacteria on food or in the environment.[48,49] Reducing rBGH use would serve to reduce antibiotic use in dairy cattle.

Scientific committees for Health Canada and the European Commission have also raised concerns about the potential effects of rBGH on cancer.[50,51] Insulin-like growth factor-1 (IGF-1) is a necessary growth hormone present and identical in both cows and humans. However, elevated IGF-1 levels in human blood are associated with higher rates of colon, breast, and prostate cancers.[52-54] Based on data submitted by Monsanto, the FDA determined that rBGH use raises levels of IGF-1 in cow's sera and cow's milk.[55] These data also show that IGF-1 survives pasteurization.[56] Animal models show that most IGF-1 in cow's milk survives digestion, reaching the bloodstream where it may promote cancer.[57-59] The U.N.'s main food safety body, the Codex Alimentarius Commission, determined in 1999 that rBGH could not be declared safe for human health.[60]

In recent years, more and more US public health organizations have taken formal stances opposing the drug, including Oregon Physicians for Social Responsibility (2003), Health Care Without Harm (2005), and the American Nurses Association (2008).[61-63] In the past three years, more than 230 US hospitals have signed a pledge committing to serve rBGH-free dairy products.[64]

A 2008 national poll showed that more than 90% of consumers favor labeling of rBGH-free products.[65] Responding to this concern, many large retail establishments—including Walmart—have phased out their milk brands produced using rBGH.[66] Milk and many other dairy products from cows not treated with rBGH are now widely available; rBGH use fell from 22% of US farms in 2003 to 15% in 2007.[67] Use of the synthetic hormone is still common practice on many large dairy operations, however. In 2007, nearly 43% of large herds were treated with rBGH.[67]

In February 2007, Monsanto appealed unsuccessfully to the FDA and the Federal Trade Commission to restrict the labeling of rBGH-free milk. Since then, policy makers in eight states have attempted to ban or restrict the labeling of rBGH-free dairy products through bills or administrative rules. All failed except in Ohio, where the proposed rules are being challenged in court.

Medical authorities and foreign governments have documented scientific public health concerns associated with rBGH use. As long as the FDA allows rBGH to remain on the market, consumers should have the "right to know" if it is present or absent in dairy products they consume. This right to know about hazardous or controversial substances has been defended in APHA Policy 2002–5.[68]

A Precautionary Approach to Hormone Growth Promoters in Beef and Dairy Cattle Production

Consistent with its explicit endorsement of the precautionary principle, the American Public Health Association is therefore opposed to the use of hormone growth promoters in beef and dairy cattle production, and strongly recommends the following:

- The FDA act with public health precaution to ban their use on the basis of certain exposure and possibility of human health risks, pending long-term epidemiological data demonstrating such exposures to be without harm to workers and/or the population as a whole.

- Hospitals, schools, and other institutions, especially those serving children, preferentially purchase food products from beef and dairy cattle produced without such hormones.

- Companies producing and retailers offering products produced without rBGH or other hormones retain the right to label such products in an easily readable and understandable fashion so that consumers in the free marketplace can be equipped to make an informed choice about which brands to buy.

- APHA support increased federal research to better delineate mechanisms of harm from hormone-disrupting chemicals in food and the environment, and to assess the cumulative public health impact from low-level exposure to multiple such chemicals, including to fetuses and children.

Notes

1. Colborn T, Dumanoski D, Myes JP. 1996. *Our stolen future.* New York, Plume, Penguin Books.

2. International Agency for Research on Cancer. 2007. Combined estrogen-progestogen contraceptive and combined estrogen-progestogen menopausal therapy. *IARC Monographs on the Evaluation of Carcinogenic Risks to Humans.* 91.

3. Swan SH. Intrauterine exposure to diethylstilbestrol: Long-term effects in humans. *APMIS.* 2000 December;108(12):793–804.

4. EXTOXNET website. *Questions about endocrine disruptors, a pesticide information project of Cornell University, Michigan State University, Oregon State University, and*

University of California at Davis. Accessed May 21, 2009, at http://extoxnet.orst .edu/faqs/pesticide/endocrine.htm.

5. Reigart R, Cummins S. Limit hormone-disrupting chemical exposure. *AAP News* 1996;12:17.

6. Centers for Disease Control and Prevention. *Health risks and related concerns for DES daughters.* Accessed March 11, 2008, at www.cdc.gov/DES/hcp/information /daughters/risks_daughters.html.

7. Diamanti-Kandarakis E, Bourguignon JP, Giudice LC, Hauser R, Prins GS, Soto AM, Zoeller RT, Gore AC. Endocrine-disrupting chemicals: An Endocrine Society scientific statement. *Endocrine Reviews* 2009;30(4):293–342.

8. Reigart R, Cummins S. Limit hormone-disrupting chemical exposure. *AAP News* 1996;12(4):17

9. Grandjean P, Bellinger D, Berman A, Cordler S, Davey-Smith G, Eskenazi B, Gee B, Gray K, Hanson M, van den Hazel P, Heindel JJ, Heinzow B, Hertz-Picciotto I, Hu H, Huang T T-K, Jensen TK, Landrigan PJ, McMillen IC, Murata K, Ritz B, Schoeters G, Skakkebæk NE, Skerfving S, Weihe P. The Faroes statement: Human health effects of developmental exposure to chemicals in our environment. *Basic & Clinical Pharmacology & Toxicology* 2008;102:73–75.

10. Cowin PA, Foster P, Pedersen J, Hedwards S, McPherson SJ, Risbridger GP. Early onset endocrine disruptor induced prostatitis in the rat. *Environment Health Perspect.* 2008;116:923–929.

11. Gray LE, Wilson VS, Stoker TS, Lambright C, Furr J, Noriega N, Howdeshell K, Ankley GT, Guillette LJ. 2006. Adverse effects of environmental antiandrogens and androgens on reproductive development in mammals. *International Journal of Andrology* 29:96–104.

12. vom Saal FS, Belcher SM, Guillette LJ, Hauser R, Myers JP, Prins GS, Welshons WV, Heindel JJ, et al. Chapel Hill bisphenol A expert panel consensus statement: Integration of mechanisms, effects in animals and potential impact to human health at current exposure levels. *Reprod Toxicol.* 2007;24:131–138.

13. Meeker JD, Calafat AM, Hauser R. Di(2-ethylhexyl) phthalate metabolites may alter thyroid hormone levels in men. *Environ Health Perspect.* 2007 July;115(7): 1029–1034.

14. Crofton KE, Craft ES, Hedge JM, Gennings C, Simmons JE, Carchman RA, Carter Jr. WH, DeVito MJ. Thyroid hormone disrupting chemicals: Evidence for dose-dependent additivity or synergism. *Environ Health Perspect.* 2005;113(11): 1549–1554.

15. Davey JC, Nomikos AP, Wungjiranirun M, Sherman JR, Ingram L, Batki C, Lariviere JP, Hamilton JW. Arsenic as an endocrine disruptor: Arsenic disrupts retinoic acid receptor- and thyroid hormone receptor-mediated gene regulation and thyroid hormone-mediated amphibian tail metamorphosis. *Environ Health Perspect.* 2008; 116(2):165–172.

16. Ruhlen RL, Howdeshell KL, Mao J, Taylor JA, Bronson FH, Newbold RR, Welshons WV, vom Saal FS. Low phytoestrogen levels in feed increase fetal serum estradiol resulting in the "fetal estrogenization syndrome" and obesity in CD - 1 mice. *Environ Health Perspect.* 2008;116:322–328.

17. Smink A, Ribas-Fito N, Garcia R, Torrent M, Mendez MA, Grimalt JO, Sunyer J. Exposure to hexachlorobenzene during pregnancy increases the risk of overweight in children aged 6 years. *Acta Paediatr.* 2008 Oct;97(10):1465-9. Epub 2008 Jul 28.

18. Hugo, ER, Brandebourg TD, Woo JG, Loftus J, Alexander JW Ben-Jonathan N. Bisphenol A at environmentally relevant doses inhibits adiponectin release from human adipose tissue explants and adipocytes. *Environ Health Perspect.* 2008. doi:10.1289/ehp.11537. Accessed August 14, 2008, at http://dx.doi.org/.

19. Lang IA, Galloway TS, Scarlett A, Henley WE, Depledge M, Wallace RB, Melzer D. Association of urinary bisphenol A concentration with medical disorders and laboratory abnormalities in adults. *JAMA.* 2008;300(11):1303–1310.

20. Rier S, Foster WG. Environmental dioxins and endometriosis. *Toxicological Sciences* 2002;70:161–170.

21. Newbold RR, Jefferson WR, Banks EP. Long-term adverse effects of neonatal exposure to bisphenol A on the murine female reproductive tract. *Reproductive Toxicology* 2007;24:253–258.

22. Hauser R, Meeker JD, Duty S, Silva MJ, Calafat AM. Altered semen quality in relation to urinary concentrations of phthalate monoester and oxidative metabolites. *Epidemiology* 2006;17:682–691.

23. Swan, SH, Kruse RL, Fan L, Barr DB, Drobnis EZ, Redmon JB, Wang C, Brazil C, Overstreet JW, and the Study for the Future of Families Research Group. Semen quality in relation to biomarkers of pesticide exposure. *Environ Health Perspect.* 2003;111:1478–1484.

24. Aksglaede L, Sorensen K, Petersen JH, Skakkebaek NE, Juul A. Recent decline in age at breast development: The Copenhagen puberty study. *Pediatrics* 2009;123: e932–e939.

25. Swan SH, Liu F, Overstreet JW, Brazil C, Skakkebæk NE. Semen quality of fertile US males in relation to their mothers' beef consumption during pregnancy. *Hum Reprod.* 2007;22(6):1497–1502.

26. APHA Policy #200011. *The precautionary principle and children's health.* January 1, 2000. Accessed June 2, 2009, at http://www.apha.org/advocacy/policy/policysearch/default.htm?id=216.

27. APHA Policy #20009. *Support for international action to eliminate persistent organic pollutants.* January 1, 2000. Accessed June 2, 2009, at http://www.apha.org/advocacy/policy/policysearch/default.htm?id=214.

28. Office of Technology Assessment. *Drugs in livestock feed* (NTIS order #PB-298450) (138–139). Washington, DC: US Government Printing Office; 1979. Accessed October 6, 2008, at www.princeton.edu/~ota/disk3/1979/7905/790504.PDF.

29. Meyer HH. Biochemistry and physiology of anabolic hormones used for improvement of meat production. *APMIS*. 2001;09:1–8.

30. Orr R. *Growth-promoting hormones in cattle*. International Food Safety Network, Kansas State University, 2001. Accessed November 7, 2009, at http://foodsafety .k-state.edu/en/article-details.php?a=4&c=19&sc=162&id=308.

31. Lange IG, Daxenberger A, Schiffer B, Witters H, Ibarreta D, Meyer HHD. Sex hormones originating from different livestock production systems: Fate and potential disrupting activity in the environment. *Anal Chim Acta*. 2002;473: 27–37.

32. Henricks DM, Gray SL, Owenby JJ, et al. Residues from anabolic preparations after good veterinary practice. *APMIS*. 2001;109:273–283.

33. Stephany RW. Hormones in meat: Different approaches in the EU and in the USA. *APMIS*. 2001;109:S357–S363.

34. Schiffer B, Daxenberger A, Meyer K, Meyer HHD. The fate of trenbolone acetate and melengestrol acetate after application as growth promoters in cattle: Environmental studies. *Environ Health Perspect* http://www.ncbi.nlm.nih.gov/pmc/articles /PMC1240476/2001;109:1145–1151.

35. Soto AM, Calabro JM, Prechtl NV, Yau AY, Orlando EF, Daxenberger A, Kolok AS, Guiletter LJ, Bizec B, Lange IG, Sonnenschein C. Androgenic and estrogenic activity in water bodies receiving cattle feedlot effluent in eastern Nebraska, USA. *Environ Health Perspect*. 2004;112:346–352.

36. European Commissions. *Scientific Committee on Veterinary Measures Relating to Public Health: Assessment of potential risks to human health from hormone residues in bovine meat and meat products*. April 30, 1999. Accessed May 22, 2009, at http://ec.europa.eu/food/fs/sc/scv/out21_en.pdf.

37. vom Saal, FS, Belcher SM, Guillette LJ, Hauser R, Myers JP, Prins GS, Welshons WV, Heindel JJ, et al. Chapel Hill bisphenol A expert panel consensus statement: Integration of mechanisms, effects in animals and potential impact to human health at current exposure levels. *Reprod Toxicol*. 2007;24:131–138.

38. Dohoo I, et al, A meta-analysis review of the effects of recombinant bovine somatotropin. *Canadian Journal of Veterinary Research* 2003;67(4):241–251.

39. Dohoo I, et al. *Report of the Canadian Veterinary Medical Association expert panel on rBST*. November 1998, http://www.hc-sc.gc.ca/dhp-mps/vet/issues-enjeux /rbst-stbr/rep_cvma-rap_acdv_tc-tm-eng.php.

40. Broom D, et al. *Report of the (European Union) Scientific Committee on Animal Health and Animal Welfare on aspects of the use of bovine somatotropin*. March 1999, http://ec.europa.eu/food/fs/sc/scah/out21_en.pdf.

41. Japan Ministry of Health, Labour and Welfare. *Ministerial ordinance on milk and milk products concerning compositional standards*. February 5, 2004.

42. Food Standards Australia and New Zealand. *A risk profile of dairy products in Australia: Food standards Australia, New Zealand*. http://www.google.com/url? sa=t&rct=j&q=&esrc=s&source=web&cd=4&ved=0CDwQFjAD&url=http%3A

%2F%2Fwww.comlaw.gov.au%2FDetails%2FF2006L03270%2Fc7851162-dbfc
-4ef4-9d08-499c25dbf23f&ei=b0CeT--8D8baiQKN4LFh&usg=AFQjCNGhUMkURh
M9rzGSOGzsOiXs5pIBaA&sig2=VF08TLslLq74mcGYMoUU2A. August 9, 2006.

43. Bauman D, et al. Production response to bovine somatotropin in northeast dairy
    herds. *Journal of Dairy Science* 1999;82:2564–2573.

44. Kronfeld DS. Recombinant bovine somatotropin and animal welfare. *Journal of the
    American Veterinary Medical Association* 2000;11(216):1719–1722.

45. United States Food and Drug Administration. *Freedom of information summary for
    Posilac®*. November 1993, Section 6-j. http://www.fda.gov/downloads/Animal
    Veterinary/Products/ApprovedAnimalDrugProducts/FOIADrugSummaries
    /ucm050022.pdf.

46. See, for example, Siebert L, et al. *Letter to Governor Kathleen Sebelius.* April 8, 2009.
    Accessed November 7, 2009, at http://www.consumersunion.org/pub/core_food
    _safety/010910.html.

47. Zwald AG, et al. Management practices and reported antimicrobial usage on
    conventional and organic dairy farms. *Journal of Dairy Science* 2004;87:191–201.

48. Aarestrup FM, Wegener HC, Collignon P. Resistance in bacteria of the food chain:
    Epidemiology and control strategies. *Expert Rev. Anti Infect. Ther.* 2008;6(5):
    733–750.

49. APHA. *Antibiotic resistance factsheet.* March 2003. Accessed June 2, 2009, at www
    .apha.org/advocacy/reports/facts/advocacyfactantibiotic.htm?NRMODE=
    Published&NRNODEGUID=%7b994096E5–45B0–46B5-B757- D61D499A16B3%
    7d&NRORIGINALURL=%2fadvocacy%2freports%2ffacts%2fadvocacyfactantibi
    otic&NRCACHEHINT=NoModifyGuest&PF=true167 168 169.

50. Health Canada. *rBST gaps analysis report.* http://www.integrativehealthcare.net
    /GapsAnalysisReport.pdf April 21, 1998.

51. The European Commission. Food safety: From the farm to the fork. *Report on public
    health aspects of the uses of bovine somatotropin.* http://www.scribd.com/doc
    /4101096/A-New-Technological-Era-for-American-Agriculture March 15–16, 1999.

52. Yu H, Rohan T. Role of the insulin-like growth factor family in cancer development
    and progression. *Journal of the National Cancer Institute* 2000;92(18):1472–1489.

53. Moschos S, Mantzoros C. The role of the IGF system in cancer: From basic to clinical
    studies and clinical applications. *Oncology* 2002;63(4):317–332.

54. Roddam AW, Allen NE, Appelby P, Key TJ, Ferrucci L, et al. Insulin-like growth
    factors, their binding proteins, and prostate cancer risk: Analysis of individual
    patient data from 12 prospective studies. *Ann Intern Med.* 2008 October 7;49(7):
    461–471, W83–88.

55. United States Food and Drug Administration. *Freedom of information summary for
    Posilac®*. November 1993, Section 7a-f http://www.fda.gov/downloads/Animal
    Veterinary/Products/ApprovedAnimalDrugProducts/FOIADrugSummaries
    /ucm050022.pdf.

56. Juskevich JC, Guyer CG. Bovine growth hormone: Human food safety evaluation. *Science* 1990;249:875–884.

57. Kimura T, et al. Gastrointestinal absorption of recombinant human insulin-like growth factor-1 in rats. *Journal of Pharmacology and Experimental Therapeutics* 1997;283:611–618.

58. Xian C, et al, Degradation of IGF-1 in the adult rat gastrointestinal tract is limited by a specific antiserum or the dietary protein casein. *Journal of Endocrinology* 1995; 146:215–225.

59. Anderle P, et al. In vitro assessment of intestinal IGF-1 stability. *Journal of Pharmaceutical Sciences* 2002;91:1.

60. Codex Alimentarius Commission. *Report: Twenty-third session*. June 28–July 3, 1999. FAO Headquarters, Rome, pp. 3–14.

61. Health Care Without Harm. http://www.google.com/url?sa=t&rct=j&q=&esrc= s&source=web&cd=4&ved=0CFQQFjAD&url=http%3A%2F%2Fwww.psr.org %2Fchapters%2Foregon%2Fsafe-food%2Fhcwh-rbgh-statement.doc&ei= 2EKeT5C0A-SPiALi6YjuDQ&usg=AFQjCNGRRGoybkgejDFbkvL_1cMx97zWhw& sig2=MH_raZ72AajaFYky58RkDQ.

62. Oregon Physicians for Social Responsibility. www.psr.org/site/PageServer?page name=oregon_safefood.

63. American Nurses Association. *Press release*. July 1, 2008. www.nursingworld.org /FunctionalMenuCategories/MediaResources/PressReleases/2008PR.aspx.

64. Health Care Without Harm website. Accessed June 6, 2009, at http://www.noharm .org/us/food/pledge.

65. Consumer Reports National Research Center. *Food labeling poll.* http://www .consumersunion.org/pub/core_food_safety/006298.html. November 2008.

66. Walmart Stores. *Walmart offers private label milk produced without artificial growth hormone.* March 23, 2008. Accessed November 7, 2009, at http://walmartstores .com/FactsNews/NewsRoom/8147.aspx.

67. United States Department of Agriculture. *Dairy 2007.* http://www.aphis.usda.gov /animal_health/nahms/dairy/downloads/dairy07/Dairy07_ir_Facilities.pdf. October 2007.

68. APHA policy # 2002–5. *Preserving right-to-know information and encouraging hazard reduction to reduce the risk of exposure to toxic substances.* 2002. Accessed June 2, 2009, at http://www.apha.org/advocacy/policy/policysearch/default .htm?id=279.

Part Six

Environmental Health

As far as we know, human beings, more than seven billion of us, are the only forms of higher intelligence to inhabit the universe. Our intelligence has resulted in our achieving the biblically promised dominion over the earth and its other creatures, but due to hubris, greed, and the triumph of competition over cooperation, we have done tremendous damage.

We are currently stressing our fragile planet beyond the breaking point through overpopulation, air and water pollution, deforestation, global warming, unsustainable agricultural and fishing practices, and, among the wealthier nations, overconsumption ("affluenza"). High levels of often-unnecessary consumption have not made Americans any happier; as studies show we are working more, taking fewer vacations, feeling more frustrated, have fewer friends, and suffer lower levels of life satisfaction as our social capital erodes, even as new technologies promise increased connectivity to each other and to our world. Consider that antidepressant use doubled between 1993 and 2005, and one out of ten Americans over age six currently takes a psychotropic medication.[1]

Our Declaration of Independence states, "All men are created equal."[2] In practice however, as noted by George Orwell, "some people are more equal than others."[3] Our national and global political and economic institutions primarily serve the interests of the wealthy. This increases the maldistribution of wealth that contributes to creating inferior schools, higher levels of hunger, and worsens health indicators among the lower socioeconomic classes. Our global imbalance between the haves and the have-nots mirrors that noted centuries ago by Voltaire, who recognized that "the comfort of the rich rests upon an abundance of the poor."[4]

We reap the rewards of certain technologies (e.g., more efficient transportation, methods of food preparation, and access to information and on-demand entertainment), yet suffer the consequences of disasters wrought by other technologies (e.g., heavy metal pollution as in Minamata Bay, Japan; chemical factory explosions as in Bhopal, India; nuclear reactor meltdowns as in Chernobyl, USSR [now Ukraine]; and oil spills consequent to the Exxon Valdez crash and the BP drilling rig explosion in the Gulf of Mexico). Our willingness to adopt new technologies without appropriate testing and precaution can have dramatic, unintended consequences.

Our health care system contributes significantly to carbon emissions and waste generation.[5] The six thousand US hospitals generate two million tons of waste per year, clinics and doctors' offices an additional 700,000 tons; 850,000 tons are incinerated, of which only 15 percent is infectious waste, that is, that requires burning. Incinerated pollutants include dioxin, mercury, cadmium, and lead, all significant toxins. Each day one hospital bed generates between sixteen and twenty-three pounds of waste.

Our global ecological footprint already exceeds by 50 percent the carrying capacity of our planet. As developing nations begin to adopt the habits of excessive consumption and massive waste production seen in the United States, many fear the collapse of contemporary civilizations through depletion of natural resources leading to famine, war, or both, a frightening demise predicted centuries ago by Thomas Malthus. We are living during the largest mass extinction since the demise of the dinosaurs sixty-five million years ago, and if we are not careful and proactive, we may number among those species lost forever to history.

As time runs out, options for resolution and remediation of environmental destruction have become increasingly limited. Yet the resilience of the human spirit and the struggle for survival still give hope to those who wish for a healthy planet. Many are altering their own lives for enhanced sustainability. Inventors are devising inexpensive devices using renewable raw materials to improve the lives of the poor. Important new laws and international agreements, albeit limited in scope and enforcement, have been signed. These include the Montreal Protocol to phase out CFCs (chlorofluorocarbons) and the POPS (Persistent Organic Pollutants) and REACH (Registration, Evaluation, Authorisation, and Restriction of Chemicals) treaties. The power and voice of green groups is increasing and coalitions are being formed among scientists, environmental activists, and members of various religions. Although many would argue that it is not right to put any price on nature, economists have begun to incorporate calculations of the worth of clean air, watersheds, forest cover, soil quality, and other factors when analyzing the financial costs and consequences of decisions to build new dams, mines, or power plants. By joining together in groups and broader coalitions, health professionals can add their expertise and enthusiasm to that of such individuals in order to preserve the health of our planet and its people.

This section describes the nature and extent of human activities that contribute to environmental degradation and social injustice, two phenomena that interact synergistically. Focusing on education and activism, Chapter Twenty-Two (by Martin Donohoe) provides an overview of major causes and consequences of environmental degradation, specifically on the contribution of various social injustices. It offers numerous suggestions for health professionals (and others) to improve our world. Chapter Twenty-Three (by Martin Donohoe) looks specifically at global warming, its causes and myriad consequences, and the need for rapid action at the personal, national, and international levels to reverse climate change before we reach a critical tipping point. Chapter Twenty-Four (by Martin Donohoe) looks at the destructive human rights and environmental consequences of symbols of love, specifically gold, diamonds, and flowers. These items carry symbolic weight as tokens of affection (due significantly to clever marketing), yet represent to millions horrific suffering and are root causes of war and ecological destruction. Chapter Twenty-Five (by Andrew Jameton) presents an analysis of energy use by the health care system along with a proposal for dramatically reducing its carbon footprint. Those seeking further information should see the environmental health and the gold/diamonds/flowers pages of the Public Health and Social Justice website at http://phsj.org/environmental-health/ and http://phsj.org/gold-diamonds -flowers/.

Responding to the US government's inquiry about buying land from Native Americans (an ironic request, given how much was taken through forced migrations and famines and outright war), Chief Seattle said, "The earth is our mother. Whatever befalls the earth befalls the sons of the earth. The earth does not belong to man, man belongs to the earth. All things are connected like the blood that unites us all. Man did not weave the web of life, he is merely a strand in it. Whatever he does to the web, he does to himself."[6] Wallace Stegner argued for environmental preservation for aesthetic and spiritual reasons: "We simply need ... wild country available to us, even if we never do more than drive to its edge and look in. For it can be a means of reassuring ourselves of our sanity as creatures, a part of the geography of hope."[7] This is true, but with overwhelming scientific data suggesting a major crisis, we must make significant changes quickly to preserve our environment or our very survival as a species is at risk.

Notes

1. Olfson, M., & Marcus, S. C. National patterns in antidepressant medication treatment. *Archives of General Psychiatry*, 2009, 66(8), 848–856. Retrieved from http://archpsyc.ama-assn.org/cgi/content/abstract/66/8/848.

2. Declaration of Independence. July 4, 1776. Retrieved from http://www.ushistory.org/declaration/document/.

3. Orwell, G. *Animal farm* (New York: New American Library/Penguin Putnam), 1946.

4. Voltaire (Francois-Marie Arouet). Quote. Good Reads. Retrieved from http://www.goodreads.com/quotes/show/53246.

5. Pierce, J., & Jameton, A. *The ethics of environmentally responsible health care* (New York: Oxford University Press), 2004.

6. Chief Seattle. Quote. Finest Quotes. Retrieved from http://www.finestquotes.com/author_quotes-author-Chief%20Seattle-page-0.htm. [There is some question as to the authenticity of Chief Seattle's words. See http://www.snopes.com/quotes/seattle.asp.]

7. Stegner, W. *Wilderness letter*. Written to the Outdoor Recreation Resources Review Commission. December 3, 1960. Retrieved from http://wilderness.org/content/wilderness-letter.

Chapter 22

Roles and Responsibilities of Health Care Professionals in Combating Environmental Degradation and Social Injustice

Education and Activism

Martin Donohoe

Introduction

Health care professionals share a responsibility to recognize the causes and health consequences of environmental degradation and social injustice, and to oppose those forces which contribute to the spread of poverty, inequality, racism, human rights abuses, and ecosystem destruction. Today our world faces a growing crisis due to the health consequences of environmental degradation and social injustice. As a result of our training, health care professionals are in a unique position to recognize the causes of this crisis. Because of our privileged positions in society, since we ourselves are in part responsible for these problems, and because our raison d'être is to promote health and fight injustice, we share a responsibility, individually and collectively, to oppose those forces which contribute to the spread of poverty, inequality, racism, human rights abuses, and ecosystem destruction. We can accomplish this through changes in our own lives, through education and policy making, and by speaking out and working against the forces of injustice.

Causes and Health Consequences of Environmental Degradation and Social Injustice

Causes of environmental degradation include overpopulation, pollution, deforestation, global warming and associated weather extremes, unsustainable agricultural and fishing practices, overconsumption ("affluenza"), an increasing maldistribution of wealth—nationally and internationally—and militarization and war. Consequences include increasing poverty and overcrowding, famine, destruction of vital ecosystems, species loss, medical illnesses (particularly infectious diseases), and widespread, preventable suffering due to military conflict.[1]

The world's population has grown exponentially, reaching six billion in 1998.[2] Poverty, impaired access to reproductive health care services, and the social, legal, educational, economic, and political marginalization of women are driving this explosive increase, which primarily affects Africa, Asia, and Latin America. Compounding this problem are urbanization and a world migrant population of almost fifty million individuals, primarily war refugees and those fleeing environmental catastrophes.[3] This Malthusian increase in population has stressed the world's ecosystems through unsustainable agricultural and fishing practices and air and water pollution.[4]

Worldwide, over one billion people live in abject poverty, consuming less than 2,150 calories per day or earning less than 500 dollars (US) per year.[5] Over one billion people have no access to clean drinking water, two billion have no electricity, and three billion lack adequate sanitation services. Two million children die each year of preventable diarrheal disease, and every two days hunger-related causes kill as many people as died in the atomic bomb explosion at Hiroshima.[6] Tens of thousands of children die every day from malnutrition and disease, roughly the same as a hundred exploding jumbo jets full of children.[7] Soil erosion exceeds soil formation,[8] almost half of the world's farmland is seriously degraded due to destructive agricultural practices,[9] and water use has tripled in the last fifty years, depleting aquifers and necessitating the development of large-scale irrigation projects like China's Three Gorges Dam.[10] Untreated sewage from factory farms pollutes waterways,[11] and excessive agricultural antibiotic use has contributed to the spread of antibiotic-resistant food-borne pathogens among humans.[12] Widespread factory-trawler fishing has seriously depleted many of the world's major fisheries, necessitating fish farming, which in turn causes harm to local estuaries and harbors. Cyanide and dynamite fishing have accelerated the global warming–induced destruction of coral reefs, upon which most of the world's ecosystems ultimately depend.[13]

Industrialization and the accelerating worldwide demand for fuel-inefficient automobiles have polluted our air and hastened global warming and the destruction of the protective ozone layer.[14] Air pollution levels have been strongly linked to morbidity and mortality from cardiopulmonary and cerebrovascular disease.[15] Global warming, a consequence of increasing atmospheric carbon dioxide and other pollutants produced mostly by the world's wealthiest nations,[16] has been associated with increasing average worldwide temperatures, the melting of polar icecaps and glaciers, and augmentation of the destructive effects of extreme weather patterns such as El Niño and La Niña.[17] Deforestation, spurred by overpopulation, poverty, unsustainable farming practices, and rapacious logging, to satisfy increasing demand for paper products, has in turn augmented global warming, degraded soil quality, and contributed heavily to species loss. Haiti, Mauritania, and Ethiopia have been completely deforested, and previously lush island countries like Thailand and the Philippines have been transformed into net importers of forest products.[18]

We are currently living in the midst of the largest species extinction since that of the dinosaurs sixty-five million years ago.[19] Of the 50,000 known vertebrate species, seven out of ten birds, one quarter of mammals, half of the 232 primate species, one third of fish species, and between one fifth and one quarter of reptile and amphibian species are threatened with extinction.[20] Because over half of the top 150 prescription drugs are derived from or patterned directly after natural products, and since less than 0.5 percent of known flowering species have been surveyed for their medicinal value, a major consequence of this mass extinction is the loss of a potentially valuable pharmacopoeia.[21]

Most garbage, produced as a byproduct of First World overconsumption, is either recyclable or compostable. Our landfills are overflowing, contributing toxic leachate to our water supply, necessitating increased incineration of toxic waste and the desperate attempts of garbage-saturated areas to export their waste to financially needy states, Native American reservations, and countries that already suffer disproportionately from the effects of ecosystem degradation and poverty.[22]

The health consequences of these phenomena and others include the decimation of the African subcontinent by the acquired immunodeficiency syndrome (AIDS);[23] the persistence and in some cases resurgence of many preventable, or at least treatable, diseases like malaria, tuberculosis, viral encephalitis, cholera, hantavirus, schistosomiasis, influenza, trypanosomiasis, onchocerciasis, dengue, leishmanasis, rabies, hookworm, and yellow fever;[24] millions of pesticide-induced illnesses;[25] and the stunted neurological development of millions of children due to lead emissions, a particular problem in countries like China and Russia where automobile use is skyrocketing and leaded gas remains the most commonly used fuel.[26] At the same time, despite their missions as institutions for the prevention and treatment of disease, hospitals contribute significant amounts of dioxins, mercury, cadmium, and lead to local environments, in part through the incineration of polyvinyl chloride, which is found in medical supplies such as intravenous bags and tubing.[27]

Contributors to Environmental Degradation and Social Injustice

The wealthy, particularly those in large industrialized countries, are the greatest contributors to worldwide environmental degradation. For example, while the United States contains just 5 percent of the world's population, it is responsible for 25 percent of the world's energy consumption, 33 percent of its paper use, and 72 percent of all hazardous waste production.[28] The worldwide gap between rich and poor doubled over the last thirty years and continues to grow rapidly. In the United States, the richest 1 percent of the population owns 48 percent of the country's wealth, while the poorest 80 percent owns just 6 percent (the widest gap of any industrialized nation). Worldwide, the top 358 billionaires are worth the combined income of the bottom 2.5 billion people (or 45 percent of the world's population).[29]

Real wages for the average American worker have decreased, job security is down, workers receive fewer benefits and possess less retirement savings, household and total credit card debt have blossomed, and a continually increasing number of Americans lack health, life, and disability insurance.[30] The United States lags behind most other industrialized nations in major health indicators, leading many to question the so-called superiority of the US health care system.[31]

A majority of the world's one hundred largest economies are now transnational corporations, which are answerable to their shareholders (with most shares being held by a small percentage of wealthy individuals), as opposed to countries, which ultimately answer to their citizens.[32] Ninety percent of transnational corporations are headquartered in the northern hemisphere, exacerbating the wealth and resource disparity between the northern and southern hemispheres. Through tax law loopholes, the transfer of assets overseas and fraud, corporations are gaining increasing power.[33] Through lobbying, campaign contributions, control of a media, which limits public debate on topics of environmental importance, and in some cases human rights abuses, corporations, in their pursuit of greater profits, fight to weaken environmental and occupational safety and health standards and to dismantle social legislation designed to protect the public's health.[34] Corporations have also benefited from various legal developments: environmental audit laws, which absolve them of much of their responsibility for ecologically destructive activities; food disparagement laws, which may override the US First Amendment protections on freedom of speech in certain states; strategic lawsuits against private parties (SLAPP suits), designed to harass environmental groups and deplete their financial resources through threatened or actual litigation;[35] and support of so-called tort reform, designed to limit product liability risks. Further, corporations can benefit from moving of production facilities to countries where cheap labor is plentiful and environmental; occupational, safety, health, and human rights protections are minimal; and the intimidation and harassment of whistleblowers and union members are ignored.[36]

Despite comprising one of the most profitable industries in the United States, pharmaceutical companies continue to charge exorbitant prices for anti-AIDS drugs and have effectively lobbied and threatened trade sanctions against developing countries in order to prevent the production and importation of much cheaper, generic versions of these life-saving medications.[37] Biotechnology companies have dramatically increased production and exportation of genetically modified foodstuffs, despite worrisome potential sequelae of their use.[38]

Corporate agendas are furthered by the World Trade Organization and by policies of the World Bank and International Monetary Fund, which promote privatization of social resources and export-oriented development. This contributes further to natural resource depletion and pollution and tends to concentrate wealth in the hands of fewer and fewer individuals, while the health and welfare needs of the average citizen are neglected. Many countries in sub-Saharan Africa and central America face asphyxiating foreign debts, which miniscule levels of foreign aid and charitable donations have reduced only slightly.[39] The Malthusian consequences of overpopulation, ecosystem destruction, and growing disparities in wealth are both local and international conflicts. These conflicts contribute to suffering indirectly, through the diversion of resources away from countries' educational, social, and health care needs, and directly, through forced migrations, destruction of agricultural settlements and forced famine, weapons, such as missiles and landmines (which kill indiscriminately) and genocide.[40] The fate of our species hangs in the balance given the ever-present threats of chemical, biological, and nuclear warfare.[41]

Astronomical military budgets divert much-needed capital away from countries' educational, social, and health care needs.[42] Dwight Eisenhower recognized this, saying, "The problem in defense spending is to figure out how far you should go without destroying from within that which you are trying to defend from without." He added, "Every gun that is made, every warship launched, every rocket fired, signifies in the final sense a theft from those who hunger and are not fed, those who are cold and not clothed."[43]

Environmental Sexism and Racism

Women suffer disproportionately from the effects of poverty, famine, and human rights abuses through impaired access to employment, education, reproductive (and other basic) health services, salary inequities, political and legal marginalization, divorce restrictions, and direct violence.[44] More than two thirds of the world's poorest citizens are women.[45] In the United States, African Americans and Hispanics suffer disproportionately from the effects of poverty and environmental destruction. They are more likely to live in heavily polluted inner cities, work in industries where they suffer exposures to toxic chemicals, live in close proximity to waste dumps and incinerators (for example the "cancer belt" between Baton Rouge and New Orleans, Louisiana), and suffer the consequences of impaired access to health care.[46]

Confronting Environmental Degradation and Social Injustice

The Role of Government and Industry

There are many ways in which government, industry, and the individual can combat the degradation of our environment and social injustice. Health professionals too should have a responsibility to recognize the links between human health care and global social issues. Government policy should encourage (or require) industry to take measures in the reduction, reutilization, and recycling of raw materials and there should be stronger environmental, occupational, safety, and health requirements for industry. Government should eliminate tax breaks and subsidies to polluting industries and increase tax benefits and research funding for renewable technologies. There should also be financial support for research and development of alternative, less-polluting fuels and more sustainable, safe methods of food production.[47] Government and industry need to ensure sustainable management of our natural resources. Government must enforce stronger legislation to punish environmental scofflaws and revise economic analyses to account for the contributions of natural resources to the world's economies.[48] Incorporating environmental effects into both corporate and governmental comparative risk assessments and subjecting these assessments to public scrutiny would give greater transparency to issues affecting our environment. There should be support of ecumenical efforts by the world's major religions to promote environmentalism through a framework of shared values,[49] and aid to non-governmental organizations which fight for environmental and social justice, while de-emphasizing the role of states, which for many reasons are constrained in acting altruistically, and hence are often impotent in the face of our deepening global crisis.[50]

On a societal level, augmenting the status of women by strengthening family planning programs and equalizing access to educational opportunities and legal and political representation;[51] forgiveness of Third World debt and support of local economies; and encouraging the poor and minorities to exercise their rights to full participation in the political process, especially through voting, would minimize the most glaring social disparities having a harmful effect on global health issues today.

The Role of the Individual

As individuals, we can support "green" products and organizations, financially and through volunteerism; invest in "socially responsible" or "green" mutual funds;[52] decrease our meat intake and avoid over-fished species;[53] purchase organic fruits and vegetables and organic, shade-grown coffee; use less paper; avoid gas-guzzling vehicles and opt for walking, bicycling, public transportation, or carpooling; shun gold, silver, and diamonds originating in countries known for environmental, civil, and human rights abuses;[54] select "green electricity" and a "green burial";[55] compost and recycle organic wastes and become mindful of their energy use and waste production.

Health professionals have inadequately addressed, individually and collectively, the links among human health, environmental degradation, and social injustice. We can and should use our privileged positions to educate students and colleagues, inform the public, and, through investment of our time and money, as well as via direct action, work to promote change which will improve the health of our planet and its inhabitants.[56]

Rudolph Virchow as Social Justice Activist

The life of the famous pathologist Rudolph Virchow stands as a worthy example of how we can fulfill these goals.[57] Best known for establishing the cell doctrine in pathology, Virchow also elucidated much of the pathophysiology of thrombosis, pulmonary embolism, leukocytosis, and leukemia. Yet Virchow's contributions to social medicine were equally valuable. He recognized that "if a disease is an expression of individual life under unfavorable conditions, then epidemics must be indicative of disturbances of mass life."[58] He argued that typhus, cholera, tuberculosis, scurvy, some mental diseases, and cretinism were among those maladies that result from the unequal distribution of civilization's advantages.[59] Virchow asserted the moral un-neutrality of medicine.[60] To him, physicians were the natural advocates of the poor.[61] He wrote, "If medicine is really to accomplish its great task, it must intervene in political and social life. It must point out the hindrances that impede the normal social functioning of vital processes, and effect their removal."[62] Virchow served as a member of state and local government for over thirty years and founded a journal entitled *Medical Reform*. Both in the legislature and through this periodical, he spoke out for public provision of medical care for the indigent, for the prohibition of child labor, for universal education, and for free and unlimited democracy. He instituted programs for improving water and sewage systems, for stricter food inspection and for revamping the old, ineffective hospital organisation.[63] He elevated standards "for the training of nurses [and set] new criteria of hygiene for the public schools."[64] His study of cross-cultural cranial capacities helped to invalidate, albeit briefly, the pernicious myth of German racial purity. Other professionals, including Thomas Hodgkin, Margaret Sanger, Albert Schweitzer, and Florence Nightingale, have led inspiring lives of social activism—innumerable individuals today labor, often anonymously, in support of the disenfranchised.

The Role of the Health Care Institutions

Collectively, health care organizations should come out strongly in favor of environmental protections and universal access to food, clothing, housing, education, a living wage, political and legal representation, and health care.[65] They should stand against corporate and governmental policies, which harm the environment and adversely affect the health of many, in order to enrich the few. We must be ever-vigilant in the face of repeated attempts by local and national legislatures to roll back pre-existing environmental regulations. Individuals and groups can make their positions known through actively seeking media exposure,[66] public speaking engagements, alliances with like-minded groups, writing op-ed columns and letters to influential legislators, volunteerism, and even running for public office.

Health care institutions should improve medical waste management through better segregation of infectious material; worker safety training; safer disposal methods; reuse and recycling programs; and by phasing out mercury-containing and polyvinyl chloride-containing compounds.[67] Investigators should be encouraged to carry out studies looking at ways to cut waste in delivery of medical care.[68] Modification of medical and nursing schools' affirmative action policies to include a focus on social class as well as race may contribute to improved care for the underserved because of the tendency of a physicians' socio-economic origins to correlate with their patterns of service to the disadvantaged. Furthermore, physician-patient communication would be enhanced based on shared experience.[69] As epidemiology continues to evolve from a science that identifies risk factors for disease to one that analyses the systems that generate patterns of disease,[70] public health programs should keep focusing on and emphasizing issues of social justice.[71]

Hospitals must be especially wary of corporate contracts which limit academic freedom and/or the dissemination of research findings vital to the public's health.[72] Scientific and ethics organizations and health professions schools should counter corporations' deliberate attempts to obfuscate environmental issues—sponsored environmental education curriculums for public schools; deceptive advertising; the vigorous promotion of faulty science by corporate front groups and "astroturfing"—the creation of artificial "grassroots coalitions," which may contain only a few members.[73] In the United States, companies capitalize on citizens' environmental ignorance, which is in part a byproduct of a public education system in disarray, particularly in poor and minority neighborhoods, which suffer disproportionately due to under-funded school systems.[74] Health care organizations should divest themselves of stock holdings in harmful products such as tobacco,[75] and advocate for strong laws and treaties to curb tobacco use.[76] They should support evidence-based humanitarian interventions[77] and work toward solutions to poverty, such as replacing the current minimum wage with a federally mandated living wage. Finally, strong advocacy for peace, decreased militarization, and increased international cooperation is essential in these dangerous times.[78]

Education in Health Professions and the Medical Humanities

Schools for health professions need to devote significantly more curricular time to teaching students and trainees, in creative ways, about the causes and health consequences of environmental degradation, poverty, racism, and other forms of social injustice. Medical schools must respond more aggressively to the Institute of Medicine's 1995 recommendations regarding increases to training in the prevention and treatment of diseases related to the environment. These schools need to re-emphasize the role of social class as a contributor to morbidity and mortality.[79]

Curricular surveys have shown that environmental ethics is largely ignored in US medical schools.[80] Furthermore, medical schools do not adequately address the medical aspects of human rights' issues in required courses,[81] despite broad recognition of the important role that medical professionals can play in the prevention of international torture and in the treatment of its survivors.[82] Medical and nursing school curriculums also inadequately cover the roles of providers in combating militarization and genocide.[83] Schools should educate health professionals regarding the consequences of chemical, biological, and nuclear warfare, so that they in turn can help educate the public and its leaders about the devastating effects weapons of mass destruction would have on the earth and its inhabitants.[84]

Topics related to environmental ethics and social justice can be taught from both scientific and ethical perspectives and would likely be more interesting if they incorporated history and the humanities. For instance, a session on toxic pollution could discuss the leak of methyl isocyanate gas during a factory explosion in Bhopal, India,[85] the nuclear power plant explosion in Chernobyl,[86] and the Exxon Valdez oil spill of 1989.[87] William Eugene and Aileen Smith's photoessay on the health consequences of methyl mercury poisoning in Minimata Bay, Japan,[88] powerfully communicates the depth and poignancy of suffering among those exposed prenatally and as adults. A session on deforestation could relate the events leading to the desertification of Easter Island.[89] George Orwell's "How the Poor Die"[90] and Anton Chekhov's "Ward No. Six"[91] offer timeless descriptions of some of the horrific conditions which even today can be found in inadequately funded public hospitals. Upton Sinclair's *The Jungle*[92] relates the experience of a poor immigrant family in the United States — the novel's revolting descriptions of Chicago's meat packing plants spurred public pressure on Congress to pass the Pure Food and Drug Act of 1906. Henrik Ibsen's *An Enemy of the People*[93] portrays how a doctor battled with city officials to clean up the local water supply. William Carlos Williams's "The Paid Nurse"[94] describes a community physician's disdain at the inadequate treatment provided to a victim of an industrial accident by a company physician.[95] Earnest J Gaines's *The Sky Is Gray*[96] relates the story of a poor, single African American farm mother trying to obtain dental care for her ill child in a racist Southern farm town. Doris Lessing's *An Old Woman and Her Cat*[97] provides a moving fictional entrée into the world of society's dispossessed, through its description of the daily struggles of an aged gypsy and her adopted alley cat trying to cope with life on the streets of London. Exposing medical professionals to the realities of historical events and evocative literature that highlights the human suffering caused by environmental disasters and social disparity can promote a more personal human understanding and inspire health professionals to use their role to take action against injustice.[98]

Compulsory community service volunteer work and mentored service-learning projects would immerse students in their communities, giving them greater insight to the health and social problems facing patients,[99] as well as an opportunity to conduct activist-oriented research.[100]

Conclusions

Regrettably, discourse regarding environmental issues by our elected and industrial leaders is marked by ignorance and oversimplification, and is often influenced by campaign contributions from individual and corporate polluters: "The most precious thing in the world is capital."[101]

Ralph Waldo Emerson, on the other hand, eloquently attacked isolationism and the accumulation of capital: "As long as civilization is essentially one of property, of fences, of exclusiveness, it will be mocked by delusions. Our riches will leave us sick; there will be bitterness in our laughter, and our wine will burn our mouths. Only that good profits which we can taste with all doors open, and which serves all men."[102] George Bernard Shaw wrote that "the worst sin toward our fellow creatures is not to hate them, but to be indifferent to them: that is the essence of inhumanity."[103] And Pastor Niemoller's "First They Came for the Jews" powerfully exhorts us to speak out on behalf of the disenfranchised, especially since one day we may join their ranks:

First they came for the Jews

First they came for the Jews
and I did not speak out —

> because I was not a Jew.
> Then they came for the communists
> and I did not speak out—
> because I was not a communist.
> Then they came for the trade unionists
> and I did not speak out—
> because I was not a trade unionist.
> Then they came for me—
> and there was no one left
> to speak out for me.[104]

While the litany of environmental destruction and social injustice presented herein could provoke overpowering depression, we must avoid succumbing to nihilism or cynicism.[105] Philip Noel-Baker, in his 1959 acceptance speech for the Nobel Peace Prize, said, "Defeatism about the future is a crime. The danger is not in trying to do too much, but in trying to do too little."[106] Elie Wiesel's Nobel speech echoes the sentiment, "There may be times when we are powerless to prevent injustice, but there must never be a time when we fail to protest. The Talmud tells us that by saving a single human being, man can save the world."[107] And, Margaret Mead's reminder, "Never doubt that a small group of thoughtful, committed citizens can change the world; indeed it is the only thing that ever has,"[108] should motivate us to struggle, both individually and collectively. Doctor Evgeny Chazov, in his Nobel speech of 1985 representing International Physicians for the Prevention of Nuclear War, said, "If we are to succeed, our vision must possess millions of people. We must convince each generation that they are but transient passengers on this planet earth."[109] Finally, let us act not primarily for ourselves, but for each other,[110] and mainly for generations to come; for, as the Native American saying reminds us, "We have not inherited the Earth from our ancestors, but have borrowed it from our children."

Notes

1. Donohoe MT, Causes and health consequences of environmental degradation and social injustice. *Social Science and Medicine*, vol. 56, no. 3, pp. 573–587.

2. Bonngaarts J, Population policy options in the developing world. *Science*, vol. 263, pp. 771–776; Delacroix M, Planet Earth. *Blue*, vol. 3, no. 2, pp. 65–69.

3. Delacroix M, Planet Earth; Parfit M, Making tracks: Migration in the 1990s. *National Geographic*, October 1998, pp. 6–35; McConahay MJ, No place to call home. *Sierra*, November/December 2000, pp. 66–72; Bacon D, Editorial on refugees. *The Nation*, March 20, 2000, p. 7.

4. Benchly P, What will be the catch of the day? *Time*, November 8, 1999, pp.104–105; Samet JM, Dominici F, Curriero FC, et al., Fine particulate air

pollution and mortality in 20 US cities, 1987–1994. *New England Journal of Medicine,* vol. 343, no. 24, 2000, pp. 1742–1749.

5. Ackerman S, The ever-present yet nonexistent poor. *Extra!,* January/February 1999, pp. 9–10.

6. Ackerman S, The ever-present nonexistent poor; Donohoe MT, Atomic anniversary is sobering one: Citizens need to act now to counter the continuing nuclear threat [editorial]. *Portland Tribune,* August 20, 2002, p. A7.

7. Cole KC, Calculated risks. *Skeptical Inquirer,* September/October 1998, pp. 32–36.

8. Land. *The Amicus Journal,* vol. 24, no. 4, 2000, p. 26.

9. Rivera R, Farmland. *The Amicus Journal,* vol. 22, no. 3, 2000, p. 8.

10. Schildgen B, China drowns? *Sierra,* November/December 2000, p. 92.

11. Silverstein K, Meat factories. *Sierra,* January/February 1999, pp. 28–35, 110–112; Harrison P, et al., Surveillance for possible estuary-associated syndrome—six states, 1998–1999. *MMWR, (Morbidity and Mortality Weekly Report),* vol. 49, no. 17, May 5, 2000, pp. 372–374, available at http://www.cdc.gov/mmwr /preview/mmwrhtml/mm4917a4.htm.

12. Smith KE, Besser JM, Hedberg CW, et al., Quinolone-resistant *Campylobachter jejuni* infections in Minnesota, 1992–1998. *New England Journal of Medicine,* vol. 340, no. 20, 1999, pp. 1525–1532; Marwick C, Animal feed antibiotic use raises drug resistance fear. *Journal of American Medical Association,* vol. 282, no. 2, 1999, pp. 120–122; Donohoe MT, Factory farms as primary polluter. *Z Magazine,* January 2003, pp. 28–30, available at http://zcommunications.org/zmag /viewArticle/13737.

13. Chadwick DH, Coral in peril. *National Geographic,* January 1999, pp. 31–37; Nash JM, Wrecking the reefs. *Time,* September 30, 1996, pp. 60–61.

14. Kay JH, Car sick country. *Sierra,* July/August 1999, pp. 42–43, 77; Mark J. Cool moves. *Nucleus,* Fall 1997, p. 4.

15. Miller KA, Siscovick DS, Sheppard L, Sheperd K, Sullivan JH, Anderson GL, Kaufman JD, Long-term exposure to air pollution and incidence of cardiovascular events in women. *New England Journal of Medicine,* vol. 356, 2007, pp. 447–458; Dockery DW, Stone PH, Cardiovascular risks from fine particulate air pollution. *New England Journal of Medicine,* vol. 356, 2007, pp. 511–513; Bobak M, Leon DA, Air pollution and infant mortality in the Czech Republic, 1986–1988. *The Lancet,* vol. 340, 1992, pp. 1010–1014; Ponka A, Virtanen M, Low-level air pollution and hospital admissions for cardiac and cerebrovascular diseases in Helsinki. *American Journal of Public Health,* vol. 86, no. 9, 1996, pp. 1273–1280; Morgan G, Corbett S, Wlodarczyk J, Air pollution and hospital admissions in Sydney, Australia, 1990–1994. *American Journal of Public Health,* vol. 88, no. 12, 1998, pp. 1761–1766; Morris RD, Naumara EN, Muasmghe RL, Ambient air pollution and hospitalization for congestive heart failure among elderly people in seven large US cities. *American Journal of Public Health,* vol. 85, no. 10, pp. 1361–1365; Dockery DW, Pope CA, Xu X, et al., An association between air

pollution and mortality in six US cities. *New England Journal of Medicine*, vol. 329, no. 24, pp. 1753–1759.

16. Dockery, et al., An association between air pollution and mortality; Donohoe MT, Global warming: A public health crisis demanding immediate action. *World Affairs Journal*, vol. 11, no. 2, 2007, pp. 44–58 (adapted from Donohoe MT, Global warming: A public health crisis demanding immediate action [part I], *Medscape Public Health and Prevention*, 2007, available at http://www.medscape.com /viewarticle/548985 [posted January 12, 2007] and Donohoe MT, Global warming: A public health crisis demanding immediate action [part II], *Medscape Public Health and Prevention*, 2007, available at http://www.medscape.com /viewarticle/549292 [posted January 16, 2007]).

17. Donohoe MT, Global warming: A public health crisis; Nash JM, The fury of El Nino. *Time*, February 16, 1998, pp. 67–73, available at http://www.time.com /time/magazine/article/0,9171,987825,00.html.

18. Shapiro RL, The effects of tropical deforestation on human health. *The PSR Quarterly*, vol. 3, no. 3, September 1993, pp. 126–135.

19. Quammen D, Planet of weeds: Tallying the losses of earth's animals and plants. *Harper's Magazine*, October 1998, pp. 57–68, available at http://www.harpers .org/archive/1998/10/0059715.

20. Wilson EO, Vanishing before our eyes. *Time*, April 26, 2000, pp. 29–34, available at http://www.time.com/time/magazine/article/0,9171,996747,00.html; Tuxill J, Bright C, Losing strands in the web of life. In: Brown LR, Flavin C, French H, et al., *State of the world 1998*. Washington, DC: Worldwatch Institute Publications, 1998; Donohoe MT, Arthritis, shark cartilage, and the protection of threatened species [letter]. *Journal of American Medical Association*, vol. 284, no. 10, 2000, p. 1241.

21. Grifo F, Rosenthal J (eds.), *Biodiversity and human health*. Washington, DC: Island Press, 1997.

22. Amato I, Can we make garbage disappear? *Time*, November 8, 1999, available at http://www.time.com/time/magazine/article/0,9171,992527,00.html; Gavzer B, Take out the trash, and put it … where? *Parade Magazine*, June 13, 1999, pp. 4–6.

23. Lemonick MD, Little hope, less help. *Time*, July 24, 2000, pp. 38–39, available at http://www.time.com/time/magazine/article/0,9171,997525,00.html.

24. Patz A, Epstein PR, Burke TA, Bulbus JM, Global climate change and emerging infectious disease. *Journal of the American Medical Association*, vol. 274, no. 3, 1996, pp. 217–223.

25. Hansen E, Donohoe MT, Health issues of migrant and seasonal farm workers. *Journal of Health Care for the Poor and Underserved*, vol. 14, no. 2, 2003, pp. 153–164; Mellon M, Rissler J, McCamant F, Sustainable agriculture. Briefing paper, *Union of Concerned Scientists*, May 1995.

26. Hattam J, Get the lead out. *Sierra*, April/May 1998, pp. 21–25; Kittman JL, The secret history of lead. *The Nation*, March 20, 2000, pp. 11–44.

27. Environmental Working Group, An analysis of pollution prevention in America's top hospitals, available at http://www.ewg.org/reports/greening; Natural Resources Defense Council, Rx for toxic trouble. *The Amicus Journal*, vol. 20, no. 1, Spring 1998, p. 47.

28. Donohoe, Causes and health consequences of environmental degradation.

29. Pappas G, Queen S, Hadden W, et al., The increasing disparity in mortality between socioeconomic groups in the United States, 1960 and 1986. *New England Journal of Medicine*, vol. 329, 1993, pp. 103–109; Lantz PM, House JS, Lepkowsky JM, et al., Socioeconomic factors, health behaviours, and mortality. *Journal of the American Medical Association*, vol. 279, 1998, pp. 1703–1708; Adler NE, Boyce T, Chesney MA, Socioeconomic inequalities in health: No easy solution. *Journal of the American Medical Association*, vol. 269, 1993, pp. 3140–3145.

30. Oregon Public Broadcasting and KCTS/Seattle, *Affluenza*. Public Broadcasting System (PBS), televised September 20, 1997; Weissman R, Molchiber R, A moment of silence. *Focus on the Corporation*, May 4, 1999, pp. 1–3; Starfield B, Is US health really the best in the world? *Journal of the American Medical Association*, vol. 284, no. 4, 2000, pp. 483–485; Passaro V, Who'll stop the drain? *Harper's Magazine*, August 1998, pp. 35–42, available at http://www.harpers.org/archive/1998/08/0059656.

31. Starfield B, Is US health really the best in the world?

32. Montague P, Taking a giant stop. *Center for Health, Environment and Justice Newsletter*, Winter 1997, pp. 8–9.

33. Bartlett DL, Steele JB, Corporate welfare. *Time*, November 9, 1998, pp. 36–79; Johnston DC, Corporations' taxes are falling even as individuals' burden rises. *New York Times*, February 20, 2000, available at http://query.nytimes.com/gst/fullpage.html?res=9C01E4DC1730F933A15751C0A9669C8B63&sec=&spon=&&scp=2&sq=Johnston%20Corporations%92%20taxes%20&st=cse.

34. Chernoff PA, Sentencing environmental offenders. *The PSR Quarterly*, vol. 3, 1993, pp. 183–186.

35. Soley L, *Censorship Inc.: The corporate threat to free speech in the United States*. New York: Monthly Review Press, 2002.

36. Beder S, *Global Spin: The corporate assault on environmentalism*. White River Junction, VT: Green Books & Chelsea Publishing Company, 1997; Nader R, Smith WJ, *No contest: Corporate lawyers and the perversion of justice in America*. New York: Random House, 1996.

37. Chirac P, Von Schoen-Angerer T, Kaper T, Ford N, AIDS: Patent rights versus patient's rights. *The Lancet*, vol. 356, 2000, p. 502.

38. Lappe M, Bailey B, *Against the grain: Biotechnology and the corporate takeover of your food*, Monroe, ME: Common Courage Press, 1998; Nash JM, Grains of hope. *Time*, July 31, 2000, pp. 39–45; Donohoe MT, Genetically modified foods: Health and environmental risks and the corporate agribusiness agenda. *Z Magazine*, December 2006, pp. 35–40; Donohoe MT, Measure 27—labelling law for

genetically engineered foods: A call for openness and food safety. *The Oregonian,* October 28, 2002, web publication, see www.oregonlive.com/opinion.

39. Ramo JC, The real agenda of debt relief. *Time,* July 24, 2000, p. 40; Pooley E, The IMF: Dr. death? *Time,* April 24, 2000, available at http://www.time.com/time /magazine/article/0,9171,996693-1,00.html; Ellsworth GA, Cassel CK, International arms trade: A barrier to democracy and to public health. *PSR Quarterly,* vol. 2, 1992, pp. 223–228; Lack of donations hurting the world's poorest countries. *The Nation's Health,* October 2000, p. 14; Loewen JW, *Lies my teacher told me: Everything your American history textbook got wrong.* New York: Touchstone/Simon & Schuster, 1995.

40. Garfield RM, Neuget AI, Epidemiologic analysis of warfare: A historical review. *Journal of the American Medical Association,* vol. 266, 1991, pp. 688–692; Orient JM, Chemical and biological warfare: Should defenses be researched and deployed? *Journal of the American Medical Association,* vol. 262, pp. 644, 648; Sidel VW, Shahi GS, The impact of military activities on development, environment, and health. In: Shahi G, Levy B, Binger A, Kjellstrom T, Lawrence R (eds.), *International perspectives on environment, development, and health: Toward a sustainable world.* New York: Springer Publishing Company, 1997, pp. 283–312; Thomas W, *Scorched earth: The military's assault on the environment.* Philadelphia: New Society Publishers, 1995; Sidel VW, Farewell to arms: The impact of the arms race on the human condition. *PSR Quarterly,* vol. 3, 1993, pp. 18–26; Toole MJ, Waldman RJ, Refugees and displaced persons: War, hunger, and public health. *Journal of the American Medical Association,* vol. 270, 1993, pp. 600–605; Ris HW, Effects of the arms race on health and human services. *Journal of Adolescent Health Care,* vol. 9, 1988, pp. 235–240.

41. Forrow L, Blair BG, Helfand I, et al., Accidental nuclear war—a post-cold war assessment. *New England Journal of Medicine,* vol. 338, 1998, pp.1326–1331; Forrow L, Sidel VW, Medicine and nuclear war: From Hiroshima to mutual assured destruction to abolition 2000. *Journal of the American Medical Association,* vol. 280, no. 5, 1998, pp. 456–461.

42. Donohoe, Atomic anniversary is sobering one.

43. Eisenhower DD, *The chance for peace.* Address delivered before the American Society of Newspaper Editors, Washington, DC, April 16, 1953, Public Papers of the President of the United States, Dwight David Eisenhower, 1953, p. 182. http://www.informationclearinghouse.info/article9743.htm.

44. Heise LL, Raikes A, Watts CH, Zwi AB Violence against women: A neglected public health issue in less developed countries. *Social Science and Medicine,* vol. 39, 1994, pp. 1165–1179; Donohoe MT, Individual and societal forms of violence against women in the United States and the developing world: An overview. *Current Women's Health Reports,* vol. 2, no. 5, 2002, pp. 313–319; Donohoe MT, Teen pregnancy: A call for sound science and public policy. In: Frick L (ed.), *Current controversies in teen pregnancy and parenting.* Farmington Hills, MI: Greenhaven Press/Thomson Gale, 2006 (reprinted from Donohoe MT, Teen pregnancy: A call for sound science and public policy. *Z Magazine,* April 2003, pp. 14–16, available

at http://www.zmag.org/zmag/viewArticle/13738); Donohoe MT, Violence against women: Epidemiology, recognition, and management of partner abuse and sexual assault. *Hospital Physician,* vol. 40, no. 10, 2004, pp. 24–31; Donohoe MT, Violence and human rights abuses against women in the developing world. *Medscape Ob/Gyn and Women's Health,* vol. 8, no. 2, 2003, available at http://www.medscape.com/viewarticle/464255 [posted November 26, 2003]; Donohoe MT, Increase in obstacles to abortion: The American perspective in 2004. *Journal of American Medical Women's Association,* vol. 60, no. 1, 2005, pp. 16–25, available at http://amwa-doc.org/index.cfm?objectid=1B138032-D567-0B25 -57EE86AC69902184; Donohoe MT, Obstacles to abortion in the United States. *Medscape Ob/Gyn and Women's Health,* vol. 10, no. 2, 2005, available at http://www.medscape.com/viewarticle/507404 [posted July 7, 2005]; Donohoe MT, Female genital cutting: Epidemiology, consequences, and female empowerment as a means of cultural change, *Medscape Ob/Gyn and Women's Health,* vol. 11, no. 2, 2006, available at http://www.medscape.com/viewarticle /546497 [posted November 6, 2006]; Adams KE, Donohoe MT, Reproductive rights—commentary: Provider willingness to prescribe emergency contraception. *Virtual Mentor: American Medical Association Journal of Ethics,* vol. 6, no. 9 September 2004, available at http://virtualmentor.ama-assn.org/2004/09/ccas2 -0409.html; Donohoe MT, Parental notification and consent laws for teen abortions: Overview and 2006 ballot measures. *Medscape Ob/Gyn and Women's Health,* 2007, available at http://www.medscape.com/viewarticle/549316 [posted February 9, 2007; accessed November 17, 2008]; Donohoe MT, Violence against women in the military. *Medscape Ob/Gyn and Women's Health,* vol. 10, no. 2, 2005, available at http://www.medscape.com/viewarticle/512380 [posted September 13, 2005].

45. Women's health, earth's health. *Sierra,* November/December 2000, p. 74.

46. Mackillop WJ, Zhang-Salomons J, Boyd CJ, Groome PA, Associations between community income and cancer incidence in Canada and the United States. *Cancer,* vol. 89, no. 4, 2000, pp. 901–912.

47. Donohoe MT, Factory farms, antibiotics, and anthrax. *Z Magazine,* January 2003, pp. 28–30, available at http://zcommunications.org/zmag/viewArticle/13737; McCally M, Donohoe MT, Dangers of food irradiation. *New England Journal of Medicine,* vol. 351, no. 4, 2004, pp. 402–403.

48. Quammen D, Planet of weeds: Tallying the losses of earth's animals and plants. *Harper's Magazine,* October 1998, pp. 57–68, available at http://www.harpers .org/archive/1998/10/0059715; Faces of environmentalism. *Sierra,* November/ December 1997, p. 27, available at http://www.sierraclub.org/sierra/199709 /lol.asp#face; Heal G, *Nature and the marketplace: Capturing the value of ecosystem services.* Washington, DC: Island Press, 2000.

49. Asmus P, Getting religion. *The Amicus Journal,* vol. 22, no. 3, 2000, pp. 32–33.

50. Wong Y, Impotence and intransigence: State behavior in the throes of deepening global crisis. *Politics and Life Sciences,* vol. 13, no. 1, 1994, pp. 3–14.

51. See references in note 45 as well as *Women and the environment in developing countries.* Union of Concerned Scientists position paper. Available at http://eric .ed.gov/ERICWebPortal/custom/portlets/recordDetails/detailmini.jsp?_nfpb= true&_&ERICExtSearch_SearchValue_0=ED388459&ERICExtSearch_SearchType _0=no&accno=ED388459; Briggs N, Illiteracy and maternal health: Educate or die. *The Lancet,* vol. 341, 1993, pp. 1063–1064.

52. Rose S, Responsible investing. Is it living up to its promise? *Sierra,* November/ December 2000, pp. 26, 28, 93, available at http://www.sierraclub.org/sierra /200011/hearth.asp.

53. Donohoe MT, Arthritis, shark cartilage, and the protection of threatened species' [letter]. *Journal of American Medical Association,* vol. 284, no. 10, 2000, p. 1241; Speer L, Feeding frenzy. *The Amicus Journal,* Spring 2000, p. 47, available at http://www.accessmylibrary.com/coms2/summary_0286-9344589_ITM.

54. Donohoe MT, Flowers, diamonds, and gold: The destructive human rights and environmental consequences of symbols of love. *Human Rights Quarterly,* vol. 30, 2008, pp. 164–182.

55. Asmus, Getting religion; Nogee A, Buy green power. *Nucleus,* Spring, 1998, p. 4; Clemmer S, State of play. *Nucleus,* Spring 1998, p. 2.

56. Donohoe, Causes and health consequences of environmental degradation.

57. Donohoe MT, Advice for young investigators: Historical perspectives on scientific research. *Advances Health Sciences Education,* vol. 8, no. 2, 2003, pp. 167–171.

58. Nuland SB, *Doctors: The biography of medicine.* New York: Vintage Books, 1988, p. 316.

59. Nuland, *Doctors: The biography of medicine,* p. 316.

60. Eisenberg L, Rudolph Virchow: The physician as politician. *Medicine and War,* no. 2, 1986, pp. 243–250.

61. Virchow R, *Collected essays on public health and epidemiology,* vol. 1. Canton, MA: Science History Publications, 1985.

62. Nuland, *Doctors: The biography of medicine,* p. 316.

63. Nuland, *Doctors: The biography of medicine,* p. 316.

64. Nuland, *Doctors: The biography of medicine,* p. 316.

65. Donohoe MT, Luxury primary care, academic medical centers, and the erosion of science and professional ethics. *Journal of General Internal Medicine,* vol. 19, 2004, pp. 90–94.

66. Donohoe MT, SGIM and the media [letter]. *Journal of General Internal Medicine,* vol. 10, 1995, p. 532.

67. The Nightingale Institute for Health and the Environment, *Eleven recommendations for improving medical waste management.* Burlington, VT, December 1997, available at http://www.nihe.org/elevreng.html; Tieszen ME, Gruenberg JC, A quantitative, qualitative, and critical assessment of surgical waste. *Journal of the American Medical Association,* vol. 267, 1992,

pp. 2765–2768; Rosenblatt WH, Ariyan C, Silverman DG, Case-by-case assessment of recoverable materials for overseas donation from 1318 surgical procedures. *Journal of the American Medical Association*, vol. 269, 1993, pp. 2647–2649.

68. Donohoe MT, Matthews H, Wasted paper in pharmaceutical samples. *New England Journal of Medicine*, vol. 340, no. 20, 1999, p. 1600. In a model program at the University of Nebraska, Doctors Andrew Jameton and Jessica Pierce have developed the Green Health Center which provides high quality health care consistent with ecological sustainability and fairness, see Jameton A, Pierce J, The Green Health Center, www.unmc.edu/green/; Pierce J, Jameton A, *The ethics of environmentally responsible health care.* New York: Oxford University Press, 2004.

69. Magnus SA, Mick SS, Medical schools, affirmative action, and the neglected role of social class. *American Journal of Public Health*, vol. 90, no. 8, 2000, pp. 1197–1201.

70. UN Environment Programme, *Global environmental outlook.* Nairobi: UNEP, 2000.

71. Beauchamp DE, Public health as social justice. *Inquiry*, vol. 13, March, 1976, pp. 3–41.

72. McCrary SV, Anderson CB, Jakovljevic J, et al., A national survey of policies on disclosure of conflicts of interest in biomedical research. *New England Journal of Medicine*, vol. 343, no. 22, 2000, pp. 1621–1626; Donohoe MT, Health services research and industry [letter]. *Journal of the American Medical Association*, vol. 278, 1997, pp. 896–897.

73. Beder, *Global spin.*

74. Lapham LH, Notebook: School bells. *Harper's Magazine*, August 2000, pp. 7–9, available at http://www.harpers.org/archive/2000/08/0066885; Sagan C, *The demon-haunted world: Science as a candle in the dark.* New York: Random House, 1996; Selcraig B, Mining. *Sierra*, May/June 1998, pp. 60–65, 86, 89–91; Baxandall P, Rosengarten D, Put up or shut up. *Dollars and Sense*, September/October 2000, p. 4; Edwards TM, What Johnny can't read. *Time*, December 1998, p. 46.

75. Himmelstein DU, Woolhandler S, Boyd JW, Investment of health insurers and mutual funds in tobacco stocks. *Journal of the American Medical Association*, vol. 284, no. 6, 2000, p. 697.

76. Donohoe MT, Cigarettes: The other weapons of mass destruction. *Medscape Ob/Gyn and Women's Health*, vol. 10, no. 1, 2005, available at http://www.medscape.com/viewarticle/501586 [posted April 5, 2005]; Donohoe MT, US attempts to scuttle World Health Organization's international tobacco treaty. *The Oregonian*, February 14, 2003, web publication, see www.oregonlive.com/opinion.

77. Lamont-Gregory, Henry CJ, Ryan TJ, Evidence-based humanitarian relief interventions. *The Lancet*, vol. 346, 1995, pp. 312–313.

78. Donohoe MT, Internists, epidemics, outbreaks, and bioterrorist attacks. *Journal of General Internal Medicine* vol. 22, no. 9, 2007, p. 1380, available at http://www.springerlink.com/content/v2r74824uv349208/fulltext.pdf; Donohoe MT, Bioterrorism curricula too limited. *Academic Medicine*, April 14, 2004; Donohoe

MT, Prevention of the acute radiation emergencies. *Annals of Internal Medicine,* July 6, 2004, available at http://www.annals.org/cgi/eletters/140/12/1037#180.

79. Faulkner LR, McCurdy RL, Teaching medical students social responsibility: The right thing to do. *Academic Medicine,* vol. 75, 2000, pp. 346–350; Donohoe MT, Exploring the human condition: Literature and public health issues. In: Hawkins AH, McEntyre MC (eds.), *Teaching literature and medicine.* New York: Modern Language Association, 2000; Donohoe MT, Danielson S, A community-based approach to the medical humanities. *Medical Education,* vol. 38, no. 2, 2004, pp. 204–217; Donohoe MT, Literature and social injustice: Stories of the disenfranchised. *Medscape Ob/Gyn and Women's Health,* vol. 10, no. 1, 2005, available at http://www.medscape.com/viewarticle/496358 [posted January 7, 2005].

80. DuBois JM, Burkemper J, Ethics education in US medical schools: A study of syllabi. *Academic Medicine,* vol. 77, no. 5, 2002, pp. 432–437.

81. Sonis J, Gorenflo DW, Jha P, Williams C, Teaching of human rights in US medical schools. *Journal of the American Medical Association,* vol. 276, no. 20, 1996, pp. 1676–1678.

82. American College of Physicians, The role of the physician and the medical profession in the prevention of international torture and in the treatment of its survivors. *Annals of Internal Medicine,* vol. 122, no. 8, 1995, pp. 607–613.

83. Willis BM, Levy BS, Recognizing the public health impact of genocide. *Journal of the American Medical Association,* vol. 284, no. 5, 2000, pp. 612–614.

84. See references in note 79 as well as, McCally M, Cassel CK, Norgrove L, Medical education and nuclear war. *The Lancet,* vol. 2, 1988, pp. 834–837; McCally M, Diensbier Z, Jansen A, et al., An international survey of medical school programmes on nuclear war. *Medical Education,* vol. 19, 1985, pp. 364–367; Winder AE, Stanitis MA, Nuclear education in public health and nursing. *American Journal of Public Health,* vol. 78, no. 8, 1988, pp. 967–968.

85. Kumar S, India: The second Bhopal tragedy. *The Lancet,* vol. 341, 1993, pp. 1205–1206.

86. Stone R, The long shadow of Chernobyl. *National Geographic,* April 2006, available at http://www7.nationalgeographic.com/ngm/0604/feature1/.

87. Natural Resources Defense Council Staff, Exxon Valdez, ten years later. *The Amicus Journal,* Summer 1999, p. 10.

88. Powell PP, Minamata disease: A story of mercury's malevolence. *Southern Medical Journal,* vol. 84, no. 11, 1991, pp. 1352–1358.

89. Papich B, A heady adventure (Easter Island). *Los Angeles Times,* October 24, 1999, pp. L1, L11–L13.

90. Orwell G, How the poor die. In: Orwell S, Angus I (eds.), *The collected essays, journalism and letters of George Orwell.* Harmondsworth, UK: Penguin, 1970, also available at http://www.orwell.ru/library/articles/Poor_Die/english/e_pdie.

91. Chekhov A, *Ward no. 6 and other stories, 1892–1895*, translated by Wilks R. London: Penguin, 2002.

92. Sinclair U, *The jungle*. New York: Signet/Penguin, 1990.

93. Ibsen H, An enemy of the people. In: Ibsen H, *Four great plays by Henrik Ibsen*, translated by Farquharson Sharp R. New York: Bantam, 1959.

94. Williams WC, The paid nurse. In: Williams WC, *The doctor stories*, New York: New Directions, 1984.

95. Donohoe MT, William Carlos Williams, MD: Lessons for physicians from his life and writings. *The Pharos*, Winter, 2004, pp. 12–17, available at http://www .alphaomegaalpha.org/PDFs/Pharos/Articles/2004Winter/Donohoe.htm.

96. Gaines EJ, The sky is gray. In: Secundy MG (ed.), *Trials, tribulations, and celebrations: African-American perspectives on health, illness, aging, and loss.* Yarmouth, ME: Inter-cultural, 1992.

97. Lessing D, An old woman and her cat. In: *The Doris Lessing reader.* New York: A Knopf, 1988.

98. Useful selections for sessions relating to war include the posthumously published poem by Mark Twain, *The war prayer.* New York: Harper and Row, 1970; Dalton Trumbo, *Johnny got his gun.* New York: Bantam, 1939; the apocalyptic science fiction classic by Walter Miller, *A canticle for Leibowitz.* Philadelphia: Lippincott, 1960; the collection of poems edited by Michael Harrison and Christopher Stewart-Clark (eds.), *Peace and war.* Oxford, UK: Oxford University Press, 1989. Works on the Holocaust by Premo Levi, *Survival in Auschwitz.* New York: Touchstone, 1958, also by Elie Weisel, *Night.* New York: Bantam, 1982; poems by Wilfred Owen, *War poems and others*, ed. by Hibberd D. Sydney: Random House Australia, 1986; for a powerful description of the experience of torture see, Jacobo Timmerman, *Prisoner without a name, cell without a number.* New York: Knopf, 1981.

99. Donohoe and Danielson, A community-based approach to the medical humanities.

100. Public Citizen's Health Research Group. *Activist-oriented research course initiative,* available at http://www.citizen.org/hrg/activistcour/index.cfm.

101. Quote from Richard Lawson, president of the National Mining Association. *The Amicus Journal,* Spring 2000, p. 7.

102. Quote by Ralph Waldo Emerson in Safransky S, *Sunbeams: A book of quotations.* Berkeley, CA: North Atlantic Books, 1990, see http://www.yourdictionary.com/civilization.

103. Quote by George Bernard Shaw, as cited in the *Journal of the American Medical Association*, vol. 284, no. 4, 2000, p. 4.

104. Niemoller P, First they came for the Jews. In: McKosker K, Alberry N (eds.), *A poem a day.* South Royalton, VT: Steerforth Press, 1996, p. 15.

105. Loeb PR, *Soul of a citizen: Living with conviction in a cynical time.* New York: St Martin's Griffin, 1999.

106. Abrams I (ed.), *The words of peace: Selections from the speeches of the winners of the Nobel Peace Prize.* New York: Newmarket Press, 1990.

107. Abrams, *The words of peace.*

108. Abrams, *The words of peace.*

109. Abrams, *The words of peace.*

110. Benatar SR, Daar A, Singer PA, Global health ethics: The rationale for mutual caring. *International Affairs,* vol. 79, 2003, pp. 107–138.

Chapter 23

Global Warming

A Public Health Crisis Demanding Immediate Action

Martin Donohoe

Causes of Global Warming

Climate Change and the Greenhouse Effect

While cooling and heating shifts in the Earth's climate occur with somewhat predicable frequency on geological time scales, it is now accepted that we are in the midst of a dramatic and rapid warming of the planet, consequent to the combustion of fossil fuels (Report of the Intergovernmental Panel on Climate Change, 2007, available at http://www.ipcc.ch; Gore, A, *An Inconvenient Truth*, New York: Rodale/Melcher Media, 2006; Donohoe, MT, "Causes and Health Consequences of Environmental Degradation and Social Injustice," *Social Science and Medicine*, Vol. 56[3], 2003; and Donohoe, MT, "Roles and Responsibilities of Health Professionals in Confronting the Health Consequences of Environmental Degradation and Social Injustice: Education and Activism. Monash Bioethics Review, 2008;27 (Nos. 1 and 2):65-82).

This warming, which began with the advent of industrialization in the late nineteenth and early twentieth centuries, has accelerated over the last few decades and bodes ill for the Earth's ecosystems and for human health.

The planetary temperature has increased one degree Celsius over the last century, a number that might seem small yet has dramatic consequences (Report of the Stern Commission on Climate Change, United Kingdom, available at http://www.cfr.org/uk/stern-commission-uk-global-warming/p12017. The last 24 years have been the hottest in the last century and a half and 2006 was the hottest year since record keeping began in 1856. If no action is taken to reduce carbon emissions, the concentration of atmospheric greenhouse gasses could reach double its pre-industrial level within the next 30 years, leading to a temperature rise of at least 2°C (ibid). Estimates from the International Panel on Climate Change place the rise as high as 10°C over the next century (Intergovernmental Panel Report, ibid).

The greenhouse effect refers to the tendency of carbon dioxide, methane, nitrous oxide, sulphur compounds and chlorofluorocarbons to trap that portion of the sun's heat energy, which is reflected off the Earth (Staff–Union of Concerned Scientists [UCS], "Frequently Asked Questions [FAQs] about Global Warming," available at http://www.ucsusa.org). Without the greenhouse effect, the Earth's average surface temperature would be -18°C instead of 15°C and our frozen planet could not sustain human life (Staff–UCS, FAQs, ibid). The presence of the major greenhouse gasses is a consequence of both natural processes like cellular respiration and manmade technologies like the burning of fossil fuels and methane production from agricultural activities like growing rice and raising cattle (Staff–UCS, FAQs, ibid).

Industrialization and Automobiles

Since pre-industrial times, the atmospheric concentration of carbon dioxide has increased 31 percent (Gore, ibid). The major cause of increased greenhouse gas production is the burning of fossil fuels such as coal, oil and natural gas. Transportation, electricity generation and heating and cooling for industrial processes contribute almost equally (Staff–UCS, FAQs, ibid).

Industrialization and the accelerating worldwide demand for fuel-inefficient automobiles have polluted our air and hastened global warming and the destruction of the protective ozone layer. Large industrialized countries are the greatest contributors to global warming. The top one-fifth of the world's nations account for over 60 percent of global CO_2 emissions, while the lowest one-fifth, just 2 percent (Staff–UCS, FAQs, ibid). While the United States contains just 5 percent of the world's population, it is responsible for 25 percent of the world's energy consumption, 33 percent of its paper use and 72 percent of all hazardous waste production (Donohoe, MT, "Causes and Health Consequences of Environmental Degradation and Social Injustice," ibid). On the other hand, the countries likely to be most affected by global warming are those least responsible for the increases in global temperature, primarily the developing nations of the southern hemisphere.

To focus on automobiles—for every gallon of gasoline manufactured, distributed and then burned in a vehicle, 25 pounds of carbon dioxide are produced (Alexander, GJ and Kanner, RE, "Air Pollution: From Irritating to Life-Threatening," IM—Internal Medicine, October 1995). In the US there is one car for every two people, in Mexico one for every eight and in China one for every 100. The global automobile population is expected to double in the next 25 to 50 years and the number of miles driven per person will grow as urban sprawl leads to longer commute distances (Mark, J and Morey, C, "Rolling Smokestacks," *Nucleus* [Union of Concerned Scientists], Summer 2000 and Staff, "Driving Ourselves Crazy," *Amicus Journal*, Summer 1999). US fuel economy standards have changed very little since the Model T, in large part due to lobbying by automobile manufacturers and the oil industry (Donohoe, MT, ibid).

The Military, Oil, and Global Warming

The world's militaries are the planet's single largest polluter, responsible for 8 percent of global air pollution and 6 percent of raw materials use (Sidel, VW and Shahi, GS, "The Impact of Military Activities on Development, Environment and Health," in Shahi, GS, Levy, BS, Binger, A, Kjeustrom, T and Lawrence, R (Eds.), *International Perspectives on Environment, Development and Health: Toward A Sustainable World*, New York: Springer Publishing Company, 1997). Even prior to the current wars in Iraq and Afghanistan, the US Defense Department was the world's largest consumer of oil and the Pentagon generated half a billion tons of toxic waste per year, more than the five top chemical companies combined (Thomas, W, *Scorched Earth: The Military's Assault on the Environment*, Philadelphia: New Society Publishers, 1995). Ironically, the Pentagon has deemed global warming a "vastly greater threat than terrorism" with enormous consequences for US national security and the potential to cause global anarchy (Townsend, M and Harris, P, "Now the Pentagon Tells Bush: Climate Change Will Destroy Us," *The Guardian*, February 22, 2004, available at http://observer.guardian.co.uk). Oil production fuels civil and international armed conflicts and is associated with human rights abuses in Nigeria, Myanmar and elsewhere. Such violence in turn exacerbates world hunger and increases infant mortality, as financial and scientific resources are diverted toward militarism and away from the amelioration of poverty.

Deforestation

Deforestation, spurred by overpopulation, poverty, unsustainable farming practices and rapacious logging to satisfy an increasing demand for paper products, has in turn augmented global warming, degraded soil quality and contributed heavily to species loss (Intergovernmental Panel Report, ibid; Gore, ibid; and Donohoe, M T, ibid). Deforestation destroys the plant life, which serves as the planet's carbon dioxide sink. Half of all tropical forests have been destroyed; by 2010, three-quarters may be lost (Donohoe, MT, ibid). In addition, 20 to

50 percent of global wetlands have been destroyed (Donohoe, MT, ibid). The areas most affected by deforestation are the Amazon, Sub-Saharan Africa, the Philippines and most recently the Pacific Northwest and British Columbia (the "Amazon of the North"). The factors that lead to deforestation are the need for new agricultural settlements, spurred by overpopulation, poverty and unsustainable farming practices; urban sprawl; logging for building materials and paper; cattle ranching and drug cultivation in countries like Peru, Bolivia and Columbia (Donohoe, MT, ibid). With deforestation and global warming come shifts in the ranges and behaviors of plant and animal species. One example is the increase in the range of mosquitoes, which carry malaria to higher elevations, contributing to a rise in the prevalence of this deadly killer disease.

Combustion for Cooking and Heating

Another important contributor to global warming and pollution is the combustion, by almost three billion people worldwide, of coal and biomass (wood, charcoal, crop residues and animal dung) for cooking, heating and food preservation (Ezzati, M and Kammen, D, "The Health Impacts of Exposure to Indoor Air Pollution from Solid Fuels in Developing Countries: Knowledge, Gaps and Data Needs," *Environmental Health Perspectives*, Vol.110 [11], 2002). Health consequences of released pollutants are magnified when such combustion is carried out in enclosed spaces, which is common.

Consequences of Global Warming

Melting and Flooding

There are many actual and potential adverse effects of global warming. Its consequences include the melting of polar icecaps and glaciers and the rise of global sea levels (Intergovernmental Panel Report, ibid; Gore, ibid; Stern Commission Report, ibid; Staff–UCS, FAQs, ibid). Over the next 100 years, sea levels are predicted to rise between 9 and 88 centimeters, which is likely to result in greater coastal erosion, flooding during storms and may inundate Male (the capital of the Maldives) and South Pacific islands like Tuvalu and Vanuatu. Low-lying countries like Bangladesh will be threatened and aquifers in New Orleans and San Francisco may be destroyed. Large portions of the Antarctic ice shelf have caved into the sea and the Greenland ice sheet is rapidly receding. With less ice to reflect sunlight, the Earth absorbs more heat, which accelerates melting. If the layer of permafrost covering the Siberian tundra continues to melt, huge amounts of carbon dioxide could be released, further accelerating global warming.

Extreme Weather Events

Global warming augments the effects of extreme weather patterns, including El Niño and La Niña, and may have contributed to the recent dramatic increase in severe hurricanes and costly flood damage in the US (Intergovernmental Panel Report, ibid; Gore, ibid; Stern Commission Report, ibid; and Staff–UCS, FAQs, ibid). Due to the added effects of global warming, overpopulation and water pollution, we are running out of fresh water, a resource over which future wars will likely be fought (Leslie, J, "Running Dry—What Happens When the World No Longer has Enough Freshwater?" *Harper's Magazine*, July 2000).

Air Pollution and Ramifications for Human Health

Numerous studies have documented the links between global warming, greenhouse gasses, air pollution, ozone depletion and acute and chronic health problems. Greenhouse gasses are major contributors to air pollution, whose levels have been strongly linked to morbidity and mortality from cardiopulmonary and cerebrovascular diseases, lung cancer and infant mortality in the US (Samet, JM, Dominici, F, Curriero, FC, et al., "Fine Particulate Air Pollution and Mortality in 20 US Cities, 1987–1994," *New England Journal of Medicine*, Vol. 343[24], 2000; Dockery, DW, Pope, CA, Xu, X, et al., "An Association between Air Pollution and Mortality in Six US Cities," *New England Journal of Medicine*, Vol. 329[24], 1993; Ponka, A and Virtanen, M, "Low-Level Air Pollution and Hospital Admissions for Cardiac and Cerebrovascular Diseases in Helsinki," *American Journal of Public Health*, Vol. 86[9], 1996; and Bobak, M and Leon DA, "Air Pollution and Infant Mortality in the Czech Republic, 1986–88," *The Lancet*, Vol. 340, 1992). Rising temperatures increase smog and ground level ozone, increasing symptoms in those suffering from asthma and chronic obstructive pulmonary disease. Higher levels of carbon dioxide favor the growth of ragweed and other pollen-producing plants, which exacerbates allergies. Furthermore, due to the pollution-induced destruction of the ozone in the upper atmosphere (as well as cooling of the upper atmosphere, a consequence of more heat being trapped in the lower atmosphere), the ozone layer, which protects us from the sun's harmful ultraviolet radiation, is being depleted. This has led to an increase in cataracts, a consequence of ultraviolet-light induced damage to the eye's lens and a predicted increase in the lifetime risk of malignant melanoma, the most virulent form of skin cancer (Whited, JD and Grichnik, JM, "Does This Patient Have Melanoma?" *Journal of the American Medical Association*, Vol. 279[9], 1998). Finally, with higher temperatures come more heat waves, resulting in more deaths from hyperthermia, although deaths from hypothermia should drop. Scientists at the World Health Organization have estimated that about 160,000 people die each year from the side effects of global warming and that this number could double by 2020 (Staff, "Global Warming Deaths on the Rise," available at http://www.wired.com/medtech/health/news/2003/09/60640).

Corporations, the Media and Unsound Science

Corporate Attacks on Global Warming Science

Through lobbying, campaign contributions, control of a media which limits public debate on topics of environmental importance and in some cases human rights abuses, corporations, in their pursuit of greater profits, have fought to weaken environmental legislation designed to protect the public's health, such as industrial emissions and fuel economy standards (Donohoe, MT, ibid). The early twenty-first century has seen a tremendous increase in the influence of corporations on national policy, with a revolving door between industry, lobbying groups and governmental agencies responsible for safeguarding the environment and protecting public health (Donohoe, MT, ibid). Pre-eminent scientists have protested the current US administration's misuse of science, including classification of data and rewriting of important policy statements, to minimize health concerns (Union of Concerned Scientists, Scientific Integrity Project, available at http://www.ucsusa.org/scientific_integrity/).

Media Misinformation

Many corporations whose activities contribute to global warming and which stand to gain financially from the perpetuation of the status quo, hide behind "greenwash" public relations and advertising campaigns designed to present themselves as eco-friendly (Beder, S, *Global Spin: The Corporate Assault on Environmentalism*, White River Junction, VT: Green Books and Chelsea Green Publishing Company, 1997). They grant large amounts of money to the few "scientists" who dispute global warming. These "scientists" at the behest of their corporate benefactors, often communicate through front groups, such as the American Council on Science and Health (ACSH) and the Foundation for Clean Air Progress. Companies also lobby legislators through the creation of artificial "grassroots coalitions," which may only contain a few members, a phenomenon known as "astroturfing" (Donohoe, MT, ibid).

In 2005, the American Association of Petroleum Geologists gave its journalism award to author Michael Crichton, a physician whose book *State of Fear* (HarperCollins, 2004) questions the existence of human-caused global warming (American Association of Petroleum Geologists Explorer Awardees, available at http://www.aapg.org; Dean C. "Truth? Fiction? Journalism? Award Goes to ..." New York *Times* 2006 (Feb 9). Available at http://www.nytimes.com/2006/02/09/national/09prize.html. Crichton also received the 2005 "Sound Science Medal" from the ACSH. The ACSH, which grants this inappropriately named award, is one of the most visible, well-funded purveyors of pseudoscience and misinformation regarding the health risks of environmental degradation. The group has a history of strong ties to corporate polluters. Its president, Dr. Elizabeth Whelan, praised Crichton for confronting "the threat of pseudoscience ... in this case, the belief that careless human activity (the burning of fossil fuels) has made the world too dangerously warm, causing death-dealing weather changes and human misery" (Whelan, EM, "Novel Debunks Environ-Dogma," available at http://www.acsh.org/healthissues /newsID.1060/healthissue_detail.asp). ACSH has referred to those who describe the serious health and environmental consequences of global warming and who call for fossil fuel restrictions as "doomsayers" and "fearmongers" ("Public Health Panel Rips Draconian Measures Pushed by Global Warming Doomsayers," American Council on Science and Health Press Release, December 14, 1997). This year, Senator James Inhofe (R, Oklahoma) called "the threat of catastrophic global warming ... the greatest hoax ever perpetrated on the American people" (Mann, M, Rahmstorf, S, Schmidt, G, Steig, E and Connolley, W, "Senator Inhofe on Climate Change," available at http://www.realclimate.org /index.php/archives/2005/01/senator-inhofe/). Such anti-science declarations are an affront to respected climate scientists worldwide.

There is a dearth of environmental coverage in the media, in part a consequence of major news outlets being owned by corporations with extensive histories of environmental destruction (Donohoe, MT, ibid). For instance, General Electric (the nation's number one corporate polluter, responsible for more Superfund sites than any other company), owns NBC (Donohoe, MT, "GE—Bringing Bad Things to Life: Cradle to Grave Health Care and the Alliance between General Electric Medical Systems and New York Presbyterian Hospital," *Synthesis/Regeneration,* Fall 2006).

Whenever the mainstream media have covered global warming, until very recently, they have portrayed it as a scientific uncertainty. Of a sample of over 900 articles dealing with climate change and published in peer-reviewed, scientific journals between 1993 and 2003, none expressed doubt as to the existence or major cause of global warming (Oreskes, N, "The Scientific Consensus on Climate Change," *Science,* Vol. 306, 2004). On the other hand, an analysis of articles in the most influential American dailies (the *New York Times,* the *Washington Post,* the *LA Times* and the *Wall Street Journal*) over a similar period found that 53 percent expressed doubt as to the cause of global warming and many gave the impression that mainstream scientists still doubted the existence of global warming (Michaels, D and Monforton, C, "Manufacturing Uncertainty: Contested Science and the Protection of the Public's Health and Environment," *American Journal of Public Health,* Vol. 95, 2005). The manufacture of controversy, the repositioning of global warming as theory rather than fact by the public relations campaigns of a small but well-funded cadre of special interests in the fossil fuels industry, is reminiscent of the tobacco companies' campaign to create doubt about the role of cigarettes in causing diseases (Michaels and Monforton, ibid).

Sponsored Environmental Curricula

Many polluting companies capitalize on Americans' environmental ignorance, which is in part a byproduct of a public education system in disarray, particularly in poor and minority neighbourhoods, which suffer disproportionately due to under-funded school systems (Donohoe, MT, ibid). For example, a majority of Americans believe that electricity in the US is produced in non-polluting ways; only 25 percent are aware that the majority (70 percent) comes from oil, coal and wood (McManus, R, "Myth Buster: Popular Fiction," *Sierra* Magazine, May–June 1999, available at http://www.sierraclub.org).

To fill the void left by the absence of environmental education programmers, corporations have distributed free, sponsored environmental educational materials to public schools. These materials are produced and supported by a loose coalition of corporate polluters, lapdog "scientists," anti-regulatory zealots and misguided parents (Selcraig, B, "Reading, 'Riting and Ravaging," *Sierra* Magazine, May–June 1998). Examples include Exxon's "Energy Cube," which states, "gasoline is simply solar power hidden in decayed matter" and "offshore drilling creates reefs for fish." International papers proclaim, "Clear cutting promotes the growth of trees that require full sunlight and allows efficient site preparation for the next crop" (Donohoe, MT, ibid).

Confronting Global Warming

A multi-faceted approach to the problems of environmental degradation includes shifting from a throwaway economy to a re-use/recycle economy and reevaluating economic inputs and outputs by including the contributions of natural phenomena and processes to human health (Donohoe, MT, ibid). To reduce their contribution to global warming, private citizens can properly insulate their homes, use energy-efficient lighting, take public transportation and stop receiving catalogues and junk mail (Direct Marketing Association's Consumer Assistance, available at http://www.dmaconsumers.org) and purchase locally produced goods, including foodstuffs, to minimize the pollution associated with the transportation of such products from distant locations.

Governments and corporations can reduce global emissions by increasing energy efficiency standards, sharing technologies, encouraging the use of renewable energy sources, eliminating coal and oil subsidies and protecting forests. Some have advocated emissions trading, in which polluting companies "purchase" pollution credits from less-polluting companies, with the goal of decreasing overall industry-wide emissions. However, such trading offers less incentive to polluters to develop and adopt technological innovations to curb their individual contributions to global warming. Stronger clean air and water standards and the elimination of fossil fuel industry tax breaks and subsidies could save billions of dollars and thousands of lives each year. Tax breaks and subsidies for research and development of renewable energy should be increased and the tax system restructured to decrease levies on work and savings and increase levies on destructive activities, such as carbon emissions and toxic waste generation. Alternatives to electrical-coal-oil-nuclear and natural gas-based power include solar energy, wind turbines, geothermal power, tidal/wave power, hydropower and co-generation (harnessing waste heat), all of which would decrease air pollution and the risk of accidental or deliberate catastrophes (Donohoe, MT, ibid).

Alternatives to automobiles include electric cars and electric trolley systems; natural gas and/or gasohol (which generates less carbon dioxide than regular gasoline); solar cars; and hydrogen-powered cars, whose byproduct is water. Electric cars were marginalized and electric trolley systems dismantled, as was much of the existing public transportation and network, by a triumvirate of oil, chemical and tire companies in the early twentieth century. Their actions led to their convictions under the Sherman Anti-Trust Act (Donohoe, MT, ibid). Trains, which are fifteen times more energy-efficient per passenger than automobiles, should be utilized more. Unfortunately, federal funding for Amtrak, the American national rail system, has declined dramatically. Some individuals car-pool or car share, while millions of Americans telecommute, that is work from home. Telecommuting leads to decreased absenteeism, job turnover and need for office space, improved worker productivity and saves between six and twelve thousand dollars per worker per year (Erickson, K, "Home Work: The Green Routine of Telecommuting," *Sierra* Magazine, September–October 1998). Still others ride bicycles or walk to work.

Improvements in the status of women, including the strengthening of family planning programmers and improved/equal access to educational opportunities and legal and political representation will produce a more equitable world and are likely to decrease the demand for large families, which spurs overpopulation (Donohoe, MT, "Individual and Societal Forms of Violence Against Women in the United States and the Developing World: An Overview," *Current Women's Health Reports*, Vol. 2[5], 2002; Donohoe, MT, "Violence and Human Rights Abuses Against Women in the Developing World," *Medscape Ob/Gyn and Women's Health*, Vol. 8[2], 2003, available at http://www.medscape.com/viewarticle/464255). To help developing nations become self-sufficient, the World Bank and the International Monetary Fund need to alter their policies and promote the production of local food crops rather than crops destined for export to developed nations (Donohoe, MT, "Genetically Modified Foods: Health and Environmental Risks and the Corporate Agribusiness Agenda," *Z Magazine*, December 2006, available at our chapter 20 or at http://phsj.org/wp-content/uploads/2007/10/GMOs-and

-Biopharming-Z-Mag-+-sidebars.doc). Debt forgiveness will also help lift many nations out of poverty, with limited impact on the financial status of the world's richest nations (Donohoe, MT, ibid).

Global cooperation through international treaties is critical for decreasing global warming. The Montreal Protocol has been fairly successful in phasing out chlorofluorocarbon use (Gore, ibid). This treaty and the international "Earth Summits" in Rio de Janeiro and Kyoto represent the beginnings of global cooperation. The US, however, has resisted international efforts to reverse global warming. On February 16, 2005, the Kyoto Protocol, an international treaty, which legally binds developed nations to limit their output of fossil fuel emissions and other harmful gases in the upcoming century, took effect in the 141 countries that ratified it. The US has refused to ratify the Kyoto Protocol and has not formulated a workable plan to achieve the goals of the Protocol. Even so, many US cities have taken the lead and passed legislation to meet Kyoto standards (Staff, "Cool Cities: Solving Global Warming One City at a Time," available at http://www.coolcities.us) and Sweden has pledged to become the world's first oil-free economy by 2020.

While the economic costs of global warming may constitute up to 20 percent of the world's gross domestic product (GDP) each year, an investment of just 1 percent of the annual world GDP by 2050 could reduce emissions significantly and head-off the worst projected impacts of global warming (Stern Commission Report, ibid). Given the enormous economic and social consequences of global warming, it is essential that we act now to ameliorate and reverse climate change.

The Role of Health Professionals

As a result of their training, health professionals are in a unique position to recognize the causes and consequences of the global warming crisis. Because of their privileged position in society, since they themselves are in part responsible for these problems and because their raison d'être is to promote health and fight injustice, health professionals share a responsibility to oppose, individually and collectively, those forces which contribute to the spread of global warming.

Conclusions

The rapid, human-caused warming of the Earth over the last century carries serious consequences for our environment and health. Urgent action on the part of individuals, health professionals, public interest groups, governments and corporations is required to confront this serious threat to global health. We must constantly remind others, through our words and deeds, of the Native American saying, "We have not inherited the Earth from our ancestors, but have borrowed it from our children."

Chapter 24

Flowers, Diamonds, and Gold

The Destructive Public Health, Human Rights, and Environmental Consequences of Symbols of Love

Martin Donohoe

Introduction: Cupid's Poisonous and Deadly Arrow

On Valentine's Day, anniversaries, and throughout the year, suitors and lovers buy cut flowers and diamond and gold jewelry for the objects of their affection. Their purchases are in part a consequence of timely traditions maintained by aggressive marketing. Most buyers are unaware that in gifting their lovers with these aesthetically beautiful symbols, they are supporting industries which damage the environment, utilize forced labor, cause serious acute and chronic health problems, and contribute to violent conflicts. This article reviews the health and environmental consequences of, and the human rights abuses associated with, the production of cut flowers, gold, and diamonds. Recommendations to improve the safety of production standards are offered as well as alternative gift suggestions for those wishing to show their affection in ways which do not promote environmental degradation, human suffering, and death.

Flowers

Buds and Thorns

Flowers have a long history of religious, folk, heraldic, and national symbolism. Today, they are given as symbols of love, friendship, and filial devotion, particularly on St. Valentine's and Mother's Days. However, the beauty of cut flowers masks a system of growth and production marked by environmental degradation, labor abuses, and the exposure of almost 200,000 people in the developing world, to a variety of toxic chemicals.[1] Compensation is poor, relative to the risks involved. For instance, on an average day, one woman working in a Colombian carnation field will pick over 400 top-grade flowers. Four such flowers will cost just under $4.00 at a US florist, more than the worker earns in a day.[2]

The Floriculture Industry

The $30 billion cut-flower industry traditionally has been based in Holland and Colombia, but now encompasses Kenya, Zimbabwe, Ecuador, India, Mexico, China, and Malaysia. Dole Fresh Flowers (a division of Dole Foods Company, Inc.) is the world's largest producer.[3] The United States, Japan, and Germany are the major consuming nations.[4] Germany and the United States are the largest import markets; most flowers headed for Germany come from the Netherlands, while those destined for the United States originate in Europe and Central and South America. Ecuador and Colombia together account for the origin of almost half of all flowers sold in the United States.[5] Floriculture now employs about 190,000 people in the developing world.[6] Roses are the main product traded internationally. Most profits flow to multinational corporations, headquartered outside the producing country.[7] Given the profitability of floriculture and its serious adverse effects on human health and the environment in the developing world, it seems safe to argue that these companies inadequately re-invest profits in local economies.

Worker Health

The floriculture industry's predominantly female workforce is paid low wages with no benefits and short contract cycles.[8] Child labor, dismissal from employment due to pregnancy, and long hours of unpaid overtime are common, especially before holidays such as St. Valentine's Day and Mother's Day.[9]

The industry claims that its jobs are more stable than those in traditional farming, which may produce export crops subject to unstable price cycles. However, the use of land for floriculture rather than for growing crops for local food consumption contributes to malnutrition and increased food costs for locals.[10] Flower production requires large quantities of irrigation water, contributing to a drop in water tables in many flower-producing regions around the world.[11]

Flowers are the most pesticide-intensive crop.[12] They are grown and picked in warm, enclosed greenhouses, which keep pests out but result in high ambient levels of pesticides. One-fifth of the fertilizers, insecticides, fungicides, nematocides, and plant growth regulators used in floriculture in developing countries are banned or untested in the United States.[13] Many are known carcinogens. Flowers carry up to fifty times the amount of pesticides allowed on foods, yet flowers entering the United States, while checked carefully by the Department of Agriculture for pests, are not inspected for pesticides because they are not considered food.[14]

Over 50 percent of workers report at least one symptom of pesticide exposure.[15] Acute organophosphate pesticide exposure causes increased salivation, tearing, blurred vision, nausea, vomiting, abdominal cramps, urinary and fecal incontinence, increased bronchial secretions, coughing, wheezing, and sweating. In rare cases "involving more severe acute intoxication, dyspnea, bradycardia, heart block, hypotension, pulmonary edema, paralysis, convulsions, or death may occur."[16]

Floriculture workers also experience allergic reactions; dermatitis; heat-related illnesses; asthma, hypersensitivity pneumonitis, and emphysema; repetitive stress injury and accelerated osteoarthritis; hepatotoxicity; acute and chronic bronchitis; urinary tract infections (resulting from urinary retention, a consequence of limited bathroom breaks); bacterial and fungal cellulitis resulting from skin pricks acquired from de-thorning roses; increased risk of cancers of multiple organs; permanent neurological deficits, such as peripheral neuropathy and deficits in motor skills, memory (or attention); mental health problems; chromosomal defects; and other cancers.[17]

Some pesticides outlawed in the United States but still used abroad are persistent organic pollutants, which may have endocrine, reproductive, and oncogenic effects on pregnant women, fetuses, and growing children.[18] Greenhouse work has been associated with decreased sperm counts in men, delayed time in conception, and increased prevalence of spontaneous abortion, prematurity, and congenital malformations (among children conceived after either parent started working in floriculture).[19] In particular, prolonged standing and bending, overexertion, dehydration, poor nutrition, and pesticide exposure contribute to increased risk of spontaneous abortion, premature delivery, fetal malformation and growth retardation, and abnormal postnatal development.[20] Lack of prenatal care, while not unique to floriculture employees in the developing world, augments these problems.

Floriculture workers usually do not recognize pesticide exposure as the cause of their symptoms. Defects in safe handling practices are common, including failures in labeling and handling toxic materials; storage, application, and safe disposal of pesticides; educating workers on the dangers of pesticide exposure; provision of protective gear; and proper dosing and application of pesticides. Material data safety sheets are generally unavailable, and protective equipment, when supplied, may be old or non-functional.[21] "Reuse of pesticide-saturated greenhouse plastic for domestic purposes such as covering houses" is not uncommon.[22] Workers carry pesticides home on their clothes, which they may wash in the same sink used for bathing children and food preparation. The doctors treating these affected patients often do not inform them that their illnesses may be due to pesticide exposure, either because of a lack of knowledge or dual loyalties when they are employed by the floriculture company.[23]

Diamonds

History and Production

Diamonds (from the Greek *adamas*, meaning unconquerable or indestructible) are transparent gems made from carbon early in the earth's history under extremes of pressure and temperature.[24] They have at various times stood for wealth, power, love, and magical powers. Diamonds are used to produce jewelry and in industry, where they are valued for their hardness and durability.

Alluvial diamonds were discovered in India around 800 BC but it was not until the discovery of massive diamond deposits in South Africa in 1866 that commercial mining began in earnest. Today diamonds are mined in at least twenty nations, with the bulk coming from Australia, Zaire, Botswana, Russia, and South Africa. The major diamond trade centers are Antwerp, Tel Aviv, New York, and Mumbai (Bombay), while most cutting is done in Tel Aviv, Mumbai, New York, and Thailand. Major retail markets include the United States and Japan. Forty-eight percent of diamond jewelry is sold in the United States.[25]

Marketing

The idea of the diamond engagement ring was introduced in 1477, when Archduke Maximilian of Austria gave one to Mary of Burgundy, but the practice really did not catch on until 1939. That year, the De Beers company, founded in 1888 by Cecil Rhodes, hired N.W. Ayer and Company to make diamonds "a psychological necessity ... the larger and finer the diamond, the greater the expression of love."[26] Within three years, 80 percent of engagements in the United States were consecrated with diamond rings.[27] In 1947, the slogan "A Diamond Is Forever" was born. Jewelers were instructed to pressure men—who buy 90 percent of all diamonds—to spend at least two months' salary on a ring. In 1999, *Advertising Age Magazine* declared the "Diamond

Is Forever" slogan the most effective of the twentieth century, recognized by 90 percent of Americans. In 2003, De Beers began a new campaign to market diamonds to single women with the slogan, "Your left hand says 'we,' your right hand says 'me.'"[28]

Profits and Losses

The 120 million carats of rough diamonds mined for jewelry each year weigh a total of twenty-four tons. They cost less than $2 billion to extract, yet ultimately sell for over $50 billion.[29] The overwhelming majority of profits do not reach the millions of diggers and miners, who earn only a subsistence living from alluvial and mine-based diamonds. Desperately poor and hoping to strike it rich in this "casino economy," most leave their homes to work under dangerous, unhealthy conditions, yet still earn a pittance.[30] Middlemen, diamond dealers, and exporters earn the lion's share of diamond mining income; a high proportion are foreign nationals, most of whom tend to reinvest very little in the industry or the country.[31]

Human Rights Abuses, Conflict, and Terrorism

Diamond mine owners violate indigenous peoples' rights by joining with local and national governments in activities that have the effect of destroying traditional homelands and forcing resettlement.[32] Mining hastens the environmental degradation of places already facing ecosystem pressures such as war, overpopulation, deforestation, unsustainable agricultural and fishing practices, and rapidly dwindling supplies of clean water.[33]

Over the past decade, diamonds have been used by rebel armies in Angola, Sierra Leone, and the Democratic Republic of the Congo to pay for weapons used to fight some of Sub-Saharan Africa's most brutal civil wars. The Revolutionary United Front (RUF) in Sierra Leone killed and mutilated tens of thousands of people through its "signature tactic" involving amputation of hands, arms, legs, lips, and ears with machetes and axes, a tactic that was used to gain control over diamond mines. With the financial support of the diamond industry's trading centers, and backed by child soldiers forcibly conscripted and drugged to blunt their fear, reluctance to fight, and innate revulsion to killing, the RUF made millions off of diamonds that were extracted by thousands of prisoner-laborers.[34] Miners, worked to exhaustion, exposed to human immunodeficiency virus (HIV) and acquired immunodeficiency syndrome (AIDS) from camp sex-slaves, frequently were executed for suspected theft, lack of production, or simply for sport.[35]

Osama bin Laden's terrorist network, al Qaeda, responsible for attacks on the World Trade Center in New York and the London Underground, has profited from sales of diamonds originating in Kenya, Tanzania, Liberia, and Sierra Leone. Both al Qaeda and the terror group Hezbollah have used rough diamonds as a means of funding terror cells; to hide money targeted by financial sanctions; to launder the profits of criminal activity; and to convert cash into a commodity that holds its value and is easily transportable.[36] According to the US State Department, smuggled and illicit conflict diamonds may amount to as much as 15 percent of diamond jewelry sold internationally.[37]

Gold

History

In addition to its aesthetic value, gold has played a dominant role throughout history in the growth of empires and the evolution of the world's financial institutions.[37] In 4000 BC, cultures in eastern and central Europe first used gold to fashion decorative objects. By 1500 BC, gold had become the recognized standard medium of exchange for international trade. In the mid-1800s, the discovery of gold in California and South Africa led to gold rushes which transformed the economies and demographics of these areas.[38]

Today the world's top five gold producers are South Africa, the United States, Australia, Indonesia, and China. The approximately 2,500 tons of gold mined each year are valued at $21 billion.[39] Approximately 85 percent gets turned into jewelry.[40] Wedding rings typically are made from gold, but throughout history the wedding band has been formulated from a variety of minerals.[41] As with diamonds, aggressive marketing has played a significant role in popularizing the gold wedding ring.

Because of its special chemical and physical properties (including malleability, ductility, thermal conductivity, durability, and resistance to corrosion), the remaining 10–20 percent of mined gold is used to produce electronics and telecommunications equipment, lasers and optical instruments, aircraft engines, and dental alloys.[42] Historically, gold was used by Catherine de Medici and others as a poison, while today it is used to relieve joint pain and stiffness in rheumatoid arthritis patients.

In the United States, a piece of gold jewelry typically sells for at least four times the value of the gold itself.[43] Currently three times more gold sits in bank vaults, in jewelry boxes, and with private investors than is identified in underground reserves.[44] This is enough gold to meet current consumer demand for seventeen years.[45]

The World's Most Deadly Industry

Mining is the world's most deadly industry. Forty workers are killed each day, and scores more injured, in extracting minerals, including gold, from the earth.[46] Over the last century, tens of thousands have been killed working in mines,[47] while union-busting and human rights abuses have helped maintain cheap labor forces.[48]

Local communities bear the costs of mining in the form of environmental damage and pollution, loss of traditional livelihoods, long-term economic problems, and deteriorating public health.[49] Hundreds of thousands of people worldwide have been uprooted to make room for gold mining projects.[50] Just as with diamond mining, sexually transmitted diseases (including HIV/AIDS) are rampant among the poorly paid miners in gold mining communities.[51] Male miners spread these diseases to their spouses upon periodic return visits to their home communities.[52]

The Resource Curse

Dependence upon gold mining slows and even reduces economic growth while increasing poverty and encouraging governmental corruption, a phenomenon that economists have dubbed "the resource curse."[53] With increasing dependence on gold exports comes a slower per capita growth rate. The benefits of gold mining usually go to investors overseas and the central government, with little of the profit passed back to the community.[54]

Rural and indigenous peoples suffer greatly, as they often lack legal title to lands they have occupied for many generations. They may be evicted without prior consultation, meaningful compensation, or the offer of equivalent lands elsewhere. In Tarkwa, Ghana, more than 30,000 people have been displaced by gold mining operations.[55]

Much of the gold mined in the United States is extracted from public lands, the rights to which domestic and foreign mining companies can purchase, under the archaic Mining Law of 1872, for between $2.50 and $5.00 per acre.[56] Government subsidies to the gold mining industry in the United States and abroad provide cheap fuel, road-building, and other infrastructure, as well as reclamation and cleanup. This makes mining highly profitable to the extracting companies, but leaves local communities impoverished and stuck with multi-million to multi-billion dollar costs for environmental cleanup once the companies have moved on.[57] For example, Galactic Resources, Inc. stuck US taxpayers with a $200 million bill to clean up the cyanide-poisoned Alamosa River watershed when it declared bankruptcy and walked away from its Summitville gold mine in Colorado in 1992.[58]

Likewise, Nevada's Carlin Trend mining operations have damaged the land of native Western Shoshones.[59] Nevertheless, the US government has ignored a 2002 ruling of the Inter-American Commission on Human Rights, which held that the United States violated the fundamental rights of the Western Shoshones to property, due process, and equality under the law.[60] Similarly,

Spirit Mountain, a sacred site of the Assinboine and Gros Ventre tribes of Montana, was polluted by the Zortman-Landusky open-pit, cyanide-leach gold mine after its residents were forced by the US government to abandon the area. Zortman-Landusky was closed in 1998, when its owner, Pegasus Gold, declared bankruptcy.[61]

Nearly one-quarter of active gold mining and exploration sites overlap with regions of high conservation value, such as national parks and world heritage sites.[62] In the United States, only a $65 million government buyout prevented Crown Butte Mining Resources, Ltd. from opening a gold, silver, and copper mine just four kilometers (2.5 miles) from the border of Yellowstone, the world's oldest national park.[63]

Gold + Cyanide + Mercury

''The gold produced for a single, .33 ounce, 18 karat gold ring leaves in its wake at least eighteen tons of mine waste.''[64] Gold is leached from ore using cyanide. Waste ore and rock leach cyanide and other toxic metals, contaminating ground-water and sometimes sitting in large toxic lakes held in place by tenuous dams.[65] When the tailings dam at the Omai gold mine in Guyana (one of the largest open-pit mines in the world) failed in 1995, the release of three billion cubic liters of cyanide-laden tailings into the Omai River rendered the downstream thirty-two miles, home to 23,000 people, an ''environmental disaster zone.''[66] In 2000, the tailings dam from the Baia Mare gold mine in Romania spilled 100,000 metric tons of toxic wastewater, killing fish, harming fish-eating animals such as otters and eagles, and poisoning the drinking water of 2.5 million people in the Danube River watershed.[67] Gold mine-related coastal dumping in other areas damages estuaries and coral reefs.[68]

The ''Amazonian Gold Rush,'' which began in the late 1970s, has resulted in the release of at least 2,000 tons of mercury, used to capture gold particles as an amalgam, into local waterways.[69] Mercury is converted to methylmer-cury in the environment, leading to elevated levels of methylmercury in the locals' predominantly fish-based diet. Exposure to methylmercury causes decreases in neurocognitive function and memory in local children, who are exposed pre- and post-natally.[70] Both adults and children develop sensory disturbances, tremors, and balance problems.[71] Some have been diagnosed with mild Minamata Disease,[72] a form of methylmercury poisoning originally described in heavily fished Minamata Bay, Japan, where the Chisso Corpora-tion dumped large amounts of methylmercury in the mid-twentieth century.[73] In the United States, fish in the Sacramento River and San Francisco Bay still show elevated levels of mercury, acquired in part as a result of the nine-teenth century Gold Rush. During the Gold Rush, about 7,600 tons of mercury, which was used instead of cyanide to purify gold, entered California's lakes, streams, and rivers, and San Francisco Bay just from mining in the central mother lode.[74]

Mercury pollution also has contributed to the spread of malaria. Mercury may lower immunity to malaria; still pools of water resulting from mining serve as breeding grounds for malaria-carrying mosquitos; and miners from other areas import new strains of the disease, to which indigenous peoples have not built up immunity. Such strains of malaria contributed to the deaths of thousands of Yanomami Indians in Brazil in the late 1960s and early 1970s.[75]

Other Environmental Harms

Once gold is extracted, its processing continues to harm the environment. Gold smelting uses large amounts of energy and releases 142 tons of sulfur dioxide annually (13 percent of the world's total output), along with nitrogen dioxide and other components of air pollution and acid rain. Chronic asthma, skin diseases, and lead poisoning are common ailments found in those who live and work in mining communities.[76]

The United States Environmental Protection Agency estimates that 40 percent of western US watersheds are affected by gold mining pollution. There are more than twenty-five mines, some of them active, on the US Superfund list (meaning that they are among the most contaminated areas in the country).[77] Mine pollution ruins farmlands and strains local food resources. Open-pit gold mines also have led to water table declines of as much as 300 meters, a consequence of the enormous quantities of water which must be pumped into the ore to release the mineral.[78]

Women and Children Last

Water pollution in the developing world forces women, who are predominantly responsible for water collection, to walk increasing distances to find potable water. By displacing agriculture, a field in which women play a major role, gold mining removes women from the labor force and concentrates economic power in the hands of men, which in turn diminishes the financial resources and educational, political, and legal opportunities of women. Those few women who obtain low-level clerical positions at mines often face severe discrimination and sexual harassment, and may be fired if they become pregnant. Gold mines also frequently utilize child labor.[79]

Human Rights Abuses and Terrorism

Just as diamonds have been linked with monies for terrorism, so has gold mining. Allan Laird, a former executive of Echo Bay Mines Limited, told ABC

News that the company paid off the militant Islamist separatist group Abu Sayyaf, which is affiliated with al Qaeda, in exchange for protection of the company's gold mine in the Philippines.[80]

The Grasberg gold mine, the largest in the world, is owned by US-based Freeport McMoRan. Situated on land seized from the Amunge and Kamoro people, it dumps 110,000 tons of cyanide-laced waste into local rivers each day. Its operators have been implicated in human rights violations, including forced evictions, murders, rape, torture, extra-judicial killings, and arbitrary detentions, abetted by the Indonesian military, which Freeport McMoRan has paid millions of dollars.[81]

Markets Versus Morals

To maintain the status quo, the mining industry maintains strong ties with governments, including the United States, where industry lobbyists contributed almost $21 million to US political campaigns between 1997 and 2001.[82] Gold mining subsidies in many countries make it cheaper to extract new gold than to recycle existing gold.[83]

Recent proposals to cancel the crushing debts of the poorest countries to the International Monetary Fund (IMF) and World Bank require the sale of IMF gold as a component of the debt-forgiveness package. However, despite an IMF plan that would ensure IMF gold sales have no net impact on the world gold market, the gold industry is blocking the debt-forgiveness agreement.[84]

Alternatives and Solutions

Flowers

In the 1990s, in response to boycotts in Germany and increased consumer awareness, Europeans devised a series of voluntary eco-labels, none of which were particularly effective.[85] These did not take hold with American consumers. Several non-governmental organizations are working to develop voluntary standards relating to cut flowers produced in a humane, ecologically sustainable manner. The Food First Information and Action Network, as part of its "flower campaign," has issued an "international code of conduct" urging the floriculture industry to conform to International Labor Organization standards, the United Nations Declaration of Human Rights, and basic environmental standards.[86] Many businesses have yet to adopt the code. Nevertheless, purchasers of flowers can purchase locally or internationally produced, organically grown, labor-friendly bouquets (e.g., at some Whole Foods Market natural and organic food chain stores or through www.organicbouquet.com), or grow and pick their own.

Recently, activist Gerald Prolman, working with growers in the United States and Latin America, seed suppliers, and supermarkets, has developed the Veriflora certification system. The basic principles of Veriflora are organic production with phase-out of pesticides, fair labor practices, water conservation, safe waste management, fair wages, overtime pay, and the workers' right to organize. Veriflora certification also requires companies to mitigate any environmental damage they may have caused in the past. Unannounced audits will ensure compliance. The Society of American Florists has not yet endorsed Veriflora. While supermarkets account for only 29 percent of overall flower sales in the United States (versus 47 percent for florists), supermarkets have been gaining market share steadily at the expense of florists. Because there are just fifty major supermarket companies (versus 1,200 wholesalers and 30,000 florists), Prolman is focusing his efforts more on supermarkets. Consumer education and pressure on supermarkets and florists, including querying managers, boycotts, and protests, might lead to more rapid adoption of environmentally and socially sound production practices among their suppliers.[87]

Diamonds

To the traditional queries of diamond purchasers—cut, color, clarity, and carat weight—should be added a fifth: conflict. Buyers should avoid purchasing diamonds that jewelers cannot certify as conflict-free. Alternatives to diamonds include cubic zirconium and synthetic (or cultured) diamonds, produced by General Electric (a company with a record of environmental, labor, and human rights abuses) and De Beers (which has been charged and fined for anti-trust activities in the United States), as well as Gemesis Corporation and Apollo Diamond, Inc.[88] Such alternatives' only "flaw" is their slightly yellow hue.[89] Another company, LifeGem, creates diamonds from carbon captured during the cremation of human and animal remains.[90]

The diamond industry and the United Nations General Assembly have lent their support to a system of rough controls, the Kimberley Process Certification Scheme, to protect legitimate diamonds and isolate "blood diamonds" from the international market.[91] Governments would license miners; diamond traders would export their goods in sealed, tamper-proof containers; and interlocking computer databases in exporting and importing countries would catch discrepancies. For such controls to be successful, countries involved in cutting and finishing diamonds (primarily Belgium, India, and Israel) and the major importers of cut diamonds and jewelry (such as the United States) would have to enact strict customs regulations, backed by thorough inspections and harsh penalties against rogue importers.[92]

In the United States, the Clean Diamonds Trade Act of 2003 mandates participation in the Kimberley Process Certification scheme by requiring that all countries exporting diamonds to the United States have in place these rough controls. Money from fines (up to $10,000 for civil and $50,000 for criminal penalties) and seized contraband is earmarked for assistance of victims of armed conflict.[93]

Despite the diamond industry's stated commitment to a system of self-regulation to prevent trade in conflict diamonds, Amnesty International and Global Witness recently found that fewer than one in five companies responding in writing to their survey were able to provide a meaningful account of their policies, and less than half of diamond jewelry retailers visited were able to give consumers meaningful assurances that their diamonds were conflict-free.[94]

Those who decide to purchase diamonds should query their jewelers aggressively and demand documentation of the diamonds' conflict-free status. As with flowers, consumer education, boycotts, and protests could lead to more rapid changes in the diamond industry.

Gold

Consumers can take the "no dirty gold" pledge to demand an alternative to gold that was produced at the expense of communities, workers, and the environment. The "no dirty gold" campaign, online at http://www.nodirtygold.org/take_action.cfm, asks that mining companies not operate in areas of armed or militarized conflict, and calls on jewelry and other retailers to not use gold that comes from conflict areas or involves human rights violations.[95]

Earlier this year, eleven of the world's top jewelry retailers pledged to move away from "dirty gold" sales and called on mining corporations to ensure that gold is produced in more socially and environmentally responsible ways. The eleven firms are Zale Corporation, the Signet Group (the parent firm of Sterling and Kay Jewelers), Tiffany and Company, Helzberg Diamonds, Fortunoff, Cartier, Piaget, Fred Meyer Jewelers, Van Cleef and Arpels, TurningPoint, and Michael's Jewelers. Leading firms cited as "lagging behind" on commitments to responsible gold sourcing are Rolex, JCPenney, Walmart, Whitehall Jewelers, Jostens, QVC, and Sears/K-Mart.[96]

Students can boycott class ring sales and marrying couples can consider other visible tokens of their shared commitment. Shareholders in mining companies can push an activist agenda through resolutions and protests at annual stockholders' meetings. Continued consumer pressure on retail outlets and governments to eschew dirty gold ultimately may lead to a system similar to the Kimberley Process. The International Labor Organization's Convention No. 169 Concerning Indigenous and Tribal Peoples in Independent Countries, which has been signed and ratified by seventeen countries, requires governments to allow for a culturally relevant system of consultation before indigenous lands are appropriated for mining, and that indigenous peoples participate in the benefits of such mining.[97] None of the top gold mining countries have ratified this treaty.[98] Finally, mining companies and governments should invest more money to develop biological and chemical treatments to decrease or destroy the cyanide in gold mill effluents, particularly for use in the developing world.[99]

Alternative Tokens of Affection

Consumers should reconsider the entire concept of purchasing cut flowers, gold, and diamonds as symbols of their affection. These symbols are not universal and have not been constant throughout history, but rather are cultural constructs extensively perpetuated by the persuasive marketing efforts of multinational corporations. The visible reminders of one's love should not also represent environmental destruction, violence, the subjugation of native peoples, child labor, and human rights abuses.

Substitute gifts include cards (ideally printed on recycled paper), poems, photos, collages, videos, art, home improvement projects, homemade meals, and donations to charities. Consider alternatives to the traditional diamond engagement and gold wedding rings, such as recycled or vintage gold: old gold can be melted down and made into new jewelry. Other options include eco-jewelry made from recycled or homemade glass and coconut beads.[100] Purchasing handicrafts constructed by indigenous peoples from outlets that return the profits to the artisans and their communities provides wide-ranging social and economic benefits. Such tokens of affection will be rendered more meaningful through their lack of association with death and destruction and because they symbolize justice and hope for the future.

Notes

1. David Tenenbaum, Would a Rose Not Smell as Sweet? Problems Stem from the Cut Flower Industry, 110 *Environ. Health Perspect.* A240, A241 (2002).

2. Kevin Watkins, Deadly Blooms, *The Guardian*, August 29, 2001, available at http://society.guardian.co.uk/societyguardian/story/0,7843,543351,00.html. These issues were dramatized briefly in the poignant and powerful 2004 film, *Maria Full of Grace*.

3. Tenenbaum, *supra* note 1, at A246.

4. International Labor Organization (ILO), *Working Paper on the World Cut Flower Industry: Trends and Prospects,* SAP 2.80/WP.139 (September 28, 2000), available at http://www.ilo.org/public/english/dialogue/sector/papers/ctflower/index.htm.

5. Ross Wehner, Flower Power: With an Entrepreneur's Jump Start, the Organic Market Blossoms, *E/The Environmental Magazine*, November–December 2004.

6. Tenenbaum, *supra* note 1, at A241.

7. Watkins, *supra* note 2.

8. Elizabeth A. Stanton, Flowers for Mother's Day? *Dollars and Sense: The Magazine of Economic Justice,* May/June 2003, available at http://www.dollarsandsense.org/0503stanton.html.

9. Id.

10. Tenenbaum, *supra* note 1, at A245.

11. Watkins, *supra* note 2.

12. Wehner, *supra* note 5.

13. Tenenbaum, *supra* note 1, at A242; Stanton, *supra* note 8.

14. Tenenbaum, *supra* note 1, at A242–A243; Wehner, *supra* note 5; Stanton, *supra* note 8.

15. Tenenbaum, *supra* note 1, at A243.

16. Eric Hansen & Martin T. Donohoe, Health Issues of Migrant and Seasonal Farmworkers, 14 *J. Health Care for the Poor and Underserved* 153, 157 (2003); Martin T. Donohoe, Trouble in the Fields: Effects of Migrant and Seasonal Farm Labor on Women's Health and Well-Being, 9 *Medscape Ob/Gyn and Women's Health* (2004), available at http://www.medscape.com/viewarticle/470445.

17. Linda Rosenstock, Matthew Keifer, William E. Daniell, Robert McConnell & Keith Claypoole, Chronic Central Nervous System Effects of Acute Organophosphate Pesticide Intoxication, 338 *The Lancet* 223, 223–228 (1991); Shelia Hoar Zahm & Mary H. Ward, Pesticides and Childhood Cancer, 106 (Supp. 3) *Environ. Health Perspect.* 893, 893–898, 904–905 (1998); Ted Schettler, Gina Solomon, Maria Valenti & Annette Huddle, Generations at Risk, *Reproductive Health and the Environment* 107, 115–125 (1999); Lola Roldán-Tapia, Tesifón Parrón & Fernando Sánchez-Santed, Neuropsychological Effects of Long-Term Exposure to Organophosphate Pesticides, 27 *Neurotoxicol. & Teratol.* 259, 259–60, 263–264 (2005); Eduard Monsó, Ramón Magarolas, Isabel Badorrey, Katja Radon, Dennis Nowak & Josep Morera, Occupational Asthma in Greenhouse Flower and Ornamental Plant Growers, 165 *Am. J. Respir. & Crit. Care Med.* 954, 954–958 (2002); B. F. Lander, L. E. Knudsen, M. O. Gamborg, H. Jarnentaus & H. Norppa, Chromosome Aberrations in Pesticide-Exposed Greenhouse Workers, 26 *Scandinavian J. Work, Env't & Health* 436 (2000); Eduard Monsó, Occupational Asthma in Greenhouse Workers, 10 *Curr. Opin. in Pulm. Med.* 147, 149 (2004); E. Paulsen, J. Søgaard & K. E. Andersen, Occupational Dermatitis in Danish Gardeners and Greenhouse Workers: (I) Prevalence and Possible Risk Factors, 37 *Contact Dermatitis* 263, 263–264, 268–269 (1997). See generally Grace J. A. Ohayo-Mitoko, Hans Kromhout, Philip N. Karumba & Jan S. M. Boleij, Identification of Determinants of Pesticide Exposure Among Kenyan Agricultural Workers Using Empirical Modeling, 43 *Ann. Occup. Hyg.* 519 (1999).

18. Carlos Sonnenschein & Ana M. Soto, An Updated Review of Environmental Estrogen and Androgen Mimics and Antagonists, 65 *J. Steroid Biochem. & Molec. Biol.* 143, 144–147, 149 (1998); Schettler et al., *supra* note 17, at 107–111,

113–120, 122–125. See generally Rosenstock et al., *supra* note 17, at 223–228; Zahm & Ward, *supra* note 17, at 893–905.

19. Annette Abell, Erik Ernst & Jens Peter Bonde, Semen Quality and Sexual Hormones in Greenhouse Workers, 26 *Scandinavian J. Work, Env't & Health* 492 (2000); Grazia Petrelli & Irene Figa-Talamanca, Reduction in Fertility in Male Greenhouse Workers Exposed to Pesticides, 17 *Eur. J. Epidemiol.* 675 (2001); Markku Sallmen, Jyrki Liesivuori, Helena Taskinen, Marja-Liisa Lindbohm, Ahti Anttila, Lea Aalto & Kari Hemminki, Time to Pregnancy Among the Wives of Finnish Greenhouse Workers, 29 *Scandinavian J. Work, Env't & Health* 85 (2003); Annette Abell, Svend Juul & Jens Peter Bonde, Time to Pregnancy Among Female Greenhouse Workers, 26 *Scandinavian J. Work, Env't & Health* 131 (2000); Sandra Gomez-Arroyo, Yooko Diaz-Sanchez, M. Angel Meneses-Perez, Rafael Villalobos-Pietrini & Jorge De Leon-Rodriguez, Cytogenetic Biomonitoring in a Mexican Floriculture Worker Group Exposed to Pesticides, 466 *Mutation Res.* 117 (2000); Tenenbaum, *supra* note 1.

20. Tenenbaum, *supra* note 1, at A245; Hansen & Donohoe, *supra* note 16, at 158; Donohoe, *Trouble in the Fields, supra* note 16; Schettler, *supra* note 17, at 16–18.

21. Tenenbaum, *supra* note 1, at A244.

22. Tenenbaum, *supra* note 1, at 243.

23. *Id.*

24. Anthony M. Evans, *Ore Geology and Industrial Minerals: An Introduction* 104, 110–112 (3d ed. 1993).

25. Andrew Cockburn, Diamonds: The Real Story, *National Geographic,* March 2002, at 21.

26. Sarah Wilkins, For Richer or Poorer: Rocking the World, *Mother Jones* 24 (January/February 2005), available at http://www.motherjones.com/news/exhibit/2005/01/exhibit.html.

27. *Id.*

28. *Id.*

29. Cockburn, *supra* note 25, at 13.

30. Global Witness & Partnership Africa Canada, *Rich Man, Poor Man: Development Diamonds and Poverty Diamonds: The Potential for Change in the Artisanal Alluvial Diamond Fields of Africa* (October 22, 2004) at 1, 6, available at http://www.globalwitness.org/media_library_detail.php/127/en/rich_man_poor_man.

31. *Id.*

32. Tom Price, Exiles of the Kalahari, *Mother Jones* 30 (January/February 2005), available at http://www.motherjones.com/news/dispatch/2005/01/01_800.html. See Elizabeth Stanton, Center for Popular Economics, *Field Guide to the US Economy, Econ-Atrocity: Ten Reasons Why You Should Never Accept a Diamond Ring from Anyone, Under Any Circumstances, Even if They Really Want to Give You One* (February 14, 2002), available at http://www.populareconomics.org/2002

/02/econ-atrocity-ten-reasons-why-you-should-never-accept-a-diamond-ring-from-anyone-under-any-circumstances-even-if-they-really-want-to-give-you-one/.

33. Martin Donohoe, Causes and Health Consequences of Environmental Degradation and Social Injustice, 56 *Soc. Sci. & Med.* 573–587 (2003); Martin T. Donohoe, *The Roles and Responsibilities of Medical Educators, Ethicists and Humanists in Confronting the Health Consequences of Environmental Degradation and Social Injustice* (2007) (unpublished manuscript, on file with Health and Human Rights).

34. Physicians for Human Rights, *War-Related Sexual Violence in Sierra Leone: A Population-Based Assessment* 1–2, 17–22 (2002), available at http://physicians forhumanrights.org/library/documents/reports/sexual-violence-sierra-leone.pdf; Stanton, Econ-Atrocity, *supra* note 32. See also World Diamond Council, *What Are Conflict Diamonds? Background,* available at http://www.diamondfacts.org /conflict/background.html; United Methodist Committee on Relief, *Do You Know Where Your Diamond Has Been?* available at http://gbgm-umc.org/UMcor /emergency/conflictdiamonds.stm; United Methodist Committee on Relief, *Diamonds Fund Cycle of Violence in Africa,* available at http://gbgm-umc.org /UMcor/stories/doyouknow.stm.

35. Human Rights Watch, *Children's Rights: Child Soldiers* (2004), available at http:// www.hrw.org/campaigns/crp/index.htm; Human Rights Watch, *Sowing Terror: Atrocities Against Civilians in Sierra Leone* (1998), available at http://www.hrw .org/reports98/sierra; Hans Veeken, Sierra Leone: People Displaced Because of Diamonds, 309 *Brit. Med. J.* 523 (1994); Global Witness & Partnership Africa Canada, *supra* note 30, at 6; Stanton, Econ-Atrocity, *supra* note 32.

36. Greg Campbell, Blood Diamonds, *Amnesty International Magazine* (Fall 2002), available at http://www.amnestyusa.org/Fall_/Blood_Diamonds/page.do? id=1105119&n1=2&n2=19&n3=338; *Global Witness, for a Few Dollars More: How Al Qaeda Moved into the Diamond Trade* (April 17, 2003) at 6–15, 20–27, 28–32, available at http://www.globalwitness.org/media_library_detail.php/109/en /for_a_few_dollars_more.37. United States General Accounting Office, Report to Congressional Requesters, *International Trade: Critical Issues Remain in Deterring Conflict Diamond Trade* (June 2002), available at http://www.gao.gov/new .items/d02678.pdf.

37. World Trust Gold Services, *As Good as Gold: A Standard for the Ages,* available at http://streettracksgoldshares.com/pdf/history_of_gold.pdf.

38. Natl Mining Assn., *The History of Gold,* available at http://www.nma.org/pdf /gold/gold_history.pdf; Rebecca Solnit, The New Gold Rush-Gold Mining in Nevada, *Sierra Magazine,* July–August 2000, at 86.

39. Payal Sampat, Worldwatch Institute, *Scrapping Mining Dependence* (2003).

40. Solnit, *supra* note 39.

41. Matt Jacks, *The History of the Wedding Ring—A Recognizable Symbol of Love,* available at http://www.thehistoryof.net/history-of-the-wedding-ring.html.

42. Scott Fields, Tarnishing the Earth: Gold Mining's Dirty Secret, 109 *Environ. Health Perspect.* A474 (2001); *Gold Jewelry: From Open Pit to Wedding Band,* Worldwatch Institute, available at http://www.worldwatch.org/node/1491.

43. Worldwatch Institute, *Gold Jewelry: From Open Pit to Wedding Band,* available at http://www.worldwatch.org/node/1491.

44. Sampat, *supra* note 40.

45. *Id.*

46. *Id.*

47. *Id.*

48. Earthworks & Oxfam America, *Dirty Metals: Mining, Communities and the Environment* 26 (2004), available at http://www.nodirtygold.org/pubs /DirtyMetals.pdf.

49. Earthworks & Oxfam America, *supra* note 49.

50. Sampat, *supra* note 40.

51. Catherine Campbell & Brian Williams, Beyond the Biomedical and Behavioural: Towards an Integrated Approach to HIV Prevention in the Southern African Mining Industry, 48 *Soc. Sci. Med.* 1624, 1626 (1999).

52. Sampat, *supra* note 40.

53. *Id.* at 120.

54. *Id.*

55. Earthworks & Oxfam America, *supra* note 49, at 18.

56. US Public Interest Research Group, *Campaign to Cut Polluter Pork* (2002), available at http://www.pirg.org/enviro/pork/index.htm.

57. Sampat, *supra* note 40; Earthworks & Oxfam America, *supra* note 49, at 29.

58. Earthworks & Oxfam America, *supra* note 49, at 29.

59. *Id.* at 16.

60. *Id.* at 23.

61. Earthworks & Oxfam America, *supra* note 49, at 22.

62. Id. at 15.

63. *No Dirty Gold, Threatened Natural Areas,* available at http://www.nodirtygold .org/threatened_natural_areas.cfm; Earthworks & Oxfam America, *supra* note 49, at 14–15.

64. *Gold Jewelry: From Open Pit to Wedding Band, supra* note 44.

65. Ronald Eisler & Stanley N. Wiemeyer, Cyanide Hazards to Plants and Animals from Gold Mining and Related Water Issues, 183 *Rev. Envtl. Contamination & Toxicol.* 21 (2004); Earthworks & Oxfam America, *supra* note 49, at 2, 9.

66. Earthworks & Oxfam America, *supra* note 49, at 5.

67. *Id.* at 29.

68. *Id.* at 6.

69. Fields, *supra* note 43, at A478.

70. Phillipe Grandjean, Roberta F. White, Anne Nielsen, David Cleary & Elisabeth C. de Oliveira Santos, Methylmercury Neurotoxicity in Amazonian Children Downstream from Gold Mining, 107 *Environ. Health Perspect.* 587 (1999); Ana Amelia Boischio & Diane S. Henshel, Risk Assessment of Mercury Exposure Through Fish Consumption by the Riverside People in the Madeira Basin, Amazon, 1991, 17 *Neurotoxicology* 169 (1996); *Id.*, at 169–175.

71. Masazumi Harada et al., Mercury Pollution in the Tapajos River Basin, Amazon: Mercury Level of Head Hair and Health Effects, 27 *Environment Intl.* 285 (2001).

72. Martin Lodenius & Olaf Malm, Mercury in the Amazon, 157 *Rev. Envtl. Contamination & Toxicol.* 25, 46 (1998).

73. Pamela Paradis Powell, Minamata Disease: A Story of Mercury's Malevolence, 84 *Southern Med. J.* 1352 (1991); M. Harada, Minamata Disease: Methylmercury Poisoning in Japan Caused by Environmental Pollution, 25 *Critical Rev. Toxicol.* 1 (1995). Minamata disease was documented with great poignancy in an award-winning photoessay by William Eugene Smith, Aileen Mioko Sprauge Smith & Ishikawa Takeshi, available at http://www.geocities.com/minoltaphotographyw /williameugenesmith.html.

74. Earthworks & Oxfam America, *supra* note 49, at 9; Solnit, *supra* note 39, at 50–57, 86; Rebecca Solnit, The New Gold Rush, *Sierra Magazine* 53, July–August 2000, at 54.

75. Fields, *supra* note 43, at A481.

76. Earthworks & Oxfam America, *supra* note 49, at 8; *Gold Jewelry: From Open Pit to Wedding Band, supra* note 44.

77. Fields, *supra* note 43, at A475.

78. Earthworks & Oxfam America *supra* note 49, at 12; Solnit, *supra* note 39.

79. Raul Harari, Francesco Forastiere & Olav Axelson, Unacceptable "Occupational" Exposure to Toxic Agents Among Children in Ecuador, 32 *Am. J. Industrial Med.* 185, 186 (1997); Earthworks & Oxfam America, *supra* note 49, at 25.

80. Marilyn Berlin Snell, The Cost of Doing Business, *Sierra Magazine,* May/June 2004, available at http://www.sierraclub.org/sierra/200405/terrorism/printable_all.asp.

81. Earthworks & Oxfam America, Dirty Metals, *supra* note 49, at 14, 19, 24.

82. Sampat, *supra* note 40, at 126.

83. Sampat, *supra* note 40, at 114.

84. Russel Mokhiber & Robert Weissman, *Sell the Gold, Free the Poor,* June 1, 2005, available at http://lists.essential.org/pipermail/corp-focus/2005/000205.html.

85. Wehner, *supra* note 5, at 19–20.

86. Tenenbaum, *supra* note 1, at A247.

87. Scientific Certification Systems, *The Veriflora Certification System*, available at http://www.scscertified.com/csrpurchasing/veriflora/docs/VeriFlora_FAQ.pdf; Wehner, *supra* note 5.

88. Martin T. Donohoe, GE — Bringing Bad Things to Life: Cradle to Grave Health Care and the Unholy Alliance Between General Electric Medical Systems and New York-Presbyterian Hospital, 41 *Synthesis/Regeneration* 31–33 (2006).

89. Sanjiv Arole, *Cultured Diamonds Are Here to Stay*, Rediff.com, March 31, 2004, available at http://inhome.rediff.com/money/2004/mar/31guest.htm.

90. Carly Wickell, *Jewelry/Accessories: Creating Diamonds from Human Ashes*, about.com, available at http://jewelry.about.com/cs/syntheticdiamonds/a/lifegem_diamond.htm.

91. Physicians for Human Rights, *supra* note 34.

92. *Id.*

93. 19 U.S.C. 3901; Global Witness & Partnership Africa Canada, *The Key to Kimberley: Internal Diamond Controls: Seven Case Studies* (22 Oct. 2004), available at http://www.globalwitness.org/media_library_detail.php/126/en/the_key_to_kimberley.

94. Press Release, Amnesty International & Global Witness, Déjà Vu: Diamond Industry Still Failing to Deliver on Promises, *AI Index POL* 34/008/2004, October 18, 2004, available at http://web.amnesty.org/library/pdf/POL340082004ENGLISH/$File/POL3400804.pdf.

95. *Gold Jewelry: From Open Pit to Wedding Band*, *supra* note 44.

96. *The Golden Rules, No Dirty Gold*, available at http://www.nodirtygold.org/goldenrules.cfm; *Retailers Who Support the Golden Rules, No Dirty Gold*, available at http://www.nodirtygold.org/supporting_retailers.cfm.

97. *Convention (No. 169) Concerning Indigenous and Tribal Peoples in Independent Countries*, adopted June 27, 1989, ILO, General Conf., 76th sess. (entered into force September 5, 1991), available at http://www.unhchr.ch/html/menu3/b/62.htm (Office of the United Nations High Commissioner for Human Rights); Earthworks & Oxfam America, *Dirty Metals, supra* note 49.

98. Int'l Labor Org., *Ratifications of ILO Convention, No. C169*, (October 3, 2007), available at http://www.ilo.org/ilolex/cgi-lex/ratifce.pl?C169.

99. Ata Akcil, Destruction of Cyanide in Gold Mill Effluents: Biological Versus Chemical Treatments, 21 *Biotechnology Advances* 501 (2003).

100. Katherine Kerlin, Diamonds Aren't Forever: Environmental Degradation and Civil War in the Gem Trade, *E/The Environmental Magazine* (2004), available at http://www.emagazine.com/view/?1078.

Chapter 25

Is a Modest Health Care System Possible?

Andrew Jameton

The health care system in the US is generally regarded by economists and activists as over-scaled and inefficient. Health care consumes nearly 15% of the US GDP (high as compared to most industrialized nations) while providing insured access only to about 85% of the population. Moreover, the provision of health care services has a relatively small effect on public health as compared to what people generally expect of it.

Substantial reductions in the overall scale of health care thus at first appear to be an excellent idea. However, health care also provides services key to the health and happiness of many individuals and vulnerable groups. So, reductions in energy consumption must be balanced against the struggle to maintain highly valued services. Moreover, whether energy consumption in health care can be reduced substantially depends on whether the 80% reductions in other economic sectors are likely to improve or reduce the health of the public.

Energy in Health Care

Some of health care's problems with energy consumption can doubtless be solved by efficiencies in other economic sectors, such as in more efficient production of electric power, but not all problems can be so easily fixed. Health care in the US (and to a lesser degree in developed nations generally) has many features that reflect high levels of energy consumption. Indeed, the modern acute care hospital—spanking clean, brightly lit, packed with imaging machinery, complex medications, and highly trained personnel—is symbolic of the humane achievements of high-energy societies. We envision health care as though we believe that high levels of energy consumption are good for health. Some of the specific high-energy features of hospitals are:[1]

- Twenty-four/seven, hospitals maintain bright lights, intensive air filtration, sealed windows, and controlled temperature levels, which involve intensive use of heating, air conditioning, and fans. Hospitals are like hotels and restaurants; they clean and process tons of food and laundry.

- Large imaging machines such as x-rays and MRIs, computers, diagnostic devices, operating rooms, intensive care units, and emergency departments use lots of electricity. Our own medical campus has three power-generating facilities.

- Health care uses energy in storing and transporting a wide range of materials and supplies as well as disposing of them and cleaning up after their use. Many hospital tools and materials are manufactured globally, and so the production network is wide and complex. Since so many therapies involve exotic materials, it is difficult to save energy by localizing the sources of materials. Indeed, the pharmaceutical industry, at the end of the 19th century, was one of the pioneering global industries.

- Pharmaceuticals are often synthesized through long chemical paths and highly purified, requiring substantial energy inputs. Cleaning up the toxic wastes of such processes requires energy all the way from manufacture to use and disposal. Chemotherapeutic agents, for instance, are often sufficiently toxic that the waste after their use needs to be transported long distances for incineration.

- Re-use of tools and materials requires more processing than normal since tools and materials must be very clean. Clean-up via incinerators or autoclave is a high-energy process.

- Hospitals are often large regional facilities requiring extensive parking lots to accommodate traveling patients. Helicopters ply the airways between traffic accidents and trauma centers. Better-paid clinicians often live in large homes in the suburbs, far from inner-city hospitals and academic medical centers, thereby increasing the energy costs of providing health care.

Because health care involves high energy consumption in so many of its functions, it is impossible to reduce its energy levels without also reducing materials consumption, together with services provided. So, in the balance of the article, I will treat the problem of reducing energy consumption largely as one of reducing the overall scale of health care materials, tools, buildings, and services.

Boiling Health Care Down to Its Essentials

The good news is that, since health care is only a minor factor in public health, it can be down-scaled without much impact on prevailing health levels. However, it provides important additional services (which I will discuss in more detail later) which will be difficult to forgo or even to provide in a more efficient manner.

Let us approach the reduction in the scale of health care by first considering a 50% reduction. Then, we can go for more. Cutting health care in half, contrary to reducing its effectiveness, is more likely to improve it. Some of the problems of bloated health care are:

- Because health care is so over-scaled, it is unmanageably complex. It has a huge administrative overload, costly in buildings, paper, computers, and personnel.

- Driven by the need for profit, new and dangerous drugs are released to market prematurely and advertised directly to patients. US patients die of medical mistakes (about half of them related to pharmaceuticals) in greater numbers than Americans die of traffic accidents. Treatment of side effects of treatment accounts, by some estimates, for about a third of all medical care.

- Harm and toxicity (remember "do no harm"?) are thus major features of health care, and in general, energy must be expended to reduce the toxicity of manufacturing and disposal processes and to repair the harm done.

- Because health care is expensive, it is more difficult for the government to finance universal access. Moreover, a costly health care system requires a giant economy to support it, and thus, unhealthy environmental damage.

Yet, cutting health care 50% won't be easy. We also need to expand access, and so lose about 15% from our 50%. Although there is agreement that half of health care is a waste, there is little agreement on which half that is; after all, every service has its constituency. And, the health care system has not so far been very successful in inducing patients to lead healthier life styles. (Why should it? It's not its job. And, we make our money on illness, not health.)

This 50% reduction in end-user energy costs may be enough, if we can reduce the background costs of health care in transportation, buildings, power production, etc. But we should also consider making more substantial reductions in the level of services since we want to get to the bare bones of what is necessary.

Health care serves important social functions besides promoting public health. One important function—the rescue of the severely ill and injured—is a key humane function of society and potentially an expensive one. Moreover, many people are vulnerable, dependent, chronically ill, and in need of health-related services to prevent their suffering and to support their inclusion in family and society. Simple assistance, such as a cane or prosthetic, or physical or speech therapy, can be very important in restoring and maintaining individuals' functions and daily activities.

So, if we have not already been charged with being inhumane for slashing health care in half, we will certainly be charged with cruelty for considering deeper cuts. Nevertheless, consider the following approach to rock-bottom energy consumption in health care.

The Modest Proposal

First, we cut health care 50% with an approach similar to the "Oregon Plan."[2] In brief, we rank order the various health care services according to their value, as rated by public meetings, and according to their energy costs. We then cut out the half that offers the least value for the highest energy costs. We establish universal access to this level of care, while at the same time prohibiting systematic provision of higher levels of care.

At the same time, we should become less sanguine about "rescue" or "saving lives" as a function of health care. We should, for example, be more concerned about providing nursing care to patients who are dying, approaching dying stages, or suffering from long-term illnesses. We should focus less on devices to cure, or to pursue the illusion of cure, and more on high-quality nursing care and comfort.

We then shift our focus in health care research, both basic and clinical, to exploring ways to conserve energy in medications, devices, and maintaining health. So, instead of focusing on finding new diseases to treat and new therapies for them, we undertake an intensive effort to reduce the energy costs of caring for and curing people. The fruits of research should make it easier to reduce energy costs further without reducing the quality of services.

Health Care Basics

In 1993, the World Bank published a major study of public health and development internationally. One of its important findings was that at the very lowest levels of national per capita income (and therefore, at the lowest levels of access to energy sources), income strongly affected public health status. As income increases at these low income levels, general healthiness rises steadily. After a certain level of income is achieved, the health status curve flattens and increased income/energy levels make little difference.[3]

There are probably a couple of things going on here. First, high levels of income cannot do much to make people safer, freer from toxins, or more athletic. Instead, higher levels of income foster harmful aspects of excess consumption—obesity, sedentary work, substance abuse, and so on. At low income levels, it matters whether a nation can provide clean water, stable access to nutritious food, safe housing, and transportation, and can clean up toxins, monitor infectious diseases, provide contraceptives, and so on. And, can provide jobs: people who have jobs and incomes also have stability, hopes, a role in society, and like psychological benefits that promote health.

Will cutting energy consumption by 80% keep society above the cusp in the curve and at an adequate and stable level of health, or will it plunge society into the perilous lower range? It is hard to know and will depend very much on our social choices with regard to every sector of the economy since everything affects health.[4] One key choice is that of income equality; without it, more people will fall into those lowest income ranges where they lack what is needed for health, and many studies show that income inequality is a major factor in poor public health.[5]

The question has been asked whether societies can maintain good public health at low levels of income, and the answer seems to be that only a few countries—such as Costa Rica, Cuba, China, and Kerala in India—have done so, and high public health status in these nations depended little on health care. They had more to do with income equality, jobs for women, a radical commitment to public welfare, and universal accessibility of such public health basics as nutrition, water, and sewage control.[6]

Health care in these nations is different from that practiced in the United States. It is more the concept of "primary care" promoted by the UN in its Alma Ata declaration and since. This approach combines access to the public health basics above with basic primary and preventive medicine for women, children, and families. Key elements are well-baby care, vaccinations, treatment of diarrhea, family planning, quarantine in periods of infection, and the like.[7] The public health functions of health care that need to be maintained are:

- Monitoring environmentally caused diseases
- Providing services that have ramifying consequences on health, such as infection control, vaccination, birth control, and education
- Providing technical advice to sewer departments, restaurants, agriculture, etc., where knowledge of human biology is needed to serve public health

These health care services generally do not necessarily require high levels of energy consumption. In comparison, high-energy health care generally represents diminishing returns as compared to such primary care measures. So, we should think more in terms of what we need to establish and sustain to maintain health rather than in terms of what we must cut back.

Some Cautions

"Alternative medicine" is not the answer, although some aspects of alternative medicine may be helpful. China, for instance, did well in its revolutionary years with traditional medicine. However, obtaining medications from natural sources has one of the same problems ethanol has: land for medications competes with food-growing land and wilderness preservation. And, ineffective medications are wasteful.

Miniaturization in medicine is not the answer. Small devices like thermometers, oximeters, pumps, pills, and so on consume little at their point of use, but they have life cycles both up- and downstream with substantial footprints. Similarly, re-use and recycling in health care tend to be energy intensive because of the need for cleanliness.

In contrast, replacing equipment with staff is an answer because, instead of using energy to maintain machines, we use energy more directly to maintain staff. So, health care should emphasize clinics, home care, and nursing care facilities more than hospitals.

Philosophically, I think we are making a shift from viewing nature as something that we should be insulated from in order to enjoy good health to a view that closeness to nature is healthy, as well as environmentally efficient. However, although nearness to nature has been shown in studies to be psychologically healthy,[8] there are physical risks, such as from mosquitoes, temperature variations, and so on.

There is now a substantial greening movement in health care. Science and Environmental Health Network has outlined basic principles of "ecological medicine" (at http://www.sehn.org). Health Care Without Harm (http://www.noharm.org/) has been promoting materials and tools that are more environmentally friendly; they have also been working on waste streams, incineration, and cleansers. And, there is a "green hospitals" movement in architecture following the principles of LEED (see the US Green Building Council at http://www.usgbc.org) and the Green Guide for Health Care (http://www.gghc.org).

These groups, however, are not working much to reduce health care overscale, and so reductions in scale could synergistically help to reduce the environmental footprint, and thereby the energy consumption, of health care.

Concluding Note: Obesity and Climate Change

A couple of points relating to energy consumption and climate change: There is a global epidemic of obesity, especially in the US. This represents an excess of food energy moving into people in relation to levels of energy output through work and exercise. The growth of obesity parallels the growth in energy consumption in society generally, and is likely aggravated by overuse of automobiles, computers, televisions, etc., which reduce activity levels overall. The "energy-saving" devices of the modern home and workplace do not really save energy; instead, they replace food-based energy expenditures with more expensive technologically based energy expenditures.

There is thus a prevailing "excess energy consumption disorder" in the developed world that is fostering both climate change and poor health related to overconsumption. Fortunately, both can be mitigated to some degree by replacing technologically based work with simpler forms of labor. It is important that as levels of needed human labor increase and displace fossil fuels, that this be accomplished in a just and healthy manner, so that everyone participates in manual labor, rather than placing the burdens of the heaviest work on the poor.

Meanwhile, if climate change cannot be significantly mitigated, the expectable results of droughts, famines, floods, heat waves, expanded ranges of tropical diseases, ocean level rise, famines, habitat loss, despeciation, and massive migration are likely to vastly reduce the health status of everyone.[9] This very real potential of global warming to stimulate a global public health disaster is one important motive for undertaking significant reductions in energy consumption in all economic sectors of society.

If business as usual continues, the tragedy likely to ensue is that while health status declines rapidly during this century's global warming, health care—because of its over-scaled energy and material consumption—will have a limited capacity to respond to these rapidly increasing health care needs. The prudent course is to reduce the scale of health care in order partly to make health care access universal, and partly to help it do its part in mitigating climate change.

Notes

1. Pierce J, Jameton A. *The Ethics of Environmentally Responsible Health Care*. Oxford: Oxford University Press; 2004.

2. Jacobs L, Marmor T, Oberlander J. The Oregon Health Plan and the political paradox of rationing: What advocates and critics have claimed and what Oregon did. *J Health Polit Policy Law* 1999 February;24(1):161–180.

3. World Bank, *The World Development Report 1993: Investing in Health*. Oxford UK: Oxford University Press; 1993, 34.

4. Evans RG, Stoddart GL. Models for population health: Consuming research, producing policy? *Am J Public Health* 2003;93:371–379.

5. Wilkinson RG, Pickett KE. Income inequality and population health: A review and explanation of the evidence. *Soc Sci Med*. 2006 Apr;62(7):1768–1784.

6. Caldwell, JC. Routes to low mortality in poor countries. *Population and Development Review* 1986;12(2):171–220.

7. World Health Organization. *Primary Health Care: Report of the International Conference on Primary Health Care,* Alma-Ata, USSR, September 6–12, 1978. Geneva: World Health Organization;1978.

8. Frumkin H. Beyond toxicity: Human health and the natural environment. *Am J Prev Med.* 2001;20:234–240.

9. Simms A, Magrath J, Reid H, The Working Group on Climate Change and Development. *Up in Smoke? Threats from, and Responses to, the Impact of Global Warming on Human Development.* International Institute for Environment and Development and New Economics Foundation, October 2003. http://www.foe.co.uk/resource/reports/up_in_smoke.pdf.

Part Seven

War and Violence

Violence is ubiquitous among animal species, and deliberate, planned violence (sometimes using crude weapons) is common among non-human primates (especially chimpanzees and gorillas). However, humans, through advances in technology, have created a world in which conflicts within and between nations can involve killing on a massive scale, one that causes immense suffering and death, environmental destruction, and could potentially wipe us out.

Organized human warfare flowered around the time agriculture began approximately ten thousand years ago, a consequence of stable populations and the division of labor into farmers, herders, crafts people, rulers, and warriors. The warriors' function was to protect a community's land and goods but they, usually at the behest of the ruling class, also invaded other communities for their land and goods.

Warfare has evolved as weapons have "improved." Around 3,500 years ago, bronze weapons and armor were developed, followed by iron battle implements 2,200 years ago. About 1,900 years ago, horses were first used in battle, increasing soldiers' mobility and hence their killing power significantly. In the ninth century, the Chinese developed bombs, followed by rockets four centuries later (although significant advances in rocketry did not take place until the nineteenth century and most dramatically in the twentieth century). The balloon, invented by the Montgolfier brothers in 1783, was first used for aerial bombing by Prussian general J.C.G. Heyne. Just a decade after the Wright brothers'

Much of the material for the introduction to this part is derived from V. Sidel & B. Levy (eds.), *War and public health* (Oxford, UK: Oxford University Press), 2008.

flight at Kitty Hawk, the airplane was employed for aerial bombing in World War I and then for the catastrophic firebombing of cities and their civilian populations in World War II (e.g., Dresden and London). On August 6, 1945, the United States dropped an atomic bomb on Hiroshima, Japan, then three days later another on Nagasaki, causing over 140,000 immediate casualties and leaving hundreds of thousands of Hibakusha to suffer the long-term consequences of radiation exposure.

Throughout history, it was widely believed that each new development in killing would be so horrible as to render war obsolete. Instead, there were 250 wars in the twentieth century, most within poor states and a substantial number involving genocide. Casualties increased exponentially, from 11 per million population worldwide in the nineteenth century to 183 per million population in the twentieth century. The percentage of casualties among civilians has increased from 10 percent to 15 percent at the start of the twentieth century to 85 percent to 90 percent today. The greatest number of conflicts and deaths have recently taken place in sub-Saharan Africa.

Consequences of war for survivors include physical and psychological trauma; famine; collapse of health care systems affecting not only the injured but also those with acute and chronic diseases; environmental degradation, including damage to water supplies, which in turn promotes infectious disease outbreaks; refugees and internally displaced persons; and increasing poverty and the debt that accrues consequent to reconstruction costs. All of these sequelae of war lead, in turn, to recurrent cycles of violence.

Today, whereas many die through small arms fire, killing at a distance has become commonplace through the use of land mines, predator drones, and long-range ballistic missiles. The United States has conducted over one thousand nuclear missile tests since 1945, many involving hydrogen bombs, whose killing power is measured in megatons as compared to the kiloton weapons used during World War II. The National Cancer Institute and the Centers for Disease Control and Prevention have estimated that eighty thousand cancers (fifteen thousand of which were fatal) have occurred in US citizens as a result of this testing.

Today, there are approximately twenty-three thousand nuclear weapons in fourteen countries. There are more than 5,200 active US warheads today and another 8,000 in Russia. One-half of the US and one-quarter of the Russian weapons are on hair-trigger alert, meaning they can be fired and reach their targets in less than one hour, causing carnage of biblical proportions, followed by nuclear winter and its attendant crop losses and famine. The spread of nuclear technology and the presence of poorly guarded caches of fissile material have put nuclear weapons into the hands of unstable dictators and even, potentially, terrorists.

Other methods of horrific mass killing that have been studied or used include chemical and biological weapons. Chemical weapons were first employed by the Athenians and Spartans, who used burning wax, pitch, and sulfur; later, Leonardo da Vinci suggested the use of arsenic and sulfur shells. In World War I, chemical weapons were used by the Italians (against the Ethiopians), the Japanese (against the Chinese), and the Germans (against the allied forces). More recently chemical weapons were used by Egypt (against South Yemen) in the 1960s and in the Iran-Iraq War during the 1980s. Chemical weapons include nerve gasses and paralytics such as sarin and VX, blistering agents such as sulfur mustard and napalm (used as a defoliant in the Vietnam war, killing many civilians in the process), and pulmonary toxicants such as chlorine and phosgene.

Biological weapons were first employed when the Assyrians poisoned wells in the sixth century BC. In 300 BC, the Greeks polluted wells, as later did the Romans, Persians, and even General Johnson (at Vicksburg in the US Civil War). Sir Jeffrey Amherst, during the French and Indian Wars, suggested "inoculat[ing] the Indians, by means of blankets [taken from victims of smallpox] ... to extirpate this execrable race."[1] In World War I, cholera, plague, glanders, and anthrax were all used. During World War II, the British (in "Operation Vegetarian") contaminated Gruinard Island (off the coast of Scotland) with linseed cakes infected with anthrax. However, their plan to kill millions of Germans and wipe out German cattle was not carried out. Today, at least seventeen countries possess biological weapons. Between 1985 and 1989, despite Iraqi president Saddam Hussein's ongoing gas attacks against the Kurds, US companies sold Iraq a number of biological agents, including the organisms that cause anthrax and botulism; even so, no evidence of weapons of mass destruction were reported found during or subsequent to the 2003 allied invasion of Iraq.

New technologies being developed to wage war include acoustic, electrical, and optical weapons. The engagement of large amounts of brainpower to the military-industrial complex (on which about two-thirds of US scientists are to some degree dependent) represents a significant diversion of intellectual resources away from solving the many other critical problems facing humankind.

Wars are often rationalized as necessary roads to progress involving the subjugation of so-called inferior peoples. Sometimes the doctrine of subjugation is formalized, as in manifest destiny. Expansion and slavery are often casually accepted as the natural consequence of colonialism, in which a "superior" nation claims the right to subjugate another, "more primitive" people, as illustrated by the following comments of Cecil Rhodes (founder of Rhodesia, the DeBeers Mining Company, and the Rhodes Scholarship), in reference to Africa: "We must find new lands from which we can easily obtain raw materials and at the same time exploit the cheap slave labour that is available from the natives of the colonies. The colonies would also provide a dumping ground for the surplus goods produced in our factories."[2]

War, and the preparation for war, often involves (usually) involuntary experimentation on large numbers of soldiers and civilians. Physicians and other health professionals, in violation of the fundamental tenets of medical ethics, have often played a role in these experiments, from the torturous use of Nazi prisoners in amputation, hypothermia, irradiation, water deprivation, and vivisection "studies" to the equally heinous "investigations" carried out on Chinese prisoners by World War II Japanese physicians, who "studied" rapid centrifugation and deliberate infections with deadly pathogens. Physicians continue to play a role in torture (including during the so-called War on Terror). Many doctors have turned to terrorism, such as George Habbas (founder of the Popular Front for the Liberation of Palestine, the organization behind the aircraft hijackings of Black September), Mohammed al-Hindi (the founder of Islamic Jihad), Ikuo Hayashi (who pleaded guilty to planting sarin gas on a Tokyo subway in 1995), Radovan Karadžić (who stands accused of genocide against Bosnian Croats and Muslims), Syrian President Bashar al-Assad (who has bombed his own citizens), and Ayman al-Zawahiri (Al Qaeda's current leader, who succeeded Osama bin Laden).

War represents the ultimate failure of civilized society. Spending on war and militarism constitutes a large percentage of nations' budgets, taking resources away from education, health care, and other social services. Scientists are diverted from other, more productive forms of research. Countries at war see a rise in hate crimes, racism, and jingoism and the erosion of civil liberties. Although weapon manufacturers profit, international cooperation suffers because international agreements are put on hold. Those promoting peace are suspected of antigovernment activities, spied on, and even locked up.

Chapter Twenty-Six (by Victor W. Sidel and Barry S. Levy) explores some of the reasons behind the dramatically increasing amounts of money spent on war and the preparation for war. The authors cover the consequences of the diversion of resources to war and militarism and away from health care and social programs and suggest that funds be diverted toward meeting human needs and addressing the root causes of armed conflict.

Chapter Twenty-Seven (by Robert Vergun, Martin Donohoe, Catherine Thomasson, and Pamela Vergun) describes briefly, yet powerfully, the disturbing medical consequences of the atomic bombings of Hiroshima and Nagasaki. The magnitude of suffering involved, which would be dwarfed by the exponentially larger power of contemporary nuclear weapons, should convince readers that the only sane response to the threat of nuclear annihilation is abolition.

Chapter Twenty-Eight is a 1949 classic by Leo Alexander (Colonel, US Armed Forces, and an advisor to the Nuremberg war crimes prosecutors). Alexander describes in horrific detail the "experiments" conducted by Nazi physicians during World War II. His chapter raises a number of provocative ethical questions relevant to contemporary human subject experimentation and to the research enterprise in general. Alexander also explores how health care professionals can turn evil and rationalize using their knowledge and skills to inflict suffering.

Killing and use in "research" are not the only way in which populations are terrorized and subjugated in war. Other methods include the use of land mines, specifically in areas of good soil, to discourage farming and thereby lead to famine; the use of slave labor, as in the concentration camps of World War II (and more recently in the 1990s' conflicts in the former Yugoslavia); and rape, a subject reviewed in Chapter Twenty-Nine (by Martin Donohoe). This last chapter focuses on twentieth-century examples of violence against, and subjugation of, women; lists the health consequences of rape in war; discusses the dangers of refugee camps, which are supposed to provide safe havens for women; reviews relevant human rights principles and international agreements; and addresses the critical role that health professionals can play in confronting the atrocity of sexual assault in war.

Readers are encouraged to explore the many other articles, frequently updated open-access slide shows, and external links on the war and peace and human subject experimentation/torture/hunger strikes pages of the Public Health and Social Justice website at http://phsj.org/war-and-peace/ and http://phsj.org/human-subject-experimentation/, respectively. Here they will find more information about these topics as well as about the specific health, environmental, and human rights consequences of war; violence against women serving in the US armed services; the medical effects of various weapons of mass destruction; an overview of human subject experimentation abuses from World War II to the present; discussions of the Geneva Conventions, human rights, and the care of active duty military personnel; and the teaching of war and peace, particularly through great literature. Here one will also find perhaps the most moving plea for peace, Mark Twain's posthumously published *The War Prayer*.[3] It is hoped that readers will be inspired to work for peace and harmony and follow the advice of Dr. Martin Luther King Jr., who wrote, "Darkness cannot drive out darkness; only light can do that. Hate cannot drive out hate; only love can do that."[4] With love and courage and persistence, perhaps we can turn swords into plowshares and focus on solving the great problems of humankind, such as poverty, hunger, homelessness, environmental destruction, and the loneliness and despair that haunt so many.

Notes

1. Education: At Amherst. *TIME,* June 14, 1926. Retrieved from http://www.time
   .com/time/printout/0,8816,751545,00.html.

2. Rhodes, C. Quote. Retrieved from http://thinkexist.com/quotation/we_must_find
   _new_lands_from_which_we_can_easily/343653.html.

3. Twain, M. (Samuel Clemens). *The war prayer* (New York: Harper Collins, 1968;
   originally published in 1923).

4. King Jr., M. L. Quote. Retrieved from http://www.mlkonline.net/quotes.html.

Chapter 26

The Health Consequences of the Diversion of Resources to War and Preparation for War

Victor W. Sidel
Barry S. Levy

A rmed conflict damages health in many ways. These include death and disability directly caused by war, destruction of the societal infrastructure that supports health and safety, forced migration of people both within their own country and as refugees to other countries, promotion of violence as a method to settle conflicts and disputes, and the long-term adverse effects on social relationships.

This special issue of *Social Medicine* examines the impact of war on human health from a geographically diverse set of countries and from diverse perspectives. Dr. Andrea Angulo Menasse, a researcher from Mexico City's Autonomous University, documents the very personal story of how the violence of the Spanish Civil War affected one family. In her case study the trauma suffered by Spanish Republicans is traced through three generations and crosses the Atlantic Ocean as the family moves and is exiled in Mexico. Dr. Sachin Ghimire from the Centre of Social Medicine and Community Health of the Jawaharlal Nehru University reports on his fieldwork in Rolpa, Nepal, the district from which the Nepal Civil War (also called the People's War) originated in 1996. Based on 80 interviews, he documents the difficulties faced by health care workers as they negotiated the sometimes deadly task of remaining in communities where control alternated between Nepalese Special Forces and the Maoist rebels. Finally, Colombian researcher, Carlos Iván Pacheco Sánchez, from the University of Rosario in Bogota, brings an epidemiologist's tools to examine the impact of the ongoing armed conflict in the border Department of Nariño. His discussion is informed by the current debate over health care in Colombia where a recent Constitutional Court decision has found that the current health care system violates the right to health. These three papers amply demonstrate the depth, breadth, and relevance of contemporary social medicine.

While the direct effects of war are usually not subtle, less frequently discussed are the adverse consequences of the diversion of human and financial resources from the provision of medical, public health, and other human services to military spending for war and the preparation for war.

As President Dwight D. Eisenhower memorably said, "Every gun that is made, every warship launched, every rocket fired signifies, in the final sense, a theft from those who hunger and are not fed, those who are cold and are not clothed." But military spending does not just divert human and financial resources from meeting basic human needs. When military spending robs resources needed to address the problems of poverty, unemployment, social injustice, ethnic and racial tensions, and other socioeconomic and sociopolitical problems, it exacerbates the underlying causes of armed conflict. In this way, it undermines the very security it is called upon to protect.

Health workers recognize the connections between population health and reductions in government spending on education, housing, job creation, poverty reduction, environmental protection, public health, and medical care. And we understand the adverse effects of diverting resources from these purposes to war and preparation for war.

After a period of declining military expenditures following the end of the Cold War, worldwide military expenditures in current US dollars grew to $1.5 trillion in 2008, a 45 percent increase from 1999. Worldwide military expenditures amount to 2.4 percent of gross domestic product (GDP) worldwide, an average of $220 annually for every human being on the planet. Fifteen countries account for 81 percent of the total expenditures, with the United States accounting for 42 percent, distantly followed by China, the United Kingdom, France, Germany, and Japan.

Military Spending in the United States

Military spending by the United States increased from $289 billion in 1998 to $534 billion in 2009; this figure does not include about $130 billion annually to fund the wars in Afghanistan and Iraq. US military spending is currently almost seven times larger than the military spending of China, the world's second largest spender on arms, and more than the combined spending of the next 14 nations. The United States and its close allies account for about 70 percent of all military spending.

US military spending is not driven by actual defense needs. Rather, it responds to a demand created by arms manufacturers, politicians, and others to maintain jobs in military industries. The debate earlier this year over spending $1.8 billion for seven additional F-22 fighter planes illustrates the problem. These were weapons the US military said it did not need. Yet, the F-22's main contractor, Lockheed Martin, and its multiple subcontracting suppliers employ 25,000 workers in 44 US states and the sale was only narrowly defeated in the US Congress.

However, $1.8 billion is small compared to the $651 billion that will be spent on "defense" during this fiscal year. Many of the weapons systems included in this spending were developed during the Cold War; their continued production serves no purpose. Congressman Barney Frank argues that a 25 percent cut in military spending would still leave the United States immeasurably stronger than any combination of countries with whom we might be engaged in war. The argument that military spending is important because it preserves jobs and helps the economy is invalid. Many economists argue that spending on military hardware is one of the most inefficient ways to use public funds to stimulate the economy.

Diversion of human and financial resources from health and human services to military purposes in the United States becomes more apparent when one considers that in 2007 the United States ranked first among countries in military expenditures and arms exports, but only 30th in life expectancy at birth and 39th in infant mortality. The United States is the world's leader in arms sales to other countries, having in 2008 signed agreements to sell armaments valued at $38 billion, or 68 percent of global arms sales. The United States was not only the leader in worldwide arms sales but also the leader of sales to nations in developing countries, signing $30 billion in weapons agreements with those nations, or 70 percent of all such deals.

The United States has already spent over $600 billion in operational costs for the wars in Iraq and Afghanistan. These costs are now almost $3 billion a week. Even if US troops are quickly withdrawn, the total cost of the wars could reach $3 trillion, making these wars the most expensive US military effort since World War II.

The National Priorities Project collects current data on the total cost of the Iraq War and on the needed social and infrastructural improvements for which resources spent on the war could have been used. The project maintains a website (http://costofwar.com/) that provides a continually incremented statement of the tax-revenue cost of the Iraq War to the entire United States and to each state and county. The website also provides comparisons to the cost of hiring public school teachers, providing health care insurance to uninsured children, building public housing units, and providing other useful programs.

Developing Countries

Diversion of resources has been an important issue for many less-developed, or developing, countries. For example, in 1990, per-capita public expenditures for military purposes in Ethiopia was $16 and for health expenditures, $1. In Sudan, $25 was spent annually for military purposes per capita, but only $1 per capita for health. And in Angola, $114 was spent annually for military purposes per capita, but only $8 per capita for health.

More recent data demonstrate that this type of disparity, although not as extreme as in the above examples, still exists for many countries. For example, India spent 3.8 percent of its gross domestic product (GDP) for military expenditures in 2005 in contrast to 0.9 percent for public expenditures on health in 2004. Comparable data for Pakistan were 3.5 and 0.4 percent; Chile, 3.8 and 2.9 percent; Angola, 5.7 and 1.5 percent; and the Syrian Arab Republic, 5.1 and 2.2 percent. In stark contrast, Costa Rica, which abolished its military forces in 1949, spent 5.1 percent of its GDP for public health expenditures in 2004 and had no military expenditures.

The human development costs of arms imports are huge, as illustrated by some choices faced by developing countries in 1992. India in that year ordered 20 MiG-29 fighter aircraft from Russia at a cost that could have provided basic education to all 15 million girls out of school. Nigeria purchased 80 battle tanks from the United Kingdom at a cost that could have immunized two million children and provided family planning services to nearly 17 million couples. And China purchased 26 combat aircraft from Russia in a deal whose total cost could have provided safe water for 1 year to 140 million people.

From 1998 to 2007, military expenditures in South America rose from $23.3 to $32.0 billion in constant 2005 US dollars, a 38 percent increase. Brazil, the leading country in military expenditures in the region, is the only Latin American country in the top 15 countries in military expenditures. It spent $15.3 billion in 2007—$80 per capita. In recent years, there have been significant arms purchases by Brazil, Chile, and Venezuela. Between 2003 and 2007, Venezuela increased its arms purchases by 73 percent. Brazil also ranks high (30th between 2003 and 2007) among all countries in supplying major conventional weapons to other nations.

What Needs to Be Done

In view of the current economic crisis in the United States and the world, military expenditures are even more inexcusable than they have been and their transfer to socially useful purposes is even more necessary. The 2009 US budget presented by the Obama administration is an important first step in cutting military spending, but the US public's desire for "change" includes change from a half-century or more of unfettered militarism, unnecessary wars, and defense budgets, bloated far beyond legitimate defense needs, which are distortions of humane and healthy social responsibility.

Funds now used for military expenditures could be used in more socially responsible ways—not only to better meet human needs, but also to address the root causes of armed conflict. This special issue is being published on the first anniversary of the report of the WHO Commission on the Social Determinants of Health. The Commission issued a challenge to the international community that it eliminate health disparities within a generation. This is a bold vision and it will require resources. We assert that, rather than purchasing weapons and fighting wars, meeting the Commission's challenge is a far better way for countries to use their human and financial resources.

Chapter 27

A Brief Summary of the Medical Impacts of Hiroshima

Robert Vergun   Martin Donohoe   Catherine Thomasson
                                                Pamela Vergun

An estimated 140,000 people died in Hiroshima and 70,000 in Nagasaki by the end of 1945 as a result of the atomic bombs. Within the eight days Sadako Okuda spent searching for her niece and nephew immediately after the atomic explosion in Hiroshima, approximately 80,000 people died in that city.

The nuclear explosion created a fireball of superheated gas that emitted intense thermal radiation. At the hypocenter—the location below the explosion of the atomic bomb over Hiroshima—ground temperatures reached 3,000 to 4,000 degrees Celsius (approximately 5,400 to 7,200 degrees Fahrenheit). This was roughly equivalent to 50% to 70% of the temperature at the sun's surface. The Hiroshima bomb released the equivalent of about 15 kilotons of TNT[1] and therefore most people close to the hypocenter were literally blown apart by the power of the blast. However, the vast majority of deaths in Hiroshima were related to thermal injuries as a result of the extreme heat of the bomb, complicated by suffocation as the firestorm consumed all available oxygen in the air.

This summary was prepared in order to relate the research on medical impacts to the specific first-hand observations of Sadako Okuda and other *hibakusha,* and heavily draws upon Committee for the Compilation of Materials on Damage Caused by the Atomic Bombs in Hiroshima and Nagasaki. (1981). *Hiroshima and Nagasaki: The Physical, Medical, and Social Effects of the Atomic Bombings,* published in English by Hiroshima City and Nagasaki City (original Japanese report published in 1979 by Iwanami Shoten Publishers), pp. 30, 107, 113, 115, 118, 121, 126, 131–136, 140, 205. The eight-day mortality figure of 80,000 was estimated by Dr. Robert Vergun based upon the finding in this report that the number of deaths within each successive six-day period after the explosion decreased by approximately 50% (p. 107).

The primary thermal injuries were flash burns, which appeared on areas of the body that were unprotected from the rays of the thermal radiation, for example areas not covered by clothing. The other type of thermal injuries or burns were secondary ones, so called because these were injuries that came about indirectly, for example, as a result of the fires spreading through the buildings of the city. Many victims were besieged by flames and had difficulty escaping from the buildings burning and collapsing all around them. Some were blinded by radiation or deafened by the pressures of the blast.

People and objects that were situated very close to ground zero were instantaneously vaporized. Near the hypocenter of the explosion, the heat radiation threw permanent shadows of the people and objects onto surfaces like sidewalks that had been behind them.[2] Many of the victims near the hypocenter in the central district who received severe thermal burns suffered loosened skin that fell off in flaps. In addition, a brief and sudden but extreme fall in air pressure near the hypocenter caused people's eyeballs to pop out of their bodies. Sadako Okuda describes these victims in her memoir.

Because of extensive burns and high fevers, victims begged and pleaded for water. This situation was made worse because of the difficulty of getting water after the bombing, coupled with the sweltering humid heat of even an ordinary Hiroshima August day. According to Sadako's account, as well as the accounts of other survivors, there were rumors circulating in Hiroshima following the blast that providing water to these victims would kill them. Most Japanese soldiers, medical providers, and ordinary Hiroshima citizens did not understand the nature of the radiation and the injuries of the victims during the immediate hours and days following the blast. One possibility is that some people dissuaded others from providing water to the victims because of the belief that the ingestion of water would increase blood flow, which in turn would increase bleeding in these victims. While this may be the case, the most comprehensive and detailed compilation of the medical impacts of the atomic attack does not mention the consumption of water as a significant cause of acute death among Hiroshima victims.[3] Another possibility was the valid concern that the water itself was poisoned (by radiation, broken sewer systems, debris in the river), but the extent of many people's injuries was so great that poisoned water may not have hastened death by more than a few hours.

Many of the victims with thermal injuries also suffered crush injuries, lacerations (from shattered glass fragments, for example), bruises, and other wounds that failed to heal because of the harmful effects of the bomb's radioactivity on the body's immune and defense mechanisms. In particular, the radioactivity caused damage to bone marrow, suppressing not only the body's ability to produce white blood cells (leaving these immune-suppressed individuals extremely vulnerable to infection), but also suppressing platelet production (resulting in severe hemorrhage).

Deaths caused by infections that originated near broken, hemorrhaging skin were widespread in the days and weeks following the blast. Slow deaths caused by uncontrolled hemorrhaging in the mouth and pharynx areas were not uncommon, as Sadako Okuda witnessed.

Most health care professionals had been transported to the front and many who remained were killed or wounded in the blast. Thus, shortages of health care professionals, shortages of medicine, the destruction of transportation infrastructure and medical facilities, and pre-existing malnutrition from food shortages that existed in Hiroshima before the atomic bomb was dropped all combined to greatly aggravate the situation. For the vast majority of victims, even palliative care with narcotics for pain relief was unavailable. The horror of the devastation surrounding them surely must have compounded their final agonies.

Roughly 70% of Hiroshima's population that did not immediately die from the blast began to suffer nausea, vomiting, and/or lack of desire to eat within the first 24 hours. Radiation resulted in the death of cells (necrosis) throughout the body. Intestinal cell necrosis resulted in significant diarrhea in about 20% to 40% of the city's population. Gastrointestinal injuries generally impair the body's ability to absorb nutrients and therefore worsen the effects of malnutrition.

Among those who survived the first few weeks, 40% to 55% of Hiroshima victims began to experience hair falling out at the roots (epilation).

Ten to fifteen years after the explosion, almost one-fourth of survivors in Hiroshima developed cataracts. The most notable long-term impact, however, was the development of cancers.[4] Five to ten years after the explosion, doctors in Japan started seeing high rates of mortality from leukemia. Hiroshima and Nagasaki victims alive after five years who had experienced significant radiation exposure from the blast (equivalent to those less than 1.5 miles from the hypocenter) were about 50% more likely to die from leukemia compared to the general population in Japan.

Ten to fifteen years after the bombing there were high rates of mortality from other cancers (e.g., lung, stomach, liver, colon, bladder, thyroid, skin, multiple myeloma, breast, ovarian). Women who were 10 years old at the time of the blast and experienced significant radiation exposure were 25% more likely to die from cancers (other than leukemia) compared to non-exposed, age-matched women in the general population.

Among persons exposed in utero, about 25% who survived infancy suffered severe lifetime mental disability associated with abnormally small head circumferences (microcephaly).

All those who survived had a high risk of developing post-traumatic stress and other psychiatric illnesses. The costs of providing medical care and social services to victims of Hiroshima were borne by a Japanese economy weakened by the war.

Three days following the Hiroshima blast, a larger, 22 kiloton atomic bomb was dropped on Nagasaki, resulting in 70,000 deaths and similar short- and long-term health and societal consequences.

This summary cannot adequately survey all of the medical impacts of the atomic bombs dropped on Hiroshima and Nagasaki.[5] However, in discussing the historical, sociological, and political background surrounding the decision to drop the bomb, we should not lose sight of the magnitude of devastation seen in the raw numbers of people who were killed and injured in Hiroshima and Nagasaki. Furthermore, since we live in a world where the megatonnage of nuclear weapons vastly exceeds that of the Hiroshima and Nagasaki bombs combined, it is imperative that we work for peace and the abolition of these weapons of horrific suffering and mass destruction.

Notes

1. Malik, John S. (1985). "The Yields of the Hiroshima and Nagasaki Nuclear Explosions," *Los Alamos Report*, LA-8819.

2. Liebow, Averill A. (1970). *Encounter with Disaster: A Medical Diary of Hiroshima, 1945*. New York: W.W. Norton and Company, p. 124.

3. Committee for the Compilation of Materials on Damage Caused by the Atomic Bombs in Hiroshima and Nagasaki. (1981). *Hiroshima and Nagasaki: The Physical, Medical, and Social Effects of the Atomic Bombings*, published in English by Hiroshima City and Nagasaki City (original Japanese report published in 1979 by Iwanami Shoten Publishers).

4. Committee for the Compilation of Materials on Damage Caused by the Atomic Bombs in Hiroshima and Nagasaki. (1981). pp. 131, 218–219, 238–241. See also Pierce, D.A., Y. Shimizu, D.I Preston, M. Vaeth, and K. Mabuchi. (1996). "Studies of the Mortality of A-bomb Survivors: Part I (Cancer: 1950–1990)," *Radiation Research*, vol. 146, pp. 1–27; Thompson, D.E., K. Mabuchi, E. Ron, M. Soda, M. Tokunaga, S. Ochikubo, S. Sugimoto, T. Ikeda, M. Terasaki, S. Izumi, and D.L. Preston. (1994). "Cancer Incidence in Atomic Bomb Survivors: Part II (Solid Tumors: 1958–1987)," *Radiation Research*, vol. 137, pp. S17–S67; Preston, D.L., S. Kusumi, M. Tomonaga, S. Izumi, E. Ron, A. Kuramoto, N. Kamada, H. Dohy, T. Matsuo, H. Nonaka, D.E. Thompson, M. Soda, and K. Mabuchi. (1994). "Cancer Incidence in Atomic Bomb Survivors: Part III (Leukemia, Lymphoma and Multiple Myeloma: 1950–1987)," *Radiation Research*, vol. 137, pp. S68–S97. See also the website of the Hiroshima Peace Museum, www.pcf.city.hiroshima.jp.

5. For example, it refers only very briefly to the mental health impacts on Hiroshima survivors. For more on those impacts, see Lifton, Robert. (1991). *Death in Life: Survivors of Hiroshima*. Chapel Hill: University of North Carolina Press (reissued).

Chapter 28

Medical Science Under Dictatorship

Leo Alexander

Science under dictatorship becomes subordinated to the guiding philosophy of the dictatorship. Irrespective of other ideologic trappings, the guiding philosophic principle of recent dictatorships, including that of the Nazis, has been Hegelian in that what has been considered "rational utility" and corresponding doctrine and planning has replaced moral, ethical and religious values. Nazi propaganda was highly effective in perverting public opinion and public conscience, in a remarkably short time. In the medical profession this expressed itself in a rapid decline in standards of professional ethics. Medical science in Nazi Germany collaborated with this Hegelian trend particularly in the following enterprises: the mass extermination of the chronically sick in the interest of saving "useless" expenses to the community as a whole; the mass extermination of those considered socially disturbing or racially and ideologically unwanted; the individual, inconspicuous extermination of those considered disloyal within the ruling group; and the ruthless use of "human experimental material" for medico-military research.

This paper discusses the origins of these activities, as well as their consequences upon the body social, and the motivation of those participating in them.

Preparatory Propaganda

Even before the Nazis took open charge in Germany, a propaganda barrage was directed against the traditional compassionate nineteenth-century attitudes toward the chronically ill, and for the adoption of a utilitarian, Hegelian point of view. Sterilization and euthanasia of persons with chronic mental illnesses was discussed at a meeting of Bavarian psychiatrists in 1931.[1] By 1936 extermination of the physically or socially unfit was so openly accepted that its practice was mentioned incidentally in an article published in an official German medical journal.[2]

Lay opinion was not neglected in this campaign. Adults were propagandized by motion pictures, one of which, entitled "I Accuse," deals entirely with euthanasia. This film depicts the life history of a woman suffering from multiple sclerosis; in it her husband, a doctor, finally kills her to the accompaniment of soft piano music rendered by a sympathetic colleague in an adjoining room. Acceptance of this ideology was implanted even in the children. A widely used high-school mathematics text, *Mathematics in the Service of National Political Education*,[3] includes problems stated in distorted terms of the cost of caring for and rehabilitating "the chronically sick and crippled, the criminal and the insane.

Euthanasia

The first direct order for euthanasia was issued by Hitler on September 1, 1939, and an organization was set up to execute the program. Dr. Karl Brandt headed the medical section, and Phillip Bouhler the administrative section. All state institutions were required to report on patients who had been ill five years or more and who were unable to work, by filling out questionnaires giving name, race, marital status, nationality, next of kin, whether regularly visited and by whom, who bore financial responsibility and so forth. The decision regarding which patients should be killed was made entirely on the basis of this brief information by expert consultants, most of whom were professors of psychiatry in the key universities. These consultants never saw the patients themselves. The thoroughness of their scrutiny can be appraised by the work of one expert, who between November 14 and December 1, 1940, evaluated 2,109 questionnaires.

These questionnaires were collected by a "Realm's Work Committee of Institutions for Cure and Care."[4] A parallel organization devoted exclusively to the killing of children was known by the similarly euphemistic name of "Realm's Committee for Scientific Approach to Severe Illness Due to Heredity and Constitution." The "Charitable Transport Company for the Sick" transported patients to the killing centers, and the "Charitable Foundation for Institutional Care" was in charge of collecting the cost of the killings from the relatives, without, however, informing them what the charges were for; in the death certificates the cause of death was falsified.

What these activities meant to the population at large was well expressed by a few hardy souls who dared to protest. A member of the court of appeals at Frankfurt-am-Main wrote in December 1939:

There is constant discussion of the question of the destruction of socially unfit life—in the places where there are mental institutions, in neighboring towns, sometimes over a large area, throughout the Rhineland, for example. The people have come to recognize the vehicles in which the patients are taken from their original institution to the intermediate institution and from there to the liquidation institution. I am told that when they see these buses even the children call out: "They're taking some more people to be gassed." From Limburg it is reported that every day from one to three buses which, shades drawn, pass through on the way from Weilmunster to Hadamar, delivering inmates to the liquidation institution there. According to the stories the arrivals are immediately stripped to the skin, dressed in paper shirts, and forthwith taken to a gas chamber, where they are liquidated with hydro-cyanic acid gas and an added anesthetic. The bodies are reported to be moved to a combustion chamber by means of a conveyor belt, six bodies to a furnace. The resulting ashes are then distributed into six urns which are shipped to the families. The heavy smoke from the crematory building is said to be visible over Hadamar every day. There is talk, furthermore, that in some cases heads and other portions of the body are removed for anatomical examination. The people working at this liquidation job in the institutions are said to be assigned from other areas and are shunned completely by the populace. This personnel is described as frequenting the bars at night and drinking heavily. Quite apart from these overt incidents that exercise the imagination of the people, they are disquieted by the question of whether old folk who have worked hard all their lives and may merely have come into their dotage are also being liquidated. There is talk that the homes for the aged are to be cleaned out too. The people are said to be waiting for legislative regulation providing some orderly method that will insure especially that the aged feeble-minded are not included in the program.

Here one sees what "euthanasia" means in actual practice. According to the records, 275,000 people were put to death in these killing centers. Ghastly as this seems, it should be realized that this program was merely the entering wedge for exterminations for far greater scope in the political program for genocide of conquered nations and the racially unwanted. The methods used and personnel trained in the killing centers for the chronically sick became the nucleus of the much larger centers on the East, where the plan was to kill all Jews and Poles and to cut down the Russian population by 30,000,000.

The original program developed by Nazi hot-heads included also the genocide of the English, with the provision that the English males were to be used as laborers in the vacated territories in the East, there to be worked to death, whereas the English females were to be brought into Germany to improve the qualities of the German race. (This was indeed a peculiar admission of the part of the German eugenists.)

In Germany the exterminations included the mentally defective, psychotics (particularly schizophrenics), epileptics and patients suffering from infirmities of old age and from various organic neurologic disorders such as infantile paralysis, Parkinsonism, multiple sclerosis and brain tumors. The technical arrangements, methods and training of the killer personnel were under the direction of a committee of physicians and other experts headed by Dr. Karl Brandt. The mass killings were first carried out with carbon monoxide gas, but later cyanide gas ("cyclon B") was found to be more effective. The idea of camouflaging the gas chambers as shower baths was developed by Brack, who testified before Judge Sebring that the patients walked in calmly, deposited their towels and stood with their little pieces of soap under the shower outlets, waiting for the water to start running. This statement was ample rebuttal of his claim that only the most severely regressed patients among the mentally sick and only the moribund ones among the physically sick were exterminated. In truth, all those unable to work and considered nonrehabilitable were killed.

All but their squeal was utilized. However, the program grew so big that even scientists who hoped to benefit from the treasure of material supplied by this totalitarian method were disappointed. A neuropathologist, Dr. Hallervorden, who had obtained 500 brains from the killing centers for the insane, gave me a vivid first-hand account.[5] The Charitable Transport Company for the Sick brought the brains in batches of 150 to 250 at a time. Hallervorden stated:

> There was wonderful material among those brains, beautiful mental defectives, malformations and early infantile diseases. I accepted those brains of course. Where they came from and how they came to me was really none of my business.

In addition to the material he wanted, all kinds of other cases were mixed in, such as patients suffering from various types of Parkinsonism, simple depressions, involutional depressions and brain tumors, and all kinds of other illnesses, including psychopathy that had been difficult to handle:

> These were selected from the various wards of the institutions according to an excessively simple and quick method. Most institutions did not have enough physicians, and what physicians there were either too busy or did not care, and they delegated the selection to the nurses and attendants. Whoever looked sick or was otherwise a problem was put on a list and was transported to the killing center. The worst thing about this business was that it produced a certain brutalization of the nursing personnel. They got to simply picking out those whom they did not like, and the doctors had so many patients that they did not even know them, and put their names on the list.

Of the patients thus killed, only the brains were sent to Dr. Hallervorden; they were killed in such large numbers that autopsies of the bodies were not feasible. That, in Dr. Hallervorden's opinion, greatly reduced the scientific value of the material. The brains, however, were always well fixed and suspended in formalin, exactly according to his instructions. He thinks that the cause of psychiatry was permanently injured by these activities, and that psychiatrists have lost the respect of the German people forever. Dr. Hallervorden concluded: "Still, there were interesting cases in this material."

In general only previously hospitalized patients were exterminated for reasons of illness. An exception is a program carried out in a northwestern district of Poland, the "Warthegau," where a health survey of the entire population was made by an "S.S. X-Ray Battalion" headed by Professor Hohlfelder, radiologist of the University of Frankfurt-am-main. Persons found to be infected with tuberculosis were carted off to special extermination centers.

It is rather significant that the German people were considered by their Nazi leaders more ready to accept the exterminations of the sick than those for political reasons. It was for that reason that the first exterminations of the latter group were carried out under the guise of sickness. So-called "psychiatric experts" were dispatched to survey the inmates of camps with the specific order to pick out members of racial minorities and political offenders from occupied territories and to dispatch them to killing centers with specially made diagnoses such as that of "inveterate German hater" applied to a number of prisoners who had been active in the Czech underground.

Certain classes of patients with mental diseases who were capable of performing labor, particularly members of the armed forces suffering from psychopathy or neurosis, were sent to concentration camps to be worked to death, or to be reassigned to punishment battalions and to be exterminated in the process of removal of mine fields.[6]

A large number of those marked for death for political or racial reasons were made available for "medical" experiments involving the use of involuntary human subjects. From 1942 on, such experiments carried out in concentration camps were openly presented at medical meetings. This program included "terminal human experiments," a term introduced by Dr. Rascher to denote an experiment so designed that its successful conclusion depended upon the test person's being put to death.

The Science of Annihilation

A large part of this research was devoted to the science of destroying and preventing life, for which I have proposed the term "ktenology," the science of killing.[7-9] In the course of this ktenologic research, methods of mass killing and mass sterilization were investigated and developed for use against non-German peoples or Germans who were considered useless.

Sterilization methods were widely investigated, but proved impractical in experiments conducted in concentration camps. A rapid method developed for sterilization of females, which could be accomplished in the course of a regular health examination, was the intra-uterine injection of various chemicals. Numerous mixtures were tried, some with iodopine and others containing barium; another was most likely silver nitrate with iodized oil, because the result could be ascertained by x-ray examination. The injections were extremely painful, and a number of women died in the course of the experiments. Professor Karl Clauberg reported that he had developed a method at the Auschwitz concentration camp by which he could sterilize 1,000 women in one day.

Another method of sterilization, or rather castration, was proposed by Viktor Brack especially for conquered populations. His idea was that x-ray machinery could be built into desks at which the people would have to sit, ostensibly to fill out a questionnaire requiring five minutes; they would be sterilized without being aware of it. This method failed because experiments carried out on 100 male prisoners brought out the fact that severe x-ray burns were produced on all subjects. In the course of this research, which was carried out by Dr. Horst Schuman, the testicles of the victims were removed for histologic examination two weeks later. I myself examined 4 castrated survivors of this ghastly experiment. Three had extensive necrosis of the skin near the genitalia, and the other an extensive necrosis of the urethra. Other experiments in sterilization used an extract of the plant caladium seguinum, which had been shown in animal studies by Madaus and his co-workers[10,11] to cause selective necrosis of the germinal cells of the testicles as well as the ovary.

The development of methods for rapid and inconspicuous individual execution was the objective of another large part of the ktenologic research. These methods were to be applied to members of the ruling group, including the SS itself, who were suspected of disloyalty. This, of course, is an essential requirement in a dictatorship, in which ''cut-throat competition'' becomes a grim reality, and any hint of faintheartedness or lack of enthusiasm for the methods of totalitarian rule is considered a threat to the entire group.

Poisons were the subject of many of these experiments. A research team at the Buchenwald concentration camp, consisting of Drs. Joachim Mrugowsky, Erwin Ding-Schuler and Waldemar Hoven, developed the most widely used means of individual execution under the guise of medical treatment—namely, the intravenous injection of phenol or gasoline. Several alkaloids were also investigated, among them aconitine, which was used by Dr. Hoven to kill several imprisoned former fellow SS men who were potential witnesses against the camp commander, Koch, then under investigation by the SS. At the Dachau concentration camp Dr. Rascher developed the standard cyanide capsules, which could be easily bitten through, either deliberately or accidentally, if mixed with certain foods, and which, ironically enough, later became the means with which Himmler and Goering killed themselves. In connection with these poison experiments there is an interesting incident of characteristic sociologic significance. When Dr. Hoven was under trial by the SS the investigating SS judge, Dr. Morgen, proved Hoven's guilt by feeding the poison found in Dr. Hoven's possession to a number of Russian prisoners of war; these men died with the same symptoms as the SS men murdered by Dr. Hoven. This worthy judge was rather proud of this efficient method of proving Dr. Hoven's guilt and appeared entirely unaware of the fact that in the process he had committed murder himself.

Poisons, however, proved too obvious or detectable to be used for the elimination of high-ranking Nazi party personnel who had come into disfavor, or of prominent prisoners whose deaths should appear to stem from natural causes. Phenol or gasoline, for instance, left a telltale odor with the corpses. For this reason a number of more subtle methods were devised. One of these was artificial production of septicemia. An intramuscular injection of 1 cc. of pus, containing numerous chains of streptococci, was the first step. The site of injection was usually the inside of the thigh, close to the adductor canal. When an abscess formed it was tapped, and 3 cc. of the creamy pus removed was injected intravenously into the patient's opposite arm. If the patient then died from septicemia, the autopsy proved that death was caused by the same organism that had caused the abscess. These experiments were carried out in many concentration camps. At Dachau camp the subjects were almost exclusively Polish Catholic priests. However, since this method did not always cause death, sometimes resulting merely in a local abscess, it was considered inefficient, and research was continued with other means but along the same lines.

The final triumph of the part of ktenologic research aimed at finding a method of inconspicuous execution that would produce autopsy findings indicative of death from natural causes was the development of repeated intravenous injections of suspensions of live tubercle bacilli, which brought on acute miliary tuberculosis within a few weeks. This method was produced by Professor Dr. Heissmeyer, who was one of Dr. Gebhardt's associates at the SS hospital of Hohenlychen. As a means of further camouflage, so that the SS at large would not suspect the purpose of these experiments, the preliminary tests for the efficacy of this method were performed exclusively on children imprisoned in the Neuengamme concentration camp.

For use in "medical" executions of prisoners and of members of the SS and other branches of the German armed forces the use of simple lethal injections, particularly phenol injections, remained the instrument of choice. Whatever methods he used, the physician gradually became the unofficial executioner, for the sake of convenience, informality and relative secrecy. Even on German submarines it was the physician's duty to execute the troublemakers among the crew by lethal injections.

Medical science has for some time been an instrument of military power in that it preserved the health and fighting efficiency of troops. This essentially defensive purpose is not inconsistent with the ethical principles of medicine. In World War I the German empire had enlisted medical science as an instrument of aggressive military power by putting it to use in the development of gas warfare. It was left to the Nazi dictatorship to make medical science into an instrument of political power—a formidable, essential tool in the complete and effective manipulation of totalitarian control. This should be a warning to all civilized nations, and particularly to individuals who are blinded by the "efficiency" of a totalitarian rule, under whatever name.

This entire body of research as reported so far served the master crime to which the Nazi dictatorship was committed—namely, the genocide of non-German peoples and the elimination by killing, in groups or singly, of Germans who were considered useless or disloyal. In effecting the two parts of this program, Himmler demanded and received the co-operation of physicians and of German medical science. The result was a significant advance in the science of killing, or ktenology.

Medico-Military Research

Another chapter in Nazi scientific research was that aimed to aid the military forces. Many of these ideas originated with Himmler, who fancied himself a scientist.

When Himmler learned that the cause of death of most SS men on the battlefield was hemorrhage, he instructed Dr. Sigmund Rascher to search for a blood coagulant that might be given before the men went into action. Rascher tested this coagulant when it was developed by clocking the number of drops emanating from freshly cut amputation stumps of living and conscious prisoners at the crematorium of Dachau concentration camp and by shooting Russian prisoners of war through the spleen.

Live dissections were a feature of another experimental study designed to show the effects of explosive decompression.[12-14] A mobile decompression chamber was used. It was found that when subjects were made to descend from altitudes of 40,000 to 60,000 feet without oxygen, severe symptoms of cerebral dysfunction occurred—at first convulsions, then unconsciousness in which the body was hanging limp and later, after wakening, temporary blindness, paralysis or severe confusional twilight states. Rascher, who wanted to find out whether these symptoms were due to anoxic changes or to other causes, did what appeared to him the most simple thing: he placed the subjects of the experiment under water and dissected them while the heart was still beating, demonstrating air embolism in the blood vessels of the heart, liver, chest wall and brain.

Another part of Dr. Rascher's research, carried out in collaboration with Holzlochner and Finke, concerned shock from exposure to cold.[15] It was known that military personnel generally did not survive immersion in the North Sea for more than 60 to 100 minutes. Rascher therefore attempted to duplicate these conditions at Dachau concentration camp and used about 300 prisoners in experiments on shock from exposure to cold; of these 80 or 90 were killed. (The figures do not include persons killed during mass experiments on exposure to cold outdoors.) In one report on this work Rascher asked permission to shift these experiments from Dachau to Auschwitz, a larger camp where they might cause less disturbance because the subjects shrieked from pain when their extremities froze white. The results, like so many of those obtained in the Nazi research program, are not dependable. In his report Rascher stated that it took from 53 to 100 minutes to kill a human being by immersion in ice water—a time closely in agreement with the known survival period in the North Sea. Inspection of his own experimental records and statements made to me by his close associates showed that it actually took from 80 minutes to five or six hours to kill an undressed person in such a manner, whereas a man in full aviator's dress took six or seven hours to kill. Obviously, Rascher dressed up his findings to forestall criticism, although any scientific man should have known that during actual exposure many other factors, including greater convection of heat due to the motion of water, would affect the time of survival.

Another series of experiments gave results that might have been an important medical contribution if an important lead had not been ignored. The efficacy of various vaccines and drugs against typhus was tested at the Buchenwald and Natzweiler concentration camps. Prevaccinated persons and nonvaccinated controls were injected with live typhus rickettsias, and the death rates of the two series compared. After a certain number of passages, the Matelska strain of typhus rickettsia proved to become avirulent for man. Instead of seizing upon this as a possibility to develop a live vaccine, the experimenters, including the chief consultant, Professor Gerhard Rose, who should have known better, were merely annoyed at the fact that the controls did not die either, discarded this strain and continued testing their relatively ineffective dead vaccines against a new virulent strain. This incident shows that the basic unconscious motivation and attitude has a great influence in determining the scientist's awareness of the phenomena that pass through his vision.

Sometimes human subjects were used for tests that were totally unnecessary, or whose results could have been predicted by simple chemical experiments. For example, 90 gypsies were given unaltered sea water and sea water whose taste was camouflaged as their sole source of fluid, apparently to test the well known fact that such hypertonic saline solutions given as the only source of supply of fluid will cause severe physical disturbance or death within six to twelve days. These persons were subjected to the tortures of the damned, with death resulting in at least two cases.

Heteroplastic transplantation experiments were carried out by Professor Dr. Karl Gebhardt at Himmler's suggestion. Whole limbs—shoulder, arm or leg—were amputated from live prisoners at Ravensbrucck concentration camp, wrapped in sterile moist dressings and sent by automobile to the SS hospital at Hohenlychen, where Professor Gebhardt busied himself with a futile attempt at heteroplastic transplantation. In the meantime the prisoners deprived of limb were usually killed by lethal injection.

One would not be dealing with German science if one did not run into manifestations of the collector's spirit. By February 1942, it was assumed in German scientific circles that the Jewish race was about to be completely exterminated, and alarm was expressed over the fact that only very few specimens of skulls and skeletons of Jews were at the disposal of science. It was therefore proposed that a collection, 150 body casts and skeletons of Jews, be preserved for perusal by future students of anthropology. Dr. August Hirt, professor of anatomy at the University of Strassburg, declared himself interested in establishing such a collection at his anatomic institute. He suggested that captured Jewish officers of the Russian armed forces be included, as well as females from Auschwitz concentration camp; that they be brought alive to Natzweiler concentration camp near Strassburg; and that after "their subsequently induced death — care should be taken that the heads not be damaged [sic]" the bodies be turned over to him at the anatomic institute of the University of Strassburg. This was done. The entire collection of bodies and the correspondence pertaining to it fell into the hands of the United States Army.

One of the most revolting experiments was the testing of sulfonamides against gas gangrene by Professor Gebhardt and his collaborators, for which young women captured from the Polish Resistance Movement served as subjects. Necrosis was produced in a muscle of the leg by ligation and the wound was infected with various types of gas-gangrene bacilli; frequently, dirt, pieces of wood and glass splinters were added to the wound. Some of these victims died, and others sustained severe mutilating deformities of the leg.

Motivation

An important feature of the experiments performed in concentration camps is the fact that they not only represented a ruthless and callous pursuit of legitimate scientific goals but also were motivated by rather sinister practical ulterior political and personal purposes, arising out of the requirements and problems of the administration of totalitarian rule.

Why did men like Professor Gebhardt lend themselves to such experiments? The reasons are fairly simple and practical, no surprise to anyone familiar with the evidence of fear, hostility, suspicion, rivalry and intrigue, the fratricidal struggle euphemistically termed the "self-selection of leaders," that went on within the ranks of the ruling Nazi party and the SS. The answer was fairly simple and logical. Dr. Gebhardt performed these experiments to clear himself of the suspicion that he had been contributing to the death of SS General Reinhard ("The Hangman") Heydrich, either negligently or deliberately, by failing to treat his wound infection with sulfonamides. After Heydrich died from gas gangrene, Himmler himself told Dr. Gebhardt that the only way in which he could prove that Heydrich's death was "fate-determined" was by carrying out a "large-scale experiment" in prisoners, which would prove or disprove that people died from gas gangrene irrespective of whether they were treated sulfonamides or not.

Dr. Sigmund Rascher did not become the notorious vivisectionist of Dachau concentration camp and the willing tool of Himmler's research interests until he had been forbidden to use the facilities of the Pathological Institute of the University of Munich because he was suspected of having Communist sympathies. Then he was ready to go all out and to do anything merely to regain acceptance by the Nazi party and the SS.

These cases illustrate a method consciously and methodically used in the SS, an age-old method used by criminal gangs everywhere: that of making suspects of disloyalty clear themselves by participation in a crime that would definitely and irrevocably tie them to the organization. In the SS this process of reinforcement of group cohesion was called "Blutkitt" (blood-cement), a term that Hitler himself is said to have obtained from a book on Genghis Khan in which this technic was emphasized.

The important lesson here is that this motivation, with which one is familiar in ordinary crimes, applies also to war crimes and to ideologically conditioned crimes against humanity—namely, that fear and cowardice, especially fear of punishment or of ostracism by the group, are often more important motives than simple ferocity or aggressiveness.

The Early Change in Medical Attitudes

Whatever proportions these crimes finally assumed, it became evident to all who investigated them that they had started from small beginnings. The beginnings at first were merely a subtle shift in emphasis in the basic attitude of the physicians. It started with the acceptance of the attitude, basic in the euthanasia movement, that there is such a thing as life not worthy to be lived. This attitude in its early stages concerned itself merely with the severely and chronically sick. Gradually the sphere of those to be included in this category was enlarged to encompass the socially unproductive, the ideologically unwanted, the racially unwanted and finally all non-Germans. But it is important to realize that the infinitely small wedged-in lever from which this entire trend of mind received its impetus was the attitude toward the nonrehabilitable sick.

It is, therefore, this subtle shift in emphasis of the physicians' attitude that one must thoroughly investigate. It is a recent significant trend in medicine, including psychiatry, to regard prevention as more important than cure. Observation and recognition of early signs and symptoms have become the basis for prevention of further advance of disease.[16]

In looking for these early signs one may well retrace the early steps of propaganda on the part of the Nazis in Germany as well as in the countries that they overran and in which they attempted to gain supporters by means of indoctrination, seduction and propaganda.

The Example of Successful Resistance by the Physicians of the Netherlands

There is no doubt that in Germany itself the first and most effective step of propaganda within the medical profession was the propaganda barrage against the useless, incurably sick described above. Similar, even more subtle efforts were made in some of the occupied countries. It is to the everlasting honour of the medical profession of Holland that they recognized the earliest and most subtle phases of this attempt and rejected it. When the Seiss-Inquart, Reich Commissar for the Occupied Netherlands Territories, wanted to draw the Dutch physicians into the orbit of the activities of the German medical profession, he did not tell them, "You must send your chronic patients to death factories at government request in your offices," but he couched his order in most careful and superficially acceptable terms. One of the paragraphs in the order of the Reich Commissar of the Netherlands Territories concerning the Netherlands doctors of 19 December 1941 reads as follow:

> It is the duty of the doctor, through advice and effort conscientiously and to his best ability to assist as helper the person entrusted to his care in the maintenance, improvement and re-establishment of his vitality, physical efficiency and health. The accomplishment of this duty is a public task.

The physicians of Holland rejected this order unanimously because they saw what it actually meant—namely, the concentration of their efforts on mere rehabilitation of the sick for useful labour, and abolition of medical secrecy. Although on the surface the new order appeared not too grossly unacceptable, the Dutch physicians decided that it is the first although slight, step away from principle that is the most important one. The Dutch physicians declared that they would not obey this order. When Seiss-Inquart threatened them with revocation of their licenses, they returned their licenses, removed their shingles and, while seeing their own patients secretly, no longer wrote death or birth certificates. Seiss-Inquart retraced his steps and tried to cajole them still to no effect. Then he arrested 100 Dutch physicians and sent them to concentration camps.

The medical profession remained adamant and quietly took care of their widows and orphans, but would not give in. Thus it came about that not a single euthanasia or non-therapeutic sterilization was recommended or participated in by any Dutch physician. They had the foresight to resist before the first step was taken, and they acted unanimously and won out in the end.

It is obvious that if the medical profession of a small nation under the conqueror's heel could resist so effectively the German medical profession could likewise have resisted had they not taken the fatal first step.

It is the first seemingly innocent step away from principle that frequently decides a career of crime. Corrosion begins in microscopic proportions.

The Situation in the United States

The question that this fact prompts is whether there are any danger signs that American physicians have also been infected with Hegelian, cold-blooded, utilitarian philosophy and whether early traces of it can be detected in their medical thinking that may make them vulnerable to departures of the type that occurred in Germany. Basic attitudes must be examined dispassionately. The original concept of medicine and nursing was not based on any rational or feasible likelihood that they could actually cure and restore but rather on an essentially maternal or religious idea. The Good Samaritan had no thought of nor did he actually care whether he could restore working capacity. He was merely motivated by the compassion in alleviating suffering. Bernal[17] states that prior to the advent of scientific medicine, the physician's main function was to give hope to the patient and to relieve his relatives of responsibility. Gradually, in all civilized countries, medicine has moved away from this position, strangely enough in direct proportion to man's actual ability to perform feats that would have been plain miracles in days of old. However, with this increased efficiency based on scientific development went a subtle change in attitude. Physicians have become dangerously close to being mere technicians of rehabilitation. This essentially Hegelian rational attitude has led them to make certain distinctions in the handling of acute and chronic diseases. The patient with the latter carries an obvious stigma as the one less likely to be fully rehabilitable for social usefulness. In an increasingly utilitarian society these patients are being looked down upon with increasing definiteness as unwanted ballast. A certain amount of rather open contempt for the people who cannot be rehabilitated with present knowledge has developed. This is probably due to a good deal of unconscious hostility, because these people for whom there seem to be no effective remedies have become a threat to newly acquired delusions of omnipotence.

Hospitals like to limit themselves to the care of patients who can be fully rehabilitated, and the patient whose full rehabilitation is unlikely finds himself, at least in the best and most advanced centers of healing, as a second-class patient faced with a reluctance on the part of both the visiting and the house staff to suggest and apply therapeutic procedures that are not likely to bring about immediately striking results in terms of recovery. I wish to emphasize that this point of view did not arise primarily within the medical profession, which has always been outstanding in a highly competitive economic society for giving freely and unstintingly of its time and efforts, but was imposed by the shortage of funds available, both private and public. From the attitude of easing patients with chronic diseases away from the doors of the best types of treatment facilities available to the actual dispatching of such patients to killing centers is a long but nevertheless logical step. Resources for the so-called incurable patient have recently become practically unavailable.

There has never in history been a shortage of money for the development and manufacture of weapons of war; there is and should be none now. The disproportion of monetary support for war and that available for healing and care is an anachronism in an era that has been described as the "enlightened age of the common man" by some observers. The comparable cost of jet planes and hospital beds is too obvious for any excuse to be found for a shortage of the latter. I trust that these remarks will not be misunderstood. I believe that armament, including jet planes, is vital for the security of the republic, but adequate maintenance of standards of health and alleviation of suffering are equally vital, both from a practical point of view and from that of morale. All who took part in induction-board examinations during the war realize that the maintenance and development of national health is of as vital importance as the maintenance and development of armament.

The trend of development in the facilities available for the chronically ill outlined above will not necessarily be altered by public or state medicine. With provision of public funds in any setting of public activity the question is bound to come up, "Is it worth while to spend a certain amount of effort to restore a certain type of patient?" This rationalistic point of view has insidiously crept into the motivation of medical effort, supplanting the old Hippocratic point of view. In emergency situations, military or otherwise, such grading of effort may be pardonable. But doctors must beware lest such attitudes creep into the civilian public administration of medicine entirely outside emergency situations, because once such considerations are at all admitted, the more often and the more definitely the question is going to be asked, "Is it worth while to do this or that for this type of patient?" Evidence of the existence of such an attitude stared at me from a report on the activities of a leading public hospital unit, which stated rather proudly that certain treatments were given only when they appeared promising: "Our facilities are such that a case load of 20 patients is regularly carried ... in selecting cases for treatment careful consideration is given to the prognostic criteria, and in no instance have we instituted treatment merely to satisfy relatives or our own consciences." If only those whose treatment is worth while in terms of prognosis are to be treated, what about the other ones? The doubtful patients are the ones whose recovery appears unlikely, but frequently if treated energetically, they surprise the best prognosticators. And what shall be done during that long time lag after the disease has been called incurable and the time of death and autopsy? It is that period during which it is most difficult to find hospitals and other therapeutic organizations for the welfare and alleviation of suffering of the patient.

Under all forms of dictatorship the dictating bodies or individuals claim that all that is done is being done for the best of the people as a whole, and that for that reason they look at health merely in terms of utility, efficiency and productivity. It is natural in such a setting that eventually Hegel's principle that "what is useful is good" wins out completely. The killing center is the reductio ad absurdum of all health planning based only on rational principles and economy and not on humane compassion and divine law. To be sure, American physicians are still far from the point of thinking of killing centers, but they have arrived at a danger point in thinking, at which likelihood of full rehabilitation is considered a factor that should determine the amount of time, effort and cost to be devoted to a particular type of patient on the part of the social body upon which this decision rests. At this point Americans should remember that the enormity of a euthanasia movement is present in their own midst. To the psychiatrist it is obvious that this represents the eruption of unconscious aggression on the part of certain administrators alluded to above, as well as on the part of relatives who have been understandably frustrated by the tragedy of illness in its close interaction upon their own lives. The hostility of a father erupting against his feebleminded son is understandable and should be considered from the psychiatric point of view, but it certainly should not influence social thinking. The development of effective analgesics and pain-relieving operations has taken even the last rationalization away from the supporters of euthanasia.

The case, therefore, that I should like to make is that American medicine must realize where it stands in its fundamental premises. There can be no doubt that in a subtle way the Hegelian premise of "what is useful is right" has infected society, including the medical portion. Physicians must return to the older premises, which were the emotional foundation and driving force of an amazingly successful quest to increase powers of healing if they are not held down to earth by the pernicious attitudes of an overdone practical realism.

What occurred in Germany may have been the inexorable historic progression that the Greek historians have described as the law of the fall of civilizations and that Toynbee[18] has convincingly confirmed—namely, that there is a logical sequence from Koros to Hybris to Atc, which means from surfeit to disdainful arrogance to disaster, the surfeit being increased scientific and practical accomplishments, which, however, brought about an inclination to throw away the old motivations and values by disdainful arrogant pride in practical efficiency. Moral and physical disaster is the inevitable consequence.

Fortunately, there are developments in this democratic society that counteract these trends. Notable among them are the societies of patients afflicted with various chronic diseases that have sprung up and are dedicating themselves to guidance and information for their fellow sufferers and for the support and stimulation of medical research. Among the earliest was the mental-hygiene movement, founded by a former patient with mental disease. Then came the National Foundation for Infantile Paralysis, the tuberculosis societies, the American Epilepsy League, the National Association to Control Epilepsy, the American Cancer Society, the American Heart Association, Alcoholics Anonymous and, most recently the National Multiple Sclerosis Society. All these societies, which are coordinated with special medical societies and which received inspiration and guidance from outstanding physicians, are having an extremely wholesome effect in introducing fresh motivating power into the ivory towers of academic medicine. It is indeed interesting and an assertion of democratic vitality that these societies are activated by and for people suffering from illnesses who, under certain dictatorships, would have been slated for euthanasia.

It is thus that these new societies have taken over one of the ancient functions of medicine — namely, to give hope to the patient and to relieve his relatives. These societies need the whole-hearted support of the medical profession. Unfortunately, this support is by no means yet unanimous. A distinguished physician, investigator and teacher at an outstanding university recently told me that he was opposed to these special societies and clinics because they had nothing to offer to the patient. It would be better to wait until someone made a discovery accidentally and then start clinics. It is my opinion, however, that one cannot wait for that. The stimulus supplied by these societies is necessary to give stimulus both to public demand and to academic medicine, which at times grows stale and unproductive even in its most outstanding centers, and whose existence did nothing to prevent the executioner from having logic on his side in Germany.

Another element of this free democratic society and enterprise that has been a stimulus to new developments is the pharmaceutical industry, which, with great vision, has invested considerable effort in the sponsorship of new research.

Dictatorships can be indeed defined as systems in which there is a prevalence of thinking in destructive rather than in ameliorative terms in dealing with social problems. The ease with which destruction of life is advocated for those considered either socially useless or socially disturbing instead of educational or ameliorative measures may be the first danger sign of loss of creative liberty in thinking, which is the hallmark of democratic society. All destructiveness ultimately leads to self-destruction; the fate of the SS and of Nazi Germany is an eloquent example. The destructive principle, once unleashed, is bound to engulf the whole personality and to occupy all its relationships. Destructive urges and destructive concepts arising therefrom cannot remain limited or focused upon one subject or several subjects alone, but must inevitable spread and be directed against one's entire surrounding world, including one's own group and ultimately the self. The ameliorative point of view maintained in relation to all others is the only real means of self-preservation.

A most important need in this country is for the development of active and alert hospital centers for the treatment of chronic illnesses. They must have active staffs similar to those of the hospitals for acute illnesses, and these hospitals must be fundamentally different from the custodial repositories for derelicts, of which there are too many in existence today. Only thus can one give the right answer to divine scrutiny: Yes, we are our brothers' keepers.

Notes

1. Bumke, O. Discussion of Faltlhauser, K. Zur Frage der Sterilisierung geistig Abnormer, *Allg. Zischr. J. Psychiat.*, 96:372, 1932.

2. Dierichs, R. Beitrag zur psychischen Anstaltsbehandlung Tuberkuloser, *Zischr. f. Tuberk.*, 74:24–28, 1936.

3. Dorner, A. *Mathematik in dienste der Nationalpolitischen Erziehung: Ein Handbuch fur Lehrer, herausgegeben in Auftrage des Reichsverbandes Deutcher mathematischer Gesellschaften und Vereine.* Second edition (revised). Frankfurt: Moritz Diesterweg, 1935. Pp. 1–118. Third edition (revised), 1936. Pp. 1–118.

4. Alexander, L. *Public mental health practices in Germany, sterilization and execution of patients suffering from nervous or mental disease.* Combined Intelligence Objectives Subcommittee, Item No. 24. File, No. XXVIII-50. Pp. 1–173 (August), 1945.

5. Idem. *Neuropathology and neurophysiology, including electro-encephalography in wartime Germany.* Combined Intelligence Objectives Subcommittee, Item No. 24. File, No. XXVII-1. Pp. 1–65 (July), 1945.

6. Idem. *German military neuropsychiatry and neurosurgery.* Combined Intelligence Objectives Subcommittee, Item No. 24. File, No. XXVIII-49. Pp. 1–138 (August), 1945.

7. Idem. Sociopsychologic structure of SS: Psychiatric report of Nurnberg trials for war crimes. *Arch. Neurol. & Psychiat.* 59:622–634, 1948.

8. Idem. War crimes: Their social-psychological aspects. *Am. J. Psychiat.* 105:170–177, 1948.

9. Idem. War crimes and their motivation: Socio-psychological structure of SS and criminalization of society. *J. Crim. Law & Criminol.* 39:298–326, 1948.

10. Idem. Madaus, G., and Koch, F.E., Tierexperimentelle Studien zur Frage der medikamentosen Sterilisierung (durch Caladium seguinum ([sic] Dieffenbachia sequina). *Zischr. f. d. ges. exper. Med.* 109:68–87, 1941.

11. Madaus, G. Zauberpflanzen im Lichte experimenteller Forschung, Das Schweigrohr—Caladium seguinum. *Umschau* 24:600–602.

12. Alexander, L. *Treatment of shock from prolonged exposure to cold, especially in water.* Combined Intelligence Objectives Subcommittee, Item No. 24. File, No. XXIX-24. Pp. 1–163 (August), 1945.

13. Document 1971 a PS.

14. Document NO 220.

15. Alexander, L. *Treatment of shock from prolonged exposure to cold, especially in water.* Combined Intelligence Objectives Subcommittee, Item No. 24. File, No. XXVI-37. Pp. 1–228 (July), 1945.

16. Seiss-Inquart. *Order of the Reich Commissar for the Occupied Netherlands Territories concerning the Netherlands doctors.* (Gazette containing the orders for the Occupied Netherlands Territories), pp. 1001–1026 (December), 1941.

17. Bernal, J. D. *The social function of science.* Sixth edition. 482 pp. London: George Routledge & Sons, 1946.

18. Toynbee, A. J. *A study of history.* Abridgement of Vol. I-VI. By D. C. Somervell. 617 pp. New York: Oxford University Press, 1947.

Chapter 29

War, Rape, and Genocide

Never Again?

Martin Donohoe

Introduction

The ongoing genocide in the Sudan—where 50,000 people have been killed, more than 1 million made homeless, and where thousands of women have been gang-raped by the government-supported Janjaweed militias—has focused international attention on the issue of rape in war.[1]

History

There were 250 wars in the 20th century, and the incidence of war is rising.[2] Most conflicts are within and between small states, many in sub-Saharan Africa. At the close of the 19th century, most casualties were among soldiers; today, 85% to 90% are among civilians.[2]

Women have always been considered among the "spoils of war." Accounts of rape in war date back to ancient Greece—the archetypal abduction of Helen of Troy and the rape of the Sabine women, for example.[3] Many hundreds of thousands of women have been raped in wars in the past hundred years. Examples include the following:

- In World War II, Japanese soldiers forced between 100,000 and 200,000 women into sexual slavery. Most were from Korea, but others came from Burma, China, Holland, Indonesia, the Philippines, and Taiwan.[4] These so-called comfort women were usually sent to the front lines where they were forced into sexual slavery. Some underwent forced hysterectomies to prevent menstruation and thereby make them constantly available.[4] More than half of the women and girls died as a direct result of the treatment they received.[5] Many survivors were detained in the program for 3 to 5 years, and most were raped 5 to 20 times per day.[5] For 3 years of enslavement, this comes to a low estimate of 7,500 rapes per person. Japan has not compensated any of these victims.[5]

- Rape occurred during the Vietnam War. Perpetrators included US soldiers; few have been brought to justice.[6]

- During Bangladesh's 9-month war for independence in 1971, between 250,000 and 400,000 girls and women were raped, leading to an estimated 25,000 pregnancies.[3]

- In Rwanda, at least 250,000 women were raped in the 1994 genocide.[7]

- During the 1990s, more than 20,000 Muslim women were raped as part of an ethnic cleansing campaign in Bosnia.[7]

- Credible allegations of sexual humiliation and rape against female detainees at US facilities in Afghanistan and Iraq have been well documented.[8-11]

- Other conflicts in which rape was widespread include civil wars in the Democratic Republic of the Congo, Liberia, Sierra Leone, and Somalia.

War and "Masculinity"

The persistence of war and its accompanying sexual violence throughout history relates in part to the pervasive glorification of war and its acceptance as a means of resolving conflict.[4] This glorification is linked to antiquated definitions of appropriate masculine behavior and coming-of-age rites. The vocabulary and imagery of war are laden with denigrations of the feminine and perverse phallic imagery of weapons as extensions of male generative organs.[4] Sexual imagery is employed in advertisements for arms, which are described in terms of "hardness, penetration, and thrust."[4] Military bases are commonly associated with prostitution, which is tacitly accepted by commanding officers and local authorities.[4,7] Men dominate as the major decision makers when it comes to pursuing militarization, fighting wars, and resolving international conflicts.[4]

Violence and Rape in War

Women and girls subject to rape in war are already vulnerable, suffering from both individual and societal forms of violence.[12-15] Individual forms of violence include domestic abuse, involuntary marriage, marital rape, forced labor, dowry-related murder, bride burning, honor killings, forced abortion and prostitution, child prostitution, and sex slavery.[12-14] Examples of societal forms of violence against women, structural forms of discrimination, or deprivation that affect women as a class include poverty, limited opportunities for employment or education, divorce restrictions, salary inequities, political marginalization, and impaired access to reproductive health services.[12-14]

Rape in war includes both individual, albeit widespread, acts of sexual violence and the systematic rape of women and children as an act of genocide, a strategy to terrorize and ethnically cleanse a population.[3,16] Rape in war is usually more sadistic than rape outside of war, if that is possible. Genocidal rapes are often committed in the presence of a woman's husband and children, who are often then killed. This compounds the subjugation and humiliation of the enemy. If the woman becomes pregnant, she may be forced to bear a child that has been "ethnically cleansed" by the seed of the rapist. In Rwanda after the 1994 genocide, as many as 5,000 children were born to women as a result of rape.[16] These offspring became known as *enfants mauvais souvenir*, or children of bad memories. Many women have difficulty caring for these children, and there have been reports of abandonment and infanticide.[16]

Although less common than female sexual assault during war, men have been raped; forced to rape or commit sexual assault on others or to perform fellatio and other sexual acts on guards and each other; and suffered castrations, circumcisions, and other sexual mutilations—all under threat of torture and/or death.[17] Male prisoners of US forces at Iraq's Abu Ghraib prison suffered numerous forms of sexual humiliation, such as being forced to adopt homosexual group sex poses.[8] Under several national and state legal systems, it is a legal impossibility for a man to be raped. Healthcare providers are often inadequately trained to recognize and care for such victims.

Health Consequences

Physical sequelae of rape in war include traumatic injuries, sexually transmitted diseases (including HIV infection), and pregnancy.[3,4,16,18] Emergency contraception, antibiotics, and access to abortion are extremely limited. Short-term psychological consequences include fear and a profound sense of helplessness and desperation.[4] In the long term, patients experience depression, anxiety disorders (including posttraumatic stress disorder), multiple somatic symptoms, flashbacks, difficulty reestablishing intimate relationships, shame, persistent fears, and a blunting of enjoyment in life.[4,18]

Refugee Camps

Girls and women in refugee settings are also at risk of rape during armed conflict.[16] At border crossings, they may be forced to endure rape as a "price of passage." Refugee camp guards may rape women or force them into sex in return for protection from bandits or for basic goods, including food.[16] The presence of abusive guards within camps, and bandits just outside, makes simple tasks such as going to the latrine or gathering water or firewood (usually the woman's job) dangerous, even life-threatening.[16,19]

Human Rights Issues

Violence against women and girls violates several principles enshrined in international and regional human rights law, including the right to life, equality, security, equal protection under the law, and freedom from torture and other cruel, inhumane, or degrading treatment.

Rape was specifically identified as a war crime for the first time in the Tokyo War Crimes Trials after World War II, when commanders were held responsible for rapes committed by soldiers under their command.[3] In 1993, the United Nations Commission on Human Rights passed a resolution placing rape, for the first time, clearly within the framework of war crimes.[3] This was reinforced by the 2001 ruling of the International War Crimes Tribunal in the Hague that rape of civilians is a crime against humanity.[20] The International Criminal Tribunals for Rwanda and the former Yugoslavia have successfully prosecuted cases of rape as a war crime and as an act of genocide.[16] Other international agreements regarding the treatment of women in war include the following:

- The Convention on the Elimination of all Forms of Discrimination Against Women (CEDAW), adopted by the UN General Assembly in 1979, which calls for equality of the sexes in political, social, cultural, civil, and other fields[7]

- UN Security Council Resolution 1325 (adopted in 2000), which mandates the protection of, and respect for, the human rights of women and girls. It calls on all parties to armed conflict to take specific measures to protect women and girls from gender-based violence, particularly rape and sexual violence.[7,21]

- The International Criminal Court (ICC), established by international treaty in 2002, which codifies accountability for gender-based crimes against women during military conflict by defining sexual and gender violence of all kinds as war crimes[7]

Regrettably, the United States has not signed UNSCR 1325, nor joined 162 other countries in ratifying CEDAW.[22] Despite the fact that 139 countries have signed on to the ICC, the United States has failed to do so, in part out of fear that its own soldiers may be prosecuted for crimes against humanity, including rape.[23]

Role of Health Professionals

The medical community can play an important role in confronting the atrocity of sexual assault in war by documenting incidents of rape; using medical data to verify widespread rape; using techniques of medical science to validate victims' testimony; and treating individual victims.[3] Managing victims of sexual violence during war entails conducting a full history and physical examination; treating physical injuries and sexually transmitted diseases; offering emergency contraception and referral for abortion; providing counseling and psychological support; facilitating the reporting of rape to the appropriate authorities; gathering forensic evidence; and providing a certificate documenting findings of the rape examination (in triplicate, with a copy for the victim, the United Nations High Commission of Refugees, and the provider's medical agency).[16] Health exams should be conducted in a confidential manner by trained workers in a safe environment. Female providers should be widely available.[16]

Preventing sexual violence in camps for refugees and internally displaced people entails placing water collection points and latrines in central, well-lighted areas; ensuring that food is distributed directly to women; and housing female-headed groups and unaccompanied children in safe areas.[16] Women should be involved in designing and helping to run the camps.[16]

Conclusions and Recommendations

The world's population is growing exponentially. Simultaneously, we are destroying the earth and our common resources, such as the air we breathe and the water we drink.[24] Millions die each year of starvation and diseases wrought by the ravages of poverty. Much of the world's population lacks access to clean drinking water, sanitation, and even minimal healthcare.[24] These stressors increase chances of hostilities. Furthermore, the growing worldwide supply of small and large arms, facilitated in part by the US government on behalf of military contractors, provides readily available tools for terrorizing, maiming, and killing soldiers and civilians alike.[2]

Each war represents a failure of our species to live in harmony, a waste of precious human capital, a further scourge on the environment, and a crime against all humanity. And rape in war represents the malevolent nadir of human behavior. Given the increasing spread of technology and materials for the construction of weapons of both small- and large-scale destruction, the enormity of the social and environmental problems facing humanity, and the realistic potential for the demise of the human species, rapid change is desperately needed. Such change would include moral leadership by the United States through limiting its excessive consumption of natural resources, building alliances, and working with the United Nations to solve international disputes, and vigorously investigating its own human rights abuses (e.g., Abu Ghraib) and prosecuting those responsible (no matter how elevated their status in the government). The United States should join the other nations of the world in signing on to international agreements, such as:

- The Convention on the Elimination of Discrimination Against Women
- UN Security Council Resolution 1325
- The International Criminal Court
- The Kyoto Protocol on Climate Change
- The Convention on the Prohibition of Anti-Personnel Land Mines
- The Comprehensive Nuclear Test Ban Treaty
- The Convention on the Rights of the Child
- The Convention on Economic, Social and Cultural Rights
- The Convention for the Suppression of Traffic in Persons

Finally, the United States should join forces with the international community to apply rapidly both economic and military pressures, including the protective use of military troops, to halt genocide and mass rape when it occurs anywhere in the world. Regrettably, as the continuing massacre in the Sudan makes clear, we are once again failing to do so. Inevitably, this will be bemoaned when our current generation of "leaders" later laments, "Never again."

Notes

1. Robinson S. The tragedy of the Sudan. *Time* October 4, 2004:45–61.

2. Levy BS, Sidel VW (eds.). *War and public health—updated edition.* Washington, DC: American Public Health Association; 2000.

3. Swiss S, Giller JE. Rape as a crime of war—a medical perspective. *JAMA.* 1993;270:612–615.

4. Ashford MW, Huet-Vaughn Y. The impact of war on women. In: Levy BS, Sidel VW (eds.), *War and public health—updated edition.* Washington, DC: American Public Health Association; 2000.

5. United Nations Commission on Human Rights, 51st session, Agenda item 11. *War rape.* Available at http://www.guidetoaction.org/parker/c95-11.html. Accessed September 9, 2004.

6. Staff. Tiger Force: Elite unit savaged civilians in Vietnam. *Toledo Blade* 2003 (October 22). Available at http://www.pulitzer.org/archives/6816. Accessed September 19, 2004.

7. Marshall L. Militarism and violence against women. *Z Magazine* 2004 (April):16–18.

8. Miles SH. Abu Ghraib: Its legacy for military medicine. *Lancet* 2004;364:725–729.

9. Article 15–6 Investigation of the 800th Military Police Brigade (*The Taguba Report*). Available at http://news.findlaw.com/hdocs/docs/iraq/tagubarpt.html# FRother2.19. Accessed October 10, 2004.

10. Captain Donald J. Reese's sworn statement and interview. (Appendix to *Taguba* investigation). Available at http://www.msnbc.msn.com/id/4894001/ns /nbcnightlynews/t/us-army-report-iraqi-prisoner-abuse/#.T6OuHuvOyfY . Accessed October 10, 2004.

11. Colonel Thomas M. Pappas' sworn statement and interview. (Appendix to *Taguba* investigation). Available at http://www.usnews.com/usnews/news/articles /040709/Pappas.pdf. Accessed October 10, 2004.

12. Heise LL, Raikes A, Watts CH, et al. Violence against women: A neglected public health issue in less developed countries. *Soc Sci Med.* 1994;39:1165–1179.

13. Donohoe MT. Violence and human rights abuses against women in the developing world. *Medscape Ob/Gyn and Women's Health* 2003;8(2). Posted November 26, 2003. Available at http://www.medscape.com/viewarticle/464255.

14. Donohoe MT. Individual and societal forms of violence against women in the United States and the developing world: An overview. *Curr Women's Hlth Reports* 2002;2:313–319.

15. Donohoe MT. Violence against women: Partner abuse and sexual assault. *Hospital Physician* 2004;40(10):24-31. Available at http://www.turner-white.com /memberfile.php?PubCode=hp_oct04_partner.pdf.

16. Shanks L, Schull MJ. Rape in war: The humanitarian response. *CMAJ.* 2000;163:1152–1156.

17. Carlson ES. Sexual assault on men in war. *Lancet* 1997;349:129.

18. Amnesty International. *Rape as a tool of war.* Fact sheet. Available at http://www.amnestyusa.org/stopviolence/factsheets/rapeinwartime.html. Accessed October 12, 2004.

19. Darfur Humanitarian Emergency. *USAID.* Available at http://www.usaid.gov /locations/sub-saharan_africa/sudan/darfur.html. Accessed October 12, 2004.

20. Kafala T. What is a war crime? *BBC News* 2003 (July 31). Available at http://www.bbc.co.uk/gov/pr/fr/-/2/hi/europe/1420133.stm. Accessed September 9, 2004.

21. Ward J, Vann B. Gender-based violence in refugee settings. *Lancet* 2004;360 (Suppl. 1). Available at http://www.thelancet.com/journal/vol360/isss1 /full/llan.360.s1.medicine_and_conflict.23369.1. Accessed September 23, 2004.

22. Staff. National Organization of Women. *Armies at war use rape as a weapon.*
     Available at http://www.now.org/nnt/fall99/viewpoint.html. Accessed September
     17, 2004.

23. Official Web site. *Rome statute of the international criminal court.* Available at
     http://untreaty.un.org/ENGLISH/bible/englishinternetbible/partI/chapterXVIII
     /treaty10.asp. Accessed October 2, 2004.

24. Donohoe MT. Causes and health consequences of environmental degradation and
     social injustice. *Soc Sci Med.* 2003;56:573–587.

Part Eight

Corporations and Public Health

For-profit corporations have played an increasing and often harmful role in many spheres of life, including banking and finance, housing, media, entertainment, agriculture, and health care. Corporations are legal devices that exist for the sole purpose of providing the greatest possible financial return to their owners or investors. Economist Milton Friedman noted, "The [only] social responsibility of business is to increase its profits."[1] To do this, corporations engage in a number of activities antithetical to democracy and public health. Noam Chomsky said, "[Corporations have] no moral conscience. [They] are designed by law to be concerned only for their stockholders, and not, say, what are sometimes called their stakeholders, like the community or the work force."[2] To fulfill their purpose, corporations internalize profits while externalizing costs (including damage done to the environment or human health). Their officers and shareholders are protected from litigation through limited liability. When a corporate entity settles a lawsuit, in the absence of a whistleblower confidentiality agreements can keep vital health information from the public, leading to further injuries and even deaths.

One of the earliest corporations, the British East India Company of the seventeenth and eighteenth centuries, used the power granted it by

Much of the material in the introduction to this part is derived from Wiist, W. (ed.), *Public health or the bottom line* (Oxford, UK: Oxford University Press), 2010.

the British government to run India, dominate the Chinese opium trade, and manage a slave-trading operation out of Madagascar. Through its affiliate, the Virginia Company, it established the colony of Jamestown using conscripted labor and later pressured Britain to pass the 1773 Tea Act, designed to extend its monopoly but ultimately leading to the Boston Tea Party and the American Revolution. Monopolistic corporations run by "robber barons" controlled the railroads (Andrew Carnegie), finance (J. P. Morgan), and the oil industry (John D. Rockefeller) in the nineteenth and early twentieth centuries until their power was diminished by the trust-busting activities of President Theodore Roosevelt. In the late twentieth and early twenty-first centuries, corporations have become increasingly powerful through mergers, consolidation, political influence, litigation, and other practices described in this section's readings.

Many historical figures have warned us about the antidemocratic implications of corporate power. Thomas Jefferson attempted to include freedom from corporate monopolies in the Bill of Rights. President Abraham Lincoln feared that "corporations have been enthroned and an era of corruption in high places will follow, and the money power of the country will endeavor to prolong its reign by working upon the prejudices of the people until all wealth is aggregated in a few hands and the Republic is destroyed."[3] A decade later, President Rutherford B. Hayes warned that the United States had become "a government of corporations, by corporations, and for corporations."[3] In 1932, presidential candidate Franklin D. Roosevelt, who went on to establish significant social safety net programs for the poor and elderly, warned that if "the process of (corporate) concentration goes on at the same rate, at the end of another century we shall have all American industry controlled by a dozen corporations, and run by perhaps a hundred men."[4]

Despite such warnings, international institutions (such as the World Trade Organization and International Monetary Fund) created during the post–World War II years and international trade agreements of the last few decades have consolidated corporate control over not only the US economy, but also over the world's economy. Corporate personhood, the product of an unofficial notation by a court reporter during the 1886 US Supreme Court case *Santa Clara County* v. *Southern Pacific Railroad*, which was incorporated into future court understandings of the rights of corporations, has given corporations unprecedented power over our economy. The Court's recent decision in *Citizens United* v. *Federal Election Commission* has granted corporations immense authority to influence elections through essentially unlimited campaign donations.[5]

Today corporations have achieved extraordinary levels of domination of our public institutions. They employ a number of legal and illegal political, financial, and public relations tactics to increase their profitability. They have deliberately corrupted public education and obfuscated many scientific findings that demonstrate how their activities have damaged human health and the environment.

This section's readings illustrate just a few of the ways in which corporations harm the public health enterprise. Chapter Thirty (by Martin Donohoe) describes the extent and nature of corporate domination of the world's economy, corporate taxation, corporate crime, and how corporations corrupt democracy through increasing control over public education and via media monopolies. The chapter also describes how corporations have augmented the global North-South socioeconomic divide, in part through pressuring US government officials not to cooperate with international agreements designed to protect human rights, achieve economic justice, ensure environmental protection, and improve human health.

Chapter Thirty-One (by Jennifer R. Niebyl) exposes pharmaceutical industry practices designed to sell drugs, whose benefits they maximize and risks they minimize. Some of these drugs are marketed for "diseases" constructed less from clinical science than for marketing campaigns aimed at convincing people that normal human feelings and behaviors are somehow pathological and require chemical control. The pharmaceutical companies spend much more on marketing (to health care providers and the general public) than on research and development, and use their considerable lobbying power to influence government legislation and limit civil and criminal liability for corrupt practices.

Chapter Thirty-Two (by Martin Donohoe) examines the causes, consequences, risks, and benefits of the marketing, and the adoption by providers and patients, of costly and unscientific (yet profitable) screening tests, including full-body CT scans to screen for cancer and other asymptomatic yet potentially dangerous conditions.

Chapter Thirty-Three (by Martin Donohoe) critiques the burgeoning drug-testing industry through its analysis of random, not-for-cause screening of physicians. Backed by poor (or even nonexistent) science, such screening (and many other forms of drug testing) engender significant economic and social costs and are emblematic of myriad ways in which our privacy has been eroded by corporations and government over the last few decades.

All the readings in this section offer suggestions for combating corporate power, including through changes in health professions' schools curricula. At the societal level, strategies include boycotts, protests, litigation, cracking down on corporate crime and holding managers accountable, countermedia activities, trust-busting, limiting corporations' involvement in elections, and enacting legislation to change the nature and improve oversight of corporations. Governments have granted corporations certain rights and privileges, and governments can take them away.

Public health professionals can play a central role in changing corporate practices through research, education, and advocacy, often through partnerships with social movements (e.g., civil rights, consumer protection, environmental justice, religious, and women's and indigenous rights groups). Given the increasing power of corporations over health professions schools' and hospitals' research and patient-care agendas, these institutions should strive to maintain their independence from industry and reevaluate the growing practice whereby they sell their names to individual and corporate donors.[6] Individual citizens can vote, pressure their elected officials, run for office, alter their levels of consumption, make responsible purchasing decisions, support alternative media, and join groups dedicated to combating corporate hegemony. Further information on topics discussed in this part can be found on the Public Health and Social Justice website at http://phsj.org/activism-and-education/, http://phsj.org/pharmaceutical-industry/, http://phsj.org/unnecessary-testing -scams/, http://phsj.org/physician-drug-testing/, and http://phsj.org/research- and-industry/.

Public health operates best in a true democracy, which requires an informed and involved citizenry. An informed populace is achievable through increased funding of quality public education, available to all and free of corporate influence, and through a free press consisting of a variety of media outlets. An involved populace requires economic security and the recognition of life's fleeting nature and the value of nature and community. Public health advocates have achieved important anticorporate successes in areas such as food safety, tobacco control, and access to health care and medications, but much work remains to be done. The next section contains inspirational readings that illuminate how we can accomplish this work.

Notes

1. Friedman, M. Quote. Retrieved from http://www.goodreads.com/quotes/show/ 240845.

2. Chomsky, N. From *The Corporation*. Retrieved from http://www.imdb.com/title/ tt0379225/quotes. 3. Wiist, W. (ed.), *Public health or the bottom line* (Oxford, UK: Oxford University Press), 2010Wiist, p. 79.

3. Wiist, p. 12.

4. Wiist, p. 82.

5. Wiist , W. H. Citizens united, public health, and democracy: The Supreme Court ruling, its implications, and proposed action. *American Journal of Public Health*, 2011, *101*(7), 1172–1179.

6. Loeffler, J. S., & Halperin, E. C. Selling a medical school's name: Ethical and practical dilemmas. *JAMA.*, 2008, *300*(16), 1937–1938.

Chapter 30

Combating Corporate Control

Protecting Education, Media, Legislation, and Health Care

Martin Donohoe

Corporations have become the predominant force in business over the last century. Designed to grow, profit, and augment the wealth of their shareholders, corporations have exercised increasing influence over public education, the media, legislation, and public policy relevant to human health and well-being.

There are almost 6 million corporations worldwide; only 25 percent of these are non-profits. Ninety percent of transnational corporations are headquartered in the northern hemisphere, one indicator of the global divide between the wealthy North and the poor South. Today 500 companies control 70 percent of world trade. Fifty-three of the world's 100 largest economies are private corporations; 47 are countries. To illustrate, Walmart is larger than Israel and Greece, and AT&T is larger than Malaysia and Ireland.

The last few decades have been marked by increasing corporate consolidation and mergers. Consequences of these and other corporate activities include inflation, rising unemployment, the rise of the "permatemp," and the expatriation of jobs to overseas factories that often lack adequate occupational health and safety and environmental standards. In the US, there has been a dramatic decline in labor union membership, in part a consequence of corporate organized harassment of union organizers. During former president George W. Bush's tenure in office, critical government services were outsourced to private industry, including military duties to private mercenaries. As of now, more than half of federal jobs have been outsourced to private companies.

Worldwide there are 27 million enslaved laborers and over 250 million child laborers. In many parts of the world, including the US, a minimum wage does not correspond to a living wage—i.e., the income needed to meet basic needs of housing, food, clothing, transportation, and child care. One-quarter of current US jobs pay less than a poverty-level income. While workers struggle to get by, executive pay has grown increasingly exorbitant, especially in the US, where chief executive officer (CEO) salaries are up 500 percent since 1980. The average CEO makes 350–400 times the salary of the average US worker (versus 41 times in 1960). In Mexico the ratio is 45:1, in Britain 25:1, and in Japan 10:1. Clearly, astronomical CEO pay is not a prerequisite for innovation or profitability.

Over 40 of the poorest countries in Africa, Latin America, and Asia owe a total of almost $300 billion in foreign debt. These countries spend more each year repaying this debt than on education and health care for their citizens. To help countries pay off this debt, corporate-friendly international bodies (such as the World Trade Organization, World Bank, and International Monetary Fund) encourage the privatization of social resources and export-oriented development at the expense of the production of food and other necessities for local consumption. Wages fall; government spending on food, fuel, and farming subsidies are reduced; social services are cut; and countries strip and sell their natural resources, contributing to deforestation and pollution. The Multilateral Agreement on Investment and trade agreements such as the General Agreement on Tariffs and Trade (GATT) and the North American Free Trade Agreement (NAFTA) reinforce such policies. US foreign aid accounts for only 0.9 percent of our gross domestic product, primarily benefits US corporations, and has little ameliorating effect on developing world poverty.

Corporate Taxes and Crime

Corporate taxes are at their lowest level since World War II. Nearly one-third of all large US corporations pay no annual taxes. Reasons for inadequate corporate taxation include corporate tax breaks and loopholes, corporate welfare, underpayment, outright cheating, and sheltering capital in offshore tax havens.

The US news media, at least prior to the recent financial meltdown, has generally focused on street ("blue collar") crime, rather than corporate ("white collar") crime. However, each year in America, while we lose $3.8 billion to burglary and robbery, we lose hundreds of billions of dollars to corporate crime, including health care fraud, auto repair fraud, and securities fraud. The savings and loan frauds of the 1980s and 1990s cost between $300 billion and $500 billion; the current economic crisis involves fraud and malfeasance, which will cost taxpayers trillions of dollars.

Corporate crime is common due to the incentives involved, and the meager fines are often just considered a cost of doing business. Corporate crime is under-prosecuted and prosecutors under-funded. Incredibly, up to three-fifths of all companies settling corporate crime cases illegally deduct some or all of their settlements on their tax returns.

Corporations have also made legal redress of their crimes increasingly difficult through strategic lawsuits against private parties (SLAPP lawsuits), which are designed to harass groups promoting social justice and environmental sustainability by depleting their resources, keeping them on the defensive, and scaring them away from proactive attempts to fight corporate malfeasance. Likewise, so-called tort reform has limited access to the courts for those damaged by corporate products and practices.

Corporate Involvement in Education

Public education in the US is in disarray. US schools are ranked lowest among western nations and suffer from inadequate funding and decaying infrastructure. The national high school graduation rate has stagnated at 65–70 percent for decades and college tuition costs continue to rise, making a college education beyond the means of most young people outside of the upper-middle and upper classes.

The depth and breadth of scientific ignorance in the United States is staggering. The lack of understanding also limits Americans' ability to realize the importance of public health and environmental science, two areas which directly impact our longevity and well-being. The following are just a few examples which illustrate a poor understanding of basic science:

- As part of a science project, a junior high school student circulated a petition among his classmates asking them if they would sign to ban the chemical dihydrogen monoxide. Reasons the student gave for such a ban included the fact that this chemical is a major component in acid rain; can cause severe burns in its gaseous state; can kill you if accidentally inhaled; and has been found in tumors of terminal cancer patients. A large majority of his colleagues elected to sign the petition to ban this ubiquitous substance, commonly known as water.

- Twenty percent of Americans do not know that the earth revolves around the sun.

- One-half of US citizens do not believe in evolution and do believe that humans and dinosaurs coexisted.

- Eleven percent of US teens are unable to locate the United States on a map. Twenty-nine percent cannot find the Pacific Ocean and 58 percent cannot locate Japan.

Many schools are unable to find (or afford) quality science teachers, especially in health and in environmental science. Sensing an opportunity to mold the malleable minds of young people, corporations offer their own pre-packaged curricula, designed to portray their industries and products as eco-friendly. For instance, International Paper's sponsored environmental education materials contain statements such as "Clear-cutting promotes the growth of trees that require full sunlight and allows efficient site preparation for the next crop." Exxon's "Energy Cube" tells students that "gasoline is simply solar power hidden in decayed matter" and that "offshore drilling creates reefs for fish." The American Nuclear Society's "Activities with the Atoms Family" and Dow's "Chemipalooza" fill students' minds with the unquestioned benefits of nuclear power and industrial chemicals.

Colleges, universities, and professional schools have also been corrupted through the growing corporatization of academia, manifested by increasing private commercial funding of university research and secrecy/gag clauses which pre-empt publication of important findings which might cast an unfavorable light on a company's product or drug. Professional organizations are susceptible to becoming mouthpieces for corporate agendas. For example, the American Association of Petroleum Geologists' 2005 Notable Achievement in Journalism prize was awarded to Michael Crichton for his book, *State of Fear*, which denies the existence of global warming.

Corporate Control of the Media

Corporations have also utilized the media for their disinformation campaigns. Television advertising provides a particularly effective vehicle for corporate public relations. The average American youth spends 1,500 hours per year watching TV, versus 900 hours per year in school. By age 65, the average American will have spent 9 years watching TV. Corporate PR tactics include "astroturfing" through artificially created grassroots coalitions, which lobby elected officials on behalf of corporate-friendly legislation, and the creation of corporate front groups with eco-friendly names like the National Wilderness Institute and the Foundation for Clean Air Progress. "Greenwashing" employs public relations and ad campaigns to portray corporations as promoting alternative energy, conservation, and sound ecological and health policies, despite evidence to the contrary. Typical greenwash campaigns invoke poor people as corporate beneficiaries and characterize those who question the benefits (or note the risks) of modern technologies as "technophobic," "anti-science," and "against progress."

To compound matters, most media organizations are owned by multi-national, multi-billion dollar corporations that are involved in a number of businesses, such as forestry, defense, real estate, oil, agriculture, steel production, railways, and water and power utilities. Not surprisingly, mainstream media fail to adequately address the public health and environmental consequences of these industries. Pre-packaged corporate video news releases often replace actual on-site reporting, and some reporters' stories have been suppressed.

Media outlets have become increasingly consolidated. In 2005, just 5 corporations controlled the majority of US media, down from 50 in 1983. Independent media have struggled to pay journalists, and many newspapers have simply gone out of business.

In order to portray themselves as "fair and balanced" with respect to scientific issues, the media have in fact obfuscated the relevance of important scientific findings. Even when there is little to no doubt among qualified scientists as to the veracity and relevance of scientific data, the media will find those few "scientists" (who are often on the payroll of corporations) willing to publicly contradict information relevant to major health risks, such as the role of environmental tobacco smoke in causing heart disease and cancer and the role of saturated fatty acids in promoting obesity, diabetes, and heart disease. For example, an important study published in *Science* magazine in 2004 showed how non-scientists might easily be confused about climate change. The study's authors noted that of 928 articles published in peer-reviewed scientific journals between 1993 and 2003, none were in doubt as to the existence or cause of global warming. During the same time period, of 636 articles in the 4 most popular US daily newspapers (the *New York Times,* the *Washington Post,* the *Los Angeles Times,* and the *Wall Street Journal*), 53 percent expressed doubt as to the existence and/or primary cause of global warming.

Corporations' Effects on Democracy and US International Policy

To complement their miseducation of the public and to drive their agendas, corporations employ thousands of full-time lobbyists. Between 1998 and 2007, the pharmaceutical industry spent $1.3 billion on lobbying, more than any other industry. In 2006, business lobbying groups spent just under $2.5 billion. For comparison, all single-issue ideological groups combined (e.g., pro-choice, anti-abortion, feminist and consumer organizations, senior citizens, etc.) spent just $76 million. Such corporate influence leads to large taxpayer subsidies to polluting industries. For instance, nuclear power receives $10.5 billion per year in subsidies, coal $8 billion per year, and oil and gas $550 million per year. Estimates of returns on investments in lobbying range from $28 to $100 for every dollar spent.

Because of the tremendous influence of corporations, the US government has isolated itself from much of the international community by failing to sign and/or ratify a number of treaties relevant to human rights, social justice, and public health. These include the Kyoto Protocol on Climate Change; the International Covenant on Economic, Social, and Cultural Rights; the Comprehensive Nuclear Test Ban Treaty; the Convention on the Prohibition of Anti-Personnel Land Mines; the Convention on the Rights of the Child; the Convention on the Elimination of Discrimination Against Women; the Stockholm Convention on Persistent Organic Pollutants; the Basel Convention on the Control of Transboundary Movements of Hazardous Wastes; and the Cartagena Protocol on Biosafety. In addition, US foreign and trade policies, often exerted through international financial institutions and global trade agreements, remain at odds with the promotion of public health and social justice.

Corporate Influence on Public Health

In the US, for-profit health care delivery systems are widely cited for higher death rates, lower quality of care, and higher administrative costs. For-profit pharmaceutical corporations are criticized for spending more on marketing than on research and development, and for egregious profits consequent to high drug prices. The enormously profitable pharmaceutical industry exerts substantial influence on providers' prescribing patterns through control of continuing medical education, "seeding" (phony research) trials, statistical manipulation of data sets to produce results favorable to a company's drug, selective publication, and gifts (bribes) to practitioners. Pharmaceutical companies, through the Pharmaceutical Research and Manufacturers' Association (Pharma), effectively lobbied and threatened trade sanctions against developing countries in order to prevent production and importation of much cheaper, generic versions of life-saving anti-AIDS drugs.

For many years, health insurers have cherry-picked low-risk patients while creating barriers to coverage for sicker individuals (such as pre-existing condition exclusions and outright denials of coverage). This has shifted the costlier care of higher-risk patients onto state and federal governments (through the Medicaid and Medicare programs). Meanwhile, for-profit companies have sprung up to sponsor luxury care consortiums for the super-rich.

The US attempted to undermine the World Health Organization's Global Tobacco Treaty through Bush administration appointees with strong ties to the tobacco industry, including deputy chief of staff Karl Rove, a former lobbyist and strategist for Phillip Morris (PM); White House liaison to the business community Kirk Blalock, a former PM public relations official; Charles Black, informal advisor to George Bush during the 2000 campaign and a former

PM lobbyist; Daniel Troy, former FDA chief counsel, who represented the industry when it sued the FDA over tobacco ad regulation; and Health and Human Services secretary Tommy Thompson, who rejected his own advisory panel's recommendation to increase the federal tobacco tax and who had received $72,000 in campaign contributions from PM executives as governor of Wisconsin. The original US negotiator, Dr. Thomas Novotny, resigned after the Bush administration pressured him to lobby for the deletion of 10 of 11 provisions from the treaty, as outlined in a PM memo. (Fortunately the treaty has mostly retained its initial form. The US has signed, but not yet ratified, it.)

General Electric Medical Systems, a subsidiary of General Electric (GE), recently signed an exclusive technology transfer agreement with NY-Presbyterian Hospital, one of the largest academic health-care institutions in the United States. GE's activities include production of plastics (including toxic bisphenol A), military hardware, and nuclear power plants. GE has investments in for-profit prison enterprises, operates coal-burning power plants, and runs the Patient Channel, an advertising vehicle for drug companies (shown in hospital rooms throughout the country), which has been criticized for manipulative marketing practices.

GE has conducted unethical human subject experiments, involving testicular irradiation of prisoners, from the 1940s to 1960s; intentionally released excessive radiation from its Hanford, Washington, nuclear reactor in the 1980s, which may have contributed to increased thyroid cancer risk in "downwinders"; and is currently America's largest corporate polluter, responsible for 75 Superfund sites nationwide. Between 1947 and 1977, two of GE's capacitor manufacturing plants dumped 1.3 million pounds of polychlorinated biphenyls (PCBs) into the Hudson River, turning 200 miles of the river into a Superfund site. PCBs are probable human carcinogens with adverse effects on the liver, kidney, nervous system, and reproductive organs.

GE has tremendous influence on US environmental, energy, and health policy. GE spent millions to avoid cleaning up the Hudson River and to weaken or eliminate the Superfund law. In 2008, it spent over $19 million on lobbying. Many members of its board of directors have government ties.

GE eliminated 150,000 jobs over the last 15 years, while receiving billions in federal contracts and millions in state and local subsidies. It is one of the nation's top outsourcers of jobs. GE continues to under-fund its employee pension plan, despite very generous compensation packages for its executives, and continues to shift health care costs onto workers, despite growing profits. GE has been cited by Human Rights Watch for "systematic workers' rights violations" in the US and abroad, by the Occupational Safety and Health Administration for numerous workplace violations, and repeatedly by the Project on Government Oversight for defrauding US taxpayers.

The agreement with NY-Presbyterian Hospital provides GE with financial incentives to promote high-technology purchases; prohibits the hospital from purchasing more effective equipment from other companies; and augments the trend in academic medical centers toward the promotion and use of pricey, high-technology care at the expense of preventive care and public health measures. The greatest irony about the agreement, however, is that patients with developmental anomalies and cancers caused by GE's pollution will be diagnosed with GE scanners and treated with GE-manufactured therapeutic devices, increasing GE's bottom line.

The American Council on Science and Health, a corporate front group has exercised unduly excessive influence through the mainstream media. Its staff members, including its medical/executive director (who was convicted of Medicaid fraud), have appeared on national TV and in major newspapers criticizing public and environmental health advocates while disseminating misinformation regarding global warming; the adverse neurological effects of lead exposure; the endocrine-disrupting effects of PCBs; the effects of agricultural antibiotics on food-borne, antibiotic-resistant human infections; the health risks of trans fatty acids; the health consequences of exposure to dioxins and pesticides; and the health risks posed by diesel exhaust fumes, arsenic in drinking water, and phthalates in medical devices and children's toys. Its methods have included ad hominem attacks and threats of litigation against respected scientists.

For-profit companies such as Corrections Corporation of America, GEO Group (formerly Wackenhut), and Correctional Medical Services have become increasingly involved in the for-profit incarceration business. Many have been accused of running substandard prisons. Other companies with investments in for-profit prisons include Westinghouse, AT&T, Sprint, MCI, Smith Barney, American Express, Merrill Lynch, Shearson-Lehman, Allstate, and GE.

Forty percent of prison health care in 34 states is provided by for-profit companies. This care is often substandard. For example, Correctional Medical Systems (the largest and least expensive provider) has been the subject of numerous lawsuits and investigations for poor care, negligence, patient dumping, and opaque accounting of taxpayer dollars. Prison Health Services was cited by New York state for negligence and unnecessary prisoner deaths, and is the subject of over 1,000 lawsuits.

The medical technologies industry has successfully promoted a variety of unproven and potentially harmful imaging modalities, such as screening whole-body computed tomography (CT) scans. These costly studies expose asymptomatic, fearful, and credulous victims to significant amounts of unnecessary, cancer-causing radiation, as well as invasive follow-up tests with their attendant risks.

In 2002, corporate agribusiness conducted a successful campaign against Oregon's Proposition 27, which would have required labeling of genetically modified (GM) foods. The bill was soundly defeated, 70 percent to 30 percent, despite public opinion polls showing 85–95 percent of the population in favor of such labeling. Proponents of the bill were outspent $5.5 million to $200,000, with most of the opposition funding coming from agribusiness giants headquartered outside Oregon. Opponents hid behind "advocacy groups" with scientific-sounding names and spread deliberate misinformation regarding the financial ramifications of the bill.

Big agriculture has also lobbied aggressively for pre-emptive anti-labeling laws relevant to GM crops and recombinant bovine growth hormone (rBGH) in milk. Monsanto, Dupont, Novartis Seeds, Aventis CropScience, and Bayer CropScience actively support the spread of GM crops to the developing world, at the expense of less risky, more productive forms of farming. They have deliberately kept GM seeds from non-corporate academic researchers, limiting their ability to conduct studies relevant to the health and environmental consequences of the spread of GM crops. Corporate agribusiness also has been at the forefront of promoting agriculture bills which provide generous subsidies to large, polluting industrial farms.

To fight the influence by corporations will require activity on a number of fronts, including:

- Fair, truly representative elections, with publicly financed campaigns, open debates, free air time for candidates, and consideration of proportional representation, instant runoff voting, cumulative voting, and range(rating) voting. By the same token, given low US voter turnout relative to other democracies, and the especially low turnout among the poor and racial minorities, it is incumbent upon those most affected by poverty to exercise their right to full suffrage.

- Increased funding of public education, combined with independent scientific review of school curricula, prohibitions on the use of sponsored curricula, and the establishment of safeguards regarding corporate involvement in academic research in order to improve the quality and veracity of public education. Education through college should be free to anyone who qualifies for admission.

- Enactment of a single-payer national health plan, providing comprehensive preventive, physical, and mental health care.

- Reconfiguration of the tax system to decrease taxes on work and savings, while increasing taxes on destructive activities such as carbon emissions and toxic waste generation.

- The passage of living wage laws and increased protection for unions to improve the status of workers.

- Diversion of excessive (and wasteful) military spending toward social programs.

- The passage of laws relevant to corporate activities based on the precautionary principle, which include financial analyses that incorporate the costs of activities on human health and the environment.

- Dramatically increased enforcement budgets for combating corporate crime.

- Subjecting convicted corporate criminals to large fines, which cannot simply be written off as "a cost of doing business," as well as serious jail time.

- Individual lifestyle modifications (such as decreasing consumption and supporting local, sustainable producers), community service, activism, letter-writing campaigns, direct protests, whistleblowing, and boycotts are all effective ways for citizens to hold corporations accountable. Joining activist organizations, directly lobbying legislators, and running for office are other effective approaches.

- Higher standards of independent journalism and the support of alternative media.

In addition, medical and public health education will need to change if we are to achieve better health care. Patient and physician dissatisfaction with our current fragmented health-care system is growing. Many medical students and residents display increasingly cynical attitudes as their training progresses and educators have expressed concern about the adequacy of students' humanistic and moral development. Interest in primary care among medical students has also been declining. Tending to physical symptoms often overshadows health professionals' attention to the psychological, economic, social, and cultural factors that prompt many clinic visits and cause as much functional impairment as physical complaints.

Increasing numbers of physicians from all fields have stopped seeing patients with certain types of insurance, complain of fatigue and burnout, and feel that medicine has lost its soul. Some doctors are even leaving the profession. The proportion of physicians providing charity care has declined over the last decade, while most academic medical centers have opened luxury care clinics for the wealthy.

The schism between schools of public health and medical schools that dates back to the early 20th century—with medical schools becoming more focused on biochemical mechanisms of disease and drug therapies than on societal issues—has yet to be healed. Furthermore, the lack of collaboration between nursing schools and medical schools has created an environment not conducive to collaborative learning. This makes post-training collaborative practice, which is critical to solving population-level health problems, more challenging. Medical education provides little in the way of public health training, despite the Institute of Medicine's recommendation that one-quarter to one-half of medical students earn the equivalent of a master's of public health degree.

Medical ethics currently overemphasizes dilemmas involving expensive technologies (e.g., gene therapy, cloning, face transplants), while under-emphasizing the psychological, cultural, socioeconomic, occupational, and environmental contributors to health and disease. This is in part due to the availability of funding for ethics projects relevant to high-technology interventions, but also due to the perceived intractability of public health problems and fear of criticizing corporate structures and agreements commonly found in academic medical centers. While major ethics organizations are increasingly confronting issues relevant to social justice, their response has been inadequate, and many ethicists risk their funding and/or their jobs if they speak out too forcefully.

Medical workers and other scientists should better use the media to confront abuses of science by corporations and governments and to better educate the public regarding the pernicious effects of corporations on public health. Institutional ethics committees should more thoroughly evaluate university financial agreements with private companies and oppose those which infringe on academic freedom or which align the university with organizations whose activities harm the very patients they are serving.

Finally, it is time for us to question the appropriateness of the profit motive in medical research. A generous and publicly funded research agenda focused on the critical needs of the suffering (as opposed to an industry-driven agenda focused on profitable procedures and me-too drugs designed primarily for diseases of the developed world) is possible, given the right combination of social and political will. Lifting the veil of secrecy surrounding medical research would foster cooperation between scientists and speed the development and dissemination of new, reasonably priced treatments, bringing social and economic benefits greatly exceeding the public's investment. Such a system would be rational, open, and egalitarian, all positive qualities which a just health care system should embody.

Chapter 31

The Pharmaceutical Industry

Friend or Foe?

Jennifer R. Niebyl

Thank you for inviting me to be here today. It is a great honor to be president of the American Gynecological and Obstetrical Society.

First, I would like to thank my escorts, who have been my mentors and colleagues for many years. They are as follows: Richard Berkowitz, MD, Steven Gabbe, MD, Irwin Merkatz, MD, John Queenan, MD, Gloria Sarto, MD, PhD, and Joe Leigh Simpson, MD. I would also like to acknowledge the late Dr J. Donald Woodruff, who brought me to my very first meeting of this organization, and who was my mentor at Johns Hopkins Hospital.

In this address I intend to show you the degree to which the drug industry is profit motivated and ultimately responsible to shareholders. However, we, as physicians, have primary responsibility to our patients. I want to remind you that drug representatives are sales people, not educators. They live by quotas and they track the prescribing habits of physicians to whom they market their drugs. Gifts, meals, samples, seminars, and advertising all influence our prescribing habits. In addition, I will briefly mention some issues about the Food and Drug Administration (FDA). It is paid by the pharmaceutical industry to approve drugs and has limited resources for postmarketing supervision of companies with regard to misleading advertising, or side effects of drugs discovered after FDA approval.

Drug representatives may find speakers, pay speakers, bring lunch, and bring gifts and samples. All of these behaviors influence physician prescribing and drive up the drug costs for hospitals and patients. That is, of course, why the drug companies pay for them.

Industry responds by pointing out that prescription drugs are expensive because they are valuable, and that they have large research and development costs. Indeed, drugs may enhance quality of life and lengthen life, and marketing may sometimes influence physicians to prescribe otherwise underprescribed drugs. However, the costs of drugs in this country are significantly increased because of the large marketing budget and profit margin of the drug industry.

Much of what I am going to say today came from the book by Dr. Marcia Angell, *The Truth About the Drug Companies: How They Deceive Us and What to Do About It.*[1] She is the former editor-in-chief of the *New England Journal of Medicine*, a physician trained in both internal medicine and pathology.

In 2003 in the United States we spent $250 billion on outpatient prescription drugs. That figure is growing 12% per year, and is the fastest growing part of health care costs. For example, the price of Claritin was raised 13 times over 5 years, a 50% increase, 4 times the rate of inflation.

I will use the term "Big Pharma" to refer to PhRMA, the Pharmaceutical Research and Manufacturers of America. This is the industry's trade association, an organization of all the drug companies around the world, including 5 giant European companies. In the United States, the pharmaceutical industry enjoys the rapid approval of drugs by the FDA and free pricing with no price controls. They also have long periods of exclusive marketing rights, and huge tax breaks.

Increased drug expenditures have come from 3 sources: 39% from increased numbers of prescriptions, 37% from the increased cost of drugs, and 24% from the shift to more expensive drugs.[2]

The average price per drug per year currently is approximately $1,500. Industry charges Medicare recipients without supplemental insurance more than HMOs or the Veterans' Administration, as the latter can buy in bulk. However, the Medicare Reform Bill of 2003 forbids Medicare to bargain for lower prices.

In fact, research and development is actually a small part of the budget of drug companies. It is approximately 14% of sales, while profit is 18% of sales. The pharmaceutical industry makes vast expenditures for marketing and administration at 36% of sales. They have 1 sales person for every 4.7 physicians, and spend $8,000-$15,000 per physician per year. Thus, prices could actually be cut significantly without threatening research and development. The major sources of innovation of new drugs are the National Institutes of Health (NIH), academic medical centers, and biotechnology companies. Many of the "new" drugs are actually just variations of older drugs, commonly referred to as "me-too" drugs. That is why we have 6 different statins that are very similar to each other, and 6 different selective serotonin reuptake inhibitors.[3]

Among drug company employees in the year 2000, the following was the distribution of tasks: marketing 39%, production and quality control 26%, research and development 22%, administration 11%, and distribution 2%.[2] Drug company jobs in marketing have significantly increased in recent years, whereas, drug company jobs in research have remained flat.

Big Pharma has been the most profitable industry for 2 decades in the United States, more profitable than oil. The drug industry median profit as a percent of revenue was 18.7% in 2000, compared with the other industry median profit as a percent of revenue of 5%.[4]

The pharmaceutical industry uses its wealth and power to influence the US Congress, the FDA, academic medical centers, and physicians in practice. They have 2 lobbyists for every congressman and spent $100 million on lobbying in 2006. They are the largest lobby of all industries in Washington, DC.

Companies may control the publication of data and may not allow publication if the data are not favorable to their drug. They also regularly lead physicians to believe that drugs are more effective and safer than reality. In 1 study of drug representative statements to doctors, 11% were inaccurate, always in favor of the drug being marketed.[5]

Few companies rely on their own research for new drugs. One-third of drugs are now licensed from universities, the NIH, or small biotechnology companies. Medical schools and faculty may enter into lucrative financial arrangements with drug companies. Another issue to be addressed is that brand name companies pay generic companies to delay release of generic drugs. Bristol-Myers Squibb paid $40 million to delay the release of the generic Plavix.

An example is the zidovudine (AZT) story. In 1983 the NIH and the Pasteur Institute in Paris discovered that AIDS was caused by a retrovirus. In 1985 the NIH screened antiviral agents at the National Cancer Institute (NCI) and Duke University and AZT was shown to be effective in clinical trials. Burroughs Well-come patented it for treatment of AIDS and charged $10,000 per year. Thus, the drug company charged high prices for a drug that it neither developed nor discovered. Another example is Taxol (paclitaxel). Research on this drug was supported by or conducted at the NCI with $183 million of tax dollars. In 1991 Bristol-Myers Squibb signed a cooperative research and development agreement with the NCI to supply paclitaxel. Then the pacific yew tree became in short supply, and in 1994 Florida State University synthesized Taxol. It was subsequently licensed to Bristol-Myers Squibb for royalties, which generated $1–$2 billion per year for Bristol-Myers Squibb and tens of millions in annual royalties for Florida State University. Bristol-Myers Squibb charges high prices for a drug it neither discovered nor developed.[1] Thus, Big Pharma is not an engine of innovation, but a vast marketing machine. It is not a free market success story, but lives off government-funded research and monopoly rights. An 800-lb. gorilla can do anything it wants to do.

Most of the "me-too" drugs are new versions of already marketed drugs. Of the 83 drugs per year approved from 1998–2002, only 32% were new molecular entities, and only 14% received priority review from the FDA.[1] Of the top 5 selling drugs in 1995, 16 of 17 key scientific papers leading to their discovery and development came from outside the industry. Fifteen percent of all relevant research came from the industry, 55% from NIH-funded laboratories, and 30% from foreign academic institutions.[1]

Seventy-seven percent of 415 new drugs approved by the FDA from 1998–2002 were "me-too" drugs. They do not have to be shown to be any better than drugs already on the market. The companies just have to show that the drugs are effective compared with placebo. They do not have to show that they are as effective as the old drug or more effective than the old drug. They can compare different doses or different clinical scenarios, such as an extended release formulation to make the new drug look different. The costs can be significantly different. Sarafem brand of fluoxetine costs $167, compared with generic fluoxetine, which is $25.[6] Interestingly, price is almost never mentioned in the advertising.

The story of the purple pill, or Nexium, is eye opening. Prilosec was about to go off patent in 2001, a potential loss to AstraZeneca. Prilosec is a mixture of 2 isomers of omeprazole. The company patented the active isomer as Nexium, and launched a massive advertising campaign for "the purple pill." They spent half a billion dollars in 2001. Prilosec generic is over-the-counter at a fraction of the cost of Nexium, $21 vs. $153.[6] In clinical trials, they compared 40 mg of Nexium with 20 mg of Prilosec, to make Nexium look better.[1] Thomas Scully, administrative head of Medicare and Medicaid, told a group of doctors, "You should be embarrassed if you prescribe Nexium. It increases costs with no medical benefits."[7]

FDA-approved generic drugs contain the same active ingredients as the innovator drug. The inactive ingredients may vary, but the active ingredients need to be identical in strength, dosage form, and route of administration. They must have the same use indications, be bioequivalent, and meet the same batch requirements for identity, strength, purity, and quality. They must be manufactured under the same standards of the FDA's good manufacturing practice regulations required for innovator products. In 2006, the University of Iowa implemented a health plan in which the employees have no co-pay if they use generic drugs. In the first year of the plan, generic use increased from 46% to 67% of prescriptions, and the health plan saved $2.5 million (personal communication from Richard Saunders, director, University of Iowa Benefits Office, Iowa City, IA, October 4, 2007).

Another example of cost savings with generic drugs would be prevention of recurrent herpes in pregnancy. Giving 1000 mg of Valtrex a day for 30 days at the end of pregnancy would cost $316. Giving 400 mg of Zovirax 3 times a day would cost $363, but giving 400 mg of acyclovir (generic) 3 times a day would cost $43. Thus, a Valtrex prescription costs 7 times as much as generic acyclovir.[6]

Another example of marketing an isomer is Clarinex vs. Claritin (desloratadine vs. loratidine). Claritin went off patent at the end of 2002. Sales of $2.7 billion in 2001 were one-third of Schering-Plough's revenues. Therefore, they had the FDA approve a Claritin metabolite, desloratadine, and they had it approved for year-round allergies, as well as seasonal allergies.[1] They marketed Clarinex at $91 as an improvement, although it is identical to loratidine at $22.[6]

Very few studies are funded by federal dollars. The NIH funded an antihypertensive and heart attacks trial involving 42,000 people over an 8-year period. Patients were randomly assigned to calcium channel blockers, alpha blockers, ACE inhibitors, and hydrochlorothiazide. The study concluded that there were fewer cases of heart failure and stroke with hydrochlorothiazide and increased heart failure with doxazosin (Cardura), and that diuretics were the best first choice to treat hypertension.[8]

Companies favor "me-too" drugs for chronic illness with a large market such as statins, antidepressants, and drugs for GERD. If a drug is not profitable, they can stop making it. There may be shortages of antivenins and steroids, and they do not develop drugs for tropical diseases, because the countries are too poor to buy the drugs. "Me-too" drugs are heavily marketed.

Clinical trials are often funded at academic centers or physicians' offices. The companies may design the trials, keep the data, analyze the data, and decide on publication. For investigators participating in these trials it is critical to retain control of the data analysis and decision for publication. Companies also fund contract research organizations. In 1990, 80% of industry-funded studies were done at academic institutions, and this had dropped to 40% in 2000 because of lower costs at contract research organizations.[9] Industry-sponsored research is 4 times more likely to be favorable to a product as NIH-sponsored research.[9]

There may often be bias in comparative trials. The investigators may enroll young subjects who get fewer side effects. They may compare the new drug with an older drug at too low a dose. The study may be only short term, when long term use is recommended. The companies may present only the part of the data that looks good and withhold publication of negative results. The studies are often powered inadequately to assess safety.

Marketing has escalated in many areas, including direct-to-consumer advertising, sales pitches to doctors in offices with free lunches and free samples, advertising in medical journals, and promotion masquerading as educational activities. Companies have prepared manuscripts for publication, and then sought authors to sign them (and edit them some) for significant financial reward.

Promotional spending on prescription drugs started in 1996 at $9 billion per year and increased to $21 billion per year in 2002. This includes samples in physicians' offices, 56%; detailing to doctors, 25%; direct-to-consumer advertising, 13%; hospital detailing, 4%; and journal ads, 2%. Direct-to-consumer advertising on prescription drugs increased from $0.8 billion in 1996 to $2.5 billion in the year 2000. Direct-to-consumer advertising is prohibited in Europe and costs are lower. In 1997 the FDA loosened the rules for advertising so that the companies only have to mention major risks and give a website to address other risks. If the ads are misleading, the company may get a letter, but often after the campaign has run its course. The FDA has very few staff to address misleading advertising.

However, the advertisements are effective. Doctors do respond to requests from patients to prescribe drugs they have seen advertised. Seventeen of 20 advertising campaigns were actually started within 1 year of FDA approval of the drug. The Institute of Medicine has recommended restriction of direct-to-consumer advertising until after more time on the market.[10]

Free samples are always of the newest, most expensive, patent-protected drugs. When a sample is exhausted, physicians often renew the drug, even if it is not their usual choice of therapy. Physicians will give samples as first-line therapy, even if it not their usual drug of choice. Of note, in 1 study, one-third of samples were used by physicians, families, and staff.[11]

Continuing medical education (CME) may be sponsored by private medical education companies, which are funded by the drug companies. They prepare teaching materials, including PowerPoint presentations, favoring the drug they are promoting. Doctors have been given lavish dinners and junkets to vacation spots to hear about drugs. Thought leaders are asked to be on speakers' bureaus. If the company can convince a physician to promote its drug, the return on investment is 2 times that of having a drug representative promote the drug.

A controversial topic is the role of lunches for faculty and residents. It is clear that gifts, even small, influence our prescribing behavior. The companies monitor our prescribing habits. There are electronic prescription tracking databases maintained by pharmacies. The representatives know what we are prescribing when they come and talk to us, and they know how to influence us to change our prescribing habits. After the lunches, the representatives collect data on the change in the numbers of prescriptions for the drug they have marketed. They receive bonuses based on sales quotas. The drug representatives are always attractive, friendly, and want to personalize the message to the physician. They offer food, flattery, and friendship.[12]

How common are physician-industry relationships? In 2001 physicians met with drug representatives on the average of four times per month. Ninety-two percent of physicians had received drug samples, 61% had received free meals, tickets, or travel, 13% had received financial benefits, and 12% had received incentives for participation in clinical trials.[13]

In 2002 the Pharmaceutical Research and Manufacturers of America published a new code of conduct. They emphasized that voluntary interactions between representatives and physicians should benefit patients, enhance the practice of medicine, and cost less than $100. They discouraged tickets to entertainment, sports, and events, which were clearly for the personal benefit of the physician. They discouraged goods not for patients' benefit. They discouraged token consulting and advisory board relationships. The American Medical Association and the American College of Physicians adopted similar codes.[14] However, despite these guidelines, doctors are still regularly seeing drug sales representatives. From 2003–2004, 83% received food in the workplace; 78% received drug samples; 41% received travel, CME, or lodging; 18% had consulting relationships; 16% were speakers; and 9% were on an advisory board. In total, 94% of physicians had relationships with industry.[14]

One argument has been made that advertising is part of our society, so we should not be concerned about it. However, gifts are in some ways different from advertising. Gifts cost money and influence behavior, like other advertising. However, gifts create an obligation, a need to reciprocate, which is what creates a conflict of interest. Gifts create a sense of entitlement, unlike advertising, and may erode professional values, unlike advertising.

When internal medicine housestaff were asked about the influence of pharmaceutical promotions on their prescribing practices, 61% said that they were not influenced at all, 38% said they were influenced a little, and 1% a lot. When they were asked if other physicians were influenced, 16% thought that other physicians were not influenced at all, 51% thought they were influenced a little, and 32% a lot.[15]

Gifts impose a sense of indebtedness. They create an obligation to reciprocate, conscious or not, and that influences behavior. The feelings of obligation are not related to the size of the gift.[16] In a randomized trial, in a restaurant in Ithaca, NY, when the waiters and waitresses presented the bill alone, compared with a bill with a chocolate on it, tips increased from 15%–18% when the chocolate was included with the bill.[17]

Do we really need the gifts? Meetings with pharmaceutical representatives are associated with requests by physicians to add drugs to the formulary. They also lead to nonrational and costly prescribing. Even small gifts influence prescribing and the profit potential for the company significantly outweighs the value of the gifts. Many physicians will claim that that they are not influenced by the trinkets and pens. A survey of 117 first- and second-year residents at a university-based internal medicine training program assessed attitudes toward 9 types of promotion. Most thought that conference lunches, dinner lectures, articles, and pens were appropriate, but fewer thought that social events, textbooks, or luggage were appropriate.[15] However, among respondents who considered an activity inappropriate, a significant percentage did participate or would have participated. Of note, our patients are more likely to consider a gift influential than are other physicians. Approximately 50% of patients thought that dinners and trips for physicians were influential on physicians' prescribing habits.[18] Wouldn't you be embarrassed if a patient asked you, "Are you prescribing drug X for me because that is what is written on your pen?"

The American Association of Medical Colleges (AAMC)[19] has published a policy on conflicts of interest and asked academic medical centers to take the lead. They want to dispel the myth that small gifts have no influence. They want to inform us that drug prescriptions increase after physicians attend company-sponsored symposia, accept free samples, or see sales representatives. Just disclosing a conflict does not eliminate a conflict of interest.[19]

The recommendations of the AAMC are as follows:

1. Ban all gifts. Ban free meals, travel to meetings, and payment for CME.
2. Ban free samples to physicians. Provide vouchers for low-income patients.
3. Exclude professionals with financial relationships with drug manufacturers from pharmacy and therapeutic committees and the FDA advisory committees.
4. Faculty should not serve as members of speakers' bureaus.

I congratulate the institutions that have already implemented these measures: Yale University, University of Michigan, University of Pennsylvania, Stanford, and University of California-Davis, and others perhaps of which I am not aware.

Currently, there are wide differences between institutions in terms of educational policies and interactions with drug representatives. Some have allowed no contact with faculty or residents. Some have highly structured and limited contact, but comprehensive policies are rare and most policies are limited and offer little guidance. Therefore, we have a significant educational opportunity to inform our residents and medical students about the potential influence of industry on physician prescribing.

Finally, I want to say a few words about the FDA. In the 1980s the pharmaceutical companies complained that it took a long time to have their proposed drugs approved. The FDA Prescription Drug User Fee Act was passed in 1993, and so the industry started paying salaries at the FDA to review drug company submissions, so-called user fees. They now comprise 40% of the budget of the FDA,[20] increasing from 9 million dollars in 1993 to 205 million dollars in 2004. Initially, only a small portion of the fees was used to evaluate postmarketing side effects (5%), but with the renewal of this bill in September

2007 more money is allocated for this because of the Vioxx postmarketing problems. A recent review of postapproval drug studies revealed that 71% were not yet started, 15% were in progress, 3% were behind schedule, and only 11% were completed.[20] So, most follow-up studies of safety are currently not performed in a timely fashion.

Who is the client of the FDA? Is it the pharmaceutical industry or the people of the United States? The drug companies are still major funders of the agency meant to regulate them.

The following is a partial summary of the recommendations for reform by Dr. Marcia Angell:[1]

Reform no. 1: Shift emphasis from "me-too" to innovative drugs. Require new drugs to be compared with old ones, not just with placebos.

Reform no. 2: Strengthen the FDA to regulate drugs. Remove FDA from the industry payroll. Shift drug resources from drug approval to monitoring drug safety, inspecting plants, and ensuring truthful advertising. Eliminate experts on advisory committees with financial ties to industry. Increase FDA funding from government.

Reform no. 3: Create an NIH institute to oversee clinical testing of drugs before FDA approval. Stop biased research by companies. The NIH should administer trials of prescription drugs. Research should be performed by independent investigators.

Reform no. 4: Get Big Pharma out of medical education. The drug companies are in the business to sell drugs for profit. Industry information comes with bias and misinformation. The message is always that new drugs are better than the old ones. There should be no private medical education industry hired by drug companies. We as physicians need to take control of education about drugs. Marketing is often masquerading as education. We need to regulate direct-to-consumer advertising.

Reform no. 5: Establish reasonable and uniform pricing. Profits could be adequate with lower prices if marketing was reduced. The Medicare Reform Bill of 2003 should be replaced by a guarantee to all Medicare beneficiaries of appropriate coverage of drug costs, a medical formulary, and government negotiated payments to industry.

Reform no. 6: Disallow gifts to physicians. Ban free lunches, drug samples, food, pens, and notepads. We need to remove real or perceived conflict of interest.

In conclusion, industry is responsible to shareholders, but we have primary responsibility to our patients. Gifts, meals, and samples influence our prescribing. The FDA has limited resources to regulate industry, and we as physicians need to take control of medical education about drugs.

Notes

1. Angell M. *The truth about the drug companies, how they deceive us and what to do about it.* New York: Random House; 2004: 58, 59, 65, 75, 78, 79.

2. Public Citizen's Congress Watch. Drug Industry Most Profitable Again: New Fortune 500 Report Confirms "Druggernaut" Tops Other Industries In Profitability Last Year. Available at http://www.citizen.org/documents/4.11.PDF. Accessed on November 21, 2007.

3. Darves B. *Too close for comfort? How some physicians are re-examining their dealings with drug detailers.* Philadelphia: American College of Physicians Observer; 2003: 1.

4. Competition and pricing issues in the pharmaceutical market, PRIME Institute, University of Minnesota. *Fortune Magazine* April 2000, Fortune 500. Available at http://money.cnn.com/magazines/fortune/fortune500_archive/full/2000/. Accessed on November 21, 2007.

5. Ziegler MG, Lew P, Singer BC. The accuracy of drug information from pharmaceutical sales representatives. *JAMA.* 1995;273:1296–1298.

6. www.drugstore.com. Accessed on November 21, 2007.

7. Two new fronts in heartburn market battle. *New York Times* August 20, 2003:C12.

8. Furberg C. The ALLHAT Officers and Coordinators for the ALLHAT collaborative research group: Major outcomes in high-risk hypertensive patients randomized to angiotensin-converting enzyme inhibitor or calcium channel blocker vs. diuretic. The antihypertensive and lipid-lowering treatment to prevent heart attack trial (ALLHAT). *JAMA.* 2002;288:2981–2997.

9. Bodenheimer T. Uneasy alliance—clinical investigators and the pharmaceutical industry. *N Engl J Med.* 2000;342;1539–1544.

10. Donohue JM, Cevasco M, Rosenthal MB. A decade of direct-to-consumer advertising of prescription drugs. *N Engl J Med.* 2007;357:673–681.

11. Coyle SL. Physician-industry relations: Part 1, individual physicians. *Ann Intern Med.* 2002;136:398.

12. Wazana A. Physicians and the pharmaceutical industry. Is a gift ever just a gift? *JAMA.* 2000;283:373–380.

13. Wazana A. *National survey of physicians: Part II, doctors and prescription drugs.* Washington, DC: Kaiser Family Foundation; 2002.

14. Campbell EG, Gruen RL, Mountford J, Miller LG, Cleary PD, Blumenthal D. A national survey of physician-industry relationships. *N Engl J Med.* 2007;356:1742–1750.

15. Steinman MA, Shlipak MG, McPhee SJ. Of principles and pens: Attitudes and practices of medicine housestaff toward pharmaceutical industry promotions. *Am J Med.* 2001;110:551–557.

16. Katz D, Caplan AL, Merz JF. All gifts large and small. *Am J Bioethics* 2003;3(3): 39–46.

17. Strohmetz DB, Rind B, Fisher R, Lynn M. Sweetening the till: The use of candy to increase restaurant tipping. *J Appl Soc Psychol.* 2002;32:300–309.

18. Gibbons RV, Landry FJ, Blouch DL, Jones DL, Williams FK, Lucey CR, et al. A comparison of physicians' and patients' attitudes toward pharmaceutical industry gifts. *J Gen Int Med.* 1998;13:151–154.

19. Brennan TA, Rothman DJ, Blank L, Blumenthal D, Chimonas SC, Cohen JJ, et al. Health industry practices that create conflicts of interest: A policy proposal for academic medical centers. *JAMA.* 2006;295:429–433.

20. Avorn J. Paying for drug approvals — who's using whom? *N Engl J Med.* 2007;356: 1697–1700.

Unnecessary Testing in Obstetrics, Gynecology, and General Medicine

Causes and Consequences of the Unwarranted Use of Costly and Unscientific (yet Profitable) Screening Modalities

Martin Donohoe

Overview

Unnecessary testing is becoming increasingly common in medical practice and consumer demand for certain types of tests have escalated. Such testing is expensive, diverts patient and provider time and attention from addressing evidence-based screening, can provide unwarranted reassurance or cause unnecessary anxiety, and can lead to further interventions that may carry risks of physical harm and even death. This chapter will provide an overview of unnecessary testing, using examples from obstetrics, gynecology, and general medicine.

There is a large body of evidence-based literature describing the extent, reasons for, and consequences of inappropriate use of laboratory tests, especially in the hospital setting. However, this column will focus primarily on more expensive screening tests, such as full-body scans, which are often marketed directly to unwitting consumers.

Evidence-Based Screening

Space limitation precludes a thorough discussion of an evidence-based approach to screening tests, but this section provides a brief overview of criteria for appropriate screening. Tests to screen for disease in the pre-symptomatic stages should meet certain criteria before being recommended. These criteria include the following:[1,2]

- The disease being screened for must be reasonably common and have a significant effect on either duration or quality of life.

- Acceptable, effective treatment must exist, and the condition must have an asymptomatic period during which detection and treatment can improve outcome.

- Treatment during the asymptomatic period must be superior to treatment once symptoms occur.

- The screening test must be safe, affordable, and have adequate sensitivity (i.e., the test is usually positive in those with disease) and specificity (the test is usually negative in those without disease).

Examples of gynecologic- or obstetrically related screening tests meeting these criteria include Pap smears, mammography, oral glucose tolerance testing during pregnancy, and universal testing of newborns for certain congenital disorders.[3,4] Other general tests of proven value include blood pressure monitoring for those older than 21 years of age, cholesterol tests for those 35 to 65 years of age, and abdominal ultrasounds for persons (especially men) with coronary risk factors and/or positive family history to screen for abdominal aortic aneurysms.

Regrettably, many well-established screening tests are underused, especially among nonwhites, those of lower socioeconomic status (SES), and those with inadequate or no health insurance.[5] Such underuse has been clearly linked with increased risk for adverse outcome. For example, SES differences in access to and use of screening mammography have been associated with advanced stage at time of breast cancer diagnosis and lower survival rates, especially among African Americans.[6] SES differences in the use of prenatal testing for trisomy 21 have also been associated with disparities in the live-birth prevalence of Down syndrome. Because incidence of this disease does not vary according to SES, it has been demonstrated that early prenatal diagnosis leads to a higher rate of elective termination of pregnancy by individuals of higher SES.[7]

Unnecessary Testing by Clinicians and Independent Companies

Certain once-broadly accepted monitoring tests that were used routinely have not been supported by outcome data. Examples from obstetric practice include electronic fetal heart rate monitoring and fetal pulse oximetry. Routine electronic fetal heart rate monitoring has not been demonstrated to decrease the rate of cerebral palsy, but has been linked to increases in the overall rate of cesarean delivery.[8,9] It has also been determined that routine use of fetal pulse oximetry is not associated with either reduced rates of cesarean delivery or improvement in the condition of newborns.[10] Although these tests are not recommended for routine assessment, they remain in use in many hospitals in the United States.

Other monitoring tests may be misused. One example of this is fetal ultrasonography. Although it is helpful in estimating gestational age, identifying twin pregnancies, and detecting genetic anomalies, the American College of Obstetrics and Gynecology (ACOG) position is that routine ultrasonographic screening during pregnancy is not mandatory. They deem routine use reasonable when requested by a patient.[11] Most women in the United States undergo at least 1 or 2 ultrasounds during pregnancy; this level of exposure has never been associated with significant risk and use may provide significant benefits. However, some expectant couples have followed the lead of actors Tom Cruise and Katie Holmes and purchased (for costs ranging between $15,000 and $200,000) their own ultrasound machines, which they use daily.[12]

There are some data (mostly from other vertebrates) suggesting that prolonged and frequent use of fetal ultrasound can cause abnormalities in fetal brain development, behavior, and body weight.[13] Even though such findings have not been substantiated in humans,[13] the US Food and Drug Administration (FDA) considers promotion, selling, or leasing of ultrasound equipment for the purpose of making "keepsake fetal videos" an unapproved use of a medical device.[14] Such use may also violate state laws and regulations.

Full Body Screening

Unnecessary testing has been promoted by both well-intentioned medical practitioners and outright quacks for centuries. Due to lack of health literacy and/or a powerful need for reassurance, many individuals are willing to pay—sometime exorbitant amounts—for screening tests that lack scientific merit. Regrettably, numerous companies have recently been created to meet the demand. For example, Biophysical 250 charges $3,400 "to screen for hundreds of diseases and conditions ... including cancer, cardiovascular disease, metabolic disorders, autoimmune disease, viral and bacterial disease and hormonal imbalance."[15]

Full-body screening, via computed tomography (CT) scanning, became increasingly popular after television talk show host Oprah Winfrey underwent testing in 2001.[16] The number of self-referral body-imaging centers, where such scans are often performed, totaled 161 in 2003, up from 88 in 2001.[17] One company, Ultra Life, offers "real time color ultrasound" of various organs, or for those inclined, a $500 "full body scan."[18]

Companies offering "metabolic screens" and whole-body scans tend to market in areas of higher SES. They prey on fear of heart disease and cancer, and on an individual's natural desire to detect health problems early in hopes of achieving a cure, or at least avoiding potentially disfiguring or toxic therapies.

Some companies also market testing devices such as body composition analyzers and bone densitometers directly to healthcare providers. Having such equipment available no doubt increases use and, when such testing is reimbursable, contributes to practice income. Education programs may be offered to assist clinicians in "optimizing the clinic visit." Under certain circumstances, this could be interpreted as "optimizing receipts through the use of procedures of questionable utility performed under dubious circumstances."

A 2004 survey of 500 Americans found that 85% would choose a full-body CT scan over $1,000 cash.[19] It is certainly problematic that these scans can deliver a radiation dose nearly 100 times that of a typical mammogram.[20] A single scan exposes the person being scanned to a level of radiation linked to increased cancer mortality in low-dose atomic bomb survivors from Hiroshima and Nagasaki.[20] Undergoing such scans annually would substantially increase one's lifetime risk of malignancy. Of course, this is not meant to imply that one should avoid medically indicated diagnostic CT scans of particular organs.

Naturopathic Testing

Many "naturopathic" approaches to diagnostic testing exist, including iridology; pulse and tongue diagnosis; electrodiagnosis; hair, urine, and stool analyses; applied kinesiology; and some forms of acupuncture.[21,22] Often, such testing leads to recommendations for treatment with unproven and/or dangerous supplements. Avoidance of standard prescription drugs and surgical treatments in favor of alternative treatment such as colonic irrigation, cranioelectrical stimulation, detoxification diets, and chelation therapy may occur.[21,22]

Most alternative practitioners do not encourage patients to forgo standard medical treatment, but instead offer naturopathic treatment as an adjunct. However, the risk that a patient may choose an unproven alternative remedy over a proven effective traditional therapy could lead to unnecessary harm, as could possible harmful interactions between traditional and non-traditional therapies.[23]

Risks of Unnecessary Testing

Before considering a full-body scan or other non-proven screening test, individuals should be made aware of the potential risks. False-positive test results are extremely common among individuals with no signs or symptoms of disease; multiple tests increase the likelihood of false-positive results. Such alarming yet incorrect test results can lead to further unnecessary investigations, additional patient costs, heightened anxiety, and risk to future insurability. Conversely, true positive results can lead to the overdiagnosis of conditions that would not have become clinically significant, thus leading to further risky interventions.[1]

Examples of potentially harmful screening methods and possible outcomes include the following:

- Pelvic ultrasounds on asymptomatic women to search for ovarian cancer could lead to unnecessary laparoscopies and biopsies, with attendant complications
- Screening all current and former smokers in the United States for lung cancer with a CT scan would identify more than 180 million lung nodules, the vast majority of which would be benign. Millions of patients with nodules could needlessly undergo invasive needle lung biopsies and/or removal of parts of their lungs, resulting in many cases of impaired breathing, pneumothorax, hemorrhage, infection, and even death.

Even commonly recommended tests carry a sometimes large risk of a false-positive result. For example, among women in their early 40s with abnormal mammograms, it was shown that approximately 57 women without cancer underwent further diagnostic workup for every 1 woman found to have a malignancy.[24]

Unnecessary Testing, Luxury Care, and the Erosion of Science and Medical Ethics

One area where over-testing is rife is luxury primary care, also known as concierge care, boutique medicine, retainer practice, executive healthcare, or premium practice.[25-27] Luxury care contributes to the erosion of the scientific practice of medicine by offering "clients" screening tests that are often not indicated and can cause more harm than good.

There is no evidence documenting a higher quality of care in concierge practices, and little data support the clinical or cost-effectiveness of many of the tests typically offered by such practices to their asymptomatic clients. Examples include percent body fat measurements, chest radiographs in smokers and nonsmokers aged 35 years and older to screen for lung cancer, electron-beam CT scans and stress echocardiograms to look for evidence of coronary artery disease, and abdominal-pelvic ultrasounds to screen for ovarian or liver cancer.[24,25,28,29] Other examples, such as mammography starting at age 35 and genetic testing, are also controversial.

Although clients pay for these tests, technicians and equipment time are diverted to produce immediate results. Because patients jump the queue in the radiology and phlebotomy suites, tests for other patients with more appropriate/urgent needs may be delayed. Regrettably, such luxury practices are often associated with, and actively promoted by, academic medical centers. Such association sullies these institutions' images as arbiters of evidence-based medicine and facilitates an erosion of professional ethics by perpetuating a two-tiered system of care within institutions that have been the traditional healthcare providers to the indigent and where clinicians in training learn professional ethics.

The use of clinically unjustifiable tests also erodes the scientific underpinnings of medical practice and sends a mixed message to trainees and patients about when and why to use diagnostic studies.[30] Such use also runs counter to physicians' ethical obligations "to contribute to the responsible stewardship of health care resources."[31] Some might argue that if patients are willing to pay for scientifically unsupported testing, they should be allowed to do so. However, such a "buffet" approach to diagnosis over-medicalizes healthcare and makes a mockery of evidence-based medicine.

Pseudoscience and Anti-Science

Without adequate science and health education and knowledge, individuals may lack the skepticism necessary to refuse unwarranted testing. Public education, including science and health education, has suffered from decaying infrastructure, funding cuts, sponsored "educational" curricula produced by corporations, and high student-teacher ratios.[32-36] At least some of the increase in unnecessary testing is due to the general erosion of science under the current federal administration, as manifested through the following:

- Appointments to key scientific bodies based on corporate connections and political or religious ideology, rather than scientific expertise
- Excessive corporate influence over legislation
- The rewriting and even suppression of scientific policy statements[31-36]

Recognizing Health Scams

Health scams are ubiquitous on the Internet and even in traditional media. Warning signs of bogus science include:[37,38]

- Claims pitched directly to the media, rather than via publication in peer-reviewed journals
- The discoverer says that a powerful establishment is trying to suppress his or her work.

- Appeals to false authorities, emotion, or magical thinking
- The scientific effect involved is at the very limit of detection.
- Evidence for the test or treatment is anecdotal and relies on subjective validation.
- The promoter states a belief is credible because it has endured for centuries.
- The need to propose new laws of nature to explain an observation

Patients should be encouraged to query their healthcare providers about sources of reliable information and to consult providers before obtaining screening and/or diagnostic tests or undergoing alternative treatments (including the use of "supplements" and "nutraceuticals"). The US Food and Drug Administration has warned consumers against purchasing medical devices from the Internet, including laboratory diagnostic kits to detect serious illnesses.[39]

Conclusion

Unnecessary testing is common among both traditional and alternative medical providers. Improved science and health education, more nuanced and responsible communication of medical information by the media, enhanced scientific integrity of governmental bodies, eliminating—or at least limiting the expansion of—luxury care, and better communication between patients and healthcare providers would all help contribute to increased use of appropriate, less harmful screening practices and to enhanced health outcomes.

Notes

1. Fletcher SW. Evidence-based approach to prevention. *UpToDate* 2006 (January). Available at http://utdol.com/utd/content/topic.do?topicKey=screenpm/6460&view=text. Accessed March 23, 2007; subscription required.

2. Jackson JL, Berbano E. Total body imaging. *UpToDate* 2006 (August). Available at http://utdol.com/utd/content/topic.do?topicKey=genr_med/14732&view=text. Accessed March 23, 2007; subscription required.

3. Fletcher SW. Screening average risk women for breast cancer. *UpToDate* 2006 (September). Available at http://utdol.com/utd/content/topic.do?topicKey=screenpm/3044&view=text. Accessed March 23, 2007; subscription required.

4. Caliskan E, Kayikcioglu F, Ozturk N, Koc S, Haberal A. A population-based risk factor scoring will decrease unnecessary testing for the diagnosis of gestational diabetes mellitus. *Acta Obstet Gynecol Scand.* 2004;83:524–530. Abstract.

5. Donohoe MT. Comparing generalist and specialty care: Discrepancies, deficiencies, and excesses. In: Isaacs SL, Knickman J, eds. *Generalist medicine and the US health*

care system. San Francisco: Robert Wood Johnson Foundation/Jossey-Bass, 2004. Reprinted from *Arch Intern Med.* 1998;158:1596–1608.

6. Li CI. Racial and ethnic disparities in breast cancer stage, treatment, and survival in the United States. *Ethn Dis.* 2005;15:S5–S9.

7. Khoshnood B, De Vigan C, Vodovar, Breart G, Goffinet F, Blondel B. Advances in medical technology and creation of disparities: The case of Down syndrome. *Am J Public Health* 2006;96:2139–2144. Abstract.

8. Greene MF. Obstetricians still await a deus ex machine. *N Engl J Med.* 2006;355:2247–2248. Abstract.

9. Clark SL, Hankins GDV. Temporal and demographic trends in cerebral palsy—fact and fiction. *Am J Obstet Gynecol.* 2003;188:628–633. Abstract.

10. Bloom SL, Spong CY, Thom E, et al. Fetal pulse oximetry and cesarean delivery. *N Engl J Med.* 2006;355:2195–2202. Abstract.

11. Sfakianaki AK, Copel J. Routine prenatal ultrasonography as a screening tool. *UpToDate* 2006 (March). Available at http://utdol.com/utd/content/topic.do?topicKey=antenatl/18708&view=text. Accessed March 23, 2007; subscription required.

12. Kritz F. Doctors not fans of Tom Cruise's baby gifts. *MSNBC* 2005 (December 6). Available at http://www.msnbc.msn.com/id/10309963/. Accessed December 30, 2006.

13. Volkin L, Dargan RS. Study shows potential dangers of ultrasound in fetal development. *American Society of Radiologic Technologists* 2006 (August 14). Available at http://www.asrt.org/content/News/IndustryNewsBriefs/Sono/studyshows062408.aspx. Accessed December 28, 2006.

14. US Food and Drug Administration. Fetal keepsake videos. *Center for Devices and Radiological Health* 2005 (August). Available at http://www.fda.gov/ohrms/dockets/dockets/04p0329/04p-0329-ts00002-02-Intro.pdf. Accessed December 29, 2006.

15. Biophysical 250. *What can Biophysical 250 tell you?* Available at http://www.biophysicalcorp.com/assessments/biophysical250.aspx. Accessed December 29, 2006.

16. Winfrey O. New medical tests. *The Oprah Winfrey Show.* Available at http://www.oprah.com/tows/pastshows/tows_past_20010312.jhtml. Accessed December 29, 2006.

17. Kalish GM, Bhargavan M, Sunshine JH, Forman HP. Self-referred whole-body imaging: Where are we now. *Radiology* 2004;233:353–358. Abstract.

18. Ultra Life Body Scan. Available at http://www.ultralifebodyscan.com/. Accessed December 29, 2006.

19. Schwartz LM, Woloshin S, Fowler FJ Jr, Welch HG. Enthusiasm for cancer screening in the United States. *JAMA.* 2004;291:71–78. Abstract.

20. Hampton T. Full-body CT scans scale up cancer risk. *JAMA.* 2004;292:1669–1670.

21. Atwood KC. Naturopathy: A critical appraisal. *Medscape Gen Med.* 2003;5(4). Available at http://www.medscape.com/viewarticle/465994_print. Accessed November 16, 2006.

22. Atwood KC. Naturopathy, pseudoscience, and medicine: Myths, pseudoscience, and medicine: Myths and fallacies vs. truth. *Medscape Gen Med.* 2004;6. Available at http://www.medscape.com/viewarticle/471156_print. Accessed November 16, 2006.

23. Adams KE, Cohen MH, Eisenberg D, Jonsen AR. Ethical considerations of complementary and alternative medical therapies in conventional medical settings. *Ann Intern Med.* 2002;137:660–664. Abstract.

24. Carney PA, Miglioretti CL, Yankaskas BC, et al. Individual and combined effects of age, breast density, and hormone replacement therapy use on the accuracy of screening mammography. *Ann Intern Med.* 2003;138:168–175. Abstract.

25. Donohoe MT. Luxury primary care, academic medical centers, and the erosion of science and professional ethics. *J Gen Intern Med.* 2004;19:90–94. Abstract.

26. Donohoe MT. Retainer practice: Scientific issues, social justice, and ethical perspectives. *American Medical Association Virtual Mentor* 2004;6. Available at http://www.ama-assn.org/ama/pub/category/12249.html. Accessed December 29, 2006.

27. Donohoe MT. Standard vs. luxury care. In: Buetow S and Kenealy T, Eds. *Ideological Debates in Family Medicine.* New York, Nova Science Publishers, Inc., 2007, pages 187-201.

28. Connolly C. The wealth care system: When CEOs and VIPs need health care, they get the best money can buy. A reporter finds out just how good that is. *Washington Post* 2002 (May 28). Available at http://www.washingtonpost.com/wp-dyn /articles/A7559–2002May24.html. Accessed December 29, 2006.

29. Connolly C. Healers for the well-heeled: 'Concierge' care sparks a debate on HMOs, medicine and morals. *Washington Post* 2002 (May 28);A01. Available at http://www.washingtonpost.com/wp-dyn/articles/A18426–2002May27.html. Accessed December 29, 2006.

30. Cohen JJ. Missions of a medical school: A North American perspective. *Acad Med.* 1999;74:S27–S30. Abstract.

31. American College of Physicians. Ethics manual. *Ann Intern Med.* 1998;128:576–594. Abstract.

32. Rosenstock L, Lee LJ. Attacks on science: The risks to evidence-based policy. *Am J Public Health* 2002;92:14–18. Abstract.

33. Donohoe MT. Causes and health consequences of environmental degradation and social injustice. *Soc Sci Med.* 2003;56:573–587. Abstract.

34. Donohoe MT. Teen pregnancy: A call for sound science and public policy. *Z Magazine* 2003;16:14–16. Available at http://zmagsite.zmag.org/Apr2003 /donohoe0403.html. Accessed December 29, 2006.

35. Donohoe MT. Increase in obstacles to abortion: The American perspective in 2004. *J Am Med Womens Assn.* 2005;60:16–25. Available at http://www.amwa-doc.org/index.cfm?objectid=1B138032-D567-0B25-57EE86AC69902184. Accessed March 23, 2007.

36. Donohoe MT. Obstacles to abortion in the United States. *Medscape Ob/Gyn Womens Health* 2005;10. Available at http://www.medscape.com/viewarticle/507404. Accessed March 23, 2007.

37. Coker R. Distinguishing science and pseudoscience. *Quackwatch* 2001 (May). Available at http://quackwatch.org/01QuackeryRelatedTopics/pseudo.html. Accessed December 29, 2006.

38. Park RL. Seven warning signs of bogus science. *Quackwatch* 2003 (March). Available at http://www.quackwatch.org/01QuackeryRelatedTopics/signs.html. Accessed December 29, 2006.

39. US Food and Drug Administration. Buying medical devices online. *Center for Devices and Radiological Health* 2001 (May). Available at http://www.fda.gov/cdrh/consumer/buyingmeddevonline.html. Accessed December 29, 2007.

Chapter 33

Urine Trouble

Practical, Legal, and Ethical Issues Surrounding Mandated Drug Testing of Physicians

Martin Donohoe

Introduction

Healthcare organizations and medical schools have increasingly adopted mandatory pre-employment and random, not-for-cause drug-testing programs for physicians.[1] This article discusses the history of drug testing in the United States, the recommendations of policy-making bodies, the prevalence of substance use and abuse among physicians, and the data on the costs and benefits of such drug-testing programs.

When used appropriately, random, for-cause drug testing of physicians who have been rehabilitated of a substance-abuse disorder have been successful in maintaining abstinence and preserving doctors' careers. However, mandatory pre-employment and random, not-for-cause testing programs are based on poor science, are financially wasteful, and are unlikely to meet the programs' implicit goals of creating a safer clinical environment and diminishing errors while improving the quality of patient care. These programs usually ignore alcohol and tobacco (the major deleterious substances affecting health and performance), are often not designed to help those few doctors who abuse other substances get appropriate treatment, can create dissent among staff, and may inhibit an organization's ability to hire individuals who are unwilling to compromise their personal ethics by capitulating to what they consider to be an unjust policy.

The invasion of privacy posed by pre-employment and random, not-for-cause drug testing programs could potentially lead to other types of unwarranted testing and the dissemination of physicians' personal health data beyond the confines of their institutions. Indeed, increased drug testing is just one example of the increasing erosion of privacy in the United States. I will describe the broader problem of erosion of individual privacy and will draw parallels with recent measures designed to protect patients' privacy.

While the public has been increasingly concerned about the erosion of patients' rights to privacy, it also has expressed a desire for greater account-ability by physicians, increased disclosure regarding the overall competency of healthcare providers, enhanced standards to protect the safety of patients, and higher standards for the quality of medical care. This article will describe effective interventions that not only protect the privacy of patients and healthcare providers, but also protect patients from incompetent and impaired physicians and enhance the safety of patients and the quality of care they receive.

Drug Testing: History, Prevalence, Policies, and Recommendations

Substance use involves the taking of legal or illegal substances that does not lead to impairment of performance. Substance abuse involves a pattern of repeated, pathological use with adverse health consequences, habituation, tolerance, withdrawal symptoms, and impaired performance. "Impairment" refers to one's inability to perform competently one's duties as a result of substance use or abuse.

Drug testing in the US began in the Armed Forces in the early 1970s, when reproducible assays were first developed.[2] By the late 1970s, prisoners were being screened, and, in the early 1980s, workers were screened at defense contractors.[3] Since 1986, when President Reagan instituted an executive order requiring federal agencies to institute drug-testing programs,[4] testing has spread throughout the public and private sectors.[5] The federal Drug-Free Workplace Act (DFWA) of 1988 mandates that all recipients of federal government contracts of $25,000 or more per year, and all recipients of federal government grants, must have written drug policies on employee substance use and abuse, establish a drug-free awareness program, and make a good-faith effort to maintain a drug-free workplace.[6] However, the DFWA does not provide instructions on how to implement its provisions.[7] Under the Omnibus Transportation Employee Testing Act of 1991, employers are only required to test workers who apply for, or currently hold, safety-sensitive positions in the transportation industry. There are no other federal laws that require private businesses to have drug-testing programs.[8]

Increasing use of drug testing has been noted in industry, despite opposition from the American Civil Liberties Union (ACLU) and other organizations.[9] In 1987, 21 percent of corporate members of the American Management Association, the nation's largest management development and training organization, had instituted drug-testing programs;[10] by 1996, 81 percent of major firms in the United States tested for drugs.[11] Among Fortune 1,000 companies, there has been a 1,200 percent increase in periodic and random employee drug testing since 1987.[12]

In 1988, the American Hospital Association recommended that healthcare institutions adopt comprehensive policies to address substance abuse, including pre-employment testing, for-cause testing, and post-accident testing, regardless of job description.[13] The American College of Occupational and Environmental Medicine finds it ethically acceptable, with appropriate constraints, to screen current and prospective employees for the presence of drugs, including alcohol, that might affect their ability to perform work in a safe manner.[14] The American Medical Association (AMA) also supports pre-employment drug screening.[15]

The purported goals of physician drug testing are to create a safer climate for patient care; to protect the university or institution from malpractice and wrongful hiring lawsuits; and to promote a positive view of the institution from patients and other "healthcare consumers."[16] In our competitive healthcare marketplace, when one hospital in a community institutes an employee drug-testing policy, others follow suit to avoid a negative image, which the public, which is generally uninformed about the nature of substance-abuse testing and treatment,[17] may attach to those without such a policy. To date, no court has held an employer legally liable for not having a drug-testing program. On the other hand, employers have incurred substantial legal costs defending their drug-testing programs against workers' claims of wrongful dismissal.[18]

While only 9 to 15 percent of hospitals surveyed in the late 1980s and early 1990s required testing,[19] this percentage is increasing.[20] That this trend parallels the impressive growth of drug testing in industry is not surprising, given the increasing corporatization of American medicine. In 1999, Montoya and colleagues found that two-thirds of 44 randomly selected large teaching hospitals had formal physician drug-testing policies.[21] For-cause testing and pre-employment testing were most common; 13 percent of policies mandated random, not-for-cause testing. In general, the policies were vague on procedural details and unclear regarding responsibility for implementation of policy guidelines. Only half mentioned employee confidentiality, and less than 50 percent of these were explicit regarding access to and storage of records. All five major academic and community teaching hospitals in Portland, Oregon, where this author practices, now require pre-employment drug testing.[22]

Substance Use and Abuse by Physicians

Prevalence data on substance use and abuse by physicians and physician-trainees are marred by overreliance on convenience sampling, self-report, and variable definitions of substance-use and impairment.[23] Nevertheless, taken together, medical students do not differ significantly from age-matched peers in substance use patterns, except that they are less likely to smoke tobacco. In a survey of 23 medical schools, the AMA found that the substances most commonly used by medical students over a 30-day period were alcohol (87.5 percent), cigarettes (10 percent), marijuana (10 percent), cocaine (2.8 percent), tranquilizers (2.3 percent), and opiates (1.1 percent).[24] Less than 1 percent of respondents felt they were dependent on any substance other than tobacco. In a national survey, Hughes and colleagues found that alcohol was used by 87 percent and marijuana by 7 percent of third-year residents over the preceding 30 days, with 5 percent reporting daily alcohol use and 1.3 percent reporting daily marijuana use,[25] 1.5 percent reported using cocaine over the last month; 3.7 percent benzodiazepines (tranquilizers); none used these substances on a daily basis. The findings of a national survey conducted by Robert and colleagues, (which may have been affected by a 52 percent response rate), are as follows: about one-fourth of students at nine medical schools suffered symptoms of mental illness, including 7 to 18 percent with substance-use disorders.[26] Among house staff, emergency medicine and psychiatry residents report higher levels of substance use.[27] House staff self-medication with benzodiazepines was not uncommon in the early 1990s;[28] today, house staff who self-medicate are more likely to use antihistamines for sleep, or selective serotonin re-uptake inhibitors for depression.[29]

Practicing physicians are no more likely to abuse substances than other professionals.[30] Physicians have lower rates of use and abuse of tobacco, marijuana, cocaine, and heroin than the general population, and do not appear to be at increased risk for alcoholism.[31] However, unsupervised use of benzodiazepines and minor opiates within the past year was reported by 11.4 percent and 17.6 percent, respectively, with higher rates of opioid use seen among anesthesiologists.[32] Whether such use impairs performance, through oversedation, or improves performance, through control of anxiety and pain, depends on the user, but such self-treatment is unwise at best and unethical at worst.[33] Prevalence rates for lifetime impairment of practicing physicians by drugs or alcohol range from 2 to 14 percent.[34]

The "Science" and Costs Behind Drug Testing

Random testing is an imperfect way to identify drug abusers and is subject to both false-positive and false-negative results. Test characteristics relating to the metabolism of different substances can lead to situations in which a physician who snorts cocaine every Saturday night is likely to test negative on a Monday, whereas an individual who attends a party and is subjected to large amounts of second-hand marijuana smoke, or who unsuspectingly ingests a brownie made with cannabis, will test positive two to three days later.[35] Moderate poppy seed biscuit ingestion can cause a false-positive test for opioids,[36] ibuprofen a false-positive test for cannabinoids; and selegiline, an anti-Parkinson's disease drug, a false-positive for amphetamines.[37] Tonic water can show up as cocaine and Nyquil as an opiate or amphetamine.[38] Seriously impaired alcoholics, who far outnumber marijuana and opioid abusers, can easily be missed even though their mental and physical impairments (including withdrawal tremors, confusion/delirium, memory loss, and subtle nerve damage) are likely to cause greater morbidity. Until a Drug Enforcement Agency (DEA) ban on the use of hemp seed oil in 2003, many food products made with this ingredient contained trace amounts of tetrahydrocannabinol (THC), the active agent in marijuana. These products, which included pasta, candy bars, and salad dressings, could have caused false-positive results for marijuana.[39]

Multiple means of sabotaging drug tests and escaping detection, including adulteration, dilution, and the purchase of "drug-free urine" are described on a growing array of websites on the Internet.[40] Ingesting large quantities of liquids, taking diuretics, or adding water or household bleach to a urine specimen can sometimes mask illicit drug use.[41] While many labs test for common adulterants, and some use temperature-sensitive cups to detect nonfresh urine and check specific gravity to detect possible dilution, it is not known how well these labs are able to recognize "fixed" samples.[42]

Employee drug testing is expensive. The federal government's drug-testing program spends from $35,000 to $77,000 to find one user.[43] Most of the workers identified are occasional moderate users rather than drug abusers, and more than half test positive only for marijuana. If one out of 10 test positives is a drug abuser—what many consider to be a high estimate—then the average cost of finding one drug abuser would range from $350,000 to $770,000. If half of the detected drug abusers would have been detected anyway, through other means, the cost of using drug testing to find one otherwise hidden drug abuser would be as high as $700,000 to $1.5 million.[44] Costs are likely to be higher when physicians are tested, due to lower rates of substance use and abuse.

In fact, no solid data exist to show that drug testing deters drug use.[45] Only 8 percent of companies with drug testing have performed any cost-benefit analysis.[46] Frequently cited estimates of lost productivity due to drug use are based on data that the National Academy of Sciences has concluded are flawed: "the data ... do not provide clear evidence of the deleterious effects of drugs other than alcohol on safety and other job performance indicators."[47] Furthermore, drug testing can have a negative impact on workplace morale, and the urine collection process itself is degrading and demeaning, particularly when it involves direct observation.[48] An analysis of 63 high-technology firms in the computer equipment and data processing industry reports that drug testing actually reduced, rather than enhanced, productivity by creating an environment of distrust and paranoia, rather than one in which employees were treated with dignity and respect.[49] Some employers have dropped pre-employment screening because it unduly hindered their ability to recruit workers with the proper skills.[50]

Physicians' Attitudes Toward Drug Testing

Physicians' opinions regarding mandatory drug testing is mixed.[51] In one study of practicing physicians in the Midwest, 60 percent of the respondents said that requiring drug testing to obtain hospital privileges infringed on their rights to privacy; 38 percent lacked confidence in the testing procedure.[52] While 56 percent of the surveyed doctors said that they would submit to mandatory testing without protest, 8 percent would refuse testing, 7 percent would hospitalize their patients in another institution, and 7 percent stated that they would file a lawsuit.[53] In a 1994 survey of family practice residency directors' attitudes toward mandatory pre-employment drug testing, almost half disagreed with mandatory substance-abuse testing and said it should not be a condition of acceptance for a house officer position.[54] Program directors and medical students do not see testing as a positive aspect of a program.[55] In one study, 22 percent of senior medical students said that they would not rank, or would rank lower, a program with mandatory pre-employment drug testing.[56]

The Physicians' Dilemma: To Be or Not to Be Tested

Since no laboratory test is 100 percent specific, false-positive results are inevitable. For nondrug users, the only type of positive test that would result from their urine being examined is a false-positive test. Rational, nondrug-using physicians might not willingly choose to risk their futures in medicine from potential false-positive tests. By participating in a drug-testing program, they put their public reputation and future employability in jeopardy (and in turn may disrupt long-standing relationships with their patients), threaten the large public financial investment in their training, and risk wreaking emotional and financial havoc on their families. Even so, given financial exigencies and the ubiquity of preemployment drug testing, there is often no real choice for such persons. Furthermore, even if their initial test is later shown to be a false positive, even temporary removal from the workplace can cause undue suspicion and embarrassment, decrease income (especially for those paid per diem), and disrupt the continuity of patient care.

Testing, Treating, and Disciplining Impaired Physicians

All rational physicians are in favor of improving the health of their professional colleagues, providing treatment in the most expeditious and confidential manner for those who have exhibited strong evidence of job impairment, and ensuring the safe delivery of error-free care to their patients. Voluntary treatment programs for substance-abusing resident physicians have been supported by the Association of Program Directors in Internal Medicine,[57] and programs for substance-abusing doctors are available in every state and have been very successful.[58] This is likely due to physicians' high levels of education, motivation, and functioning, as well as possession of a professional career that provides financial and personal resources that can support and sustain treatment and recovery.[59] Nearly all (90 percent) of state licensure applications ask about substance abuse and inquire about functional impairment from substance use, not simply substance use per se.[60] If a physician self-reports and/or cooperates with treatment, state medical boards may not pursue disciplinary action.[61] Physician wellness and remediation programs have been fairly effective in ensuring the confidentiality, or at least the limited dissemination, of clients' information.[62]

In contrast, the medical profession has been slow to discipline adequately impaired or poorly performing doctors, which erodes the public's trust. Of 1,715 doctors who were disciplined for substance abuse by state medical boards between 1990 and 1999, only 32 (4 percent) had to stop practicing, even temporarily; others faced increased monitoring.[63] Stories of "bad doctors" who continue to harm patients are frequently reported in the lay press.[64] Some of these practitioners have not been adequately disciplined nor have they been stripped of their licenses or practice privileges due to impaired performance secondary to substance abuse. Increased restrictions on, and suspensions of, the licenses of these physicians is clearly warranted. Additionally, medical schools and training programs should improve and mandate curricula on physicians' impairment and substance abuse[65] and on reducing errors.[66]

The Growth of Drug and Other Pre-Employment Testing

Trends in drug testing in the healthcare sector parallel those in public education.[67] Over the past few years, in response to affirmative Supreme Court decisions, the number of schools that require expensive, mandatory drug testing has grown substantially.[68] School-based drug-testing programs promulgate misconceptions regarding drug use/abuse, increase the acceptability of drug testing in areas outside of medicine, and may enhance the public's willingness to accept the misguided notion that pre-employment and random, not-for-cause drug testing of physicians is an accurate and appropriate way to enhance patients' safety and the quality of care.

The explosive growth of drug testing in many spheres of employment has been fueled by popular misconceptions surrounding substance use and abuse, "junk science," business interests like the Institute for a Drug-Free Workplace (comprised of representatives from the United States Chamber of Commerce and corporations, including pharmaceutical and drug-testing companies),[69] and the public relations campaigns of a multi-billion dollar industry whose entrepreneurial interest lies in magnifying the severity of drug-related problems in the workplace and extolling the benefits of drug testing as a solution.[70]

In conjunction with the ascendancy of drug testing to meet the real and perceived needs of corporate employers, the following unscientific, poorly validated, and invasive (yet highly profitable) testing industries have blossomed: personality and "integrity" assessment,[71] polygraph testing,[72] background checking,[73] "snitch" programs,[74] and examination of prospective employees by substance-sniffing canines.[75]

Drug Testing and the Erosion of Privacy

Employee drug and other pre-employment testing programs erode individuals'privacy. Many drug-testing programs require one to divulge prescription and nonprescription medications that one is using, since some of these can cause false-positive or false-negative test results.[76] More than one-third of the American Management Association's members reported that they tape phone conversations, videotape employees, review voice mail, and check computer files and e-mail.[77] Companies frequently conduct database searches of applicants' credit reports, driving and court records, and workers' compensation claims.[78] Some prohibit coworkers from dating, or ban off-the-clock smoking and drinking.[79] Nearly half of the Fortune 500 companies report that they collect data on their workers without informing them; a majority share employee data with prospective creditors, landlords, and charities;[80] 35 percent check medical records before they hire or promote; and some check urine pregnancy tests, using the same sample obtained for pre-employment drug screening.[81] It is not surprising, then, that the Federal Trade Commission found that 80 percent of Americans polled said that they are worried about what happens to information that is collected about them.[82]

The slippery slope of workplace drug testing for physicians and others could lead to the analysis of employees' hair for drug use, as hair is subject to external contamination from passive exposure and different sensitivities based on hair color;[83] testing urine for metabolites of medications used to treat conditions that may impair performance, such as antidepressants, anti-Parkinsonian agents, antihistamines and cold remedies, anti-seizure medications, and drugs for coronary and cerebral vascular disease; and genetic testing for diseases that may affect the length of one's potential career, such as tests for Huntington's disease or other early-onset dementias.

Today, as many as 10 percent of companies use genetic testing for employment purposes.[84] While 37 states have enacted legislation that prohibits discrimination in employment or insurance on the basis of genetic information, these laws provide little practical protection, as the burden of proof is on the applicant and discrimination is difficult to prove.[85] Some individuals who are at risk for genetic conditions have experienced discrimination based on their risk status.[86] Currently, only 15 states have enacted laws that help protect employees from genetic discrimination in the workplace; a few other states and the federal government have legislation pending.[87] In the last year of his presidency, Bill Clinton signed an executive order prohibiting federal agencies from using genetic information in any hiring or promotion decisions.[88] Of note, the American Medical Association opposes pre-employment genetic testing.[89]

There is no way to completely safeguard that information obtained through drug-testing programs will not be shared with life, home, or health insurance companies (and, by extension, with pharmaceutical companies) or with future employers.[90] Indeed, one state's medical board's actions may be disseminated among other states' boards through the Federation of State Medical Boards,[91] and, in almost all states, may be made available to the public.[92] The National Practitioner Databank, which one day might be accessible to the general public, may contain information on actions resulting from physician impairment.[93]

It is unclear to what extent Fourth Amendment protections against unreasonable search and seizure and the Americans with Disabilities Act may protect physicians with respect to disclosure of information or testing of bodily fluids.[94] Court challenges to drug testing, based on the First, Fifth, and Fourteenth Amendments that allege violations of due process and equal protection have been generally unsuccessful.[95] It is interesting that the Canadian Human Rights Commission has disallowed random and pre-employment drug testing of public employees, calling it a human rights violation under the Canadian Human Rights Act.[96]

Ethical questions abound regarding privacy, bodily integrity, and confidentiality. These unanswered questions include Which physicians should be tested (clinicians, researchers, administrators)? How often? Who should have access to a physician's test results (and, by extension, potentially to other personal health data)? Also, if a staff physician's test results are going to be known to his division chief, department chair, and potentially to the dean and president of the university (as required by the local policies I reviewed),[97] then one might argue that the staff physician should be privy to their results (which is not the case in these policies). The physician may reason that the decisions that the division chief, department chair, dean, and president make on a daily basis affect far more people (patients, employees, and members of the community) than those that the physician makes, and that, indeed, his or her superiors are the individuals responsible for the educational, clinical, and social missions and the economic well-being of the hospital and university.

Patients' Privacy

Ironically, the trend toward increasing drug testing of healthcare and other professionals and the multiple erosions of privacy discussed above come at a time when patients are expressing increasing concerns over privacy and access to their confidential medical records.[98] A study by the Institute for Health Care Research and Policy at Georgetown University reports that between one-fifth and one-fourth of Americans polled believe that their personal medical information has been improperly disclosed by a healthcare provider, insurance plan, government agency, or employer.[99] According to the same study, one in seven Americans polled, to safeguard privacy and avoid embarrassment, stigma, or discrimination, has withheld information from healthcare providers, provided inaccurate information, doctor-hopped to avoid a consolidated medical record, paid out-of-pocket for care that is covered by insurance, or avoided care altogether.[100] A Princeton study reports that a large majority of Americans polled oppose giving doctors free access to their medical records and are concerned about government agencies and researchers violating their privacy.[101] The Health Insurance Portability and Accountability Act (HIPAA) of 1996, implemented nationwide by the US Department of Health and Human Services, attempts to address the public's concerns.[102] Unfortunately, HIPAA offers limited and burdensome protections to prevent the exchange of health information for marketing purposes.[103] Furthermore, implementation has been marred by confusion, which has complicated cooperative care among different providers who provide care simultaneously for the same patient.[104]

Conclusions

Pre-employment and random drug testing of physicians is ill-justified. Tests are expensive, are based on poor science, represent an unwarranted invasion of privacy, and are unlikely to meet the purported goals of diagnosing functional impairment, improving patient safety, and enhancing quality of care.

Patients' and doctors' desires for privacy safeguards may clash with patients' demands for increased accountability by healthcare providers. To achieve both greater privacy and enhanced accountability, the medical profession will need to be more proactive in disciplining impaired and incompetent providers, improving substance-abuse education and training, and reducing errors through continuous quality improvement and other means.

Suggested Alternatives/More Effective Ways to Improve Quality of Care

In our efforts to protect patients while safeguarding physicians' privacy, we should not rely on public relations gimmicks or costly, unscientific, and ineffective measures like preemployment and random, not-for-cause drug screening. Instead, we should promote reference checking of new staff members to appraise previous job performance; train supervisors to identify, confront, and refer impaired physicians to drug-treatment programs; pay increased attention to physicians' job and life-satisfaction (including the early identification and treatment of depressive disorders, especially common in female physicians,[105] and marital discord); and support knowledge testing (through mandatory recertification), periodic hospital recredentialing, skills appraisal by colleagues and supervisors, and intermittent impairment testing (for example, periodic evaluation of vision, reflexes, and coordination) to determine doctors' fitness to perform their jobs safely.[106] Impairment testing can uncover not only impairment from substance abuse, but also that resulting from important physical disabilities (including dementia),[107] mental illness, and sleep deprivation,[108] which should prompt treatment or work-modification for the impaired physician (or the impaired worker in any major industry, for that matter). If impairment testing suggests drug abuse, then screening, treatment, license restriction, and/or suspension, and follow-up drug testing are not only reasonable, but also likely to benefit affected physicians and their patients.

Those institutions that are truly committed to improving job safety and quality of care should instead focus their attention and resources on the system factors that cause or contribute to a majority of medical errors.[109] They could invest in computerized medication-ordering systems to avoid prescribing errors[110] and more ancillary staff to assist residents in non-educational tasks, which contribute to sleep deprivation, and in turn can lead to errors.[111] They should also enhance procedural training and oversight; encourage reporting, frank discussion, and analysis of errors; improve sign-out protocols; and reverse the trend toward downsizing registered nurses in favor of less-well-trained (and less expensive) licensed practical nurses and clinical nursing assistants.[112]

Acknowledgments

The author wishes to thank Susan Tolle, Sidney Wolfe, Peter Lurie, Linda Ward, and Betty Ward for helpful comments, and Micki Franks, Linda Ward, Betty Ward, and Rachel Adams for excellent technical assistance.

Notes

1. I.D. Montoya, J.W. Carlson, and A.J. Richard, "An Analysis of Drug Abuse Policies in Teaching Hospitals," *Journal of Behavioral Health Services & Research* 26, no. 1 (1999): 28–38; J. Tanner et al., "Substance Abuse and Mandatory Drug Testing in Health Care Institutions," *Health Care Management Review* 13, no. 4 (1998): 33–42; J.W. Fenton and J. Kinard, "A Study of Substance Abuse Testing in Patient Care Facilities," *Health Care Management Review* 18, no. 4 (1993): 87–95; S.J. Lemon, D.G. Sienko, and P.C. Alguire, "Physicians' Attitudes Toward Mandatory Workplace Urine Drug Testing," *Archives of Internal Medicine* 152 (1992): 2238–2242; H.F. Laufenburg and B.A. Barton, "Attitudes of Family Practice Residency Program Directors Toward Mandatory Pre-Employment Drug Testing," *Family Medicine* 29, no. 9 (1997): 625–628; W.H. Bellica, S. Miller, and C.K. Thomas, *Preemployment Drug Testing of Residents* (Phoenix: Family Practice Center, University of Arizona, 1993); A.F. Painter et al., "Potential Influences of Residencies' Health Risk Policies on Ranking by Ohio Applicants," *Academic Medicine* 67 (1992): 340–341.

2. Tanner et al., see note 1 above; P. Cassidy, "Pee First, Ask Questions Later," *In These Times* (December 2002): 1–4, http://www.inthesetimes.com/issue/27/04/views1.shtml (accessed June 1, 2003).

3. Cassidy, ibid.

4. Members of the National Academy of Science's Committee on Drug Use in the Workplace, *Executive Order 12564* (September 1986).

5. L.L. Matlby, *Drug Testing: A Bad Investment,* 1st ed. (New York: American Civil Liberties Union, 1999), http://www.aclu.org/FilesPDFs/drugtesting.pdf (accessed May 18, 2000).

6. Drug-Free Workplace Act of 1988, 41 U.S.C. §§701–707 (1988).

7. Montoya, see note 1 above; ibid.

8. See note 5 above.

9. See note 5 above; J.W. Fenton, "Negligent Hiring and Retention: Some Evidence of Hospital Vulnerability," *Health Care Management Review* 16 (1991): 73–81.

10. Fenton, ibid.

11. See note 5 above.

12. Montoya, see note 1 above.

13. American Hospital Association Board of Trustees, *Management Advisory, Human Resources: Substance Abuse Policies for Health Care Institutions* (Chicago: American Hospital Association, 1992).

14. American College of Occupational and Environmental Medicine. *Ethical Aspects of Drug Testing*, February 04, 2009 (updated from 2006). Available at http://www.acoem.org/EthicalAspectsOfDrugTesting.aspx.

15. D. Orentlicher, "Drug Testing of Physicians," *Journal of the American Medical Association* 264, no. 8 (1990): 1039–1040.

16. Montoya, see note 1 above; Fenton, see note 9 above.

17. R.F. Blendon and J.T. Young, "The Public and the War on Illicit Drugs," *Journal of the American Medical Association* 279, no. 11 (1998): 827–832.

18. See note 5 above.

19. Tanner, see note 1 above; Fenton and Kinard, see note 1 above.

20. Montoya, see note 1 above.

21. Ibid.

22. M.T. Donohoe, "Survey of Drug-Testing Policies of the Five Teaching Hospitals in Portland, Oregon" (unpublished data, 2001).

23. P.G. O'Connor and A. Spickard, "Physician Impairment by Substance Abuse," *Medical Clinics of North America* 81, no. 4 (1997): 1037–1052; L.G. Croen et al., "A Longitudinal Study of Substance Use and Abuse in a Single Class of Medical Students," *Academic Medicine* 72, no. 5 (1997): 376–381.

24. D.C. Baldwin et al., "Substance Use Among Senior Medical Students: A Survey of 23 Medical Schools," *Journal of the American Medical Association* 265 (1991): 2074–2078.

25. P.H. Hughes et al., "Resident Physician Substance Abuse in the United States," *Journal of the American Medical Association* 265 (1991): 2069–2073.

26. L.W. Robert et al., "Perceptions of Academic Vulnerability Associated with Personal Illness: A Study of 1,027 Students at Nine Medical Schools," *Comprehensive Psychiatry* 42, no. 1 (2001): 1–15.

27. See note 25 above.

28. See note 14 above.

29. J.A. Underwood and K.A. McGarry, "The Use of Psychotropic Medications Among Medical Resident Physicians," *Journal of General Internal Medicine* 15, suppl. 1 (2000): 47.

30. W.E. McAuliffe et al., "Alcohol Use and Abuse in Random Samples of Physicians and Medical Students," *American Journal of Public Health* 81, no. 2 (1992): 177–182; E.V. Boisaubin and R.E. Levine, "Identifying and Assisting the Impaired Physician," *American Journal of Medical Science* 322, no. 1 (2001): 31–36.

31. J.V. Booth et al., "Substance Abuse Among Physicians: A Survey of Academic Anesthesiology Programs," *Anesthesia and Analgesia* 95, no. 4 (2002): 1024–1030; P.H. Hughes et al., "Prevalence of Substance Abuse Among US Physicians," *Journal of the American Medical Association* 267 (1992): 2333–2339.

32. Hughes et al., ibid.

33. Council on Ethical and Judicial Affairs, American Medical Association, *Ethics Manual*, http://www.ama-assn.org/ama/pub/category/8288.html; American College of Physicians, *Ethics Manual* (Philadelphia: American College of Physicians, 1998).

34. Boisaubin and Levine, see note 30 above; Hughes et al., see note 31 above; R.D. Moore, L. Mead, and T.A. Pearson, "Youthful Precursors of Alcohol Abuse in

Physicians," *American Journal of Medicine* 88 (1990): 332–336; Medical Board of California Diversion Program, *Mission Statement* (Sacramento: Medical Board of California, 1995).

35. E. Cone et al., "Passive Inhalation of Marijuana Smoke: Urinalysis and Room Air Levels of 9-Tetra-Hydrocannabinol and Its Metabolites in Human Body Fluids," *Journal of Analytical Toxicology* 11 (1987): 89–96; A.R. Forrest, "Ethical Aspects of Workplace Urine Screening for Drug Abuse," *Journal of Medical Ethics* 23 (1997): 12–17; J. Adams, "Pitfalls in Industrial Drug Screening," *Journal MSMA* (1998): 214–217.

36. O'Connor and Spickard, see note 23 above.

37. "ACLU in Brief: Workplace Drug Testing; Workplace Rights; Privacy in America." American Civil Liberties Union, http://www.aclu.org/library/pbr5.html (accessed May 18, 2000); "Tests for Drugs of Abuse," *Medical Letter* 44 (2003): 71–73.

38. Adams, see note 35 above; "Tests for Drugs," see note 37 above; D. Hawkins, "Trial by Vial: More Schools Give Urine Tests for Drugs—But at What Cost?" *US News and World Report* (May 1999), http://www.usnews.com/usnews/issue /990531/nycu/drugs.htm (accessed May 31, 2000).

39. R. Hodge, *Harper's Weekly Review* (December 2001), 2, http://www.harpers.org /weekly-review (accessed June 1, 2003).

40. Hawkins, see note 38 above; R.F. Crown and J.G. Rosse, "Critical Issue in Drug Testing," in *Applying Psychology in Business,* ed. J.W. Jones et al. (Lexington, Mass.: D.C. Heath and Co., 1991), 260–274; T. Chong, "Urine Luck," http://www.urineluck.com (accessed June 12, 2000); Privacy Protection Services homepage, http://www.privacypro.com/page2.htm (accessed June 12, 2000).

41. "Tests for Drugs," see note 37 above.

42. Ibid.

43. Members of the National Academy of Science's Committee on Drug Use in the Workplace, "Focus on Federal Drug Testing: Individual Employment Rights," *Bulletin of the National Academy* (1991): 4.

44. See note 5 above.

45. Ibid.

46. Ibid.

47. J. Normand, *Under the Influence? Drugs and the American Workforce* (Washington, D.C.: National Academy Press, 1994).

48. See note 5 above.

49. Ibid.

50. "Drug Testing: Cost and Effect," *Cornell/ Smithers Report on Workplace Substance Abuse Policy* 1 (1992): 1, 4.

51. Lemon, Sienko, and Alguire, see note 1 above.

52. Ibid.

53. Ibid.

54. Laufenburg and Barton, see note 1 above.

55. Laufenburg and Barton, ibid.; Bellica, Miller, and Thomas, see note 1 above.

56. Painter, see note 1 above.

57. R.D. Aach et al., "Alcohol and Other Substance Abuse and Impairment Among Physicians in Residency Training," *Annals of Internal Medicine* 117, no. 3 (1992): 267–268; Painter, ibid.; Bellica, Miller, and Thomas, see note 1 above.

58. Boisaubin and Levine, see note 30 above; R.D. Blondell, "Impaired Physicians," *Primary Care* 20 (1993): 209–219; B.W. McIntyre and M.W. Hamolsky, "The Impaired Physician and the Role of the Board of Medical Licensure and Discipline," *Rhode Island Medicine* 77 (1994): 3578; "Drug Testing," see note 50 above.

59. Boisaubin and Levine, ibid.

60. R.A. Sansone, M.W. Wiederman, and L.A. Sansone, "Physician Mental Health and Substance Abuse, What Are State Medical Licensure Applications Asking?" *Archives of Family Medicine* 8 (1999): 448–451.

61. Ibid.; T.L. Jones, "The Road to Recovery: New Law Removes One Barrier to Rehabilitation for Impaired Physicians," *Tex Med* 91 (1995): 22–24; C. O'Brien, "Mental Health Questions for Licensure: Who Benefits?" *Archives of Family Medicine* 8 (1999): 452.

62. See note 58 above.

63. Public Citizen Health Research Group, *Health Letter,* 16 (September 2000): 9.

64. D. Eisenberg and M. Sieger, "The Doctor Won't See You Now," *TIME* (June 2003): 46–60.

65. G.D. Lundberg, "New Winds Blowing for American Drug Policies," *Journal of the American Medical Association* 278 (1997): 946–947; P.D. Friedmann et al., "Screening and Intervention for Alcohol Problems, A National Survey of Primary Care Physicians and Psychiatrists," *Journal of General Internal Medicine* 15 (2000): 8491.

66. K.G. Volpp and D. Grande, "Residents' Suggestions for Reducing Errors in Teaching Hospitals," *New England Journal of Medicine* 348 (2003): 851–855.

67. Cassidy, see note 2.

68. See note 5 above; Hawkins, see note 38 above.

69. Institute for a Drug-Free Workplace, "Why Become a Member of the Institute?" http://www.drugfreeworkplace.org/membership.html (accessed May 18, 2000).

70. L. Zimmer and J.B. Jacobs, "The Business of Drug Testing: Technological Innovation and Social Control," *Contemporary Drug Problems* 19 (1992): 1–26; American Bio Medica Corporation, http://www.americanbiomedica.com/about.htm (accessed June 12, 2000); G.D. Lundberg, "Mandatory Unindicated Urine Drug Screening: Still Chemical McCarthyism," *Journal of the American Medical Association* 256, no. 21 (1986): 303–305.

71. B. Ehrenreich, "What Are They Probing For? Applying for a Job? Get Ready for a Test of Your Innermost Thoughts," *TIME* (June 2001): 86.

72. A.P. Zelicoff, "Polygraphs and the National Labs: Dangerous Ruse Undermines National Security," *Skeptical Inquirer* (July 2001): 21–23; R. Steinbrook, "The Polygraph Test—A Flawed Diagnostic Method," *New England Journal of Medicine* 327, no. 2 (1992): 122–123.

73. "Background Checks, Pre-employment Screening and More," http://www.preemploy.com (accessed July 1, 2003).

74. Ibid.; "Cedar Rapids Police Department Memo," as cited in "Harper's Index," *Harper's Magazine* (July 2001): 11.

75. "Just Say Woof," *Mother Jones* (January 2002): 21.

76. Hawkins, see note 38 above.

77. See note 5 above; Fenton, see note 9 above.

78. Matlby, ibid.; Fenton, ibid.; Economist.com, "Living in the Global Goldfish Bowl," Wysiwyg://33/Wysiwyg://33/http://www.economist.com/displayStory.cfm?Story_ID=268789 (accessed October 9, 2000); Economist.com, "The Surveillance Society," Wysiwyg://46/Wysiwyg://46/http://www.economist.com/displayStory.cfm?Story_ID= 202160 (accessed October 9, 2000); T. Sulamain, "More Companies Are Checking Credit History of Job Applicants," *Oregonian* (June 2003): C12.

79. ACLU, "Lifestyle Discrimination in the Workplace: Your Right to Privacy Under Attack," http://www.aclu.org/library/pbr1.html (accessed May 18, 2000).

80. See note 5 above; Fenton, see note 9 above; ACLU, ibid.

81. ACLU, "Worker's Rights—Genetic Discrimination in the Workplace Fact Sheet," http://www.aclu.org/issues/worker/gdfactsheet.html (accessed May 18, 2000).

82. "The Surveillance Society," see note 78 above.

83. *Forensic Drug Abuse Advisor,* (November/December 1996): 8, 10; P. Kintz, "Hair Testing and Doping Control in Sport," *Toxicology Letters* 102–103 (1998): 109–113; *Forensic Drug Abuse Advisor* 9 (April 1997): 4.

84. ACLU, see note 81 above; ACLU, "Defend Your Data: What They Do Know Can Hurt You! Your Right to Privacy and That of All Citizens Is Under Unprecedented Assault," http://www.aclu.org/privacy/ (accessed May 18, 2000).

85. C.A. Welch, "Sacred Secrets—The Privacy of Medical Records," *New England Journal of Medicine* 345 (2001): 371–372.

86. L.N. Geller et al., "Individual, Family, and Social Dimensions of Genetic Discrimination: A Case Study Analysis," *Science and Engineering Ethics* 2, no. 1 (1996).

87. ACLU, see note 81 above; Council for Responsible Genetics, http:http:www.gene-watch.org (accessed July 24, 2000).

88. "Order Bans Misuse in Hiring, Promotions—Federal Initiative Focuses on Genetic Discrimination," *Nation's Health* (April 2000): 5.

89. American Medical Association, Council on Ethical and Judicial Affairs, "Use of Genetic Testing by Employers," *Journal of the American Medical Association* 266, no. 13 (1991): 1827–1830.

90. See note 78 above.

91. C. Marick, "State Medical Boards Discipline More, Want Role in Health System Reform," *Journal of the American Medical Association* 271 (1994): 1723–1724.

92. H.S. Peyser, "Self-Incrimination on Medical Board and Licensing Applications," *Hospital and Community Psychiatry* 44 (1993): 517.

93. O'Connor and Spickard, see note 23 above.

94. Hawkins, see note 38 above; G. Smith, "How Parents Can Help Children Live Marijuana Free," *Extra!* (November/December 1998).

95. Fenton and Kinard, see note 1 above.

96. P. Armentano and A. St. Pierre, "Random Workplace Drug Testing Struck Down by Canadian Human Rights Commission," *NORML News* (July 10, 2002), http://www.chrc-ccdp.ca/news-comm/2002/NewsComm071002.asp?l=e (accessed June 1, 2003).

97. See note 22 above.

98. Institute for Health Care Research and Policy, Georgetown University, "Health Privacy Polling Data: Health Privacy Project," www.healthprivacy.org (accessed June 1, 2003); see note 64 above.

99. Institute for Health Care, ibid.

100. See note 98 above.

101. Institute for Health Freedom, *Public Attitudes Toward Medical Privacy* (Princeton, N.J.: September 2000), www.forhealthfreedom.org/Gallupsurvey/.

102. L.O. Gostin, "National Health Information Privacy: Regulations Under the Health Insurance Portability and Accountability Act," *Journal of the American Medical Association* 285 (2001): 3015–3021.

103. Ibid.

104. Health Privacy Project "Myths and Facts About the HIPAA Privacy Rule," http://www.healthprivacy.org/info-url_nocat2303/info-url_nocat_show.htm?doc_id+173435 (accessed June 10, 2003).

105. Boisaubin and Levine, see note 30 above.

106. See note 5 above; see note 15 above; G.B. Collins, "New Hope for Impaired Physicians: Helping the Physician While Protecting Patients," *Cleveland Clinical Journal of Medicine* 65, no. 2 (1998): 101–106; M.D. Johnson, T.J. Heriza, and C. St. Dennis, "How to Spot Illicit Drug Abuse in Your Patients," *Postgraduate Medicine* 106, no. 4 (1999): 199–218.

107. J. Turnbull et al., "Cognitive Difficulty in Physicians," *Academic Medicine* 75, no. 2 (2000): 177–181.

108. See note 15 above.

109. L.L. Leape, "Error in Medicine," *Journal of the American Medical Association* 272 (1994): 1851–1857.

110. D.W. Bates et al., "Effect of Computerized Physician Order Entry and a Team Intervention on Prevention of Serious Medication Errors," *Journal of the American Medical Association* 280, no. 15 (1998): 1311–1316.

111. American College of Physicians, "Internal Medicine Trainees Working Too Many Hours," *American Society of Internal Medicine Observer* (April 2000).

112. See note 66 above.

Part Nine

Achieving Social Justice in Health Care Through Education and Activism

The chapters in this final section include reflective essays on social justice and provide advice for health professionals, educators, patients, legislators, and concerned citizens who hope to improve awareness of social justice issues and to change public policy.

Chapter Thirty-Four (by Stephen Bezruchka) explains major paradigm shifts in public health in the twentieth century and calls for a new revolution in the field, with less focus on individual behaviors and more emphasis on the role of societal factors underlying health inequalities. The author suggests practical strategies for promoting public understanding of population health through print and online media, formal education, and civic engagement.

Chapter Thirty-Five (by Peter Montague and Carolyn Raffensperger) describes some ideas for a common agenda based on the golden rule to help citizens work together to build stronger communities, protect the commons, and promote democratic reforms aimed at increasing justice.

Chapter Thirty-Six (by Robert Weissman) celebrates important victories of workers, environmentalists, public health and consumer rights advocates, and others over corporate corruption and power.

Chapter Thirty-Seven (by David U. Himmelstein and Steffie Woolhandler) criticizes contemporary patchwork reforms of the US health care system and makes the case for universal coverage with a single-payer system.

Chapter Thirty-Eight (by Walter J. Lear) describes the important role of health professionals in opposing major twentieth-century wars.

Chapter Thirty-Nine (by A. H. Strelnick, Debbie Swiderski, Alice Fornari, Victoria Gorski, Eliana Korin, Philip Ozuah, Janet M. Townsend, and Peter A. Selwyn) focuses on the residency program in social medicine at Montefiore Medical Center, whose model curriculum combines interdisciplinary training in medicine and public health with service to the local community. This program and others (such as Brigham and Women's Hospital's residency in global health equity and internal medicine[1]) have set the standard for similar programs nationwide.

Chapter Forty (by Martin Donohoe) reviews the current state of training in ethics and public health and describes injustices that contribute to poor health and that are inadequately covered in traditional curricula. The chapter presents an argument for enhancing the public health education of health professions students and practitioners through the use of history, literature, and photography, with the goal of creating activists knowledgeable about, and eager to confront, the social, economic, and cultural contributors to illness.

For those wishing to teach courses in public health and social justice, please see the open-access curricula available on the course syllabi page of the Public Health and Social Justice website at http://www.phsj.org/cpirse -syllabi. Instructional, inspirational slide shows describing how health professionals can become activists are available on that website at http://phsj.org/activism-and-education/. To learn more about universal health care and a single payer system, visit the website at http://phsj.org/universal- health-caresingle-payer-system/ and http://phsj.org/literature-medicine-and -public-health/. To take action, peruse the external links page at http:// www.phsj.org/external-links, which provides the web addresses of hundreds of activist-oriented groups. Submissions of slideshows, articles, and external links are encouraged.

Note

1. Furin, J., Farmer, P., & Wolf, M., et al. A novel training model to address health problems in poor and underserved populations. *Journal of Health Care for the Poor and Underserved*, 2006, *17*, 17–24. Abstract retrieved from http://muse.jhu.edu /login?uri=/journals/journal_of_health_care_for_the_poor_and_underserved/v017 /17.1furin.pdf.

Chapter 34

Promoting Public Understanding of Population Health

Stephen Bezruchka

Introduction

This chapter addresses the need to apply the information and perspectives described in this volume to improve health. The basic premise of the book is that individual behaviors are less important for producing health than are structures that underlie inequalities in a society. This concept may be thought of as a scientific revolution or new paradigm in our thinking about health, and as with most paradigm shifts, is resisted by both scientists and the general population. Putting these ideas into action will require promoting a broader public understanding and acceptance of the basic determinants of health. The subject of this chapter provides a framework with which to proceed. Citizens of the US, being less healthy than those in other rich countries, are the target group.

What We Know About Population Health

The concept of a socioeconomic gradient, or differences in various measures of hierarchy in a society, is a property of populations, not of individuals. That hierarchical relationships lead to health disparities may be debated, but there is strong evidence supporting that link (Wilkinson, 1996, 2005). The best ways to conceptualize and measure hierarchy and health are still under study, but current knowledge, if the goal is improving health, is adequate to justify action. In essentially all developed and middle-income countries today, societies with a greater hierarchy tend to be less healthy than those with a smaller gap between social and economic classes. Geoffrey Rose (1992, p. 129) concluded his seminal monograph *The Strategy of Preventive Medicine* with "The primary determinants of disease are mainly economic and social, and therefore its remedies must also be economic and social. Medicine and politics cannot and should not be kept apart."

The societal factors that impact a population's health relate to how that population shares its resources, and to how that "sharing" determines the "caring" that goes on in that particular society. Where there is less economic disparity, there tends to be less social disparity and more support at many levels that benefit health (Wilkinson and Pickett, 2006). A wide range of terminology is used to describe these social processes: social justice, equity, trust, social capital or, simply, fairness. However it is described, the effect of the social and economic environment on the health and well-being of persons living in that environment is profound, and not adequately recognized by either the lay public or the healthcare system in the US.

Paradigm Shifts in Public Health

The material in this book describes a kind of scientific revolution as depicted by Thomas Kuhn (1962). Kuhn argued that science does not progress with a steady accumulation of knowledge, but instead undergoes periodic shifts. Such revolutions, or paradigm or worldview shifts, tend to be invisible and strongly resisted by those in the scientific community whose scholarship is threatened. Often in other scientific revolutions, such as the advent of quantum mechanics, one incident or breakthrough brings the phenomenon to public attention. History provides useful examples. The dropping of two atomic bombs by the US on Japan in 1945 presented an astounding visual image that had never been previously observed. The visual impact of those two events required a new understanding of the scope of "scientific progress" than had existed prior to that point in time. Over the next few decades, the concept of atomic energy began to reach school curricula and popular parlance. Eventually, although few citizens grasped the details of quantum mechanics behind discovery of this form of energy, many understood that vast energy could be released from splitting and fusing atoms.

A similarly earth-shaking event was the launch of the first satellite, *Sputnik*, and then the first human into space by the Soviet Union. These remarkable accomplishments captured the attention of Americans, who had always portrayed the Soviet society after the Second World War as primitive and underdeveloped compared to their own. The launching of Sputnik invigorated the teaching of science and mathematics in the US in the 1950s and 1960s. Again, although most citizens were not rocket scientists and could not have built or launched a rocket, they understood that the world was entering a revolutionary era of space travel that previously had only been the subject of science fiction.

Medical and surgical care changes in the last half-century are sometimes considered another scientific revolution, with profound impacts that have affected our understanding of what is possible from medical care. Premature infants weighing one pound at birth can live and grow to adulthood; hearts, lungs and livers can be transplanted, and severed limbs reattached. Yet the argument can be made that this scientific revolution has been heavily oversold: dramatic efforts that save individual lives and limbs have yet to improve overall population health. Among the few studies of the impact of healthcare on the health of populations, none can unequivocally demonstrate benefits to whole societies (Jamrozik and Hobbs, 2002). In fact, most of the impacts of healthcare have been relatively minor, despite the popular desire to equate the terms "health" and "healthcare." Even the sacred cow of universal healthcare has not been demonstrated to improve population health or to decrease health disparities in countries where it has been studied (Roos et al., 2006).Yet population health concepts could have much broader impact on health than technological medical advances, if they were more broadly understood.

There are many reasons for the dearth of attention to population health issues by the medical care system and its academic establishment. Achieving success in academia results from asking narrowly directed questions that can be answered in the confines of a grant-funding cycle. The published results generally conclude by asking that more research be done on a similarly narrow topic. That ritual leads to a never-ending cycle of narrow research results and academic promotions that continue until the professor retires. Increasing specialization within academic departments occurs because "knowing more about less" commands more respect than attempting to understand broader questions of causality. Issues of advocacy or even disseminating findings beyond scientific meetings are considered outside the values of the ivory tower (Bezruchka, 2008).

Because of the medical emphasis on the epidemiology of specific conditions and individual "risk factors" for illness, most people in the US think of health as determined by the usual do's and don'ts promoted by the conventional healthcare system: eat right, don't smoke, exercise, just say no, and see your doctor. These precepts are taught at all levels of society, and increasingly throughout the world—and at the individual level they are reasonable admonitions. But scholarship over the last few decades has demonstrated that the context in which these behaviors take place is an important modifier of their effects on health (Lantz et al., 1998). Smoking, for example, in a highly hierarchical society (such as the US) appears to be far more detrimental to the health of smokers than when it takes place in a society with a smaller hierarchical gradient, such as Japan (Bezruchka et al., 2008). Herein lies part of our problem in improving general understanding of the determinants of health. We must recognize that correcting this cognitive simplicity in people's minds, that healthcare and "healthy" individual behaviors equal health, will lead to profound cognitive dissonance—yet this dissonance will be required if the public is to understand health as a product primarily of socioeconomic forces, and not medical care.

Teaching the ecological or population-level factors that influence health is rarely a part of the educational programs in US schools at any level, kindergarten through university. Neither are these factors typically considered by public health departments in their discussion of policy options, nor in clinical training for medical doctors, nurses, pharmacists or other health practitioners. The American concept of "public health" is in the main defined by interventions that address the physical environment, such as pure water, sanitation and control of specific disease conditions, as well as access to health services and "health education" to improve individual behaviors. That the social environment could be a critical element in the production of health is not well understood, not acknowledged or is considered to be outside the purview of public health practice.

Public health research similarly tends to focus on various approaches to improving health services or on risk factors associated with health, in which social and economic variables are typically controlled for but not examined. Academics occasionally document steps that could be taken to turn research findings into policy, but they rarely get to the point of recommending how that might be done in practical terms. There is often also an implicit assumption that policy makers, when presented with research findings, will act benevolently (Earle et al., 2006). Even dramatic or highly significant findings typically are not presented in terms of how they might be used to shape policy, nor about the difficulty of creating understanding of such new ideas. Research findings rarely change dysfunctional social systems (Kingdon, 1995).

What, then, will be needed if we are to achieve the goal of public awareness and public concern about the social and economic determinants of health? Many of us in the health field may have to unlearn many assumptions of the old paradigm, and learn the new. Medical practitioners have had to undergo this process regularly over the years, such as when learning new surgical techniques or medical regimens. The challenge at hand for population health may be more like the process by which the germ theory of disease was accepted—which took perhaps a century. Since we have had at least a century and a half of evidence for the critical importance of social and economic factors on health, the time for a broader acceptance of those concepts may be at hand.

Public Dissemination of the New Science on Health

Dissemination of scientific revolutions or paradigms and their adoption by society runs no predetermined course. Logically, however, one might assume that after a few key leaders in the field are convinced of the key elements of the new paradigm, a subsequent challenge would be to convince influential sectors of the general public of the need to consider these new ideas, and to become convinced of their importance. Part of that process might be to point out a few examples where commonly held assumptions are starkly contradicted by "the facts"—for example, to point out that the US is less healthy as a nation than nearly all the other rich countries. This kind of simple fact is remarkably little understood, and will often lead to a series of questions as a response. Asking difficult questions in public venues can begin the process. While it would be useful to have this happen in high-profile settings—perhaps by the US president in the annual State of the Union address—smaller public venues are more realistic.

Creating public awareness is the challenging task. From an economic perspective, there is no product to sell, no magic potion, pill, weight-loss machine or life-saving medical procedure. There is no mushroom cloud, or real-time moon-landing show. There is only information that, if presented effectively, will challenge most people's perceptions of reality. To affect deeply held belief systems often takes a generation or two, so it will be important to get population health concepts into the public's eye with exposure at earlier and earlier ages. From this perspective, promoting the population health concept is similar to movements such as women's suffrage or the abolition of slavery. These were based on deeply held beliefs that were promoted from a wide range of social groups and individuals, and are still in fact in the process of completion. Some argue for the need to continue to purge racist ideas throughout the lifespan, and such efforts may be needed for understanding population health.

We as public health researchers and practitioners must take the lead in creating public awareness. To influence opinion we can create one-liners that grab the attention of the listener, and back them up with substantial statements. It is useful to keep a list of quotes and statistics with sources for this purpose, for example, "Do you want health or healthcare?", "We must organize or die." Developing the message is a matter of trial and much error. It is important in this process to recognize that even one insignificant factual error can and usually will be used to discredit our main message—so accuracy is paramount.

A major difficulty in promoting ideas that reflect social responsibility in the US is that "rugged individualism" is in effect our first language. But the language of community deserves attention, and messages must be crafted using America's other language—one based on the traditions of knowing and caring for one another (Wallack, 2003; Wallack and Lawrence, 2005). We need to adapt this language for various audiences, so that what is said to a group of homeless people will be quite different from the messages for a meeting of labor union members. The carefully focused framing of concepts has emerged as a very useful device employed by those who shape public opinion through the commercial media (Lakoff, 2006). Our role is to use similar techniques to present ideas about what makes a population healthy.

Disseminating Through Public Presentations

At a personal level, I first came to see the increased hierarchy–poorer health relationship as being important in the early 1990s, at the same time that I came to recognize the limitations of medical care in producing health. My first attempts to talk about this in public began at conferences of medical doctors in 1995. It took me a few more years of efforts to recognize that doctors had little interest in health, especially from the perspective I was presenting. The concepts had no clinical relevance to them and were rarely discussed in the professional medical setting. I continue to include doctors in talks, conferences, publications and the increasingly rare opportunity to teach medical students about population health, but I also understand that there are major limitations of this approach. Similarly, academic meetings and conferences of public health officials and workers offer important venues for presenting contributed papers, taking part in discussion panels and other formats. Public health workers are, in theory, more open to considering socioeconomic aspects of health than are clinicians. However, I still expect resistance to getting on the program if my abstract does not address topics congruent with the conventional wisdom of the group.

Many different kinds of organizations outside the medical sphere, such as church groups, parent-teacher associations, service organizations, professional organizations and community councils, present opportunities to speak to the members on some aspect of the population health topic. I have, for example, recently addressed senior citizens groups, a conference on ageing, gatherings of public health officials, Unitarian Church meetings and labor unions. Such small meetings represent wonderful opportunities to craft specific messages in effective ways and to stimulate further discussion. There is no better way to gain competence in presenting ideas of population health than to engage smaller groups where interaction can occur. For example, the PBS (Public Broadcasting Service) series, "Unnatural Causes: Is Inequality Making Us Sick?" that aired in the US in 2008 provides an opportunity to screen segments for audiences and to facilitate a discussion on the concepts. The website provides a community action toolkit and much useful material (www.unnaturalcauses.org).

A host of community service television programmers with access to various individuals and groups can be used to present new ideas. We can access the many radio programmers in cities that host citizen groups to discuss important issues, often with listener call-ins. Most talk shows present an opportunity to mention key concepts, but the editorial process typically allows for little depth of discussion. Some progressive radio stations also feature interview or talk shows that are open to discussing the topic. Once we develop a suitable framework and focus for presenting population health ideas, it is not difficult to adapt the messages to different topics. Every exposure has the potential for making useful contacts that lead to more opportunities for dissemination.

Community events with public demonstrations or marches can present a ready-made venue, including tables at conferences and meetings where flyers, posters and readings can be made available. Those with artistic skills can craft signs for demonstrations that attract attention to gain broader media exposure. Newspapers and television stations want catchy visuals and radio reporters want actualities (statements from the demonstrators) for their reports. For example, my carrying a placard stating, "WTO is bad for your health" at the 1999 Seattle demonstrations resulted in my getting interviews with the local media.

Once on a program, with a stationary audience, the standard principles of effective presentations are useful. For many groups, going "PowerPointless" may be best. Face-to-face audience engagement is easier with less visual distraction if we can command attention verbally. Telling stories is often the most effective way to communicate with non-professional audiences — as noted by the Scottish patriot, Andrew Fletcher (1653–1716), "whoever tells the stories of a nation need not care who makes its laws" (http://www.main .nc.us/cml/new_citizen/summer95.html). An effective story tends to involve individuals, require a hazard, danger or threat, a victim, an attacker, a means of doing harm, a protector and means of protection. The challenge is telling a story that deals with both individuals and populations, linking the two.

Disseminating Through the Print Media

I endeavor to disseminate population health ideas through whatever public media I can access. One simple approach to getting into the print media is by writing letters to the editor in response to health and political issues. Following standard approaches to writing effective letters (keep them short, focused, timely) will increase the likelihood of getting published. Such letters are not major vehicles for supporting paradigm shifts, but occasionally a few readers want to become better informed, and request more information. It is important to develop a concise message in one sentence. What is the problem, what can be done about it? I even practice this technique with telephone solicitors, especially those where the call is "being recorded for quality assurance purposes," since they are less likely to summarily hang up!

Population health is almost entirely a political subject, so there is plenty of scope for those inclined to make use of these channels of dissemination.

One prime challenge to optimal use of the print media is the difficulty of getting articles into newspapers and magazines with significant circulation. Personal contacts may be helpful—I was able to get a one-page story in *Newsweek* as a result of serendipitous conversations with a *Newsweek* editor over dinner at a professional meeting (Bezruchka, 2001). Stories need to be crafted in relation to current events, and a gripping lead is required. A standard approach to enlisting the general reader's sympathy is a human interest story—which is a challenge to adapt to population issues. Most publications have strict word limitations, requiring careful writing that leaves much unsaid. However, success at being published in a major newspaper or magazine may well result in hundreds of responses via email or regular mail, as well as telephone calls and other communications. I believe that it is important for us to respond to as many of these communications as possible, in the interest of cultivating every possible advocate for population health.

Writing popular books has been a traditionally successful approach to challenging the public with new ideas and promoting scientific revolutions. Although several academic and politically focused publishers are now interested in the topic, to date the published books on population health in the US have not been in a format that is likely to be read by the general public from whom, in my estimation, the battering ram for change must come.

Disseminating Through the Internet

The Internet represents the cutting edge of communication, but the extent to which it affects people's deeply held beliefs or understanding is unclear. The opportunities to participate in Internet discussions are nearly endless. Newspaper articles and various other Internet sites often have a web-commentary section for responses that can be viewed by anyone interested in the topic. Those of us who use this means of communication can spread the population health message. The responses can excoriate or support or constructively engage in a discussion, but we can expect to be strongly criticized for views we present that go beyond individual agency as the chief means of health production. On the other hand, the Internet is an accessible mechanism for people who want to be involved to make contact with and learn from like-minded others. We might eventually find this process making substantial inroads in getting our ideas greater exposure. Blogs represent another easily accessible way to craft arguments in written form.

A tremendous variety of other publishing means are available on the web. Podcasting allows voiced material to be disseminated widely, as do hosted discussions on the web with downloadable audio files. Our challenge is creating files that might be suitable for general listening, just like the music that can be downloaded. Many of us belong to listservs and we can use them to highlight news stories with our personal commentary. Using the web for information and constructive engagement may be akin to trying to slake thirst from a fire hose—but we ignore it at our peril.

Dissemination Through the Educational System

The formal educational system, from elementary through university level, represents a largely untapped resource for broadening public understanding of the determinants of health. The opportunity for us to engage in formal teaching is immense. As health professionals of all types we can teach and write for specialty journals and conferences, as well as for institutions of advanced education. Community colleges, universities and the like have few courses dealing with the health of populations but a course title such as "Global Health" can get us in the door. There are endless opportunities—online education, for example, represents a relatively new one. Recognize that it may take a year or more to set up a teaching opportunity, given the individual contacts and relationships that must be built. Formal teaching allows the unique possibility of crafting course outputs that require students themselves to take responsibility for dissemination. I tend to let the students choose the methods they will use based on the principles described earlier, but give a list of various suggestions and possible venues, such as screening "Unnatural Causes" in small groups. I continue to be surprised by the innovative and sometimes inspiring activities they carry out and find more interest among non-health career students, who tend to be less resistant to the concepts, than health career students.

Teachers at all levels are important influences on developing minds. Over the long term, promoting middle- and high-school curricula on population health may be the most effective strategy for bringing about a shift in public understanding of the socioeconomic determinants of health.

The Need for Curricular Change

"Health education" in US schools, from elementary through high school, is based on traditional concepts of individual health production. Individual behaviors are the main emphasis, and no attention is given to comparisons of health status for populations. There is certainly no mention of the relative decline of health in the US over the last 40 years. Medical care is usually overemphasized as an important factor producing health.

To ask why our health education system avoids addressing social and economic determinants of health is to invite questioning of the broader purposes of the education system. Carol Bellamy, who was director of the United Nations

Children's Fund (UNICEF) for several years, once said, "The business community needs peace to see economic growth. They need kids to be educated to be consumers and workers" (quoted in the *New York Times,* September 3, 2000). I would suggest that if the purpose of an education is to create consumers and workers, then the system is working. However, if the purpose is to instill an understanding of the world and critical thinking skills, then much needs to be done. We might look elsewhere for guidance: scholars in Australia, for example, a much healthier country than the US, promote the concept of critical health literacy (St. Leger, 2001). The three levels of health literacy that they describe involve functional elements such as factual information; interactive aspects that understand the nature of a supportive environment; and the critical element requiring civic engagement to impact social, political and economic forces that impact health. Teaching civic engagement as an element of health education is necessary if we recognize that youth represent the next generation to effect social change. Teaching young people the importance of social action, with accompanying skills, is empowering and increases self-efficacy. This framework would provide a simple yet comprehensive organizing principle for a viable school health education curriculum that truly addresses health.

Practical Strategies

I often begin a session with students by asking them to describe what they do to keep themselves healthy, and then to try to explain what they think makes people healthy in a larger community. In Seattle, classroom settings often have students from very diverse ethnic and national backgrounds. A wide range of responses from children who are African Americans, Hispanics or recent immigrants from Russia or Ethiopia illustrate the many social realities from which they come, and a sometimes profound understanding of the effects of those settings on their lives. A useful homework assignment is to ask the students to graph the top 25 or so countries in the "Health Olympics," the ranking of countries by a mortality measure such as life expectancy. Engaged students will continue graphing beyond 25 countries to discover where the US stands. Another effective teaching tool is to present a colored map of the US by county indicating life expectancy ranges and ask the students to explore possible reasons behind the geographical distribution of health that they see (Murray et al., 1998, 2006). Asking why such large disparities exist in the US prompts looking at basic concepts of population health. I then discuss with them the income distribution–mortality relationship among states. Homework can include short essay questions, true-false choices and other formats that can lead to discussions about specific issues. Facts that can be brought in may relate to issues such as why the US has the highest child poverty rates of all the rich countries, and 10–20 times the teenage birth rates of other rich countries.

We have almost endless opportunity here—in many cases the facts very nearly speak for themselves, when provided to ears that are willing to listen.

By comparing information on health-related outcomes for the US with other countries, we are forced to ask why the observed patterns occur. Why such high teenage birth rates? Or high youth homicide rates? Why so much child poverty? These data naturally lead students to discuss economic and political realities associated with the problems—without any need to explicitly mention partisan political issues.

Another teaching tool I have used, especially during a biennial Olympic year, is reader's theatre in which a "Health Olympics finish" scenario takes place (Maher, 2006). Students take on country roles, there is a race announcer and scripts are handed out to study the day before. Often focusing on three contestants, Japan, Canada and the US, students race with flag-bearing t-shirts and additional information cards that are flashed to the rest of the class. The US crosses the finish line 4.6 years after the winner in the life expectancy race. This exercise makes use of active participation and entertainment while getting a memorable message across.

Teaching methods that focus on active discussion or other participation and that do not use too many visual materials seem to work best in elementary classrooms. If an audiovisual aid such as a video is used, be sure it is entertaining as well as informative. I like to show a 10-minute video segment of a British documentary, "The Great Leveller" (part of a Channel 4 *Equinox* series screened in 1996). This fast-paced and cleverly narrated program effectively presents some of the biology behind the hierarchy-health relationship through human, baboon and macaque monkey studies.

Promoting Civic Engagement

An important element of our curricular efforts is to help students to grasp the basic concept that political decisions about distributional economic issues are critical factors that affect the health of populations. A number of population health themes have been investigated for school use. A useful wealth distribution exercise is to divide the class into quintiles, and then "give out" US household wealth as it is actually distributed, using trillion dollar notes. This visible depiction of reality often gets strong reactions from students of all ages—including "but that's not fair!"—and can lead to civic engagement, the third part of critical health literacy. The links between relative poverty and environmental contamination can be presented in a class setting by dividing students in the class into quartiles or quintiles by wealth and instructing one group, the poorest, that, no matter what happens, they are to keep mute. A symbolic bucket of toxic waste is brought into the classroom and the students have to discuss where it will go among the groups. Although the resulting decision has been quite unpredictable, it always leads to engagement and, I believe, a deeper understanding of relevant issues. A simple homework task is to talk about these ideas with friends, siblings and parents.

I have later found students who attended these classes who become active in the social justice movement—and who report that their classroom experience was what got them involved. Another element of civic engagement is to have students produce graphical materials for display. In a module entitled, "World Health and Art Activism," high school students were able to produce creative and effective posters that addressed issues such as student stress, the wealth gap, world hunger and teenage births. In another class, students drew up models displaying the hierarchy-health relationship. We can script role plays in which students learn to discuss the concepts with strangers and practice with each other or with friends and family.

One of the unexpected developments from presenting new and stimulating information is that parents can contact the classroom teacher if they want to know more about what their student has been learning. Teachers also use the lesson elements provided by guest instructors in future years so there is a stimulus for continuing population health education. After your first teaching experience at the pre-college level you may be "hooked." Use class evaluations to finetune future lessons.

Another opportunity that can offer an enrichment experience, particularly for students from more privileged schools, is actual travel to a poor country. We have worked with a school in which the students spend a month in Vietnam at the end of grade 8. Before they go we discuss issues of poverty and social factors at work in the Vietnam setting. Debriefing sessions on return are critical. One student, when asked about the "big picture" in Vietnam as he saw it, replied, "We went there and like you said, they were poor, but we also saw they were happy, and it wasn't a drug-induced kind of happiness." The actual experience of the everyday realities of poor countries can have a transformative experience at any age.

Major global events provide other opportunities for teaching this material. The 10th anniversary of the Beijing women's conference was an appropriate time to discuss gender issues in health production. Discussions about our relations with Cuba highlight the finding that it is as healthy as the US despite economic sanctions placed on it by the US—which stretch over almost 50 years. Russia's rise to house the second largest number of billionaires in the world was coupled with an immense absolute health decline. Sri Lanka has health indicators close to those of the US despite the lack of economic growth and a protracted civil war. An impressive number of world events provide teaching material for health topics.

Teaching population health concepts have now been presented at social studies teacher conferences and to various teacher-training environments.

Adoption has been limited because of the lack of sustained curriculum support as well as the lack of mainstream attention paid to our health as a society. We are in the process of doing more curriculum development and dissemination (Just Health Action, www.justhealthaction.org/).

There are few standardized lesson plans for teaching this material available in the US. A sourcebook by World Hunger Year produced by Kids Can Make a Difference presents a variety of lesson plans (Kempf, 2005). One book in the Rethinking Schools series has relevant materials (Gutstein and Peterson, 2005), but none directly related to population health. Similarly, *Teaching Economics as if People Mattered* by United for a Fair Economy presents other engaging lesson material (Giecek, 2000). There are really novel teaching tools for global health available from www.gapminder.org/.

College-Level Courses

It is remarkable how few college-level courses address the broad determinants of health—we can expect to break new ground by working in this area. Even more revolutionary are classes that require the student to apply the information in a useful way. As a part of the output of both my undergraduate and graduate courses covering population health at the University of Washington and at Seattle University, students carry out a dissemination exercise. I am impressed with the number of students who carry out teaching exercises in middle and high schools. They have gone to minority enrichment programmers, to history classes, to social studies classes, to health education classes, and discovered their own teaching styles. To help students grapple with the ideas, they are required to write a paper criticizing these concepts. I am in contact with a few other university teachers in the US attempting to teach this material, largely in anthropology, sociology and social work departments. There is more opportunity for these ideas in countries other than the US (Bezruchka, 2006). The analogous course for physicians—"social medicine"—is being taught in only a few medical schools in the US (Anderson et al., 2005). To my knowledge, few public health schools address this material, although there has recently been a growing interest in the "social determinants of health" as an academic topic.

Conclusion: A Call to Action for Public Health Professionals

We who work in traditional fields of public health in the US need to recognize that while our work may be important, health outcomes in the US suggest the need for a new approach to producing health. It is disgraceful that the wealthiest country in the world has allowed its health status to deteriorate to the present level. The way forward will require us to step out of our narrow academic and personal boundaries. We must build cohesive bridges among disciplines, social and economic classes, and between professionals and our education system.

This chapter suggests that the current scholarship around population health represents a scientific revolution in progress. There is strong resistance to new worldviews, and we in the US are no exception, particularly when it comes to the topic of health. We are faced with relearning what produces health and choosing whether or not to teach what we have chosen to learn. Having healthy grandchildren and great-grandchildren will require concerted efforts by the current generations. There is pioneering work to do in disseminating the concepts of the population health revolution.

References

Anderson, M.R., Smith, L. and Sidel, V.W. (2005). What is social medicine? *Monthly Review* 56(8): 27–34.

Bezruchka, S. (2001). Is our society making you sick? America's health lags behind that of more egalitarian nations. *Newsweek,* February 26: 14.

Bezruchka, S. (2006). Epidemiological approaches. In D. Raphael, T. Bryant and M. Rioux (eds.), *Staying alive: Critical perspectives on health, illness and health care.* Toronto: Canadian Scholars' Press: 13–33.

Bezruchka, S. (2008). Becoming a public scholar to improve the health of the US population. *Antipode* 40(3): 455–462.

Bezruchka, S., Namekata, T. and Sistram, M. (2008). Improving economic equality and health: The case of postwar Japan. *American Journal of Public Health* 98(4): 589–594.

Giecek, T.S. (2000). *Teaching economics as if people mattered: A high school curriculum guide to the new economy.* Boston: United for a Fair Economy.

Gutstein, E. and Peterson, B. (eds.). (2005). *Rethinking mathematics: Teaching social justice by the numbers.* Milwaukee: Rethinking Schools Publication.

Earle, A., Heymann, J. and Lavis, J.M. (2006). Where do we go from here? Translating research to policy. In J. Heymann, C. Hertzman, M.L. Barer and R.G. Evans (eds.), *Healthier societies: From analysis to action.* New York: Oxford University Press.

Jamrozik, K. and Hobbs M.S.T. (2002). Medical care and public health. In R. Detels, J. Mcewen, R. Beaglehole and H. Tanaka (eds.), *Oxford textbook of public health.* Oxford, UK: Oxford University Press: 215–242.

Kempf, S. (2005). *Finding solutions to hunger: Kids can make a difference.* New York: World Hunger Year.

Kingdon, J.W. (1995). Agendas, alternatives, and public policies. New York: Longman.

Kuhn, T.S. (1962). *The structure of scientific revolutions.* Chicago: University of Chicago Press.

Lakoff, G. (2006). *Thinking points: Communicating our American values and vision: A progressive's handbook.* New York: Farrar, Strauss, & Giroux.

Lantz, P.M., House, J.S., Lepowski, J.M., Williams, D.R., Mero, R.P. and Chen, J. (1998). Socioeconomic factors, health behaviors, and mortality: Results from a nationally representative prospective study of US adults. *JAMA* 279(21): 1703–1708.

Maher, J. (2006). *Most dangerous women: Bringing history to life through readers' theater.* Portsmouth, NH: Heinemann.

Murray, C.J.L., Kulkarni, S.C., Michaud, C., Tomijima, N., Bulzacchelli, M.T., Iandorio, T.J. and Ezzah, M. (2006). Eight Americas: Investigating mortality disparities across races, counties, and race-counties in the United States. *PLoS Medicine* 3(9): e260.

Murray, C.J.L., Michaud, C.M., McKenna, M.T. and Marks, J.S. (1998). *US patterns of mortality by county and race: 1965–1994,* Cambridge, MA: Burden of Disease Unit, Harvard Center for Population and Development Studies.

Roos, N.P., Brownell, M. and Menec, V. (2006). Universal medical care and health inequalities: Right objectives, insufficient tools. In J. Heymann, C. Hertzman, M.L. Barer and R.G. Evans (eds.), *Healthier societies: From analysis to action.* New York: Oxford University Press: 107–131.

Rose, G.A. (1992). *The strategy of preventive medicine.* New York: Oxford University Press.

St. Leger, L. (2001). Schools, health literacy and public health: Possibilities and challenges. *Health Promotion International* 16(2): 197–205.

Wallack, L. (2003). The role of mass media: A new direction for public health. In R. Hofrichter (ed.), *Health and social justice: Politics, ideology, and inequity in the distribution of disease.* San Francisco: Jossey-Bass: 594–625.

Wallack, L. and Lawrence, R. (2005). Talking about public health: Developing America's "second language." *American Journal of Public Health* 95(4): 567–570.

Wilkinson, R.G. (1996). *Unhealthy societies: The afflictions of inequality.* London: Routledge.

Wilkinson, R.G. (2005). *The impact of inequality: How to make sick societies healthier.* New York: New Press.

Wilkinson, R.G. and Pickett, K.E. (2006). Income inequality and population health: A review and explanation of the evidence. *Social Science & Medicine* 62(7): 1768–1784.

Chapter 35

Some Ideas for a Common Agenda

Peter Montague
Carolyn Raffensperger

Many of us could benefit if we had a few common ideas to guide our work. To provoke discussion about the elements of a common agenda, we have put together these initial thoughts. This first attempt is centered on the US because it is the place we know best. The picture we sketch here contains elements that, to some, may seem remote from the traditional work of environmental protection, environment, and health, or even public health. Perhaps few will want to engage all aspects of this picture; nevertheless, we hope there is some value in painting with broad strokes on a large canvas. Everything really *is* connected. Furthermore, we believe that people of good will, sharing a few common ideas and goals—and willing to form surprising alliances—can create a successful web of transformation.

First, we want to acknowledge some of our assumptions.

The Golden Rule

The wellspring of these ideas is a simple, universal ethic—every culture and every religion endorses the Golden Rule,[1,2] which says, "Treat others the way you want to be treated." This tells us, first, to alleviate suffering. This, in turn, leads directly to human rights—we all have a basic right to a life free of suffering, to the extent possible. The elements of such a life were laid out in the Universal Declaration of Human Rights, which the US endorsed December 10, 1948.

From the Golden Rule and the Universal Declaration: Justice

For us, the Golden Rule and the Universal Declaration together define justice. Justice is *action* that tends to manifest the Golden Rule and the Universal

Declaration; injustice is action in another direction. It is unjust, unfair, and therefore unacceptable to impose suffering on others or to stand by and allow suffering to go unnoticed or unchecked. It is unjust, unfair, and unacceptable to deprive anyone of any human right as spelled out in 1948. Justice is not passive. Justice demands action, sometimes aggressive action, conflict, and struggle. Without justice, there can be no peace. We stand with Gandhi, advocating non-violent action.

In recent years, science has confirmed what people have always known: community is essential for human well-being. We humans evolved as social creatures[3,4] who cannot thrive when separated from our circle of family, friends, acquaintances, and animal companions. Social isolation *makes us sick* and leads to *an early death.* This is one reason why racism and *white privilege* are profoundly wrong. At a minimum, they create social isolation, which leads to illness and suffering, and so they are unjust and unacceptable.

Furthermore, when we damage nature we diminish our own—and everyone's—possibilities for a life as free as possible of suffering. When we create havoc via global warming or damage to the Earth's protective ozone layer, or when we pave over fertile farmland, or exterminate the fish of the sea or the birds of the air, we *diminish everyone's possibilities* for securing life, liberty, and the pursuit of happiness (to quote the Declaration of Independence of 1776). This is unjust and unacceptable.

As Jeremy Bentham told us in 1789, animals too have a right to live a life free of suffering to the extent possible. As Bentham said, the question is not whether they can reason, or whether they can talk. Their right to live free from torment hinges on the question, can they suffer? Their suffering stands on a moral plane with ours.

However, we want to emphasize that humans are dependent upon *all* creatures, not just those that are sentient. Science now confirms the wisdom of indigenous peoples, that we are all interdependent, all humans, all species. We humans are part of, and are supported by, a biological platform of enormous complexity, which we cannot understand, but which we know with absolute certainty *nourishes and sustains us.* Even a child can see that, without it, we are lost.

Because rights and justice cannot be secured if our biological platform is shredded, we all have a right to intact natural and social environments—environments that enable us to provide for ourselves the essentials of air, water, food, shelter, and community, which we all require to prevent suffering.

The earth is our home and we have to take care of it, for the reason that we absolutely depend on it. To preserve our home without understanding all its billions of inter-related parts, we can aim to preserve every part of it. No part of creation can be presumed dispensable. We can say we know what's dispensable, but what if we're wrong? In recent years we humans came close to making the surface of the earth uninhabitable for humans because we failed to understand how CFC chemicals were damaging the ozone layer. It was a close call. Our ignorance is vast. As Albert Einstein reportedly said, "We still do not know one-thousandth of one percent of what nature has revealed to us."[5]

Because the biological platform, upon which we all depend, cannot be secured unless we are free to take action to protect it, human rights and justice are essential requirements for human survival.

Good Health Is a Fundamental Right

What is health? What conditions are necessary for health?

Aldo Leopold *defined* health as the capacity for self-renewal. The preamble to the constitution of the World Health Organization (WHO, July 22, 1946) defines health as "a state of complete well-being, physical, social, and mental, and not merely the absence of disease or infirmity." The WHO's Ottawa Charter says, "The fundamental conditions and resources for health are: peace, shelter, education, food, income, a stable eco-system, sustainable resources, social justice, and equity."

The WHO constitution also defines health as a basic human right: "The enjoyment of the highest standard of health is one of the fundamental rights of every human being without distinction of race, religion, political belief, economic or social condition." This is consistent with Article 25 of the Universal Declaration of Human Rights of 1948, which says, "Everyone has the right to a standard of living adequate for the health and well-being of himself and his/her family, including food, clothing, housing, and medical care."

The *right to health* is crucial to all other human rights.

Enjoyment of the *human right to health* is vital to all aspects of a person's life and well-being, and is crucial to the realization of all other fundamental human rights and freedoms.

Our health depends upon three environments:

1. The natural environment (air, water, soil, flora and fauna)
2. The built environment (roads, power plants, suburban sprawl, chemicals, etc.)
3. The all-important social environment (relationships of trust, mutual respect, and friendship but also poverty, racism and white privilege, sexism, homophobia, insecurity, the sense that life is out of control, and so on). The social environment creates what the United Nations calls "the social determinants of health." There is a very large body of literature indicating the importance of these determinants of a person's resilience in the face of stress.

All three environments are always intertwined in all "environmental" work and especially so in all "environment and health" work.

The Basis of Community and the Economy Is Sharing the Commons

The commons includes all the other things that we share together and that none of us owns or controls individually. The commons has been described as a river with three forks:[6]

1. Nature, which includes air, water, DNA, photosynthesis, seeds, topsoil, airwaves, minerals, animals, plants, antibiotics, oceans, fisheries, aquifers, quiet, wetlands, forests, rivers, lakes, solar energy, wind energy, ... and so on

2. Community: streets, playgrounds, the calendar, holidays, universities, libraries, museums, social insurance (e.g., social security), law, money, accounting standards, capital markets, political institutions, farmers' markets, flea markets, Craigslist, ... etc.

3. Culture: language, philosophy, religion, physics, chemistry, musical instruments, classical music, jazz, ballet, hip-hop, astronomy, electronics, the Internet, broadcast spectrum, medicine, biology, mathematics, open-source software, ... and so forth

Even the collective enterprise we call the "private sector" depends for its success upon the roads, the bridges, the water systems, the currency, the mercantile exchanges, the laws, the language, the knowledge, the understanding, and the trust that all of us, and our ancestors, have built in common.

Government has three main purposes, which cannot be separated from each other:

1. To guarantee the rights of the individual, as outlined in the Universal Declaration of 1948

2. To ensure justice

3. To protect and restore the commons, holding them in trust for this generation and for those to come

Prevention Is Essential

The 20th century has left us with an intractable legacy—toxic and radioactive wastes, proliferating weapons, global warming, nearly two million citizens imprisoned, rising rates of childhood disease and chronic illness (e.g., asthma, attention deficits, autism, diabetes, Alzheimer's). We have learned the hard way that managing large problems such as these is prohibitively expensive.

Therefore, our best hope is to create a culture of prevention—to develop a habit of always doing our best to prevent problems before they occur, rather than paying to manage them afterward. This is the *precautionary* approach, and it lies at the heart of traditional public health practice.

Just as our great-grandparents made slavery unthinkable, our challenge is to make it unthinkable to finalize any large decision without examining the alternatives we face, asking who bears the burden of proof, and anticipating ways to prevent and minimize harm.

Our Goal Together Can Be to Permanently Alter the Culture

We can aim to permanently alter the culture, not merely its laws, though laws can play an important part in both provoking and institutionalizing cultural transformation. Just as our forebears made slavery unthinkable, our goal together can be to make unsustainable life ways unthinkable.

Historically, in the US and Europe, culture has been changed by social movements—the first of them being the anti-slavery movement in England, 1787–1838. (See Adam Hochschild, *Bury the Chains,* ISBN 0618619070.) Therefore we believe that our goal of changing the culture can only succeed if it encourages, appeals to, and engages large numbers of people.

Accordingly, we believe a common agenda could be constructed from among the following ideas (plus others that we have not yet learned about):

I. Build a Multi-Issue, Multi-Racial, Multi-Ethnic Movement

1. We can make our work explicitly anti-racist. Because of European and US history, it is essential that we take a strong position against racism and white privilege. This entails a relentless, ongoing effort to change the culture of the United States. In addition to being a matter of simple justice, opposing racism is crucial politically because the New Deal coalition that governed the US from 1940 to 1980 was divided and conquered using race as the wedge issue, beginning with Senator Goldwater's presidential platform opposing civil rights laws in 1964.[7] If we ever hope to become politically influential in the US, we will need to build a multi-racial, multi-ethnic, multi-issue coalition. Understanding and confronting white privilege will be essential in any such effort.

It is worth pointing out that the various movements for health and justice in the US, taken together, make up a numerical majority in the US by at least two to one, and on many issues by far more than that. Therefore, the only way our adversaries can prevail is by dividing us. Race (and to a lesser extent class, ethnicity, national origin, religion, gender, and sexual orientation) has been the dividing wedge that our adversaries have used most effectively. (What are some other issues that our adversaries use to divide us? This seems worthy of considerable discussion.)

II. Reform the System for Choosing Candidates for Public Office

2. We can get private money out of elections. In principle, our republican democracy rests on the bedrock of "one person, one vote," not "one dollar, one vote." In the modern day, this means getting the mountains of private money out of elections, which in turn requires that *elections be publicly financed* so that every qualified individual is eligible to become a candidate for office, regardless of his or her personal wealth. (Various eligibility requirements have been proposed, such as the requirement that prospective candidates must gather a certain number of signatures to qualify as a candidate deserving of public financing.)

3. We can adopt the election system called *instant runoff voting* (IRV). In this system each voter ranks the candidates, 1, 2, 3, etc. If one candidate gets a clear majority of first-rank votes, he or she is declared the winner. However if no one candidate gets a clear majority of first-place votes, then the candidate with the least first-place votes (let's call this the "least popular candidate") is eliminated and his or her votes are re-distributed to the remaining candidates in the following way:

   Each ballot that ranked the "least popular candidate" as No. 1 is examined and the second-place choice on those ballots is the candidate who receives that particular "least popular candidate" ballot. This process of elimination goes on until there is a clear winner holding a majority of ballots.

   The system has many advantages over the current system and it is catching on across the US.

III. Protect the Commons

4. We can explicitly give all individuals the right to a safe and healthy environment. However, this alone will not suffice. We can also give these rights far higher priority than they have under current law, where they are presently trumped (for example) by the right to use one's property as one chooses for economic gain.

5. We can designate or elect guardians *ad litem* for future generations.

6. We can conduct annual audits of the commons (using consistent measures) with public reports supported by action plans for preservation, restoration, and prevention of harm.

7. We can establish a public interest research agenda that has as its first priority protecting and restoring the commons.

IV. Develop an Economy Whose Footprint Is Not Growing, or Is Even Shrinking

8. We can create an economy whose *ecological footprint* is not growing, or is even shrinking. Sustainability cannot be achieved without this bedrock idea, so it needs some elaboration and discussion.

A sustainable society is one in which the human economy provides the basics of a "good life" for everyone but the "footprint" of the economy never grows so large as to overwhelm the planet's natural ability to renew itself. As we will see, a sustainable society is also one in which justice and equity are continuously pursued.

There are two parts to the "footprint"—the number of people and their individual demands on the ecosystem.

Our current way of thinking and being in the world—premised on perpetual growth of the human footprint—is not sustainable. At present, the *human footprint is simply too large* for the planet to sustain, and the evidence is emerging all around us—global warming; destruction of the ozone layer; decimation of marine fisheries; industrial poisons in breast milk; increasing rates of chronic disease (attention deficits; asthma, diabetes, some childhood cancers); accelerating extinction of species; and so on.

Because the total human footprint is unsustainably large, both human population and individual consumption must shrink. However, the only proven way to curb human population is to (a) achieve economic growth to escape the chains of poverty and (b) achieve freedom and opportunity for women. The evidence is that, once the chains of poverty are broken, and children are no longer the only available old-age insurance, then most women with prospects choose not to bear large numbers of children.

This implies that all societies need sufficient economic growth to escape poverty—which implies the need for more roads, power plants, ports, and so on. However, given that the global human footprint is already unsustainably large, the need for growth in the global South requires footprint shrinkage in the global North. This, then, is the goal of forward-looking (precautionary) decision making: to make choices that can shrink the footprint of the global North, to make room for growth in the global South, to end poverty and liberate women so they can choose small families.

An end to growth-as-we-know-it immediately raises the issue of a just distribution of available goods (and bads). In the traditional way of thinking (at least in the US), poverty will be alleviated by economic growth—the poor are promised that, as the pie grows, even their small piece of the pie will grow apace. They need only be patient. But if the size of the pie is going to remain constant, or perhaps even shrink in some dimensions, growth can no longer serve as the safety-valve for "solving" poverty. Now we must begin to ask, "What's a fair distribution of the pie?" Thus a sustainable society not only has a sustainable footprint, but it also will never abandon the active pursuit of justice and equity.

Therefore, we need an economy that can grow (in places where growth is needed today to eliminate poverty, for example in Africa) but is not required to grow as the present economy is required to do (so that "developed" nations can achieve a constant or shrinking footprint). By "growth" we mean growth in capital stock, or growth in "throughput of materials" ("stuff"). A steady-state economy will still be dynamic and innovative. What is needed is a constant (or shrinking) "footprint" for the human economy—but within that footprint, technical and ethical innovation can be boundless.

One proposal envisions an economy based on competitive markets plus public ownership of productive facilities (factories, farms), renting them to producer co-ops, with investment capital raised by a flat tax on productive assets and distributed each year to all regions of the nation on a per-capita basis. (See David Schweickart, *After Capitalism*, ISBN 0742513009.) No doubt there are other ways to achieve the steady-state economy—all we know is that a steady-state economy (or an economy with a steady-state footprint) is essential. Perpetual growth on a finite planet is a certain recipe for a failed future.

Perhaps the nub of this issue is money lent at interest—usury in the original meaning of the word. It is payment of interest on borrowed funds that creates the requirement for economic growth. So the question could be framed as, "How can a society provide interest-free investment funds to replace and modernize infrastructure as it decays?"

9. We can organize our economy around the concept of zero waste. The present one-way torrent of materials out of the ground for single use (or nearly so), followed rapidly by reentry into the ground, will be recognized as an unsustainable absurdity. In a sustainable economy, every product will be designed for repeated re-use and the cost of its reprocessing for re-use will be included in the original sale price. (See Paul Palmer, *Getting to Zero Waste*, ISBN 0976957107.)

10. We can guarantee full employment with decent wages to end poverty. The Humphrey-Hawkins Full Employment Act of 1978 [P.L. 95–253] can serve as a model, with the added proviso that the federal government can serve as the employer of last resort. Everyone who wants to work has a right to a place in the shared enterprise.

V. Prevent Illness, Eliminate Health Disparities, Provide Universal Health Care

11. We can create a single-payer universal health care program, modeled on Canada's. This will be a health care program that seeks first to prevent illness and relies on "cures" only as secondary measures.

A central goal of any health system will be the elimination of health disparities—including disparities based on race and ethnicity, gender, and geography.

Health disparities are a human rights violation because they indicate that someone has been deprived of his or her right to health; therefore health disparities are unacceptable and must be eliminated and prevented.

NACCHO (National Association of County and City Health Officials) has defined "health disparities" as "differences in populations' health status that are avoidable and can be changed. These differences can result from social and/or economic conditions, as well as public policy. Examples include situations whereby hazardous waste sites are located in poor communities, there is a lack of affordable housing, and there is limited or no access to transportation. These and other factors adversely affect population health."

VI. Make Decisions to Prevent Harm

12. We can adopt the precautionary principle to avoid trouble and prevent harm, rather than clean up messes.

VII. Expressing an Anti-Racist Intention

13. From its early beginnings, European society has been based on racist assumptions that have produced unacknowledged systems of white privilege. Racist ideology predates capitalism and has been fundamental to the creation of much of the modern world. The US has been caught up in this mindset to an even greater degree than most European societies. The first step is to openly acknowledge the problem in its many dimensions.

14. Expressions of an explicit anti-racist intention are needed throughout the culture to counteract hundreds of years of silent violence against people of color. Anti-racism can be expressly practiced in the courts, the schools, our elections, the media, the churches, NGOs, in our funding priorities, our public health goals and practice, and on and on. Racism is not limited to individual acts of meanness, as much of the culture would have us believe. Racism is a largely invisible, embedded system of privilege that gives white people unearned assets that they can count on cashing in each day, but about which they remain largely oblivious. As Peggy McIntosh has described it, "White privilege is like an invisible weightless knapsack of special provisions, maps, passports, codebooks, visas, clothes, tools, and blank checks." White privilege is difficult for some people to acknowledge because its pervasive nature means we do not, in fact, live in the meritocracy. The deck is stacked at birth by skin color.

VIII. Restoring Justice: A Vision of the Courts for the 21st Century

15. We can develop a vision of the courts for the 21st century. Elements of this could include the following:

   a. Eliminating racist outcomes from court proceedings, with a goal of vastly reducing the number of people in prison
   b. Ending the status of corporations as persons entitled to the same rights as individuals under the Constitution, to restore individual responsibility and accountability. The term "person" in the 14th amendment should not include corporations. The goal here is democratic control of the nature and behavior of corporations, as was the norm in the US at an earlier time.
   c. Reversing the burden of proof, giving the benefit of the doubt to ecosystems, to future generations, to the luckless and the downtrodden
   d. Taking seriously our commitment to future generations, to pass along to them undamaged the world we inherited from our forebears, and establishing our priorities in the courts to allow this to happen

IX. Free Education for All

16. We can provide free education from pre-school through college. Investment in education—whether Head Start or the GI Bill of Rights—is an investment that demonstrably pays enormous dividends, generation after generation.

X. A Foreign Policy Free of Imperialism or Colonialism

17. We can adopt a foreign policy that brings an end to imperialism and colonialism. Bretton Wood institutions can be abolished and new institutions of international finance invented. The aim of military dominance of the planet and of outer space can be discarded.

XI. Organize Society to Provide Time for Democratic Engagement

18. Society can be organized to give everyone time to participate in democratic decision making. This will require a work-week shorter than 40 hours, living near the workplace to minimize travel time, and partners sharing child-rearing and household tasks. (See Gar Alperovitz, *America Beyond Capitalism*, ISBN 0471790028.)

19. Gender equity can be made a priority as a matter of fairness and justice, and because, for many people, having time for democratic participation

depends on sharing child-rearing and household tasks with a partner. Furthermore, worldwide, gender equity accompanied by opportunity and education is the only proven formula for limiting human population, as discussed above.

20. We can establish as a goal that everyone can walk to work, with incentives for city planners, urban developers, and local decision makers who meet this goal. This is important for personal health, for gender equity (couples must work near home if they are to share child-rearing and household tasks), and for democratic participation (time not wasted on commuting can become available for community engagement).

XII. The Future of These Ideas for a Common Agenda

21. This is just a beginning. Please contribute your ideas. Together all of us can be wiser and more successful than any of us alone.

Notes

1. http://www.religioustolerance.org/reciproc.htm
2. http://kvc.minbuza.nl/uk/archive/report/chapter1_3.html
3. http://www.medicalnewstoday.com/releases/38011.php
4. http://www.powells.com/biblio/1-0813339367-0
5. Einstein quoted in *The Sun* (June 2006), p. 48. Also available at http://www.brainyquote.com/quotes/keywords/nature.html.
6. Peter Barnes, *Capitalism 3.0* (San Francisco: Berrett-Kohler, 2006), p. 5.
7. Four books support this point with considerable historical detail: Dan T. Carter, *From George Wallace to Newt Gingrich: Race in the Conservative Counterrevolution, 1963–1994* (1996; ISBN 0807123668); Thomas and Mary Edsall's *Chain Reaction: The Impact of Race, Rights and Taxes on American Politics* (1992; ISBN 0393309037); Sara Diamond, *Roads to Dominion; Right Wing Movements and Political Power in the United States* (1995; ISBN 0898628644); Jean Hardisty, *Mobilizing Resentment* (1999; ISBN 0807043168).

Chapter 36

Taking On Corporate Power—and Winning

Robert Weissman

Corporate power has ascended to previously unimaginable peaks over the last 25 years.

All the more remarkable then has been incredible mobilizations of people, in communities around the planet, and between communities across borders, to confront multinational corporations.

Workers, environmentalists, public health advocates, consumer rights advocates and others have shown that, for all their power, multinational corporations can be defeated.

Campaigners and activists have succeeded at imposing meaningful restraints on corporate power. They have curbed abusive practices from bribery to predatory lending. They have imposed mandates on corporations, forcing them to take responsibility for the waste they generate and to test dangerous chemicals for health impacts. They have advanced worker rights to decent terms of work. They have created alternative sources of economic and political power, enabling generic manufacturers to compete with brand-name drug companies and generating markets for solar power.

Most victories are partial. They don't solve everything or even the entire problem campaigners seek to address. But they take the world closer to a place where people are treated with dignity, basic services are provided as a matter of right not privilege, ecological sustainability is respected, and power is democratized.

In this, the second part of our review of citizen victories over concentrated corporate power (see "Victories! Justice! The People's Triumphs over Corporate Power," *Multinational Monitor*, July/August 2005 for the first half), we again celebrate these achievements.

They are presented with the same caveats as our first 25 profiles of citizen victories: We don't claim these are the most important achievements over corporate power of the last quarter century, though we do think these were all landmark accomplishments. Nor are we making any effort to rank this list in importance—it is presented in a very rough chronological order, taking into account that many of these victories have unfolded over a long period, sometimes as long as or longer than the quarter-century lifespan of *Multinational Monitor.*

India's Generic Gambit

Its rapid economic growth in recent years notwithstanding, India remains a desperately poor country. For those with at least modest incomes, however, medicines are affordable.

The reason? The Indian Patents Act of 1970.

The Patents Act did away with product patents on pharmaceuticals and led to the development of a thriving, competitive generic pharmaceutical industry that was able to drive down the price of drugs.

"The objectives" of the 1970 law, explains B. K. Keayla, convener of the National Working Group on Patent Law in India, "were that there should be faster industrialization of the country and law should be designed to serve the public interest in a balanced manner." And the law worked, Keayla says.

Before 1970, India was dependent on multinational drug corporations and subject to the high charges demanded by the drug companies.

But the legal change contained in the 1970 patent law broke the monopoly power of Big Pharma and permitted Indian companies to develop local expertise.

Before 1970, India imported roughly 85 percent of its pharmaceuticals and made 15 percent domestically. Now the numbers have flipped, with India manufacturing approximately 85 percent of the drugs it consumes and importing the remaining 15 percent.

Low prices, driven by competition and efficient production, make drugs far more affordable in India than they would be otherwise, and have made Indian suppliers a crucial source of lower-priced pharmaceuticals for developing countries across the globe. The Indian price of ciprofloxacin, the antibiotic made famous as the best treatment for anthrax exposure, is about 1.5 percent of the cost in the United States. Indian drug makers now sell AIDS drugs for less than 2 percent of the price charged by the Big Pharma multinationals just a few years ago.

Indian drug companies such as Cipla, Ranbaxy, Hetero and Dr. Reddy now operate internationally and export around the world, including to the United States. More than 250 plants in India meet good manufacturing practice standards.

In 2005, India was required to adopt product patents for pharmaceuticals in order to be compliant with its obligations under the World Trade Organization. This means price-lowering competition for new drugs will be much delayed, unless compulsory licensing safeguards—authorizing generic competition while products remain on patent—are employed regularly.

Whether the Indian achievement in driving down pharmaceutical prices can be maintained in the future thus remains very much in question. Public health activists and the generic industry are working hard to ensure that implementation of India's WTO obligations does not erase the country's achievement in providing low-cost drugs.

Babyfood Justice

The World Health Organization (WHO) estimates that 1.5 million infants die as a result of diarrhea every year because they are not breastfed. Unsafe water used to mix infant formula can lead to infections and diarrhea, the leading killer of children worldwide. Where water is unsafe, UNICEF says that babies are 25 times more likely to die if they are bottle fed.

The babyfood companies have tricked hundreds of millions of women into bottle-feeding their babies, instead of relying on safe and health-giving breastmilk.

Recognizing that this corporate intervention into the most basic of human activities was taking millions of innocent lives of the most innocent, a number of consumer and health organizations in the 1970s vowed to take action.

In the United States, INFACT launched a boycott of the leading formula maker, Nestle.

Globally, consumer and health groups formed the International Baby Food Action Network (IBFAN). Through IBFAN's work, the World Health Assembly (the governing body of the World Health Organization, with representatives from all member countries) in 1981 adopted the International Code of Marketing of Breast-milk Substitutes.

But adopting a set of guidelines on how breastmilk substitutes should be marketed did not force any change in industry behavior. What has improved matters has been ongoing pressure from advocacy groups on babyfood manufacturers, and the adoption into law in many countries of the breastmilk substitute marketing code. At least 20 countries have implemented all or nearly all of the provisions of the code into law, according to IBFAN, with more than two dozen others adopting many provisions into law.

In 1984, the Nestle boycott was suspended, after the company promised to bring its marketing efforts into compliance with the international code. But by 1988, the boycott was back on, due to the company's unwillingness to abide by the code in good faith. The Nestle boycott is now coordinated by the UK group, Baby Milk Action.

Although significant gains have been registered, the babyfood companies continue to engage in unethical behavior. Although marketing tactics have changed, the corporate effort to undermine breastfeeding continues.

"Most baby food manufacturers are continuing their unethical promotional activities whilst claiming to abide by the International Code," reports IBFAN, which publishes a tri-annual report that monitors company compliance with the code. "They are increasingly 'investing' in health workers and health care systems, spending more money promoting their products than most governments spend on health education."

"Companies know that if they persuade a health worker to recommend their milk, they have gained a lifetime's brand loyalty. This is much more cost effective than persuading mothers individually. Advertising in hospitals implies that the product is endorsed by the health service: coupled with misinformation, this has created the false impression amongst mothers and health workers that many women cannot breastfeed."

"Even more effective is the practice of giving free or subsidized supplies of baby milk to hospitals and maternity wards. This encourages artificial infant feeding, which interferes with lactation. Once a mother leaves hospital, formula is no longer free, the company has another captive customer, and the mother and baby are denied the best start in life."

Essential Drugs

Prescription drug price, access and use are hot-button issues in the United States, where drugs make up only about 15 percent of healthcare costs.

In developing countries, by contrast, prescription drug costs make up a quarter to two-thirds of healthcare expenditures. And as much as 85 percent of prescription drug payments are out of pocket.

Given the much tighter budget constraints in poor countries, these facts mean that many people simply go without needed medicines, and many who do manage to pay suffer extreme financial burden. At the same time, thanks in no small part to heavy promotion and marketing by brand-name drug companies, lots of the money that is spent is wasted on inappropriate drugs irrationally prescribed.

Against this backdrop, health activists in the 1970s innovated the concept of an essential drugs list—a limited set of medicines selected based on disease prevalence, evidence on efficacy and safety, and comparative cost-effectiveness.

In 1977, WHO adopted its first essential drugs list of 208 medicines, a grouping found to be sufficient to treat nearly all serious communicable and non-communicable diseases.

The idea behind the list—which WHO continues to maintain and update periodically—is that governments should at least give preference to these medicines over others; encourage doctors to prescribe drugs from the list rather than alternatives that may be inappropriate, dangerous or unnecessarily costly; and find ways to supply these medicines to citizens.

Most countries now adapt the WHO list to meet their own circumstances—more than 150 have such lists. In about two thirds of cases, public sector procurement is limited to drugs on the national essential drugs list.

In no small part as a result, access to essential drugs almost doubled between 1977 to 1997, according to Margaretha Helling-Borda, a former director of WHO's Action Programme on Essential Drugs. "But one-third of the world's population still does not have regular access to essential medicines," she notes.

Nowhere was the essential drug concept used more aggressively than in Bangladesh.

There, an aggressive national drug policy went into place in 1982. Drugs that did not appear on the essential drugs list could not be imported or sold on the grounds that they were unnecessary and would require waste of national resources.

As Dr. Zafrullah Chowdhury, who helped pioneer the policy, explains, "We eliminated bad drugs with this very sweeping policy very quickly. In two months' time, we eliminated 2,000 drugs." The results were widely understood, Chowdhury says. "Overnight, people also realized that the price of the drugs had fallen by half. That was a shock. Better medicine at half the price."

Under pressure from the pharmaceutical multinationals and the US government, the Bangladesh policy would eventually be weakened—Chowdhury estimates it is 60 percent intact. But the policy remains a significant success. When the policy first went into effect, "only about 10 percent [of people in Bangladesh] had access to modern medicine. Today, more than 45 percent of the people have access to modern medicine."

Pittston Coal Strike

The class struggle does not heat up any hotter than in the coal mines.

In the late 1980s, the Pittston Coal Group decided to return violence and intimidation to the Appalachian coal fields.

The United Mine Workers of America (UMWA) recognized this for what it was, and said they were ready to engage in class warfare rather than surrender. The miners' aggressive campaign, almost entirely nonviolent in the face of a militarized company stance, succeeded in considerable part.

The UMWA contract with Pittston expired in 1988, after which the company cut off healthcare coverage for 1,500 pensioners, widows and disabled miners. The company engaged in bad-faith bargaining for more than a year, making it impossible to reach terms on a new contract.

In April 1989, the miners went on strike.

Pittston responded by hiring scabs to work the mines, and a latter-day Pinkerton security force to guard its mines. The company spent $20 million security over six months in 1989.

The company benefited as well from a friendly judiciary. Virginia state court Judge Donald McGlothlin Jr. issued an injunction limiting the number of pickets the mineworkers could post near mine entrances. When the mineworkers refused to abide by these restrictions, the judge imposed massive fines on the union, eventually totaling $64.3 million.

The UMWA responded to the Pittston provocation with a militant worker mobilization and a national solidarity campaign. They blockaded roads. Thousands of camouflage-wearing miners and their supporters were arrested. Wildcat strikes involving tens of thousands of miners broke out in support of the Pittston miners. Tens of thousands of supporters came to the UMWA's Camp Solidarity. The city of Boston withdrew its funds from Shawmut Bank, because the bank's vice chair served on the Pittston board of directors. The union organized a peaceful four-day occupation of a company preparation plant.

The high-profile campaign and refusal to buckle spurred the federal government to intervene. A federal mediator helped broker a final deal that was favorable to the miners, including on the crucial question of continuing to pay health benefits for retired and disabled miners and for widows. The UMWA was able also to win some modest revenge against its nemesis, Judge McGlothlin. In a November 1989 election, UMWA District 28 president Jackie Stump won a stunning write-in victory over the judge's father in an election for state representative, by a 2-to-1 margin. The union also ultimately escaped from the fines imposed by Judge McGlothlin, with the US Supreme Court ruling that punitive fines could only be imposed through criminal proceedings, with defendants given the right to a jury trial.

Banning the Global Waste Trade

"I think the economic logic behind dumping a load of toxic waste in the lowest wage country is impeccable and we should face up to the fact that ... underpopulated countries in Africa are vastly under-polluted."

At *Multinational Monitor*, we think this 1991 statement from Lawrence Summers, then–World Bank chief economist and currently president of Harvard University, is so remarkable that we named an award for outlandish statements or behavior after Summers.

But while Summers later said his comment was intended to be ironic and provocative, it does in fact express the logic of corporate globalization. Indeed, the 1980s saw the growth of a thriving global trade in hazardous waste, with rich countries shipping toxic waste to poor countries where it could be cheaply disposed of (and often simply dumped).

In 1986, the issue catapulted to international consciousness. The city of Philadelphia chartered a cargo ship named the Khian Sea to dispose of 14,000 tons of incinerator ash. For two years, the ship sought a country that would accept the waste. In 1988, the Khian Sea dumped 4,000 tons of its toxic load on a Haitian beach. The Haitian government ordered the dumping stopped and the toxic waste loaded back on the ship, but the Khian Sea slipped away. The ship traveled the globe looking for a place to dump its load, even changing its name along the way. But Greenpeace activists notified countries of the impending hazard and none agreed to permit the ship to dock. Eventually, the Khian Sea dumped its waste at sea.

In 1989, 118 nations signed the Basel Convention on the Control of Transboundary Movements of Hazardous Waste and Their Disposal. But environmental activists and the African countries that were recipients of so much waste denounced the treaty as ineffectual. The goal shouldn't be to control the waste trade, they argued, but to ban it. Greenpeace tracking of waste deals showed they actually increased after the Basel Convention was signed.

In 1991, the members of the Organization of African Unity sought to address the problem on their own, adopting the Bamako Convention banning the import of hazardous and nuclear waste. Other developing country groupings followed this example.

Meanwhile, developing countries insisted a global ban needed to be enacted. At the first conference of the parties to the Basel Convention, the head of the Indian delegation said, "You industrialized countries have been asking us to do many things for the global good—to stop cutting down our forests, to stop using your CFCs. Now we are asking you to do something for the global good—keep your own waste." Then, in 1994, overcoming objections from the United States, other rich countries and industry groups such as the International Chamber of Commerce, developing countries succeeded in winning amendments to the Basel treaty banning waste shipments from rich countries to developing nations.

The Basel Ban introduced a modicum of environmental justice into global affairs and transgressed dominant free trade orthodoxy. It also places pressure on rich countries to stop generating so much toxic waste.

"The progressive closure of the global escape valves for cheap and dirty solutions to our waste crisis provides incentives for industry to internalize the very real costs incurred by the act of generating toxic wastes in the first instance," explains Jim Puckett, a former Greenpeace campaigner who is now with the Seattle-based Basel Action Network.

Providing Civil Justice

Although Big Business has relentlessly attacked the US civil justice system for the last quarter century or more, the ongoing operation of the trial-by-jury system has had diverse and far-reaching impacts both in retroactively compensating people for injuries and proactively making the world safer and cleaner.

As the Center for Justice and Democracy explains, lawsuits "make us safer."

"Lawsuits deter culpable manufacturers, polluters, hospitals and other entities from repeating their negligent behavior or misconduct and give them the proper economic incentive to become safer and more responsible," the center explains in its 2002 report, "Lifesavers." Large verdicts often cause companies to improve dangerous products or end unsafe practices. The threat of adverse judgments, including the threat of punitive damages, deters companies from engaging in unsafe behavior. The documents that emerge in the "discovery" phase of litigation—when parties may demand information from their adversaries—often leads to public disclosure of unknown or under-appreciated dangers and frequently provokes a regulatory response.

Privately, at least, corporate executives acknowledge the beneficial role of lawsuits. A 1987 study based on a survey of risk managers at large US corporations, the industry-backed Conference Board found, "Where product liability [the legal doctrine making corporations responsible for harms caused by products they sell] has had a notable impact—where it has most significantly affected management decision making—has been in the quality of the products themselves. Managers say products have become safer, manufacturing procedures have been improved, and labels and use instructions have become more explicit."

In its "Lifesavers" report, the Center for Justice and Democracy lists dozens of safety reforms that have been achieved as a result of civil litigation. Among the safety reforms:

- Playtex in the mid-1980s removed its super-absorbent tampons from the market, after litigation showed they caused deadly toxic shock syndrome.

- After a Maryland court ruled in 1985 that the maker of Saturday night special handguns knew or should have known that their chief use was in committing crimes, the manufacturer, R. G. Industries was unable to obtain liability insurance and stopped manufacture of the guns in the United States. The company went out of business in 1986.

- After a 1993 lawsuit generated a huge verdict and focused national attention on how Domino's guarantee of pizza delivery within 30 minutes led delivery persons to drive recklessly, Domino's dumped its guarantee policy.

Nutrition Labeling

With obesity rates among children and adults in the United States soaring, an epidemic of type II diabetes racing out of control and growing public concern about eating healthier, but lots of confusion about which foods to choose, imagine this: things could be worse.

That they are not worse is a tribute to the Nutrition Labeling and Education Act (NLEA) of 1990, the culmination of a decade's worth of advocacy work by consumer and health organizations, led by the Center for Science in the Public Interest, to overcome opposition from the grocery manufacturers.

The NLEA is responsible for the labels on the side of packaged foods, a dramatic improvement from the skimpy labels that preceded them. Although problems remain with labels—including defined serving sizes that are often much smaller than many consumers would expect—they do a very good job of conveying what is in packaged food, as well as key nutritional information.

Consumers who use the labels do in fact make better choices about what they eat. Professor Rodolfo M. Nagaya of Texas A&M University has found that consumers who use nutrition labels get fewer calories from fat, consume less cholesterol, take in smaller amounts of sodium and eat more fiber.

The NLEA was also designed to crack down on misleading health claims regarding food. By 1989, four out of 10 new food products contained a health claim—many, such as health claims for juices that were mostly sugar and water, with no scientific justification. The Nutrition Labeling and Education Act banned deceptive health claims and established a science-based framework for determining when such claims are permitted.

The system worked very well to stop misleading health claims through the mid-1990s, but legislative and regulatory rollbacks have since hindered its effectiveness.

Still, the NLEA remains a positive framework upon which consumer groups are trying to build, including by requiring labeling of restaurant food.

One recent addition to the packaged food label is a line for trans fatty acids, most of which come from partially hydrogenated vegetable oil added to foods. Transfats very dramatically increase the risk of heart disease. The addition of the transfat line to the label is spurring food manufacturers to reformulate their products to eliminate partially hydrogenated vegetable oil. The US Food and Drug Administration (FDA) has found that removing partially hydrogenated vegetable oil from foods would save at least 10,000 lives a year in the United States.

Antarctica Off-Limits to Mining

Antarctica represents about 10 percent of the earth's surface and plays a central role in regulating the earth's weather patterns and ocean circulation systems. It is renowned for its beauty and pristine condition.

And its very pristine condition makes it desirable for mining companies.

The Antarctic Treaty, which came into force in 1961, demilitarized the Antarctic, promoted scientific cooperation and set aside disputes over territorial sovereignty. But it did not address mining issues.

In 1976, the parties to the treaty adopted a moratorium on mineral exploration. In 1981, they began negotiating over mining proposals, leading to the 1988 agreement on a convention to regulate—but permit—mining. Campaigning by Greenpeace, WWF-the Worldwide Fund for Nature, and others led Australia and France to reject the agreement.

That spurred negotiations over a comprehensive ban on mining in Antarctica. The United States, the United Kingdom and Japan argued against such a ban. Those objections were overridden. A deal was reached in 1991 to ban commercial mining for at least 50 years, and went into effect in 1998.

"Antarctica is the world's last great wilderness, a continent of awe-inspiring beauty, and a vital international scientific laboratory," said Beth Clark, director of the Washington, DC-based The Antarctica Project, after Japan, the last of the 26 Antarctic Treaty member nations, agreed to ratify the environmental protocol. "By establishing high standards for all human activities in the region, the Environmental Protocol goes a long way towards safeguarding Antarctica before it suffers from the human impacts felt over most of the rest of the earth."

Fishing-Free Reserves

It's not easy being a fish these days.

Just as aggressive development has devastated land-based species, so too have the fish taken a beating over the last century. Scientists have found that, thanks in large part to overfishing by industrialized fishing fleets, the population of large fish such as tuna, shark, cod and grouper has declined by roughly 90 percent over the last 50 years.

All kinds of fisheries management approaches are now being proposed to address the problem.

One of the most promising is the creation of marine reserves—"no-take" zones in which all animal and plant life is protected, forever.

The global leader in marine reserves may well be New Zealand. There, environmentalists waged a multi-year campaign that led to the adoption of the country's Marine Reserve Act. Today, New Zealand maintains 28 marine reserves protecting 7.6 percent of its territorial waters. It aims to take the total up to 10 percent by 2010.

No-fishing zones do wonders for fish. The global experience with marine reserves "reveals that most well-enforced marine reserves result in relatively large, rapid, and long-lasting increases in the population sizes, numbers of species, and reproductive output of marine animals and plants," according to the Partnership for Interdisciplinary Studies of Coastal Oceans (PISCO), a research consortium involving marine scientists from four universities along the US West Coast. "The average biomass, or weight of all animals and plants studied, is more than four times larger in reserves than in unprotected areas nearby. On average, the density, or number of animals in an area, triples, and the number of species is 1.7 times higher in marine reserves than in unprotected areas. In addition, the average body size of animals is 1.8 times larger in reserves than in fished areas.''

Not just the fish benefit. The public is welcomed and encouraged to enjoy marine reserves—through diving, snorkeling, taking photographs, swimming, kayaking, navigating through, picnicking on the land in the reserves ... but not through fishing. In New Zealand, and elsewhere, the marine reserves have proven an unexpected tourist attraction. They are valuable areas for scientific research. And, somewhat unexpectedly, they've proved beneficial for fishers.

Fish populations flourish in areas surrounding reserves, increasing fish catch in those places. Fishing boats now linger on the edges of marine reserves, because those are recognized as the places with the most fish.

At least 23 countries now maintain marine reserves. Most are small, with a median size of less than 1.5 square miles, but some are large and significant.

In the United States, fully protected areas are in place in Maine, Washington and California, among other areas. California protects only a tiny portion of its waters—two-tenths of a percent—but an environmental coalition is working to expand the state's marine reserves dramatically.

Marine reserves cannot be a sole solution to the problems of overfishing and other maltreatment of the seas, simply because there is little prospect of such reserves occupying a sufficient portion of planetary waters. But they can serve as a unique and important part of a comprehensive solution.

Writes New Zealand marine biologist Bill Ballantine, a leading advocate for marine reserves: "Marine reserves help maintain the intrinsic properties and processes of the sea, by keeping some areas free from all potentially disruptive human activity. The concept is proactive, not reactive. There is no need to identify each potential problem, nor to wait for problems to occur. There is no requirement to show that a particular disturbance causes any particular level of damage. Some areas are kept free of all disturbance on principle."

Forest Protection up the Supply Chain

For two decades or more, eco-activists have waged a valiant struggle to protect forests in the US Northwest and in the Canadian West. Countless protests, tree-sits and massive civil disobedience have slowed timber cutting in the region.

But by the early 1990s, a group of activists decided that confronting the tree-cutting companies wasn't enough, and would not ultimately be a successful strategy.

In a campaign focused on protecting the Clayoquot Sound on Vancouver Island in British Columbia, a new collaboration that would ultimately result in creation of the San Francisco-based ForestEthics decided on a different approach. Instead of targeting the timber cutters, they focused on the wood buyers. These companies, which maintain retail operations and care about their reputation with consumers, were much more vulnerable to citizen pressure. When these companies indicated that they no longer wanted to be buying clear-cut timber from ancient forests, the logging companies agreed to stop clear cutting.

ForestEthics has since used a similar approach to win protections for millions of acres of forest land in British Columbia and Chile.

ForestEthics and other environmental groups have also won commitments from major wood sellers, including the dominant home improvement chains Home Depot and Lowe's, not to sell wood from endangered forests and to give preference to wood products certified as sustainably harvested by the Forest Stewardship Council. And they have convinced office supply stores like Staples to stock more post-consumer recycled paper, and make it more attractive for consumers.

ForestEthics is currently focusing on catalog companies, which send out 17 billion catalogs a year, demanding they stop using virgin paper. The top target is Victoria's Secret (see www.victoriasdirtysecret.net), which mails nearly 400 million catalogs a year, using virgin fiber paper with little or no recycled content. ForestEthics charges that much of the paper is made from trees from Canada's Boreal forest, which contains 25 percent of the world's remaining intact forest.

"The Boreal forest is a key regulator of the world's climate, and it is being turned into junk mail," says Lafcadio Cortesi of ForestEthics. "Are we really supposed to stand by while Victoria's Secret turns one of the earth's few safeguards against global warming into catalogs?"

Sweating for Sweat-Free Goods

Low-paying jobs in cramped and unsafe working conditions, where worker rights are denied and managerial control is exerted through intimidation and fear, are a pervasive feature of corporate globalization.

That these facts are now so familiar is a testament to the achievements of the international campaigns against sweatshops and for worker rights. But the campaigns have achieved more than media attention. Sweatshops remain omnipresent, but on-the-ground organizing and international solidarity campaigns have scored some notable gains for workers on the global assembly line.

The global anti-sweatshop campaign probably came of age in 1996, when the New York-based National Labor Committee issued a report documenting that TV personality Kathie Lee Gifford's line of clothing, sold in Walmart stores, was made in sweatshops in Honduras. Gifford initially issued a tearful denial of the charges on her television program, "Live with Regis and Kathie Lee," creating a media sensation. She later acknowledged the charges to be true, though she denied knowing about conditions in the factories where her line of clothing was made. The charges, tearful denial and ultimate promise by Gifford to support reform created a media sensation that brought unprecedented national and international attention to the sweatshop issue.

The Kathie Lee Gifford controversy followed years of hard work by a small number of activists in the United States and other rich countries working to support workers and worker advocacy efforts in developing countries. The GAP and Nike had been two of the early targets of these activists, with the GAP agreeing in 1995 to authorize independent third-party monitoring of its overseas contracting operations. Nike has been much more grudging in acceding to demands to end sweatshops, but even it has made some significant improvements.

What these early cases highlighted was how the spread of sweatshops was the outgrowth of a global system of outsourcing and multinational efforts to escape responsibility. Increasingly, multinationals in the clothing and shoe business (as well as much higher-end products) contracted out the manufacture of their goods. They benefited from super-exploited labor in the process, but disclaimed responsibility for conditions in the factories where their products were made. The anti-sweatshop campaign's success turned on its ability to reverse that trend, to hold the brand-name companies responsible for what went on in those outsourced factories, and to sully the reputation of the brand-name enterprises with bad records.

Students on US college campuses took up the call, and launched campaigns across the country demanding that their colleges and universities take responsibility for the conditions under which t-shirts, sweatshirts and other products adorned with school logos and names were manufactured. Under the banner of United Students Against Sweatshops, they held demonstrations, wrote detailed policy papers and staged sit-ins in university office buildings.

Students' efforts led to the creation of the Workers Rights Consortium (WRC), a grouping that administers a genuine system to promote sweat-free production. Nearly 150 schools are members of the WRC. They pledge to adopt a manufacturing code of conduct and work to include the code in contracts with makers of their logo goods, and ask licensees to provide the WRC with the names and locations of all factories involved in the production of their logo goods.

Other efforts to demand high-profile brands stop relying on sweatshops continue to gain ground, and to amass bulk-buying power for sweat-free purchases. San Francisco in 2005 agreed to require city contractors to guarantee that the uniforms, computers and other goods they supply are not made in sweatshops. Los Angeles, Milwaukee, Newark, New Jersey and Albuquerque have similar laws.

Relying on vulnerable immigrant workers, sweatshops have proliferated in the United States at the same time they have grown overseas. Organizations like Sweatshop Watch have gained some important victories for mistreated workers in these assembly shops, and workers' centers have provided important legal services for them.

Like many victories and achievements, these are all imperfect. At both the national and global level, comprehensive solutions remain, so far, out of reach.

Outlawing Bribery

Pay a bribe, take a tax write off.

Until 1997, that had long been the rule in Germany and other industrialized countries. These nations had not only tolerated bribery of overseas government officials, they had effectively encouraged bribery through tax policies that treated bribes like any other business expense.

But a wave of concern about the impact of corruption, and a civil society campaign that was supported by US companies, changed that. In 1997, the Organisation of Economic Co-operation and Development (OECD), a grouping of the world's rich nations, adopted an anti-bribery convention, requiring countries to criminalize bribery of foreign public officials.

Corruption is a severe problem around the globe, but it takes its greatest toll in developing countries, where public resources are severely constrained. Not only does corruption divert public resources from productive use, it also undermines democratic governance and impedes efficient functioning of both the public and private sector, including small and large business.

Corruption flourishes throughout much of the developing world because monitoring of government is weak and poorly paid governmental officials are more susceptible to bribes. However, as Dr. Peter Eigen, chair of Transparency International, an advocacy group that monitors worldwide corruption, noted at the time the treaty was adopted, the OECD Convention recognizes that a large share of the corruption in developing countries "is the explicit product of multinational corporations, headquartered in leading industrialized countries, using massive bribery and kick-backs to buy contracts in the developing countries and the countries in transition."

US multinationals backed the OECD treaty because they already faced restrictions on overseas bribery, thanks to the US Foreign Corrupt Practices Act. With the convention, the US companies hoped to create a level playing field, in which they are not disadvantaged vis-à-vis European and Japanese competitors. The bribery treaty illustrated how unilateral restrictions on US companies can be effective, not only at curbing US corporate abuses overseas, but also at turning US multinational corporations into advocates of enacting those restrictions into international law.

Developing countries have adopted treaties against corruption as well. In 1996, the Organization of American States—which includes the nations of North and South America—adopted a Convention Against Corruption. The African Union adopted an anti-corruption treaty in 2003.

Only a naïf would say that the global corruption problem is anything close to being solved. But the adoption of anti-bribery treaties has established a worldwide norm that bribery and corruption are wrong, imposes some non-trivial restraints on bribes by multinationals and has helped energize a grassroots anti-corruption campaign led by Transparency International and others around the world.

Full-Time Strike at UPS

US workers don't go on strike very often anymore. Over the last decade, there have been just 28-and-a-half strikes a year involving more than a thousand workers.

And when workers do go on strike, it is often not on terms of their choosing, but simply a reaction to complete employer recalcitrance and refusal to bargain.

But in 1997, workers at UPS, the parcel shipping giant, showed that the strike remains a potent tool for unions that act strategically and militantly.

UPS had turned the use of part-time employees, who cost less per worker because they receive fewer or no benefits and are paid on a lower wage schedule, into a business model. Part-time workers averaged about $11 an hour, while full-timers made nearly double, about $20 an hour. In the years previous to the strike, 80 percent of the company's new hires had been part-timers.

As UPS and the teamsters union representing UPS workers went into negotiations, UPS sought to exacerbate its part-time hiring strategy with enhanced authority to contract out.

The teamsters, then under the leadership of reformer Ron Carey, were having none of this.

After five-and-a-half months of failed negotiations, the union led the workers out on strike in August. The union had mobilized UPS workers for the negotiations and a strike, sending questionnaires to members before negotiations started—and which they used to establish demands at the bargaining table—and collecting signatures backing union demands. Workers embraced the strike, with very few crossing the picket line. Full-time workers walked the line for part-timers, out of solidarity and an understanding that the increase in part-time jobs ultimately threatened their own position.

The union masterfully framed the debate and conveyed its concerns to the public. The teamsters highlighted the abuses of the UPS part-time strategy, showing how it unfairly disadvantaged workers—not a few of whom worked multiple part-time jobs at the company, but still only received part-time wages and benefits—and provoked extraordinary turnover (of more than 180,000 part-timers hired in 1996, only 40,000 were still with the company at the end of the year).

After 16 days, UPS capitulated on most of the contentious issues. It agreed to hire more full-time workers, and increase the number of full-time jobs that would be set aside for part-timers. The company also agreed to increase pay for part-timers, and backed down on pension demands for full-timers.

"Workers have shown we can stand up to corporate greed," Carey declared after the union's victory. "After 15 years of taking it on the chin, working families are telling big corporations that we will fight for the American dream."

Explains Matt Witt, a spokesperson for the teamsters during the strike and now director of the American Labor Education Center, "The UPS strike of 1997 forced one of the nation's largest and most visible corporations to shift thousands of part-time jobs with few or no benefits to regular full-time jobs with health care and pensions, in the process focusing national attention on American corporations' throwaway jobs strategy."

M.A.I. Goes M.I.A.

Some time in the 1990s, a band of corporate-oriented lawyers came up with what they thought was a neat idea: observing a growing number of treaties affording strong protection to the trade in goods, they reasoned, why not develop an international instrument that would provide robust guarantees to cross-border investments?

Multinational corporations were globalizing at an increasing pace, and investing ever more heavily in developing countries—new foreign direct investment topped $300 billion in 1995, more than 50 percent higher than the figure at the start of the decade, with almost a third of the 1995 investment going to the Third World. At the same time, financial flows were speeding up, with lots of rich country money sloshing in and out of developing countries in speculative investment.

Investors, whether manufacturing or financial corporations, were very excited about the opportunities presented by a world without investment borders. But there were nagging concerns. It hadn't been that long ago when multinational corporations saw their factories expropriated in many developing countries—and they wanted to make sure that history was not repeated. And, there were regulatory standards imposed on investors—sometimes just on foreign investors (like obligations to hire local people in top management positions), and sometimes on all investors (like requirements to meet certain environmental standards)—that interfered with profit-making.

To cure both of these perceived evils, the idea of the Multilateral Agreement on Investment (MAI) was dreamed up.

In 1995, the Organization of Economic Cooperation and Development (OECD, the grouping of rich countries) began negotiations for an MAI. The idea was to reach agreement among the rich nations, and then permit developing countries to join the deal on a take-it-or-leave-it basis.

"The MAI would guarantee the investor and the investment fair and equitable treatment and full protection and security," according to OECD documents made public after negotiations broke down in 1998.

In practice, the MAI would have afforded foreign investors not "equitable" treatment, but superior powers and privileges over domestic investors—not to mention actual citizens!—while imposing no responsibilities on them.

As Public Citizen's Global Trade Watch noted, the treaty would have provided speculators and multinational corporations:

- The right to compete against domestic companies in all economic sectors
- The right to acquire any business or property in any economic sector, including natural resources and strategic industries such as communications and defense
- The right to convert currency and move money across borders without constraints, fostering the sorts of currency crises that collapsed the Mexican peso and caused the 1997 Asian financial meltdown
- The right to move production facilities without limit or penalty, regardless of the impacts on workers or the host community
- Freedom from conditions (called performance requirements) placed on investment to counter speculation and ensure that corporations meet basic rules of conduct
- The right to sue governments for cash damages (paid from public funds) for restitution if an investor claimed its rights had been violated under the agreement

The investment agreement met a sudden demise in April 1998, when French negotiators refused to agree to provisions that they believed would threaten national cultural protections.

But underlying the collapse of the negotiations was a global civil society mobilization that would be viewed as one of the first, large-scale international campaigns to make effective use of the Internet. Advocacy groups obtained a copy of the then-secret negotiating text and posted it on the web (*Multinational Monitor* actually did the initial posting). Using the Internet, consumer, environmental, development and other organizations mobilized an international campaign that made the MAI a high-profile issue around the world. Canadian activists in particular elevated the issue to national prominence. With the veil of secrecy removed and increasing attention focused on the spectacular corporate power grab promised by the MAI, the negotiations were unsustainable, and broke down.

Saving Organic Standards

Organic food has come a long way in a short time. Just a couple decades ago, "organic" was associated with shriveled and spot-marked fruits and vegetables.

Now, it is the highest end of the markets for fruits, vegetables, meat and poultry, and has been growing in the United States at an astronomical 15–20 percent a year over the last decade. Organic sales in the United States in 2004 topped $12 billion.

Rapidly growing consumer interest in organics and environmental advocacy led in 1990 to passage of the Organic Foods Production Act.

But in late 1997 and 1998, it appeared that the US Department of Agriculture (USDA), acting at the behest of the biotech industry, chemical makers and other large agribusiness interests, would use the act to undermine the organic market.

In December 1997, USDA proposed organic labeling rules that would determine what food could be labeled organic and what could not. Although the National Organic Standards Board, an official advisory board created by the Organic Foods Production Act, had recommended application of a strict standard for organics, USDA demurred. Instead, it proposed to define organics so that crops that were genetically modified, irradiated or fertilized with sewer sludge could be labeled organic. Meat and poultry treated with considerable amounts of antibiotics, denied access to outdoors or fed up to 20 percent non-organic feed could be labeled organic.

Organic advocates greeted the USDA proposals with dismay and outrage. Labeling as "organic" food that did not meet generally recognized standards of organic would undermine consumers' commitment to organic, they feared, and make it hard or impossible even for committed consumers to purchase genuinely organic food.

"Time and time again US government officials have ignored citizens' concerns and interests. The USDA understands that the public will never accept chemically contaminated or genetically engineered foods if given any real choice in the marketplace," said Ronnie Cummins, national director of the Pure Food Campaign. "But Monsanto and the agri-toxics crowd are determined to undermine consumer choice and to cram their products down peoples' throats if necessary."

But organic advocates did not just rail against the rule. They organized.

They organized environmentalists and organic producers and organic consumers. Stores that sold organics encouraged consumers to submit comments to USDA.

Citizens sent in more than 150,000 comments to USDA, virtually all of them opposing USDA's proposals.

Faced with this mounting opposition, USDA had little choice but to concede.

It was back to the drawing board. At the end of 2000, USDA published a revised, final rule that went into effect in 2001 and was fully implemented the next year. The revised rule constituted a rejection of the agency's position on virtually all of the crucial controversies surrounding the previous proposal.

The Spread of Smokefree Spaces

"The logical appeal of smokefree air is irresistible to politicians, commentators, even some smokers," wrote an executive with the now-defunct Tobacco Institute in 1985. "It is the most effective way to reduce smoking."

And for exactly that reason, Big Tobacco for decades has made opposition to smokefree laws a top priority. The industry has funded front groups, pushed for ineffective alternatives to smokefree spaces (such as heightened ventilation standards), supported junk science challenging the evidence of harms to nonsmokers from exposure to second-hand smoke and invested millions in campaigns to oppose smokefree laws.

For many years, and to a considerable extent even still, the strength of the movement for smokefree spaces was at the grassroots level. Communities across the United States adopted smokefree rules for particular public spaces, then workplaces, then restaurants and then for all public places including bars. Big Tobacco fought these fights as best it could at the local level, while striving to pass state laws that would preempt local ordinances.

But the persistence of grassroots activists, combined with steadily increasing scientific evidence of the harms from second-hand smoke, conspired to overcome the powerful industry.

"Study after study confirms that smokefree workplace laws save lives, save money and make communities healthier, more attractive places in which to live and work," explains Cynthia Hallett, executive director of Americans for Nonsmokers' Rights (ANR), the leading advocate for smokefree areas. "Secondhand smoke is the third-leading cause of preventable death in this country, killing tens of thousands of nonsmokers each year, according to the National Cancer Institute. It is a leading cause of heart disease, lung cancer and respiratory illnesses."

The Centers for Disease Control has found that, by 2004, two thirds of US states had smokefree laws; and in the states without smokefree laws, hundreds of cities and towns have adopted their own ordinances.

In 1998, California went smokefree in bars (having made all restaurants smokefree in 1994). That move, which seemed so radical at the time, in fact started a torrent of similar efforts. More than 100 US municipalities are now smokefree in workplaces, bars and restaurants, according to an ANR tally.

Smokefree areas has been one of the only areas in which the United States was a world leader in tobacco control, but other countries are now catching up and surpassing the United States in providing protections to nonsmokers. Latvia, Vietnam, Bulgaria, Italy, Iran, Russia, Australia, Uganda, Tanzania, Norway, Thailand and Pakistan are among the many countries that have adopted some variant of national smokefree laws. In Ireland, all workplaces—including pubs!—are now smokefree.

Cochabamba Claims the Right to Water

It may at times appear that they are just doing the bidding of multinational corporations, but the zealots at the World Bank believe the gospel they preach. And their core message is: markets work better than the public sector.

So, while it may have been a conceptual leap for a regular person to come up with the idea that drinking water service to residences and businesses should be provided not by the government but by private corporations, it was an obvious step for World Bank staff.

With similar ideologues in places like Margaret Thatcher's Britain pushing for water privatization, a handful of multinational companies, mostly European, suddenly emerged to swoop in and take over municipal or national water systems in both rich and poor countries.

Although it may appear an apostasy to the World Bank, the water privatization movement has been an utter failure. It turns out that private water companies are less efficient than public ones, charging higher prices to serve fewer consumers. The water companies are generally not interested in serving the broad public—preferring instead to service elite, heavier water users—so they are both less equitable and less efficient.

Some water privatization efforts are collapsing simply because the privatizers are inefficient, and because they find that even with favorable contract arrangements they cannot make the kind of profits they desire.

But it is little solace to consumers that water service privatization efforts may, in time, fall apart, and the service revert to public control. And so a growing worldwide movement is emerging to challenge water privatization schemes before they take root and to undo privatizations already undertaken.

The movement's greatest success has been in Bolivia, where a surge of protests in Cochabamba, the country's third-largest city, kicked out Aguas de Tunari, a consortium of companies in which the US corporation Bechtel was the lead partner.

The Bolivian government had signed a sweetheart deal in 1999 with Aguas de Tunari, guaranteeing the consortium a 16 percent rate of return per year on its investment. After the company came in, water prices soared—by as much as 400 percent. Paying for water suddenly constituted a major expenditure for people and businesses.

A broad civic coalition, the Coordinator for the Defense of Water and Life, formed to oppose the privatization. Within two months of the consortium taking over the water system, the coordinator mobilized between 15,000 and 20,000 people to occupy the city's main plaza. They called a general strike and blockaded roads. Protests continued and grew over the next several months; the government responding with violence, and well over a hundred protesters were injured. In April 2000, demonstrations intensified, and a 17-year-old protester was killed. Two days later, 80,000 people were blockading the streets, demanding the law authorizing the privatization be revoked.

In the face of this broad and passionate mobilization, the consortium and the government backed down. The company simply abandoned the city, and the government proceeded to modify the law to satisfy the protesters.

Preserving Biodiversity

The 1992 Earth Summit in Rio de Janeiro in many ways represented the culmination of a surge of interest in environmental issues in the early 1990s.

Dozens of world leaders and thousands of delegates convened to debate environmental issues and adopt an ambitious plan, known as Agenda-21, for putting the planet on the path to sustainability.

But, in retrospect, the media and political concentration on that moment in Rio yielded little. The promises have been forgotten, and Agenda-21 remains little more than an interesting relic—a worthy document in many ways, but little more than an aspirational program that governments ignore.

One concrete thing that did emerge from the Earth Summit was the Convention on Biological Diversity. Now ratified by more than 175 countries (but not the United States), the convention commits nations to preserving biodiversity. Thanks to human impact on the environment, species are disappearing at somewhere between 50 and 100 times the natural rate, a figure likely to rise dramatically, thanks to forest and coral destruction and global warming, among other factors. Thousands of plants and animal species are at risk of extinction. Recognizing the complex and overwhelming threats to biodiversity, the convention calls for application of the precautionary principle—"where there is a threat of significant reduction or loss of biological diversity, lack of full scientific certainty should not be used as a reason for postponing measures to avoid or minimize such a threat."

Much of the convention calls on national governments to take steps within their own borders. It has helped prod governments to take steps to protect biodiversity, and made available some modest resources to developing countries for such purposes.

Thanks to campaigning by environmental groups and the insistence of African and other developing countries, a special protocol was adopted in 2000 to deal with a transborder issue: trade in genetically modified seed. The Cartagena Protocol on Biosafety was adopted over the heated opposition of complaints from agribusiness, the United States and other biotech-exporting countries. It addresses the twin concerns that genetically modified seed may pollute the gene pool for a crop, thus eliminating natural plants without genetically modified traits, and eradicate the "centers of origin" where cultivated crops originally grew wildly and which remain crucial for replenishing the gene pool of cultivated crops.

Operationally, the Cartagena Protocol enables governments to inform a central clearinghouse that they refuse imports of genetically modified seed, with exporting countries bound to respect such notifications. Like most other citizen victories and including especially those in the realm of international treaty-making, the Cartagena Protocol is imperfect and fails to address crucial issues (notably, exports of seed allegedly for human or animal consumption). Nonetheless, it has helped put a brake on the efforts of biotech companies to spread their products across the planet and put at risk global biodiversity, and much more.

Solar Wins at the Ballot Box

The world urgently needs solar energy developed on a massive scale, if the worst effects of global warming are to be averted.

But a government-energy industry de facto conspiracy has worked to undercut solar from both the supply and demand side. Government investments in solar R&D have been slashed (outside of the Pentagon, the US government now spends less than $100 million on solar research). Demand is limited because the unit cost of solar remains above that of subsidized fossil fuels. In this environment, independent firms have foundered; BP and Shell are now the largest solar researchers.

Activists in San Francisco decided to take action to overcome these obstacles to solar development. In 2001, with the California energy crisis fresh on voters' minds, they placed on the ballot an initiative that directed the city to spend $100 million on solar panels, energy efficiency and wind turbines for public facilities. In November 2001, with 73 percent of the vote, San Franciscans approved Proposition B, a $100 million bond initiative.

Prop B promised to pay for itself, by combining the rapidly accrued payback from investments in energy efficiency with expenditures on solar.

"Solar may be expensive, but energy efficiency is cheap," explains the Vote Solar Initiative. "Wind power is, in many places, extremely cost competitive with other energy sources. The trick is to develop some projects with shorter payback periods, bundle them with solar, and evaluate the costs on a whole-project basis."

Large-scale expenditures on solar help drive down costs, too. "In San Francisco's case," explains the Vote Solar Initiative, "the size of the project was not just for bragging rights: lowering costs through economies of scale and the promise of developing a local solar manufacturing base were practical arguments for thinking big."

Economies of scale are even more important on an aggregate basis. If enough municipalities and other large-scale energy purchasers follow the San Francisco model, solar efficiencies will grow and per-unit prices will come down.

The solar initiative won a major victory at the end of 2005, with the California Public Utilities Commission announcing plans for a "California Solar Initiative," a 10-year, $3.2 billion solar incentive program to develop 3,000 megawatts of solar across the state.

Science for Women

Drug companies don't like to do tests on women and children.

But they don't mind subjecting them to drugs for untested purposes. Or, stated differently, they don't mind doing uncontrolled tests on the general population of women and children.

Some health advocates don't think this is such a good idea.

When the drug manufacturer Wyeth sought in the early 1990s authorization to market hormone pills to women for the purpose of reducing heart disease—although there was no evidence from randomized clinical trials to show that it was effective for this purpose—the National Women's Health Network and Public Citizen's Health Research Group objected.

At the same time, women's health groups were highlighting the failure of drug companies to test pharmaceuticals on women. They were also raising questions about whether drugs and dosages tested on men had different effects on women, and about the effect of drug interactions, including for example with contraceptive pills, on women. They complained that medical researchers conducted their studies on men, though the results were generalized to men and women alike. For example, as the National Institutes of Health states, "many of the largest studies of heart disease did not include women, despite the fact that heart disease is the number one cause of death in women overall. These studies were aimed at prevention of early heart attacks and were thus focused on men, in whom heart disease manifests approximately 10 years earlier than women."

These twin concerns led to the launch of the Women's Health Initiative at the National Institutes of Health in 1992. The Women's Health Initiative featured two components: a randomized clinical trial and an observational study. The clinical study was the largest, most definitive long-term study of postmenopausal women's health ever undertaken in the United States.

The hormone prong of the study had explosive impact. Not only did long-term hormone therapy for post-menopausal women fail to reduce the risk of heart disease, it actually increased it, as well as the risk of breast cancer, stroke and pulmonary embolism.

The study disproved years of bad science peddled by Wyeth—which through elaborate marketing campaigns had succeeded in inducing millions of women to undertake long-term hormone use.

The study also revealed broader truths: the need for unvarnished, independent research into the safety and efficacy of the drugs pushed by gigantic marketing machines.

"Hormone replacement therapy is not the only therapy being over-promoted by drug companies to healthy people," says Cindy Pearson of the National Women's Health Network. "Pharmaceutical companies have bought physicians, have bought scientists and have bought clinical medicine. Science must be separated from advertising."

"The lesson we need to learn for the future is that we need unbiased research. We need to remove drug company influence from all medical education. And pharmaceutical interventions should not be inflicted on healthy people until these interventions are proven safe and effective in randomized controlled trials."

Arsenic No More

The dangers of arsenic are immortalized in everything from Shakespeare's work to Joseph Kesselring's "Arsenic and Old Lace."

But for two decades it was used as a preservative in pressure-treated wood in the United States, with the arsenic imported from China, where it is manufactured in dangerous conditions.

Arsenic-treated wood had been banned or strictly regulated in Japan, Germany, Australia and other countries, the Healthy Building Network notes. But, "despite evidence that arsenic was leaching into groundwater and contaminating land, each year nearly 6.4 billion board feet of wood treated with a chromium-copper-arsenic (CCA) formula was created, fueling the growth of a $4 billion industry."

For years, US environmentalists had urged the Environmental Protection Agency (EPA) to address the hazards of arsenic in wood, but to no avail.

That changed after a campaign spearheaded by the Healthy Building Network.

The campaign made two key moves. First, it highlighted the use of pressure-treated wood in playgrounds, and the risks to children. Studies by the Healthy Building Network and the Environmental Working Group found that an area of arsenic-treated wood the size of a four-year-old's hand contains an average of 120 times the amount of arsenic EPA allows in a 6-ounce glass of water. Some of the arsenic rubs off playground equipment onto children's hands and is absorbed and ingested when children put their hands into their mouths.

Second, the campaign looked to pressure points other than the Environmental Protection Agency. It filed a petition with the Consumer Product Safety Commission to remove arsenic-treated wood from playgrounds. It also demanded Home Depot and Lowe's—which between them sell the vast majority of pressure-treated wood in the United States—stop selling such wood.

Organized by Clean Water Action, tens of thousands of consumers sent postcards to the companies urging them to stop selling arsenic-treated wood. The campaign also launched a paid advertising campaign against Home Depot, contrasting the use of arsenic-treated wood in playgrounds with the prohibition on arsenic wood that had been instituted by most of the nation's premier zoos.

"We wanted to draw public attention to the fact that children were permitted to eat and play on poisoned wood, but it was considered too dangerous for zoo animals," says Paul Bogart of the Healthy Building Network.

The combined agitation achieved rapid success. In 2002, within a year of the campaign's initiation, the EPA announced that the manufacture and sale of arsenic-treated wood for most residential uses would cease by the end of 2003.

"The wood treatment industry and the EPA finally reached the common-sense conclusion that the best way to protect kids from arsenic wood was not to affix a poison label to it, but to eliminate it," says Bogart.

"This victory proves that when citizens demand safe choices and healthy alternatives, manufacturers, retailers and governments listen," says Lynn Thorp, of Clean Water Action.

Reaching for Sustainability

The precautionary principle is an idea whose time has come.

As the world now faces unfathomable hardship from a global warming phenomenon that could have been avoided or least drastically lessened with preventative action, there is no longer a credible case, if there ever was, against the precautionary principle.

The precautionary principle directs that where public health and environmental protection is at stake, the proponents of an activity bear the burden of showing it is safe. Rather than passively accept technological and other choices made by corporations, society should consider alternatives to proposed activities, and opt for the safest option, including the possibility of doing nothing.

It is a commonsense doctrine, already embedded in many policies, such as the requirement that pharmaceuticals be shown to be safe before being permitted on the market.

But it is one facing enormous resistance from Big Business as pressure grows to apply the precautionary principle to environmental risks.

The European Union is fast outdistancing the world in implementation of the precautionary principle.

In perhaps the most important manifestation, in May 2003, the EU formally proposed its REACH— Registration, Evaluation, Authorisation, and Restriction of Chemicals—policy. In basic outline, REACH will require companies to provide evidence regarding the toxicity of their products and information about how humans or the environment might be exposed to them. For chemicals produced in large amounts or that are especially toxic, government experts will evaluate the safety of the chemicals—a process that might lead to bans of certain uses of a chemical. Especially toxic chemicals—carcinogens, mutagens, reproductive toxicants and chemicals that persist and accumulate in the environment—will require affirmative authorization, with regulators maintaining the authority to force transitions to safer, substitute products.

This policy contrasts with past approaches in Europe—and continuing policy in the United States—which permits companies to keep dangerous chemicals on the market, absent a governmental showing that they are hazardous. Under REACH, the burden rests on industry, not government, and chemical peddlers must make an affirmative showing that they are selling a safe product.

Much of the chemical industry despises REACH and is working aggressively to thwart it, including by employing the US government to lobby to undermine it.

As a result, the policy has been weakened, and continues to be the subject of major policy disputes. The Europeans remain on track to implement REACH in 2007, but what exactly they will achieve remains very much uncertain.

Taking on Predatory Lending

Too often, poor people can't win for losing. In the perverse modern-day economy, poor people are simultaneously denied credit and offered more credit than they need.

Actually, this apparent paradox isn't so hard to understand.

While mainstream financial institutions do their best to avoid poor and minority neighborhoods in the provision of standard forms of credit ("redlining" and its variants), lenders also seek to exploit the poor by providing them with loans and credit at super-high interest rates ("predatory lending"). As predatory lending—including high-rate ("subprime") mortgage loans, payday loans and refund anticipation loans—has grown into a sophisticated, high-return and nationalized market, many of the same businesses that underserve poor neighborhoods with standard mortgages, small business loans and other forms of credit and banking services are getting into the predatory lending business.

But not without resistance from the affected communities. The Association of Community Organizations for Reform Now (ACORN) and others have been working, with considerable success, to curb the predatory lenders and to establish local and state rules to curb their abuses.

Predatory loans include mortgage loans with both high interest rates and extensive extra fees attached; payday loans—short-term loans in anticipation of a paycheck that may charge interest rates over 1,000 percent on an annual basis; and refund anticipation loans—loans from tax preparers, made in anticipation of a tax rebate, at interest rates that sometimes exceed 700 percent.

Subprime refinance and home purchase loans rose more than 1,000 percent in the 1990s, and continue to skyrocket.

The National Consumer Law Center has documented how refund anticipation loans alone drained over $1 billion in loan fees, plus $389 million in other fees, from the wallets of more than 12 million US taxpayers in 2003.

Poor people get stuck with rip-off mortgage deals because regular banks and credit agencies don't make regular mortgage services easily available, and often misdirect minority borrowers to "subprime" loans without regard to their credit record. Payday loans, refund anticipation loans and similar instruments have proliferated because mainstream lending institutions won't make available small amounts of credit for short-term need.

To forestall this organized theft from poor people, ACORN and allied organizations have taken on the predatory lenders directly and campaigned for legal protections.

Subprime lenders Ameriquest, Associates (now owned by Citigroup), Household International and its subsidiaries Household Finance and Beneficial (now owned by HSBC Holdings) and Wells Fargo are among the operations that have agreed to substantial reforms as a result of community group mobilization.

Following two years of an ACORN-led campaign—including a 2,000 person march to company headquarters in 2004, interventions at shareholder meetings, and ongoing litigation—Wells Fargo announced some notable reforms in August 2005. These included limits on certain lending charges and elimination of mandatory arbitration clauses for loan disputes.

ACORN applauded these changes. "However," said Maude Hurd, ACORN's national president, "Wells still needs to compensate the families and communities its predatory lending has hurt. In addition, these business practice changes must be made permanent and enforceable by court order. Otherwise, Wells could revert to its old ways of doing business."

In a September 2005 report, ACORN documented that, when receiving a loan from one of Wells Fargo's lending companies, African-Americans were

5.3 times more likely than whites to receive a subprime loan, and Latinos were 3.4 times more likely than whites.

Meanwhile, community groups are winning legislation in an increasing number of states and localities to restrict predatory lending. New Jersey, New Mexico, Arkansas, Texas, Connecticut and Massachusetts are among the states where activists have registered victories. Signed into law in August 2004, the Massachusetts law is among the most far-reaching laws. Its provisions include a prohibition on prepayment penalties, a requirement that borrowers receive housing counseling on the advisability of the loan, and a limitation on the amount of fees financed into the loan.

Computer TakeBack Campaign

With technology racing ahead, computers become obsolete about every three years. You can hold on for longer, but if you go much beyond five years you'll soon find your machine unable to apply the latest technological wizardry, which quickly comes into everyday usage.

As a result of this speedy obsolescence, discarded computers are piling up. Consumers and businesses in the United States now discard tens of millions of computers every year. The Environmental Protection Agency says e-waste is about 1 percent of the global trash total. Computers contain a lot of bad stuff: about 40 percent of the heavy metals, including lead, mercury and cadmium, in landfills come from electronic equipment discards.

Making matters still worse, as the Seattle-based Basel Action Network has documented, lots of computer waste is shipped to developing countries, often in the guise of "recycling," where there is limited capacity to manage the toxic components of computer waste.

Recognizing a growing problem, a coalition of environmental, health and labor organizations joined together in 2001 to launch the Computer TakeBack Campaign. The campaign developed a platform embodied in a simple theme: "Take it back, Make it clean. Recycle responsibly." In other words, computer makers should take responsibility for disposal of the computers they have sold; computers should be manufactured to reduce and then eliminate toxic components; and recycling efforts must constitute legitimate recycling, not covert disposal, with workers given proper safety protections and the right to organize.

In general, between the top two computer makers, Hewlett-Packard has been much readier to take responsibility for computer waste, with Dell a laggard. The campaign has focused on Dell, the industry leader, to force it to set a positive industry standard. A 2003 report from the Silicon Valley Toxics Coalition and the Computer TakeBack Campaign, for example, showed how HP had in place a relatively efficient and transparent recycling operation, while Dell was relying on "Unicor, a publicly subsidized prison industrial operator, [which] used practices disturbingly similar to those found in developing nations."

At Dell's 2002 shareholder meeting, Michael Dell stated that he "hasn't seen the consumer demand" for computer takeback, and saw no reason to act in the absence of consumer demand.

Thanks to the campaign's work, that would change. The campaign has extensively documented the harms from computer waste and disposal, and mobilized individual and institutional consumers to demand Dell take responsibility for disposal and/or recycling of the computers it sells; and used shareholder, publicity and a range of other tactics to put pressure on Dell. It launched Toxicdude.com (referring to Dell CEO Michael Dell) to educate college students about Dell's environmental practices and encourage them to demand better from the company.

The campaign has had an impact. Dell agreed to take back 50 percent more computers in fiscal year 2005 than in the previous year, a goal it met, and to increase that total by 50 percent in fiscal year 2006. Dell says it supports the precautionary approach, and is working to phase out use of lead and dangerous components in its machines. The company also agreed to end the use of prison labor for recycling.

Canceling Third World Debt

Since the 1980s, and earlier for some countries, much of the Third World has been mired in the debt trap: Thanks to borrowed money that was misspent on failed megaprojects or diverted by dictators for corrupt purposes, these countries accumulated sizeable foreign debts. When interest rates spiked in the 1980s, the size of debts exploded.

Many countries have struggled just to make interest payments, with no serious prospect of ever paying off the loans. Countries have paid back much more than they ever borrowed, but because of the effect of compound interest, find themselves owing ever more. And still, the countries must allocate big chunks of their annual gross domestic product, and very significant portions of government budgets, to make payments on the debt.

They also find themselves needing new loans to pay off the old ones, which means constant negotiations with the International Monetary Fund (IMF) and continual efforts to adapt economic policy to the IMF's preference for free-market fundamentalism.

Everyone who understands what is going on knows Third World debts, especially in the poorest countries, are unsustainable.

Periodically, the rich countries and the IMF and World Bank undertake efforts to recalibrate the debts, lowering the amounts owed—but always making sure that the basic debt servitude relationship persists.

As the millennium approached, groups around the world formed "jubilee" campaigns, urging a more fundamental abolition of Third World debt.

The immediate results of the Jubilee 2000 campaign—which pointed to the year 2000 as the moment for a policy response—were disappointing, with yet another debt re-write.

But the campaign did point the global spotlight on the damage caused by Third World debt. As campaigners persisted in demanding genuine debt cancellation after 2000, as more attention was focused on lowering living standards in poor African nations, and as many African countries were ravaged by HIV/AIDS and thus even less able to manage their debt burdens, momentum built again for genuine debt cancellation.

In 2005, the G-8 group of richest countries agreed to cancel the debts owed to the IMF and World Bank, as well as the African Development Bank, by many of the world's poorest nations.

The deal falls far short in the countries it covers—19 initially, plus likely 9 more (all of which have already passed through a devastating IMF/World Bank economic reorganization process)—but represents real and important progress in canceling 100 percent of debt from poor countries, without the imposition of additional harmful conditions.

It will release close to $1 billion annually in resources poor nations can use for development.

After the G-8 agreed on the debt-cancellation package, IMF staffers sought to sabotage it by excluding certain countries that had been promised a debt write off. International pressure led to the full deal being adopted in December 2005.

"We are relieved that the IMF board reversed a terrible proposal that would have delayed $650 million in debt cancellation for some of the world's most impoverished nations," says Neil Watkins, national coordinator of Jubilee USA Network.

"Pressure from debt campaigners across the United States and the globe and supportive governments led to this important reversal. We welcome the decision. We also serve clear notice that this agreement is only a first step on a long journey and we will continue to pressure world leaders to cancel the debts of all impoverished countries in the months and years ahead."

Chapter 37

US Health Care

Single-Payer or Market Reform

David U. Himmelstein
Steffie Woolhandler

Almost all agree that our health care system is dysfunctional. Forty-seven million Americans have no health insurance, resulting in more than 18,000 unnecessary deaths annually according to the Institute of Medicine.[1] Tens of millions more have inadequate coverage. Health care costs reached $7,498 per capita this year, 50% higher than in any other nation, and continue to grow rapidly. Market pressures threaten medicine's best traditions, and bureaucracy overwhelms doctors and patients. Opinion on solutions is more divided.

Discussion of health reform was muted in the 1990s after the defeat of President Clinton's Byzantine scheme for universal coverage. Now, however, the accelerating collapse of employment-based coverage under the pressure of globalization is reopening debate. Firms like General Motors and Ford are crippled by the growing burden of health costs, which add $1,500 to the price of a General Motors car versus $419 for a German Mercedes and $97 for a Japanese Toyota.[2] Recently, the big three automakers have been pushing their liability for health costs onto their unions, replacing their previous guarantee of full employee and retiree health coverage with lump sum payments to establish (underfunded) union-run health care trust funds.

Meanwhile, low-wage employers like Walmart gain competitive advantage by purchasing goods made overseas (where health benefit costs are low) and offering only the skimpiest of health coverage to their US workers. Governments face a double whammy: burgeoning benefit costs for their public employees (e.g., teachers, firemen, police) and sharply escalating costs for public programs, such as Medicaid and Medicare.

As employers attempt to shed the costs of health care, working families increasingly find care and coverage unaffordable. In 2005, 18% of middle-income adults lacked health insurance for at least part of the year, up from 13% in 2001.[3] Nearly a quarter of Americans report being unable to pay medical bills, and 13% had been contacted by a collection agency about a medical bill within the past year.[3] Eighteen percent of those with coverage (and 43% of the uninsured) failed to fill a prescription last year because of cost, and millions forgo routine preventive care, such as Papanicolaou smears, mammograms, and colon cancer screening, because of lack of coverage.[3] More than half of American families in bankruptcy courts are there, at least in part, because of medical illness or medical bills, and three quarters of the medically bankrupt had health insurance at the onset of the illness that bankrupted them.[4]

The authors advocate a fundamental change in health care financing—national health insurance (NHI)—because lesser measures, such as Medicaid expansions and government mandates that people buy private insurance, have been tried and failed. Moreover, the alternative to NHI advocated by the Bush administration—so-called consumer-directed health care (CDH)—would actually make matters worse. As discussed in detail elsewhere in this article, CDH would financially penalize older and sicker patients, deter millions from seeking needed care, shift additional medical resources to those who are already well served, further inflate bureaucracy, and do little or nothing to contain costs.

Failure of Incremental Reforms

Since the implementation of Medicare and Medicaid in the late 1960s, a welter of piecemeal reforms have aimed to reduce medical costs and expand coverage. Health maintenance organizations (HMOs) and diagnosis-related groups (DRGs) promised to moderate health spending and free up funds to expand coverage. Tens of billions have been allocated to expanding Medicaid and similar programs for children. Medicare and Medicaid have tried managed care. Tennessee promised nearly universal coverage under the TennCare program, and several states have implemented high-risk pools to insure high-cost individuals. For-profit firms, which allege that they bring business-like efficiency to health care, now own most HMOS, dialysis clinics, and nursing homes, in addition to many hospitals, and in accordance with the prescription of many economists, the health care marketplace has become increasingly competitive. Yet, none of these initiatives have put a brake on the relentless increases in the number of uninsured, the soaring costs of care, or the rising number and power of health care bureaucrats.

Mandate Model Reforms

The experience of three states with incremental reforms deserves particular attention because each tried to achieve universal health care using a "mandate model" (sometimes called "mixed model"), now advocated by leading Democrats. Such reforms couple an expansion of Medicaid (or a similar public program) with a mandate that people (or their employers) purchase private insurance coverage. This model was first proposed by Richard Nixon in 1971 and was first enacted into law in 1988 by Massachusetts Governor Michael Dukakis on the eve of his presidential bid.

The Dukakis plan levied a fine on employers who failed to purchase private coverage for their employees and included an individual mandate requiring self-employed persons and adult students to purchase their own unsubsidized coverage. In 1989, Oregon passed a similar mandate-model reform (with expanded Medicaid eligibility and an employer mandate). The Oregon plan also included a highly publicized provision rationing expensive services, such as bone marrow transplants, for Medicaid recipients. Washington state followed, with the passage of another mandate model reform (which included an individual mandate similar to the one in the Dukakis plan) in 1993.

In all three cases, politicians and major media outlets, such as the *New York Times*, trumpeted the new laws as achieving universal coverage. In all cases, it soon became evident that the costs of the new coverage were unsustainable and the laws died quiet deaths. State legislators backed away from enforcing the mandates and eventually repealed them. Even when legislators found funds to expand Medicaid, gains in coverage were offset by the continued erosion of employer-sponsored insurance. None of the three states saw a drop in the numbers of uninsured residents, even in the short term.

The latest iteration of mandate model reform was passed in 2006 by Massachusetts governor Mitt Romney and the Democratically controlled state legislature. As in the earlier reforms, Massachusetts's 2006 law expanded Medicaid, offered subsidized Medicaid-like coverage for the near poor, and imposed a fine on employers failing to cover their workers, although the 2006 law's employer fine is quite modest (at most, $295 per worker annually). The novel feature of the new law is its extensive and punitive "individual mandate"—a requirement that hundreds of thousands of middle-income uninsured persons buy their own coverage. For a 56-year-old single man earning $31,000 (i.e., more than 300% of poverty), the cheapest available plan costs $4,100 and comes with a $2,000 deductible that must be met before his providers collect anything from insurance. When the full fines kick in at the end of 2008, he could be fined $982 annually if he refuses to buy the policy. Yet, such skimpy coverage might leave him worse off than no coverage at all; illness would still bring crippling out-of-pocket costs, but the $4,100 annual premium would have emptied his bank account even before the bills start arriving. Little wonder that among those required to buy such unsubsidized coverage, only 4% had signed up as of November 1, 2007. Meanwhile, the state just announced a $147 million funding shortfall, threatening the subsidized coverage for the poor.[5]

The 2006 Massachusetts reform, like all such patchwork reforms, is already foundering on a simple problem: expanding coverage must increase costs unless resources are diverted from elsewhere in the system. With US health costs nearly double those of any other nation and rising more rapidly[6] and government budgets already stretched, large infusions of new money are unlikely to be sustainable.

Without new money, patchwork reforms can only expand coverage by siphoning resources from clinical care. Advocates of managed care and market competition once argued that their strategy could accomplish this by trimming clinical fat. Unfortunately, new layers of bureaucrats have invariably overseen the managed care "diet" prescribed for clinicians and patients. Such cost-management bureaucracies have proved not only intrusive but expensive, devouring any clinical savings. For instance, HMOs in the Medicare program now cost the taxpayers at least 12% more per enrollee than the costs of caring for similar patients under traditional Medicare.[7]

Resources seep inexorably from the bedside to administrative offices. The shortage of bedside nurses coincides with the growing number of registered nurse utilization reviewers. Productivity pressures mount for clinicians, whereas colleagues who have moved from the bedside to the executive suite rule our profession. Bureaucracy now consumes nearly a third of our health care budget.[8]

Consumer-Directed Health Care, Another Disappointment

A popular policy nostrum, CDH, is premised on the idea that Americans are too well insured, painting them as voracious medical consumers too insulated from the costs of their care. CDH proponents advocate sharply higher insurance deductibles (e.g., $5,000 for an individual or $10,000 for a family) as the stimulus needed to make Americans wiser medical consumers. In policy wonks' dreams, these high-deductible policies are coupled with health savings accounts (HSAs), which are tax-free accounts that can be used to pay the deductible and medical services, such as cosmetic surgery, that are entirely excluded from coverage. In practice, however, most employees covered by CDH plans receive little or no employer contribution to their HSA,[9] leaving many patients at risk for massive uncovered bills without savings with which to pay them.

CDH plans may benefit those who are young, healthy, and wealthy but threaten the old, sick, and poor. Under CDH, those with low medical expenses win; they get lower premiums, pay trivial out-of-pocket expenses, and perhaps accumulate some tax-advantaged savings in their HSA. Patients needing care lose, however. For instance, virtually anyone with diabetes or heart disease is sure to pay more under CDH plans. For them, the higher out-of-pocket costs required before coverage kicks in exceed any premium savings. Even those with only hypercholesterolemia or hypertension face higher costs unless they forgo needed medications or other care.

CDH incentives selectively discourage low-cost primary and preventive care, although doing nothing to reduce the high-cost care that accounts for most health spending. High deductibles cause many to think twice before opting for a routine mammogram, prostate-specific antigen (PSA) screening, cholesterol check, or colonoscopy. In the Rand Health Insurance Experiment, the only randomized trial of such health insurance arrangements, high-deductible policies caused a 17% decline in toddler immunizations, a 19% drop in Papanicolaou tests, and a 30% decrease in preventive care for men.[10] Although high deductibles caused a 30% drop in visits for minor symptoms, they also resulted in a 20% decline in visits for serious symptoms, such as loss of consciousness or exercised-induced chest pain.[10] Most patients have no way of knowing whether their chest discomfort signals indigestion or ischemia.

Although CDH discourages many patients from seeking routine low-cost care, those with severe acute illnesses have no choice. Even 1 day in the hospital pushes most patients past CDH plans' high-deductible thresholds, leaving the patient with a large bill for the first day of care but with no further incentive to be a prudent purchaser. Hence, CDH incentives inflict financial pain on the severely ill, who account for 80% of all health costs, but have little impact on the overall costs of their care.

Moreover, the risk-selection incentives inherent in CDH threaten to raise the cost of other insurance options. As younger and healthier (i.e., lower cost) patients shift to CDH plans, premiums for the sick who remain in non-CDH coverage are going to skyrocket. Already in the Federal Employee Health Benefits Program, CDH plans are segregating young men from the costlier female and older workers.[11] According to a leaked memo, Walmart board of directors considered offering CDH plans to its employees as an explicit strategy to push sicker high-cost workers to quit.[12]

CDH also seems unfair on other accounts. The tax breaks for HSAs selectively reward the wealthiest Americans. A single father who makes $16,000 annually would save $19.60 in income taxes by putting $2,000 into an HSA.[13] A similar father earning $450,000 would save $720 in taxes.

If making Americans pay more out of their pockets for care could constrain health care costs, it would already have done so; the United States already has the world's highest out-of-pocket costs for care and the highest health costs. Copayments in Switzerland, a nation near the top of the charts in health spending, have not reduced total health expenditures.[14] In Canada, charging copayments had little impact on costs; doctors less frequently saw the poor (and often sick) patients who could not pay but filled their appointment slots with more affluent patients who could.[15,16] Higher copayments for medications in Quebec resulted in increased emergency department (ED) visits, hospitalizations, and deaths for the poor and elderly.[17] Similarly, capping drug coverage for Medicare beneficiaries in the Kaiser HMO caused a sharp drop in adherence to drug therapy (in addition to an increase in lipids, blood pressure, and blood glucose) but no change in overall health costs.[18]

Moreover, CDH and HSAs add new layers of expensive health care bureaucracy. Already, insurers and investment firms are vying for the estimated $1 billion annually in fees for managing HSAs.[19] CDH would force physicians to collect fees directly from patients (many of them unable to pay), a task that is even costlier than billing insurers,[20] while still making us play by insurers' utilization review and documentation rules; failure to do so disqualifies bills from counting toward the patient's deductible.

Although CDH proponents paint a rosy picture of consumer responsiveness and personal responsibility, CDH would punish the sick and middle aged while rewarding the healthy and young. Employees would bear more of the burden, and employers would bear less. Working families would be forced to skimp on vital care, whereas the rich would enjoy tax-free tummy tucks. In addition, as in every health reform in memory, bureaucrats and insurance firms would walk off with an ever larger share of health dollars.

The Case for National Health Insurance

In contrast to CDH, a properly structured NHI program could expand coverage without increasing costs by reducing the huge health administrative apparatus that now consumes 31% of total health spending. Health care's enormous bureaucratic burden is a peculiarly American phenomenon. No nation with NHI spends even half as much administering care or tolerates the bureaucratic intrusions in clinical care that have become routine in the United States. Indeed, administrative overhead in Canada's health system, which resembles that of the United States in its emphasis on private fee-for-service-based practice, is approximately half of the US level.[8]

Our biggest HMOs keep 20%, even 25%, of premiums for their overhead and profit;[21] Canada's NHI has 1% overhead, and even US Medicare takes less than 4%.[8,22] In addition, HMOs inflict mountains of paperwork on doctors and hospitals. The average US hospital spends one quarter of its budget on billing and administration, nearly twice the average in Canada. American physicians spend nearly 8 hours per week on paperwork, and employ 1.66 clerical workers per doctor,[23] far more than in Canada.[8]

Reducing our bureaucratic apparatus to Canadian levels would save approximately 15% of current health spending, $340 billion annually, enough to cover the uninsured fully and to upgrade coverage for those who are now underinsured. Proponents of NHI,[24] disinterested civil servants,[25,26] and even skeptics[27] all agree on this point.

Unfortunately, neither piecemeal tinkering nor wholesale computerization[28] can achieve significant bureaucratic savings. The key to administrative simplicity in Canada (and other nations) is single-source payment. Canadian hospitals (mostly private nonprofit institutions) are paid a global annual budget to cover all costs, much as a fire department is funded in the United States, obviating the need for administratively complex per-patient billing. Canadian physicians (most of whom are in private practice) bill by checking a box on a simple insurance form. Fee schedules are negotiated annually between provincial medical associations and governments. All patients have the same coverage.

Unfortunately, during the 1990s, Canada's program was starved of funds by a federal government that faced budget deficits, reflecting the pressure from the wealthy to avoid paying taxes to cross-subsidize care (and other services) for the sick and poor. Whereas Canadian and US health spending was once comparable, today, Canada spends barely half (per capita) what we do.[6] Shortages of a few types of expensive high-technology care have resulted.

Nevertheless, Canada's health outcomes remain better than ours (e.g., life expectancy is 2 years longer), and most quality comparisons indicate that Canadians enjoy care at least equivalent to that for insured Americans.[6,29] Moreover, the extent of shortages and waiting lists has been greatly exaggerated.

In British Columbia, the provincial Ministry of Health posts current surgical waiting times,[30] making it possible to follow surgical waiting lists in real time. Information on waits for urologic surgery is available.[31] As of the middle of October 2007, at the highest volume urologic surgery center (Greater Victoria Hospital), 1 of the 7 urologists had no wait for a "priority 1" surgical patient. Three other surgeons listed expected waits of 1 or 2 weeks. The surgeons' wait times for lower priority cases range from 0 to 10 weeks. At the second most active urologic center, none of the 10 urologists report a wait for priority 1 patients. Lower priority patients can expect a median wait of 4 weeks, but actual waits vary depending on their choice of surgeon. It seems unlikely that waits of this magnitude constitute an important health hazard. A system structured like Canada's but with nearly double the funding (i.e., the current level of health funding available in the United States) could deliver high-quality care without the modest waits or shortages that Canadians have experienced.

The NHI that the authors and many colleagues have proposed would create a single tax-funded comprehensive insurer in each state, federally mandated but locally controlled.[32] Everyone would be fully insured for all medically necessary services, and private insurance duplicating the NHI coverage would be proscribed (as is currently the case with Medicare). The current Byzantine insurance bureaucracy with its tangle of regulations and duplicative paperwork would be dismantled. Instead, the NHI trust fund would dispense all payments, and central administrative costs would be limited by law to less than 3% of total health spending.

The NHI would negotiate an annual global budget with each hospital based on past expenditures, projected changes in costs and use, and proposed new and innovative programs. Many hospital administrative tasks would disappear. Hospitals would have no bills to keep track of, no eligibility determination, and no need to attribute costs and charges to individual patients.

Group practices and clinics could elect to be paid fees for service or receive global budgets similar to hospitals. Although HMOs that merely contract with outside providers for care would be eliminated, those that actually employ physicians and own clinical facilities could receive global budgets, fees for service, or capitation payments (with the proviso that capitation payments could not be diverted to profits or exorbitant executive compensation). As in Canada, physicians could elect to be paid on a fee-for-service basis or could receive salaries from hospitals, clinics, or HMOs.

A sound NHI program would not raise costs; administrative savings would pay for the expanded coverage. Although NHI would require new taxes, these would be fully offset by a decrease in insurance premiums and out-of-pocket costs. Moreover, the additional tax burden would be smaller than is usually appreciated, because nearly 60% of health spending is already tax supported (versus roughly 70% in Canada.[33]) In addition to Medicare, Medicaid, and other explicit public programs, our governments fund tax subsidies for private insurance, costing the federal government alone more than $188 billion annually.[34] In addition, local, state, and federal agencies that purchase private coverage for government workers account for 24.2% of total employer health insurance spending,[35] dollars that should properly be viewed as a public rather than a private health expenditure.

The NHI that the authors propose faces important political obstacles. Private insurance firms and HMOS staunchly oppose NHI, which would eliminate them along with the 8-, 9-, and even 10-figure incomes of their executives. Similarly, investor-owned hospitals and drug firms fear that NHI would curtail their profits. The pharmaceutical industry rightly fears that an NHI system would bargain for lower drug prices, as has occurred in other nations.

Practical problems in implementing NHI also loom. The financial viability of the system that the authors propose depends on achieving and maintaining administrative simplicity. The single-payer macromanagement approach to cost control (which relies on readily enforceable overall budgetary limits) is inherently less administratively complex than our current micromanagement approach, with its case-by-case scrutiny of billions of individual expenditures and encounters. Even under NHI, however, vigilance (and statutory limits) would be needed to curb the tendency of bureaucracy to reproduce and amplify itself.

NHI would reorient the way we pay for care, bringing the hundreds of billions now squandered on malignant bureaucracy back to the bedside. NHI could restore the physician-patient relationship, offer patients a free choice of physicians and hospitals, and free physicians from the hassles of insurance paperwork.

Patchwork reforms cannot simultaneously address the twin problems of cost and access. CDH is a thinly veiled program to cut back on already threadbare insurance coverage and offers no real hope of cost containment. NHI offers the only viable option for health care reform. The authors invite colleagues to join with the 14,000 members of Physicians for a National Health Program[36] in advocating for such reform.

Notes

1. Institute of Medicine. *Insuring America's health: Principles and recommendations.* Washington, DC: National Academies Press; 2004.

2. Taylor M. Applying the brakes. *Mod Healthc.* 2005;35(43):14.

3. Collins SR, Davis K, Doty MM, et al. *Gaps in health insurance: An all-American problem. Findings from the Commonwealth Fund biennial health insurance survey.* New York: Commonwealth Fund; 2006.

4. Himmelstein DU, Warren E, Thorne D, et al. Illness and injury as contributors to bankruptcy. Web exclusive; 2005. Available at http://content.healthaffairs.org /content/early/2005/02/02/hlthaff.w5.63.full.pdf+html.

5. Dembner A. Success could put health plan in the red. *Boston Globe* (November 18, 2007). Available at http://www.boston.com/news/local/articles/2007/11/18 /success_could_put_health_plan_in_the_red/?page=full. Accessed November 20, 2007.

6. Organization for Economic Cooperation and Development (OECD). *OECD health data 2005.* Computer database. Paris: OECD; 2005.

7. Miller (executive director, MEDPAC) ME. *The Medicare Advantage program.* Testimony before the Committee on the Budget, US House of Representatives. 2007. Available at http://www.medpac.gov/documents/062807_Housebudget _MedPAC_testimony_MA.pdf. Accessed October 12, 2007.

8. Woolhandler S, Campbell T, Himmelstein DU. Health care administration costs in the US and Canada. *N Engl J Med.* 2003;349:768–775.

9. EBRI/Commonwealth Fund Survey. 2006. Available at http://www.ebri.org /publications/ib/index.cfm?fa=ibDisp&content_id=3769. Accessed October 30, 2007.

10. Newhouse JP and the Insurance Experiment Group. *Free for all? Lessons from the Rand health insurance experiment.* Cambridge, MA: Harvard University Press; 1993.

11. United States Government Accountability Office. *Federal Employees Health Benefits Program: Early experience with consumer-directed health plans.* GAO-06-143. Washington, DC: US Government Printing Office; November 2005. Available at http://www.gao.gov/newitems/d06143.pdf. Accessed February 14, 2006.

12. *Supplemental benefits documentation: Board of Directors Retreat FY06 Wal-Mart Stores, Inc.* Available at http://www.nytimes.com/packages/pdf/business /26walmart.pdf. Accessed February 14, 2006.

13. Tax Policy Center. *Effective marginal federal income tax rates for a head of household with one child in 2005.* Available at http://www.taxpolicycenter.org /TaxFacts/TFDB/Content/Excel/effective_marginal_hoh1_2005.xls. Accessed February 14, 2006.

14. Conference Board of Canada. *Challenging health care system sustainability, understanding health system performance of leading countries.* 2004. Available at http://wvw.conferenceboard.ca/boardwiseii/signin.asp. Accessed October 2007.

15. Enterline PE, Salter V, McDonald AD, et al. The distribution of medical services before and after "free" medical care-the Quebec experience. *N Engl J Med.* 1973;289(22):1174–1178.

16. Beck RG, Horne JM. Utilization of publicly insured health services in Saskatchewan before, during and after copayment. *Med Care* 1980;18(8):787–806.

17. Tamblyn R, Laprise R, Hanley JA, et al. Adverse events associated with prescription drug cost-sharing among poor and elderly persons. *JAMA.* 2001;285(4):421–429.

18. Hsu J. Price M, Huang J, et al. Unintended consequences of caps on Medicare drug benefits. *N Engl J Med.* 2006;354:2349–2359.

19. Becker C. One question: Credit or debit? As health savings accounts gain in popularity, insurers and the financial services industry want to bank the cash. *Mod Healthc.* 2006;6–16.

20. Romano M. Driven to distress. *Mod Healthc.* 2006;28–30.

21. Special report. *BestWeek Life/Health.* April 12, 1999.

22. Heffler S, Levit K, Smith S, et al. Health spending growth up in 1999: Faster growth expected in the future. *Health Aff.* 2001;20(2):193–203.

23. Remler DK, Gray BM, Newhouse JP. Does managed care mean more hassles for physicians? *Inquiry* 2000;37:304–316.

24. Grumbach K, Bodenheimer T, Woolhandler S, et al. Liberal benefits conservative spending: The Physicians for a National Health Program proposal. *JAMA.* 1991;265:2549–2554.

25. US General Accounting Office. *Canadian health insurance: Lessons for the United States.* GAO/HRD-91-90.Washington, DC: US Government Printing Office; 1991.

26. Congress of the United States Congressional Budget Office. *Universal health insurance coverage using Medicare's payment rates.* Washington, DC: US Government Printing Office; 1991.

27. Sheils JF, Haught RA. *Analysis of the costs and impact of universal health care coverage under a single payer model for the state of Vermont.* Falls Church, VA: The Lewin Group Inc.; 2001.

28. Himmelstein DU, Woolhandler S. Hope and hype: Predicting the impact of electronic medical records. *Health Aff.* 2005;24(5):1121–1123.

29. Lasser KE, Himmelstein DU, Woolhandler S. Access to care, health status, and health disparities in the United States and Canada: Results of a cross-national population-based survey. *Am J Public Health* 2006;96:1300–1307.

30. Available at http://www.hlth.gov.bc.ca/waitlist/html.

31. Available at http://www.swl.hlth.gov.bc.ca/swl/swl-db/swl.WaitlistPkg .GetHospitalListBySurgSpecNLF?lEvent=UR.

32. Woolhandler S, Himmelstein DU, Angell M, et al. Proposal of the Physicians' Working Group for Single-Payer National Health Insurance. *JAMA.* 2003;290: 798–805.

33. Woolhandler S, Himmelstein DU. Paying for national health insurance—and not getting it: Taxes pay for a larger share of US health care than most Americans think they do. *Health Aff.* 2002;21(4):88–98.

34. Sheils J, Haught R. The cost of tax-exempt health benefits in 2004. *Health Aff.* Web exclusive posted. Available at http://content.healthaffairs.org/cgi/reprint/hlthaff .w4.106v1;2004. Accessed June 6, 2006.

35. Office of the Actuary. National Center for Health Statistics. *Sponsors of health care costs: Businesses, households and governments.* 1987–2004. Available at http:// www.cms.hhs.gov/NationalHealthExpendData/downloads/bhg06.pdf. Accessed June 6, 2006.

36. Available at www.PNHP.org.

Chapter 38

US Health Professionals Oppose War

Walter J. Lear

Thousands of US physicians, nurses and other health professionals have opposed the several US imperialist wars of the twentieth century. They were distressed by the violent deaths and the serious and multiple injuries to both body and mind inflicted on the people engaged in these wars. They recognized that the victims were combatants and civilian, both in the countries attacked by the US—devastatingly—and in this country—to a lesser but still agonizing extent. War destroyed not only people in the countries that were attacked, but also housing, agriculture, industry and the basic systems and infrastructures essential for healthy and humane living conditions. Both in the United States and abroad the state of war brought a curtailment of human rights and the waste of huge amounts of money that could have been better spent for proper food, education, health care and improvements of the quality of life.

The motivation of these health professionals to oppose these wars was frequently based on one or more of their religious, moral, legal and political beliefs as well as their humanitarian concerns. Among the key individuals in this movement were several physicians and nurses. They expressed their anti-war positions in a variety of ways including for a few, non-violent actions which led to arrests, convictions and time in prison.

World War I

World War I provoked a modest-sized but nonetheless militant anti-war movement. Among the anti-war movement they were shocked and enraged when Woodrow Wilson after election as president broke his pre-election promise to keep the US out of the European war.

William J. Robinson (1867–1936) was a New York City general practitioner well-known for his prolific writings, his vigorous advocacy of sexual enlightenment and birth control, and his independent radical politics. In 1903 he founded his principal journal, *Medical Critic and Guide,* which he edited and published until his death. Simultaneously he edited a number of other professional and popular journals. He wrote over thirty books, almost all dealing with marriage, abortion, venereal diseases and other aspects of "sexology."

Robinson fought US participation in World War I with his strongest resource—his journalistic expertise. The following quotes are from the first issue of *A Voice in the Wilderness* (September 1917), his quixotic, mainly self-written and self-financed anti-war journal which he published for two years. In his impassioned and acrimonious style he expresses the main theme of the journal—his abhorrence of war and his conviction that wars were undertaken primarily for the benefit of national leaders and capitalists and were a calamity for the people:

We are living in truly terrible times: The murder and mutilation of the world's manhood, of the physically best specimens of the nations, the destruction of the material resources of the world, the burning of villages and cities, the actual dying of hunger of millions of children, the indescribable anguish of those left at home, the mothers, fathers, wives, sweethearts, brothers, sisters—all these things are sufficient to break the hearts of the most indifferent, most callous, most unimaginative.

But there are other horrors. The sowing of hatred; the deliberate poisoning of the minds of a nation against its "enemies"; the successful attempt to make each belligerent nation believe that it is fighting for self-defense, for justice, for liberty, for democracy, and that its war is therefore a holy war, while its "enemy" nations are fighting an aggressive war, a war for autocracy, for world domination, for the enslavement of little nations, and that their war is therefore an unholy war; the deliberate, systematic manufacture of brutal falsehoods, the shameless ridiculing of everything humanitarian, of everything that is kind, gentle and peaceful; the regarding of war not as something essentially vicious and evil tho occasionally unavoidable, but as something essentially good and noble in itself; the fostering and fanning of the vilest passions; the glorification of the most brutal instincts; the trampling upon our most essential rights and liberties acquired by centuries of struggle; the roughshod riding of the autocrats and rowdies over everything that is humane and decent; the justification of every invasion, even if distinctly contrary to the organic law of the land; the clubbing and imprisoning of everybody who dares to express his honest convictions—these moral injuries, these wounds inflicted upon us by a chauvinistically frenzied but powerful minority, will be harder and will take longer to recover from than the purely material losses.

***

Did we go to war to make the world safe for democracy or safe from democracy?
***

Yes, we the few who remain true to the ideals of liberty, truth and humanity cannot help a feeling of despair. But while despairing we must not hold our arms and do nothing. We must not sulk and grieve in our tents. We must not let the forces of darkness and cruelty run over the world unopposed. We must not be silent, even tho our voice be a voice in the wilderness. If we are to be destroyed, let us be destroyed fighting, with our boots on.

James P. Warbasse (1866–1957) was not only a well-regarded New York City surgeon but a founder and leader of the American cooperative movement including the Rochdale Institute and the Cooperative League of the United States. He was on the executive committee of the American Union Against Militarism. Because of his pacifist views he was expelled from his county medical society. Alice Hamilton was another of the activist physicians of this period who were antiwar.

Lavinia Dock, Margaret Sanger and Lillian Wald, founders of the field of public health nursing, were also prominent in the movement opposed to US participation in World War I. They considered the elimination of violence between people and nations to be an integral and essential aspect of public health nursing. Dock focused on establishing professional nursing organizations which would be "a moral force on all the great social questions of the day"; she thought healing soldiers was "giving moral support to war which every human being should refuse to give. Does it not make war more tolerable, more possible and, by mitigating, keep it bolstered up and alive?" Sanger asserted that war and birth control were inherently incompatible as the US "obsession" with war blinded the people from seeing the health value of birth control and fostered the disparaging and delimiting definition of women as "breeders."

Wald believed that a major role of public health nursing was treating personal ills by correcting social ills; she helped found and served as president of the American Union Against Militarism. Right after the US declared war, Dock and Wald were among 1,500 women who marched down New York City's Fifth Avenue in a Women's Peace Parade.[1]

Emma Goldman trained as a nurse and midwife. But during this period she was a leading anarchist, a founder of the No-Conscription League and a vigorous and public advocate of draft resistance. For this latter activity she was tried and convicted of conspiracy under the Espionage Act. She was sentenced to two years in prison and, on release from prison, she was deported.

There follows a few excerpts from her statement to the jury in her anti-conscription trial.[2]

It is organized violence on top which creates individual violence at the bottom. It is the accumulated indignation against organized wrong, organized crime, organized injustice which drives the political offender to his act. To condemn him means to be blind to the causes which make him. I can no more do that, nor have I the right to, than the physician who would condemn the patient for his disease. The honest, earnest, sincere physician does not only prescribe medicine, he tries to find out the cause of the disease. You and I and all of us who remain indifferent to the crimes of poverty, war and human degradation, are equally responsible for the act committed by the political offender.

***

Whatever your verdict, gentlemen, it cannot possibly affect the rising tide of discontent in this country against the war which despite all boasts is a war of conquest and military power. Neither can it affect the ever increasing opposition to conscription which is a military and industrial yoke placed on the necks of the American people. Least of all will your verdict affect those to whom human life is sacred, and who will not become a party to world slaughter. Your verdict can only add to the opinion of the world as to whether or not justice and liberty are a living force in this country or a mere shadow of the past.... It must be decided sooner or later whether we are justified in telling people that we will give them democracy in Europe, when we have no democracy here. Shall free speech and free assemblage, shall criticism and opinion be destroyed? Shall it be trampled underfoot by any detective or policeman, anyone who decides upon it? Or shall free speech and free assemblage continue to be the heritage of the American people?

The War in Vietnam

The 1963–1975 protest by US citizens of the "undeclared" military partic-ipation in the civil war in Vietnam was unique in its character, size and duration. It took many forms including the nonviolent ones customary for public political movements. But it also took special forms relevant to its histor-ical context—draft resistance, military property destruction and Buddhist-style immolations. Contrary to considerable contemporary and subsequent descrip-tions, this antiwar movement was "not inspired or led by foreign powers ... not anti-American, rather it was a movement arising from profound patriotism ... not a movement of the young although young people gave it energy and some of its leaders ... not a movement of cowards ... or licentious coun-terculturals ... not a violent movement ... not a monolithic organization following the dictates of one party line. [It was a movement] representative of America's diversity."[3]

Activist health professionals were already mobilized by their participation in the Civil Rights Movement. Their organization was called the Medical Commit-tee for Human Rights (MCHR). MCHR's formal entry into the anti-Vietnam war movement was the unanimous adoption of a resolution at its 1967 convention opposing "this senseless and self-defeating war" as "the problems of Vietnam cannot be solved by military force." MCHR requested of the US government "unilateral, immediate cessation of hostilities ... negotiations with all bel-ligerents" and "arrangements for internationally supervised free elections" that would "recognize the right of the Vietnamese people to determine their own identity." The American Public Health Association and other professional health organizations had similar "peace" policies and activities. Health professionals in Boston, Chicago, New York City, San Francisco and elsewhere provided energy, money, leadership and impressive credentials to lobbying, petitions, rallies and marches. A special function of anti-war physicians in many cities was draft counseling and examinations.

One of the most extensively involved (and publicized) anti-war physicians was the pediatrician Benjamin Spock, the famous "Dr. Spock." He was arrested for civil disobedience in several of the many anti-war demonstrations he participated in. His part in 1968 anti-draft activities resulted in his indictment for counseling and abetting resistance to the draft. After a notable trial and conviction, he was given a two-year prison sentence which on appeal was rescinded. At the press conference immediately after the trial, Spock, ("a towering personification of wrath," as noted by Jessica Mitford) shouted to the nation these final words: "Wake up, America! Wake up before it is too late! Do something now!"[4]

The anti-war activities of two nurses, Susan Schnall and Jane Kennedy, were particularly notable for their creativity and daring. Susan Schnall was a MCHR chairwoman. In 1968 while wearing her Navy uniform she distributed ant-war leaflets from an airplane over military installations in the San Francisco area. She was court-martialed and discharged. Later she helped organize and staff a militarism education coffee-house adjacent to the Fort Sam Houston Army Medical Center in San Antonio, Texas.

In 1969 Jane Kennedy, a MCHR vice-chairwoman, and seven other pacifists, broke into the offices of local draft boards in Indianapolis destroying hundreds of draft files. They also entered the Dow Chemical Research Center in Midland, Michigan, destroying tapes and processing cards for military scientific research. After publicly claiming responsibility for these activities, the eight were arrested, convicted and sentenced to five year prison terms. While imprisoned Jane launched campaigns to improve prison health services and living conditions.

Howard Levy, a dermatologist, was drafted into the Army in 1967. A short time later he refused to obey an order to train Green Berets (Special Services aidmen headed for Vietnam) in dermatological skills. He understood that these skills would be used as part of the aidmen's official function to curry favor and coerce desired behavior from the "enemy" not simply as ethically proper health service. He was charged with willful disobedience and promotion of disaffection and disloyalty among the enlisted men. He was court-martialed. At his news-worthy trial, his defense argued that the political use of medicine jeopardized the internationally approved tradition of the noncombatant status of medicine. Nonetheless, he was given a dishonorable discharge and sentenced to three years of hard labor at Leavenworth military prison.

The 1991 Gulf War

The 1991 Gulf War provoked over 200 military personnel including one physician, to become conscientious objectors, disobeying military orders and requiring military reprisals. Yolanda Huet-Vaughn, a Kansas City family practitioner and mother of three children, was a captain in the US Army Medical Corps Reserve and was called to active duty service in December 1990. After refusing to serve she was classified as a "deserter," court-martialed and sentenced to thirty months in prison. Excerpts from her eloquent explanatory statement follow:[5]

> I am refusing orders to be an accomplice in what I consider an immoral, inhumane and unconstitutional act, namely an offensive military mobilization in the Middle East. My oath as a citizen-soldier to defend the Constitution, my oath as a physician to preserve life and prevent disease, and my responsibility as a human being to the preservation of this planet would be violated if I cooperate with Operation Desert Shield. I had hoped that we as people had learned the lessons of Vietnam—50,000 Americans dead and hundreds of thousands of civilians dead—and environmental disaster. What we face in the Middle East is death and destruction on a grander scale.... The majority of casualties will be civilians, as 57 percent of the population of Iraq and Kuwait are concentrated in urban centers. Of this civilian population, 47 percent are children under the age of fifteen.... As a mother I am keenly aware of the long-term medical and environmental consequences that may occur in the Middle East region and which may indeed have a global impact if war breaks out.
>
> ***
>
> From a medical point of view, the public has been misled concerning the catastrophic nature of wounds and injuries that will befall combatants and civilians. Are we as Americans willing to live through the evening news tallies of dead and wounded Americans knowing in advance that this war was avoidable? As a doctor I know that where there can be no medical cure, prevention is the only remedy. I therefore commit my medical knowledge and training to the effort to avert war by refusing orders to participate in Operation Desert Shield... I urge our political and military leaders to acknowledge the severity of these medical and environmental consequences in committing themselves to diplomatic solutions. I consider myself a patriot and have taken these actions in support of American troops who have been deployed in the Gulf region, in support of the American people, and in support of the children both here and in the Middle East who have no voice. I hope that in some small way my act of conscience will help promote peaceful resolution of the Gulf crisis.

Lessons Learned

These anti-war health professionals in their consideration of war use a disease model—they emphasize finding the cause and eliminating it. Deeply committed to the health and well-being of the people of this country and throughout the world, they identify the cause of war more or less explicitly, whether 1917 or 1991, as the quest of the powerful and wealthy for more power and more wealth. Obviously eliminating that cause is a daunting task.

Barry Levy and Victor Sidel in their timely book *War and Public Health* include in their final chapter a summary of the roles health professionals can play in preventing war and its consequences; their summary is a fitting and excellent conclusion to the lessons that emerge from the stories reported here:[6]

- Participating in surveillance and documentation of the health effects of war and of the factors that may cause war.
- Developing and implementing education and awareness-raising programs on the health effects of war.
- Advocating policies and promoting actions to prevent war and its health consequences.
- Working directly in actions to prevent war and its consequences.

Perhaps because I am an activist, I believe the greatest need is for the last two recommendations. Many, many more US health professionals should be vigorously fighting the unhealthy and immoral obsession of the US with war.

Notes

1. Temkin E. "Nurses and the Prevention of War: Public Health Nurses and the Peace Movement in World War I" in *War and Public Health* edited by Barry E. Levy and Victor W. Sidel, American Public Health Association, Washington, DC, 2006, pp. 350–359.

2. "Emma Goldman, Address to the Jury in *US* v. *Emma Goldman and Alexander Berkman* (July 9, 1917)" in H. Zinn and A. Amove (eds.), *Voices of a People's History of the United States,* Seven Stories Press, New York, 2004, pp. 292–294.

3. Zaroulis N, Sullivan G. *Who Spoke Up: American Protest Against the War in Vietnam, 1963–1975,* Doubleday Press, Garden City, NY, 1984, pp. xii–xiii.

4. Mitford J. *The Trial of Dr. Spock, the Rev. William Sloane Coffin Jr, Michael Goodman and Marcus Raskin,* Alfred A. Knopf, New York, 1969, p. 272.

5. "Yolanda Huet-Vaughn, Statement Refusing to Serve in the 1991 Gulf War (January 9, 1991" in H. Zinn and A. Amove (eds.), *Voices of a People's History of the United States,* Seven Stories Press, New York, 2004, pp. 555–557.

6. Levy, BE, Sidel VW (eds.), *War and Public Health,* American Public Health Association, Washington, DC, 2006, p. 388.

Chapter 39

The Residency Program in Social Medicine of Montefiore Medical Center

37 Years of Mission-Driven, Interdisciplinary Training in Primary Care, Population Health, and Social Medicine

A. H. Strelnick   Debbie Swiderski   Alice Fornari
Victoria Gorski   Eliana Korin   Philip Ozuah
Janet M. Townsend   Peter A. Selwyn

Beginning in 1988 with *The Future of Public Health*[1] and in subsequent publications, the Institute of Medicine (IOM) has explored the challenges facing the American health system: a strained safety net,[2] widespread health disparities,[3] a workforce that lacks diversity,[4] and a chasm-like divide between clinical medicine's focus on individual health and public health's focus on population health.[5] The IOM defined public health broadly as "what we as a society do collectively to assure the conditions in which people can be healthy,"[1] which clearly includes both individual-oriented clinical care and population-oriented public health. The IOM has also twice examined the public health workforce.[6-7] In its 1996 report, *Primary Care: America's Health in a New Era*, the IOM argued that primary care is the "logical foundation for the US health care system of the future."[8] A theme common to all of these reports is that physician education can bridge this historical divide and promote an integrated continuum from primary care to public health.

At a 1998 conference entitled "Education for More Synergistic Practice of Medicine and Public Health," Harvard historian Allan Brandt described social medicine as "situated on the San Andreas fault between medicine and public health" and described the relationship between these two as "characterized by critical tensions, covert hostilities, and at times, open warfare."[9] For some, social medicine is not a clinical but a critical and theoretical discipline responsible for prescribing a more ideal health system rather than practicing within the current one. In contrast, the Residency Program in Social Medicine (RPSM) of the Montefiore Medical Center (MMC) and Albert Einstein College of Medicine (AECOM) has been successfully training primary care physicians collaboratively in family medicine, internal medicine, and pediatrics for underserved communities within a population health and social medicine framework since 1970. For 37 years its mission, vision, and hallmarks have remained focused on improving the health of medically underserved communities even as its curriculum, organizational structure, and clinical settings have changed and evolved. In this article, we describe the RPSM as a case study of graduate medical education (GME) that has successfully integrated individual patient care and population health.

Historical Background and Context

Foundation

The Bronx is the nation's poorest urban county and New York City's poorest borough,[10] now with 1.4 million residents, more than half (51%) of whom are Latino and one third (33%) of whom are African American.[11] To serve residents of the South Bronx, the Dr. Martin Luther King, Jr., Health Center (MLKHC) was established in 1967, and its founders sought primary care physicians who could work in interdisciplinary teams with nurses, social workers, and family health workers, and who could provide comprehensive, culturally sensitive, and community-oriented care (Figure 39.1). MLKHC was then the flagship of the neighborhood health center movement, the forerunner of today's federally qualified community health centers (FQHCs). MLKHC was sponsored by the leading federal agency in President Johnson's War on Poverty, the Office of Economic Opportunity. Health centers then provided not only comprehensive health and social services, but often housing, job training, and legal services, too.[12] MLKHC's founders, unable to recruit such physicians, decided to train them on-site in collaboration with MMC. Together, the leaders of MLKHC and MMC recruited the RPSM's first residents in internal medicine and pediatrics in 1970 and then added family medicine in 1973. When Title VII of the Health Professionals Educational Assistance Act of 1976 first created federal grants to support primary care residency programs focused on underserved populations, the RPSM served as one of its models.

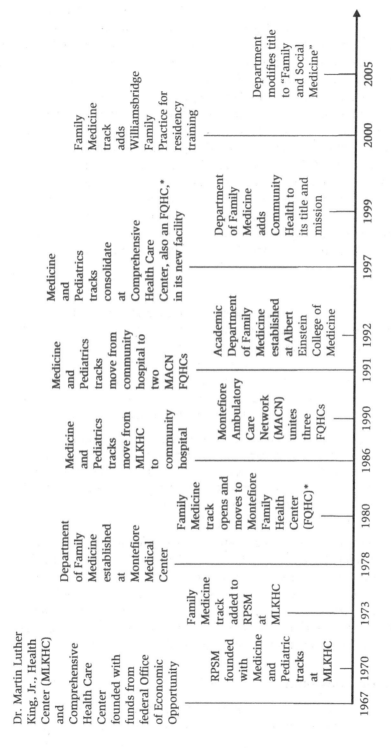

Figure 39.1. Historical Timeline for Residency Program in Social Medicine (RPSM)

*Federally qualified community health center.

In 1978, MMC's Department of Family Medicine (DFSM) was founded with the RPSM as its core, and MLKHC became organizationally independent of MMC, with its own board of directors. RPSM's family medicine track outgrew MLKHC's satellite clinic, and in 1980 it moved to its current home, the Montefiore Family Health Center (FHC). In 1992, the DFSM secured its own geographic inpatient service facility and became a full academic department at AECOM.[13] MLKHC's finances deteriorated after the severe federal budget cuts of the Reagan administration in the 1980s, so the social internal medicine and pediatrics tracks had to move, eventually consolidating at the Comprehensive Health Care Center (CHCC) in 1997. Both CHCC and FHC are FQHCs, funded through Section 330 of the US Public Health Service Act, under the aegis of the Bronx Community Health Network. The social internal medicine and pediatrics tracks are an integral part of the DFSM, as well as of their parent departments of medicine and pediatrics, which provide oversight and accreditation, organize inpatient rotations, and coordinate the National Residency Matching Program numbers.

Mission and Vision

Since its founding, the RPSM has repeatedly returned to reassess its commitment to its original mission to meet the health care needs of the medically underserved. Our founding credo was (and still remains) "Make a Difference," and our current vision statement reads, "Promoting health and social justice in the Bronx and beyond ..." Each of these serves as a call and challenge to end health care disparities and social inequities before such terms were mainstreamed by *Healthy People 2010.*[14] The current RPSM mission statement reads,

> In order to improve the health of underserved communities, our mission is to (1) train excellent primary care physicians grounded in the biopsychosocial model who are effective advocates for social change, (2) deliver quality, community-oriented primary care, (3) generate new knowledge and innovations in health care and medical education, and (4) maintain and enrich the physical, spiritual, intellectual, emotional, and material resources necessary for these tasks.

Although population and public health are not explicit terms in the mission and vision statements, they are clearly implied in the phrases *health of underserved communities, community-oriented primary care, and promoting health ... in the Bronx and beyond,* as well as in how the RPSM has emphasized the *social* in the *biopsychosocial model.* The vision statement's call for social justice and the mission statement's call for advocacy for social change also encompass the IOM definition of public health as collective action.

Hallmarks of Innovation

In reviewing "innovative generalist programs," Urbina et al.[15] identified the RPSM as the leading example of the strategy in GME, both to "develop separate tracks for primary care" and to "offer residents a common generalist curriculum." The RPSM also employs the other two innovations they describe: establishing community-based, continuity practice sites and training physicians in managed care systems. These strategies, rooted in the social innovations of the late 1960s, are embedded in the hallmarks that distinguish the RPSM: (1) mission-oriented resident recruitment and selection and self-management, (2) interdisciplinary, collaborative training among primary care professionals, (3) community-health-center-based and community-oriented primary care (COPC) education, (4) a biopsychosocial and ecological family systems curriculum, and (5) the social medicine core curriculum and projects.[16] The sixth hallmark, federal funding through Title VII grants, came in the late 1970s. These innovations are each described briefly below.

1. Mission-Oriented Resident Recruitment and Selection and Self-Management

Recruitment and Selection

A shared commitment to the underserved is an essential criterion for recruitment and selection of residents and faculty and accounts for much of the success that the RPSM has had in recruiting, training, and graduating physicians of color;[17,18] in creating a diverse faculty and staff; and in graduating physicians who make careers of practicing in underserved communities. Consistent with the evidence that minority physicians are more likely to practice in underserved communities,[19] RPSM recruitment includes explicit commitments to diversity. In addition, both the RPSM curriculum and faculty development overtly include topics about race, racism, and culture.[20] Special recruitment efforts include sending residents and faculty to staff booths and make presentations at the annual meetings of the American Medical Student Association, Boricua Latino Health Organization, and Student National Medical Association, seeking to recruit applicants who share our mission. Fourth-year student electives, such as our course, "Research-Based Health Activism," offer potential residency candidates an opportunity to learn our approach to advocacy and population health.

Self-Management

RPSM residents actively participate in the management and design of their educational program. Residents assume significant recruitment, administrative, and problem-solving responsibilities, including selecting, interviewing, and ranking applicants within and across disciplines. This participation grew both from resident activism in shaping the early training experience in collaboration with a small, then-embryonic faculty and from a common belief in self-management. Active resident participation continues as a "flattened hierarchy" that promotes the learning of community-participatory planning.

Self-management and resident participation conform to the principles of adult education[21] and help residents develop effective management, leadership, advocacy, and team skills.[22]

2. Interdisciplinary Collaborative Training Among Primary Care Professionals

Although many have called for closer collaboration among family medicine, internal medicine, and pediatrics, the RPSM remains the only integrated GME program for all three primary care specialties in the United States. Our three residencies share the following: mission, faculty, curricula (in systems-based practice and interpersonal and communication skills), community orientation, offices, support and administrative staff, and budget.

As described in the past,

> The common training experience teaches the differences between disciplines and promotes mutual respect, cooperation, and support for primary care within each discipline. Each discipline brings special strengths to conjoint learning experiences. The developmental perspective of pediatrics emphasizes health promotion, antici-patory guidance, and disease prevention; the scientific, problem-focused approach of internal medicine emphasizes differential diagnosis and proven interventions; and the contextual perspective of family medicine emphasizes relationships and interactions between doctor, patient, and family.[23]

Interdisciplinary Teams

The interdisciplinary teams developed at MLKHC included not just the primary care disciplines but also nursing, health education, dentistry, obstetrics–gynecology, pharmacy, and family health workers. Recently emphasized in the Accreditation Council for Graduate Medical Education (ACGME) core competencies[24] and Chronic Care Model,[25] teamwork grew from necessity in serving the diverse and impoverished South Bronx, and interdisciplinary teams remain central to accomplishing the RPSM mission. MLKHC's legacy of a diverse and interdisciplinary staff is now incorporated into the RPSM faculty, which has included physicians, psychologists, social workers, health educators, pharmacists, family therapists, nutritionists, family health workers, and public health professionals. Follow-up studies found that RPSM graduates who worked in teams such as these had twice the percentage of poor patients and three times the percentage of working class patients in their practices as those who did not.[23]

Clinical Partnerships

A major training innovation, which RPSM graduates report as a most valuable learning experience, is the clinical partnership whereby two residents share their hospital and health center practices.[23] This allows both to go on rounds in the hospital in the morning and one to care for their hospitalized patients during the rest of the day while his or her partner sees their shared continuity patients at the community-based FQHC. The partnership system reduces the conflicts between the demands of in- and outpatient care, facilitates compliance with resident work rules, and provides time for the social medicine projects (described following) and social medicine and psychosocial curricula (described following). Residents learn communication and negotiation skills and how to develop long-term, professional relationships. What was created initially to solve logistical and scheduling problems and to promote ambulatory continuity has proven to be a powerful pedagogical tool.

3. Community-Health-Center-Based and COPC Education

Recent initiatives to promote teaching in community health centers recognize that students and physicians trained in such settings are more likely to practice in health centers and in low-income communities.[26] The RPSM has dealt with the logistical and financial challenges of community-based continuity practice and education over its entire history. Currently, residency positions at our two FQHCs are supplemented by a third community-based clinic, the Williamsbridge Family Practice. Because of the seminal link between residency training and the community health center movement, COPC has been taught and practiced in the RPSM since its beginning,[27] and the IOM cited the Montefiore Family Health Center as one of seven models chosen as case studies for its 1984 report on COPC.[28]

4. Biopsychosocial and Ecological Family Systems Curriculum

The RPSM's behavioral science curriculum includes explicit training in the social and population components of race, ethnicity, gender, socioeconomic class, and the urban environment. Four principles are emphasized: the concept of process as reflected in human development and individual and family life cycles; the doctor-patient relationship; the person-in-situation or biopsychosocial, ecological systems model; and the context of practice.[29] The behavioral science curriculum is progressive, focused on interviewing skills and the doctor-patient relationship during the first year; health and mental health assessments at the individual, family, and community levels during the second year; and intervention skills during the third year (Figure 39.2). Most resident continuity sessions, home visits, and videotape reviews are supervised by both physician and behavioral science faculty, who teach collaboratively, thus modeling the interdisciplinary approach to patient care and clinical supervision. Attention

Residency Year / Curricular Feature	PGY-1	PGY-2	PGY-3
Social Medicine Core Courses	Medical Spanish, Community Orientation	"Evidence-Based Medicine: Epidemiology, Community Assessment and Research"	"Understanding Health Systems and Health Teams"
Longitudinal Experiences	Social Medicine Project Planning, Implementation and Presentation Social Medicine Rounds (bimonthly) Behavioral Science Case Seminars (weekly) Psychosocial clinical consultation		
Behavioral Science and Psychosocial Curriculum	Interviewing Skills Doctor-Patient Relationship in Primary Care	Psychosocial Assessments (Individual, Family and Community Foci)	Intervention Skills in Primary Care: Individual and Family Counselling and Behavior Change

Figure 39.2. Residency Program in Social Medicine: Social Medicine and Behavioral Science Curriculum by Residency Year

is focused on clinical reasoning, learning how to listen, critical pedagogy, advocacy, and reflection-in-action.[30]

The diversity of the Bronx has demanded continuous efforts to develop genuine respect and support for all types of diversity and appropriate educational experiences to enrich cultural sensitivity and promote multiculturalism. The continuity practices, home visits, and social medicine and orientation projects have led many trainees into the community, and the biopsychosocial and social medicine curricula have brought the community inside the training program.

5. Social Medicine Core Curriculum and Projects

The social medicine core curriculum has evolved over time and incorporates formal courses in medical Spanish, evidence-based medicine (EBM), and health systems, as well as a month-long orientation and ongoing seminars on the broader health system and determinants of health[31] (Figure 39.3). Social medicine projects have also evolved from laissez faire explorations to more structured and rigorous research, education, outreach, and quality-improvement initiatives.

Core Curriculum in Social Medicine

The core courses of Medical Spanish; Evidence-Based Medicine: Epidemiology, Community Assessment, and Research; and Understanding Health Systems and Health Teams are structured as month-long, block rotations, with one taken each postgraduate year. Small-group seminars are held every morning for four weeks so residents may attend their continuity practices during the afternoons. The core courses include required readings, faculty and guest lectures with discussions, resident reports or critical appraisals of literature, role-playing exercises, debates, and other methods of interactive and experiential learning. (Course syllabi are available on request.)

Both the EBM and health systems courses have been evaluated by pre- and posttest examinations of content knowledge and skills self-assessment. Among the 80 residents from the family practice and pediatric specialties who completed the EBM course from 1998 to 2005, mean examination scores increased 54% ($P < .000$); there were no differences by gender, track, or year of residency. Nine measures of self-confidence in EBM skills increased significantly ($P < .05$) for all residents, but the use of literature reviews increased significantly only for residents who applied them to their own practices. From 1996 to 2005, among 110 residents from all three specialties in the health systems course, posttest knowledge improved over pretest scores by 38% ($P < .000$), without differences by gender, track, or year of residency. There were broad, statistically significant attitudinal changes following the course as well, reflecting residents' growing appreciation of the complexity of the health system. Residents reported statistically significant ($P < .001$) more confidence in their abilities to do work in underserved communities, health policy, and COPC. (Taught by adjunct faculty, Medical Spanish does not have comparable pre-post evaluations.)

Since 1981, our social medicine rounds have been a two-credit course for students at the Columbia University Mailman School of Public Health. RPSM graduates can also receive advanced standing or graduate credits toward a master's degree in public health. Since 1996, when the transfer of academic credits to Columbia was formalized, 16 RPSM graduates have received 15 credits towards advanced degrees (15 for masters of public health [MPH] degrees and one for a doctorate of philosophy in education). Before 1996, five RPSM graduates, including the current DFSM chair, attended Columbia and earned MPH degrees. A total of 50 RPSM graduates earned MPH degrees; some graduates worked toward these before, but only one during, residency training.

Social Medicine Projects

All residents are required to complete a social medicine project of their own design; these range from qualitative and quantitative original research to health-center-based quality-improvement projects to targeted health education programs designed for the communities we serve. Projects are longitudinal, with a specific timeline for progress in each postgraduate year, and they may be conducted by an individual, partnership, or team which is mentored by faculty with appropriate expertise and undergoes regular group supervision. Financial support is provided when needed by departmental or alumni funds. Projects culminate each spring when third-year residents, as individuals, teams, or groups, present their outcomes in a series of three sequential social medicine rounds attended by faculty and peers. Among some of the social medicine projects that have led to enduring health services, successful research, and academic publications are projects that have focused on, respectively, establishing satellite, homeless, and school-based health clinics; assessing health literacy; and managing asymptomatic patients who are HIV positive.[32] In recent years we have emphasized longitudinal, mentored projects that produce results suitable for publication or presentation at professional meetings; from 2003 to 2006, residents' projects have resulted in 17 peer-reviewed publications and 36 presentations at national meetings.

First-Year Resident Community Orientation

Our month-long orientation for first-year residents is designed according to the principles of adult learning theory.[21] Framed by Engel's[33] biopsychosocial model, the orientation's overall goal is to introduce residents to the philosophy, theoretical framework, and practice of social medicine in the Bronx. Its activities are structured around three themes: community, patient care, and the physician-as-person (Figure 39.3). In recent years, faculty have identified a specific clinical focus (e.g., diabetes, obesity, violence) as a unifying theme. First-year residents from all three tracks are freed from their inpatient duties and spend an average of just two clinical sessions per week at their FQHC to attend the orientation, which includes a daylong tour of the Bronx; meetings with community-based organizations and leaders; supervised home visits; experiential small-group exercises on health beliefs and behaviors; and seminars on the history of Bronx health institutions, continuous quality improvement, narrative medicine, and COPC. A community-mapping exercise gives residents a close-up view of where their patients live, shop, socialize, and worship. A collaborative community project, based on the month's theme, serves as the orientation's main conjoint learning vehicle. Together, the residents conceive, plan, implement, and evaluate this project, which culminates in a collective social medicine rounds presentation to the RPSM community as a whole.

The orientation takes place several months into postgraduate year one, so residents might reflect on their development as physicians and the effect of training on their personal lives. Stress-management sessions are designed to help residents become more self-aware as clinicians and to help them develop professional resilience to sustain practice in underresourced settings.

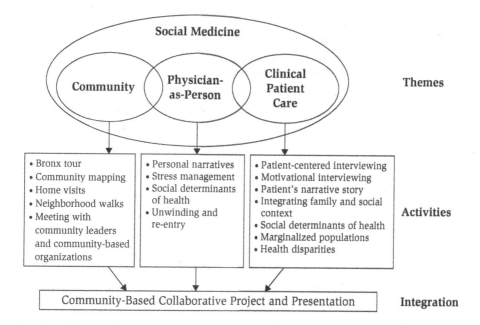

Figure 39.3. Schematic Model of Organizing Themes, Educational Activities, and Project-Based Integration of Bronx Community Orientation for Postgraduate Year One in the Residency Program in Social Medicine

Weekly Likert-style quantitative evaluations with room for comments are conducted during the orientation. At its conclusion, qualitative data are collected using a nominal group technique (a more ordered approach to brainstorming that encourages all members to contribute ideas). These two data sources reflect resident satisfaction with the orientation.[21] Resident learning is assessed through an individual self-reflective narrative exercise and the residents' conjoint project presentation. Residents are not individually evaluated, and the rotation is considered pass/fail.

The RPSM is not the only GME program to employ block rotations for orienting residents to the community;[34] to teach EBM,[35] population health,[36] or advocacy;[37] to base continuity practices in FQHCs[38] or in underserved communities;[39] to organize resident partnerships to facilitate ambulatory training;[40] or to commit itself to public service.[41] The RPSM is relatively unique, however, in combining all of these elements.

Complementary Medicines, Alternative Therapies, and Palliative Care

Education in complementary medicine and alternative therapies began in 1976 and continues today with dedicated faculty and structured electives for residents to observe acupuncture, biofeedback training, guided imagery, herbal therapies, homeopathy, hypnosis, shiatzu massage, and spinal manipulation. Self-care and patient education are emphasized, preparing RPSM graduates for the widespread use of alternative therapies by patients, especially in HIV care. We have published a book[42] and several manuals for primary care clinicians on general[43] and HIV[44] complementary care (the latter a social medicine project). Palliative care has recently been added to our curriculum, as well as to our own and hospital-wide inpatient services, so low-income, minority populations may now access them, too.

6. Grant Support Through Title VII

Because our mission is consistent with that of the primary care cluster of grant programs administered by the Bureau of Health Professions of the Health Resources and Services Administration (HRSA), the RPSM has received federal grants almost continuously for 30 years. These Title VII grants have supported curricular innovations and the tracking of our graduates' careers. They have provided resources and personnel to coordinate the social medicine curriculum, the community orientation, and residents' social medicine projects; to develop innovative clinical and quality-improvement initiatives at our health centers; and to conduct rigorous clinical evaluations using standardized patients from the community who have been trained to give feedback on resident performance in their continuity practices.

General Competencies

The RPSM has aligned its principles with the six competency areas outlined by the ACGME: patient care, medical knowledge, practice-based learning and improvement, interpersonal and communication skills, professionalism, and systems-based practice.[45] They are integrated into curriculum development, resident assessment tools, and, most importantly, faculty development. This ensures that our faculty integrate the ACGME competency areas into our mission and intertwine them in teaching, clinical supervision, and experiential learning in the residents' continuity practices, the hospital, and their communities.

Outcomes

RPSM Practice Outcomes

How does a residency program measure its impact on the careers of its graduates? The RPSM maintains an alumni database[46] to track graduates' careers, subsequent practice sites, and academic degrees because HRSA awards Title VII

Table 39.1. Residency Program in Social Medicine (RPSM) Graduates by Gender and Discipline, 1970–2006

Gender	Family medicine: No. (%)	Internal medicine: No. (%)	Pediatrics: No. (%)	Total: No. (%)
Female	136 (59)	96 (53)	95 (63)	327 (58)
Male	93 (41)	85 (47)	57 (37)	235 (42)
Total	229 (41)	181 (32)	152 (27)	562 (100)

Source: RPSM graduate database.

grants partially on the rates at which graduates enter practice in underserved communities. In addition, a formal alumni association was organized in 2005 which also facilitates tracking the careers of RPSM graduates. Our database includes current workplace, title, advanced degrees, and contact information. RPSM files an annual report with HRSA and has published our outcome data as a whole[16,23] and specifically for graduates of social pediatrics.[47]

Tables 39.1 and 39.2 present descriptive demographic data (gender and race/ethnicity) for all 562 RPSM graduates by specialty discipline from 1970 to 2006. All three disciplines graduate a majority of female residents (53%–63%) and percentages (36%–44%) well above the national average of underrepresented minorities (i.e., African American, Hispanic, American Indian, and Native Hawaiian/Pacific Islander). Half of RPSM graduates practice in New York, 20% in New England and Mid-Atlantic states, 6% in California, and 3% each in Texas and Florida (Table 39.3).

Table 39.4 summarizes a survey of social pediatrics graduates (1970–2002) that was conducted for the doctoral dissertation of its former residency director.[48] Of 147 social pediatrics graduates, 137 (93%) have at some time practiced and 103 (70%) currently practice in medically underserved areas; 119 (81%) have at one time practiced and 75 (51%) currently practice in FQHCs; and 106 (72%) have at some time practiced and 79 (54%) currently practice in health-professions-shortage areas (both federal designations). On average, the social pediatrics graduates' patients were 70% Medicaid and uninsured and 28% self-pay and privately insured.[48] Although recent comparable surveys of family and internal medicine alumni are not available, past RPSM graduate questionnaires have found no significant differences among any of the three disciplines.

To evaluate the effect of residency training over and above the self-selection process of medical graduates who are already predisposed to our goals, the RPSM employed a quasi-experimental design to compare 27 social intern medicine graduates from a five-year cohort (1978–1982) who responded

Table 39.2. Residency Program in Social Medicine (RPSM) Graduates by Ethnic or
Racial Group and Discipline, 1970–2006

Ethnic or racial group	Family medicine: No. (%)	Internal medicine: No. (%)	Pediatrics: No. (%)	Total: No. (%)
White	103 (45)	102 (56)	78 (52)	283 (50)
African American	61 (27)	35 (20)	29 (19)	125 (22)
Hispanic/ Latino	36 (16)	25 (14)	28 (18)	89 (16)
Hawaiian/ Pacific Islander	3 (1)	2 (1)	2 (1)	7 (1)
American Indian	1 (0.4)	0	0	1 (0.02)
Asian	10 (4)	7 (4)	4 (3)	21 (4)
Indian Sub-continent	14 (6)	6 (3)	7 (5)	27 (5)
Middle Eastern	1 (0.4)	4 (2)	4 (3)	9 (2)
Total	229 (41)	181 (32)	152 (27)	562 (100)

Source: RPSM graduate database.

to a follow-up, mail, postresidency survey versus those who applied to the RPSM during the same period but trained elsewhere ($N = 80$).[49] The HRSA-sponsored study demonstrated dramatically different residency training experiences between RPSM graduates and their "applicant controls" ($P < .001$). Residency curriculum elements statistically associated with primary care practice in underserved communities were many of the RPSM hallmarks—that is, continuity practice in an inner city ($P = .02$), social medicine project ($P = .005$), learning about the community of their continuity practice site ($P < .001$), epidemiology and biostatistics ($P = .07$), and Medical Spanish ($P = .01$). The study also found RPSM graduates practicing primary care with the underserved at a significantly higher rate than controls ($P = .03$). Multivariate analysis showed that both subspecialty training ($P = .001$) and higher percentages of middle class patients in residency patient panels ($P = .002$) were significantly associated with *reduced* rates of primary care practice in underserved communities, whereas minority physicians with higher percentages

Table 39.3. Residency Program in Social Medicine 1970–2006
Graduates' Current Practice Locations by State and Region, 2007

Practice location	No. (%)
New York	284 (50)
California	34 (6)
Connecticut	34 (6)
New Jersey	25 (4)
Massachusetts	23 (4)
Texas	19 (3)
Florida	17 (3)
Maryland	17 (3)
Southeastern states	37 (7)
Other Mid-Atlantic and New England states	16 (3)
Midwestern states	24 (4)
Pacific Northwest	13 (2)
Mountain and Plains states	15 (3)
Puerto Rico and International	4 (1)
Total	562 (100)

Source: RPSM graduate database.

of minority residency colleagues were significantly more likely to practice in underserved communities ($P = .04$).

Empirical evidence generated through these follow-up surveys and comparisons of RPSM graduates to applicant controls lend only inferential support to the notion that the RPSM curriculum and training hallmarks contribute causally to the career and practice choices that our graduates have made. Because randomized study designs are not feasible, finding fair comparison groups for more rigorous studies will require creative and adequately powered designs.

Leadership and Excellence

To fulfill the RPSM mission to "advocate for social change" and "generate new knowledge and innovation," our graduates have become leaders at many

Table 39.4. Practice Outcomes of Social Pediatrics Residency Graduates, 1970–2002

Practice settings	At some point: No. (%)	Current: No. (%)
Medically underserved areas	137 (93)	103 (70)
Primary care practice	129 (88)	106 (72)
Community health centers	119 (81)	75 (51)
Health professional shortage areas	106 (72)	79 (54)
Federally-funded health centers	106 (72)	72 (49)

Source: Ozuah PO, Stick SL. Practice locations of graduates of a social pediatrics residency. *JAMA.* 2003;290(9):1154. Ozuah PO. *A Study of the Outcomes of Graduate Medical Training in Social Pediatrics* [dissertation]. Lincoln: University of Nebraska, 2002.

levels. In the 2002 survey of social pediatrics graduates, 59 (41%) reported serving as leaders in regional and national professional organizations, 49 (33%) in their community health centers, 38 (26%) in their hospitals, and 38 (26%) in their medical schools, so that 85 (58%) reported serving in one or more leadership positions.[48] Current leadership positions held by RPSM alumni indicate a broad range of settings for their efforts, led by academic division and center directors and community health center medical directors (Table 39.5).

Our small program (graduating one to ten family physicians, one to six pediatricians, and one to six internists per year) and its graduates have won several national awards and have produced more than our share of prestigious Robert Wood Johnson Clinical Scholars, Kellogg National Leadership Fellows, and CDC Epidemic Intelligence Service Officers. RPSM graduates have served as medical directors at four of the seven major hospitals in the Bronx, at 23 FQHCs in seven states, and two for the National Health Service Corps. Six others have served elsewhere in the US Department of Health and Human Services, including as HRSA's current chief medical officer; another serves as staff to the Committee on Oversight and Government Reform of the U.S. House of Representatives. Five have served as vice presidents and one as president of the New York City Health and Hospitals Corporation. Seven have served as assistant deans or higher in medical and public health schools. Six have served as health department assistant commissioners, including two of the three current medical directors of district public health offices established by the New York City Department of Health and Mental Hygiene in the South Bronx, Harlem, and Central Brooklyn.

Serving Special Populations

Because of its mission, RPSM graduates have not limited their efforts just to poor neighborhoods, but they have also pursued clinical care, leadership,

Table 39.5. Leadership Roles of Residency Program in Social Medicine Graduates by Track, 2007

Venue and role	Family medicine	Internal medicine	Pediatrics	Total
Hospital				
Medical director/vice president	3	3	0	6
Department chair	5	0	2	5
Division chief/center director	7	8	7	22
Community Health center				
Medical director	8	4	5	17
Associate director	2	2	2	6
Academic				
Dean (associate/assistant)	2	1	2	5
Department chair	3	0	3	6
Division chief/center director	15	15	5	35
Public health department				
Commissioner	0	0	1	1
Associate commissioner	0	0	1	1
Assistant commissioner	2	4	1	7
Other medical directors*	8	7	5	20

Source: RPSM graduate database.

*This includes medical directors of institutes, consulting firms, geriatric centers, home care agencies, insurance companies, managed care organizations, mental retardation/developmental disorder centers, National Institutes of Health, occupational health centers, and pharmaceutical companies.

education, and research in serving other underserved populations, including those with HIV, people with addiction disorders, adults with developmental disabilities, prisoners, refugees, and those who are homeless.[34,50] RPSM graduates have also pursued population-oriented disciplines, including school health and adolescent, geriatric, and occupational medicine (Table 39.6). When the AIDS epidemic began, RPSM graduates not only cared for these patients who were often stigmatized by others, but also led the federally funded New York AIDS Education and Training Center,[51] the New York State AIDS Institute's HIV Scholars program, and seminal programs for injection drug users,[52] adolescents, and "street" youth.[53] RPSM alumni include the new president of

Table 39.6. Number of Residency Program in Social Medicine Graduates Serving Special Populations, 2007

Population	Number
HIV/AIDS	21
Homeless	12
Geriatrics	9
Adults with mental retardation and developmental disabilities	7
Occupational and environmental health	7
School-based health clinics	6
Adolescents	4
Prisoners	3

Source: Residency Program in Social Medicine alumni database.

MMC,[54] the current director of Montefiore's Adolescent AIDS Program,[55] and the DFSM chair[56] and vice chair.[57]

Advocacy: "What We ... Do Collectively to Assure the Conditions in Which People Can Be Healthy"

The RPSM affects primary care and public health policy through its faculty and graduates who have served as members or consultants to important state and national commissions, including New York State's Council on Graduate Medical Education ($N = 4$), Minority Health Council ($N = 1$), and Research Council Advisory Panel on Primary Physicians ($N = 6$), as well as on HRSA's national Council on Graduate Medical Education ($N = 5$), whose current executive secretary is an RPSM graduate. In addition, a graduate and past director of RPSM, who now directs the New York Academy of Medicine, chaired the IOM committee that published *The Future of the Public's Health in the 21st Century*.

RPSM faculty and alumni have led the national efforts to provide comprehensive family planning training, including emergency contraception and medical and surgical abortions, in family practice residency programs, now institutionalized under our Center for Reproductive Health Education in

Family Medicine.[58–61] As advocates for the discipline of social medicine,[62] RPSM graduates and faculty have established both a social medicine portal (www.socialmedicine.org) with many links to Web sites, documents, presentations, and organizations devoted to social medicine, and an online journal, *Social Medicine* (http://journals.sfu.ca/socialmedicine/index.php /socialmedicine/index).

RPSM and Its Institutional Relationships

The RPSM was conceived, grew, and continues to evolve in a relatively supportive institutional context, an example of MMC's community service mission and long social tradition that includes founding our community health centers[63] and establishing the first hospital-based departments of social services and of social medicine.[64] MMC was a finalist in 2006 for the American Hospital Association's McGaw Prize for Community Service, and it received the Association of American Medical College Community Service Award in 1994, which was recently renamed the Spencer Foreman Community Service Award for MMC's retiring president. MMC has provided resources, flexibility, and stability while RPSM suffered growing pains when residency positions or ambulatory sites were added; during difficult transitions changing ambulatory practice sites; or after losses of grants, clinical sites, or key personnel. Likewise, RPSM has served MMC as a training venue for center, division, department, and hospital-wide leaders and as a laboratory for new programs, such as the school health program and what the authors of *In Search of Excellence* called a "skunk works," an organizational enclave where autonomy and entrepreneurship are fostered.[65]

To assure Medicare indirect GME reimbursements for resident time spent seeing their continuity patients, our FQHCs are licensed under MMC's operating certificate, which has centralized the formers' administration, oriented their priorities toward productivity and quality improvement in an integrated health system rather than community health, and constrained their innovation and finances (i.e., as hospital outpatient clinics rather than freestanding centers, so that their Medicaid reimbursements are capped in New York State).

In contrast to our long-standing, reciprocal relationship and shared mission with MMC, our short-lived collaboration with a community hospital that provided both a family medicine inpatient service and ambulatory, continuity practices for internal medicine and pediatrics proved to be far less beneficial. When this hospital realigned its teaching affiliation, we learned that our missions diverged and that we had to relocate precipitously. MMC's and DFSM's affiliated FQHCs provided our safety net.

Lessons Learned

Multiple Demands of Multiple Departments

Other challenges to implementing the RPSM mission through its hallmarks have come from many quarters and have been addressed programmatically. The centrifugal disciplinary demands of the departments of medicine and pediatrics often erode residents' participation in and faculty members' commitment to RPSM's interdisciplinary education and administration, which we try to overcome with our conjoint social medicine administrative structure and activities. In addition, each specialty has adapted its own unique partnership model. Supervising faculty, fellows, and residents in other departments often do not understand resident partnerships or why RPSM residents need to leave the hospital bedside for their health centers or social medicine rounds; mitigating these misunderstandings requires continuous communication to other departments about RPSM resident responsibilities.

National Standards Applied Uniformly to the Unique RPSM

The Family Medicine Residency Review Committee (RRC) applies national norms for clinical exposure and resident productivity that do not distinguish between preparing rural and urban family physicians or between preparing physicians to care for primarily English-speaking or Spanish-speaking patients. In addition, the Internal Medicine RRC does not permit family physicians to cross-cover and supervise internal medicine residents. To meet its RRC clinical exposure and productivity requirements, family medicine has forged special arrangements for residents' obstetrical deliveries and has divided its continuity practice between two centers (i.e., FHC and Williamsbridge). Social internal medicine has joined forces with a primary care track and no longer needs family physicians to cross-cover.

Differences Among Disciplines

Differences in cultural values and leadership, teaching, and learning styles also contribute to tensions within and among the three disciplines, sometimes promoting and sometimes challenging our collaborative model along that "San Andreas fault line" between learning the specialized knowledge and skills of each specialty and the common interdisciplinary content of social medicine and population health. Organizational structure (e.g., a division of GME) and clear leadership (e.g., a director of RPSM) have supported and sustained the integrated model.

Meeting Many Recommendations

The 2003 IOM report, *Who Will Keep the Public Healthy?* recommended that all physicians learn both the ecological model of the determinants of health and 13 population-health content areas (i.e., epidemiology, bio-statistics, environmental health, health services administration, social and behavioral sciences, informatics, genomics, communication, cultural competence, community-based participatory research, global health, policy and law, and public health ethics).[6] In its 2007 report, *Training Physicians for Public Health Careers,* the IOM recommended that "each graduate medical education program identify and include the public health concepts and skills relevant to the practice of that specialty" and also move toward assessing competencies; the IOM also added leadership, clinical and community preventive services, and public health emergency preparedness to its recommended content areas.[7] With the exceptions of genomics and emergency preparedness, the RPSM's curriculum and training hallmarks meet the IOM's recommendations almost completely.

Looking Ahead

Despite a renewed recognition of a physician workforce shortage[66] and the explicit goal of eliminating health disparities in *Healthy People 2010,* federal funding through Title VII for primary care and diversity programs, such as those which have supported the RPSM, have been drastically reduced. With increased federal funding for community health centers, many of these FQHCs are now suffering staff vacancies and experiencing difficulties recruiting physicians, dentists, and other health professions to meet their patients' needs.[67,68] Besides restoring federal funding for health workforce development, states, counties, and municipal governments as well as private foundations need to focus their resources on ensuring that the health workforce reflects our growing diversity and is equipped with the skills to reduce and eliminate health disparities.

Summing Up

The RPSM continues to pursue its "distinct and visionary" mission,[69] in which population health is deeply embedded, and the program remains committed to addressing the special challenges of poverty, the urban environment, and our changing health system. The RPSM nurtures and protects the idealism that brings people to medicine and gives them the knowledge, skills, and resilience to realize their ideals and leadership potential in serving stigmatized, oppressed, and impoverished individuals and populations. With creativity and innovation have also come unintended consequences and failed experiments, but never a doubt of our guiding goals.

The RPSM demonstrates a successful, mission-driven model for GME in family medicine, internal medicine, and pediatrics that seeks to integrate individual and population health. With Title VII funding, RPSM provides inter-disciplinary and community-based primary care training enriched by mental health, nursing, public health, and social work faculty. Empirical evidence has begun to validate RPSM's training hallmarks that converge with the IOM's recommended content areas for public health. RPSM's graduates are fulfilling the mission as leaders and practitioners in underserved communities and with underserved populations across New York State and the nation. The RPSM makes a difference—in the lives of underserved people, in the careers of its graduates, and in the health system itself—and seeks to make health care an instrument of social justice.

Acknowledgments

The authors would like to thank Ms. Nicole Lewis and Ms. Deyanira Suarez for their efforts to maintain and update the RPSM alumni database.

Notes

1. Committee for the Study of the Future of Public Health, Division of Health Care Services, Institute of Medicine. *The Future of Public Health.* Washington, DC: National Academy Press; 1988.

2. Committee on the Changing Market, Managed Care, and the Future Viability of Safety Net Providers; Lewin ME, Altman S (eds.); Institute of Medicine. *America's Health Care Safety Net: Intact but Endangered.* Washington, DC: National Academy Press; 2000.

3. Smedley BD, Stith AY, Nelson AR, eds.; Committee on Understanding and Eliminating Racial and Ethnic Disparities in Health Care; Board of Health Sciences Policy; Institute of Medicine. *Unequal Treatment: Confronting Racial and Ethnic Disparities in Health Care.* Washington, DC: The National Academies Press; 2003.

4. Committee on Institutional and Policy-Level Strategies for Increasing the Diversity of the US Health Care Workforce; Board on Health Sciences Policy; Smedley BD, Butler AS, Bristow LR, eds.; Institute of Medicine. *In the Nation's Compelling Interest: Ensuring Diversity in the Health-Care Workforce.* Washington, DC: The National Academies Press; 2004.

5. Committee on Assuring the Health of the Public in the 21st Century; Board on Health Promotion and Disease Prevention; Institute of Medicine. *The Future of the Public's Health in the 21st Century.* Washington, DC: The National Academies Press; 2003.

6. Gebbie K, Rosenstock L, Hernandez LM, eds.; Committee on Educating Public Health Professionals for the 21st Century; Board on Health Promotion and Disease Prevention; Institute of Medicine. *Who Will Keep the Public Healthy? Educating Public Health Professionals for the 21st Century.* Washington, DC: The National Academies Press; 2003.

7. Committee on Training Physicians for Public Health Careers; Board on Population Health and Public Health Practice; Hernandez LM, Munthali AW, eds.; Institute of

Medicine. *Training Physicians for Public Health Careers*. Washington, DC: The National Academies Press; 2007.

8. Donaldson MS, Yordy KD, Lohr KN, Vanselow NA, eds.; Committee on the Future of Primary Care Division of Health Care Services; Institute of Medicine. *Primary Care: America's Health in a New Era*. Washington, DC: National Academy Press; 1996.

9. Brandt A, Kass A. Collaboration and competition: Tracing the historical relationship of medicine and public health in the 20th century. In: Hager M, Bondurant S, eds. *Education for More Synergistic Practice of Medicine and Public Health: A Conference Sponsored by the Josiah Macy, Jr. Foundation*. New York: Josiah Macy, Jr. Foundation; 1999.

10. Leonhardt D. US poverty rate was up last year. *New York Times* August 31, 2005. Available at http://www.nytimes.com/2005/08/31/national/31census.html. Accessed December 22, 2007.

11. US Census Bureau. *American Community Survey, 2006*. Available at http://fact finder.census.gov/prod/2007[ibs/acs-08.pdf. Accessed December 20, 2007.

12. Strelnick AH. Increasing access to health care and reducing minority health disparities: A brief history and the impact of community health centers. *N Y Univ J Legis Public Policy* 2005;8:63–80.

13. Purpura DP. Establishing an academic department of family medicine at the Albert Einstein College of Medicine. *Fam Med*. 1992;24:423–425.

14. US Department of Health and Human Services. *Healthy People 2010*. Available at http://www.healthypeople.gov/About/goals.htm. Accessed December 20, 2007.

15. Urbina C, Hickey M, McHarney-Brown C, Duban S, Kaufman A. Innovative generalist programs: Academic health care centers respond to the shortage of generalist physicians. *J Gen Int Med*. 1994;9(4 suppl. 1): S81–S89.

16. Boufford JI. Primary care residency training: The first five years. *Ann Intern Med*. 1977;87:359–368.

17. Strelnick AH. Affirmative action in medical schools. *N Engl J Med*. 1986;314: 1584–1585.

18. Strelnick AH, Massad RJ, Bateman WB, Shepherd SD. Minority students in US medical schools. *N Engl J Med*. 1986;315:67–69.

19. Saha S, Shipman SA; US Dept. of Health and Human Services; Health Resources and Services Administration; Bureau of Health Professions. *The Rationale for Diversity in the Health Professions: A Review of the Evidence*. Available at http://bhpr.hrsa.gov/healthworkforce/reports/diversity/default.htm. Accessed December 18, 2007.

20. Townsend JM, Fulchon C. Minority faculty: Recruiting, retaining, and sustaining. *Fam Med*. 1994;26(10):612–613.

21. Strelnick AH, Gold M, Dyche L, et al. Orientation to social medicine and the Bronx: An educational experience for adult learners. *Teach Learn Med*. 1998;10:101–108.

22. Massad RJ. Training for inner-city family practice: Experience of the Montefiore Medical Center. In: Birrer RB, ed. *Urban Family Medicine*. New York: Springer-Verlag; 1987.

23. Strelnick AH, Bateman WH, Jones C, et al. Graduate primary care training: A collaborative alternative for family practice, internal medicine, and pediatrics. *Ann Intern Med*. 1988;109:324–334.

24. Accreditation Council for Graduate Medical Education. *Outcomes Project*. Available at http://www.acgme.org/outcome/comp/GeneralCompetenciesStandards21307 .pdf. Accessed December 22, 2007.

25. *Improving Chronic Illness Care. The Chronic Care Model*. Available at http:// improvingchroniccare.org. Accessed December 20, 2007.

26. Prislin MD, Morohashi D, Dinh T, Sandoval J, Shimazu H. The community health center and family practice residency training. *Fam Med*. 1996;28:624–628.

27. Boufford JI. Medical education and training for community-oriented primary care. In: Connor E, Mullan F, eds.; Division of Health Care Services; Institute of Medicine. *Community-Oriented Primary Care: New Directions for Health Services Delivery— Conference Proceedings*. Washington, DC: National Academy Press; 1983:167–197.

28. Nutting PA, Connor EM, eds. Montefiore Family Health Center. In: Nutting PA, Connor EM, eds.; Division of Health Care Services; Institute of Medicine. *Community-Oriented Primary Care: A Practical Assessment—Case Studies. Volume II*. Washington, DC: National Academy Press; 1984:115–136.

29. Zayas LH, Dyche LA. Social workers training primary care physicians: Essential psychosocial principles. *Soc Work* 1992;37:247–252.

30. Schön D. *The Reflective Practitioner: How Professionals Think in Action*. New York: Basic Books; 1983.

31. Strelnick AH, Shonubi PA. Integrating community oriented primary care into training and practice: A view from the Bronx. *Fam Med*. 1986;18:205–209.

32. Hecht FM, Soloway B, Cotton DJ, Friedland GH. *HIV Infection: A Primary Care Approach*. Waltham: Pub. Division of the Massachusetts Medical Society; 1994.

33. Engel GL. Sounding board: The biopsychosocial model and medical education: Who are to be the teachers? *N Engl J Med*. 1982;306:802–805.

34. Thompson R, Haber D, Chambers C, Fanuiel L, Krohn K, Smith AJ. Orientation to community in a family practice residency program. *Fam Med*. 1998;30:24–28.

35. Thom DH, Haugen J, Sommers PS, Lovett P. Description and evaluation of an EBM curriculum using a block rotation. *BMC Med Educ*. 2004;4:19.

36. Patmas MA, Rosenberg M, Gragnola T. A rotation in population-based health for internal medicine residents. *Acad Med*. 2001;76:557.

37. Paterniti DA, Pan RJ, Smith LF, Horan NM, West DC. From physician-centered to community-oriented perspectives on health care: Assessing the efficacy of community-based training. *Acad Med*. 2006;81:347–353.

38. Zweifler J. Balancing service and education: Linking community health centers and family practice residency programs. *Fam Med.* 1993;25:306–311.

39. Eddy JM, Labuguen RH. A longitudinal community-based underserved care elective for family practice residents. *Fam Med.* 2002;34:567–569.

40. Adam P, Williamson Jr. HA., Zweig SC. Resident partnerships: A tool for enhancing ambulatory training. *Fam Med.* 1997;29:705–708.

41. Miller ST, Lancaster DJ. Transformation of an internal medicine residency program to address the health of the Tennessee public. *J Tenn Med Assoc.* 1994;87:468–471.

42. Grossman R. *The Other Medicines: An Invitation to Understanding & Using Them for Health & Healing.* Garden City, NY: Doubleday; 1985.

43. Grossman R, Lefferts S, eds. *Practitioner's Guide to Complementary Therapies.* Bronx, NY: Center for Health in Medicine, Residency Program in Social Medicine, Department of Family Medicine; 1982.

44. Mangum T. *Complementary Medical Approaches to the Treatment of HIV Disease and Immune Deficiencies.* Bronx, NY: Department of Family Medicine; 1994.

45. Accreditation Council for Graduate Medical Education. *Outcome Project.* Available at http://www.acgme.org/outcome. Accessed December 18, 2007.

46. Albert Einstein College of Medicine of Yeshiva University. Residency Program in Social Medicine database. Available at http://www.aecom.yu.edu/rpsm/search .asp. Accessed December 20, 2007.

47. Ozuah PO, Stick SL. Practice locations of graduates of a social pediatrics residency. *JAMA.* 2003;290:1154.

48. Ozuah PO. *A Study of the Outcomes of Graduate Medical Training in Social Pediatrics* [doctoral dissertation]. Lincoln: University of Nebraska; 2002.

49. Strelnick AH. *Can the Content and Setting of Residency Training Promote Primary Care Practice in Underserved Areas? Assessing the Impact of a Title VII Residency Program in Primary Care Internal Medicine* [unpublished report]. Rockville, MD: Health Resources and Services Administration, Office of Health Policy, Analysis, and Research; 1994.

50. Plescia M, Watts GR, Neibacher S, et al. A multidisciplinary health care outreach team to the homeless: The 10-year experience of the Montefiore Care for the Homeless team. *Fam Community Health* 1997;20:58–69.

51. Strelnick AH, Futterman D, Carrascal A, et al. Controversies: The role of HIV specialists. *JAMA.* 1998;279:834–835.

52. Selwyn PA, Budner N, Wasserman W, et al. Utilization of on-site primary care services among HIV-seropositive and seronegative drug users in a methadone program. *Public Health Rep.* 1993;108:492–500.

53. O'Keefe R. Adolescent sexuality. *Am Fam Phys.* 1992;46:38–45.

54. Solomont EB. Safyer tapped to lead Montefiore Medical Center. *New York Sun.* November 28, 2006. Available at http://www.nysun.com/article/67141. Accessed December 20, 2007.

55. Futterman DC. HIV and AIDS in adolescents. *Adolesc Med Clin.* 2004;15:369–391.

56. Selwyn PA. A piece of my mind: Small victories. *JAMA.* 2007;297:2455–2456.

57. Soloway B, Hecht FM. Managed care and HIV. *AIDS Clin Care.* 1997;9:67–69, 71.

58. Gold M. Abortion training in family medicine. *Fam Med.* 1996;28:287–288.

59. Lesnewski R, Prine L, Gold M. New research: Abortion training as an integral part of residency training. *Fam Med.* 2003;35:386–387.

60. Dehlendorf C, Brahmi D, Engel D, Grumback K, Joffe C, Gold M. Integrating abortion training into family medicine residency programs. *Fam Med.* 2007;39: 337–342.

61. Brahmi D, Dehlendorf C, Engel D, Grumback K, Joffe C, Gold M. A descriptive analysis of abortion training in family medicine residency programs. *Fam Med.* 2007;39:399–403.

62. Anderson M, Smith L, Sidel VW. What is social medicine? *Monthly Rev.* 2005;56: 27–34. Available at http://www.monthlyreview.org/0105anderson.htm. Accessed December 20, 2007.

63. Sidel VW. The Department of Social Medicine at Montefiore in the 1970s and 1980s. *Montefiore Med.* 1980;5:55–60.

64. Levenson D. *Montefiore: The hospital as social instrument, 1884–1984.* New York: Farrar, Straus & Giroux;1984.

65. Peters TJ, Waterman RH. *In Search of Excellence: Lessons from America's Best-Run Companies.* New York: Warner Books; 1982.

66. Salsberg E, Grover A. Physician workforce shortages: Implications and issues for academic health centers and policymakers. *Acad Med.* 2006;81:782–787.

67. Rosenblatt RA, Andrilla CH, Curtin T, Hart LG. Shortages of medical personnel at community health centers: Implications for planned expansion. *JAMA.* 2006;295: 1042–1049.

68. Lee C. Community health centers flourish, but doctors are few. Government needs to entice physicians, health officials say. *Washington Post* June 19, 2007:A02. Available at http://www.washingtonpost.com/wp-dyn/content/article/2007/06 /18/AR2007061801368.html. Accessed December 17, 2007.

69. Miller WL. Books: *Urban Family Medicine,* edited by Richard B. Birrer [book review]. *Fam Syst Med.* 1989;7:458–463.

Chapter 40

Stories and Society

Using Literature to Teach Medical Students About Public Health and Social Justice

Martin Donohoe

Introduction

This chapter presents an argument for enhancing the public health education of medical students through the use of literature, with the goal of creating activist physicians knowledgeable about, and eager to confront, the social, economic, and cultural contributors to illness. The current state of training in ethics and public health will be reviewed, followed by a description of injustices which contribute to poor health. The value of literature to public health education will be described, and specific curricular suggestions offered. While the paper focuses on medical students, its lessons are applicable to all health professionals, practitioners and students alike.

Current Medical School Training in Ethics and Public Health

Despite calls for an increased emphasis on global bioethics,[1,2] contemporary ethics training tends to focus more on fascinating dilemmas involving expensive technologies (e.g., gene therapy, assisted reproduction, cloning, prenatal genetic diagnosis and treatment, and face transplants), while inadequately addressing the psychological, cultural, socioeconomic, occupational, and environmental contributors to the health of individuals and populations.

Social issues and public health are inadequately covered in US medical schools.[3] Similarly, human rights, environmental health, women's reproductive rights, and war and militarization are marginalized.[4-18] Despite the Institute of Medicine's recommendation that 1/4 to 1/2 of medical students earn the equivalent of a master's in public health, only 10% of students at US public health schools are physicians, down from 60% in the 1960s.[19]

Barriers to social sciences instruction include lack of perceived relevance for clinical practice; limited curricular time; lack of qualified instructors; a dearth of commitment from deans and department chairs; inadequate funding; and a paucity of role models. The schism between schools of public health and medical schools that dates back to the early twentieth century—with medical schools becoming more focused on biochemical mechanisms of disease and drug therapies than on societal issues—has yet to be healed. Furthermore, the lack of collaboration between nursing schools and medical schools has created an environment not conducive to collaborative learning. This makes post-training collaborative practice, which is critical to solving population-level health problems, more challenging.

Social Injustices and Public Health

This is a time of increasing injustice in health care in the US and worldwide. Today 47 million Americans lack health insurance. Millions more are underinsured, remain in "dead-end" jobs to maintain their health insurance, or go without needed prescriptions because of skyrocketing drug prices. The increasing role played by for-profit corporations in causing and perpetuating worldwide social injustices is mirrored by the pernicious influence of for-profit entities (health maintenance organizations, hospital systems, and pharmaceutical and biotechnology companies) on the American health care system.[20-24] For-profit health care systems in the US have been widely cited for higher death rates, lower quality of care, and higher administrative costs.[25]

Patient and physician dissatisfaction with many aspects of our current fragmented health care system is growing.[25] Many medical students and residents display increasingly cynical attitudes as their training progresses, and some educators have expressed concern about the adequacy of students' humanistic and moral development.[26] Increasing dissatisfaction, cynicism, and the erosion of professional behaviors among practicing physicians and trainees have been described,[27] and interest in primary care among medical students has been declining.[28] Tending to physical symptoms often overshadows health professionals' attention to the psychological, economic, social, and cultural factors that prompt many outpatient visits and cause as much functional impairment as physical complaints.[29] Increasing numbers of physicians from all fields have stopped seeing patients with certain types of insurance, complain of fatigue and burnout, and feel that medicine has lost its soul.[27] Some doctors are even leaving the profession. While almost half of US medical schools sponsor student-run health clinics for the indigent,[30] the proportion of physicians providing charity care has declined over the last decade.[31] Meanwhile, most academic medical centers have opened luxury primary care clinics, and concierge care for the wealthy is growing.[32,33]

Despite spending a larger proportion of its gross domestic product on health care than any other nation, the US ranks 37th in overall health care system performance.[34] In the US, 20–25 percent of its children live in poverty.[9] Disparities have grown in wealth, access to care, and morbidity and mortality between rich and poor.[9,34] Racial inequalities in processes and outcomes of care persist, some seemingly explainable only by racism or poverty (itself in part a consequence of past and present racism).[9]

Differences between developed and developing nations, in terms of financial, economic, environmental and health-related resources, have further widened and are especially dramatic.[9,10] Over one billion people lack access to clean drinking water, and three billion lack adequate sanitation services. Tens of thousands of children die every day from malnutrition and disease. The worldwide gap between rich and poor doubled over the last 30 years and continues to grow rapidly.[9,10]

The United States has failed to sign and/or ratify a number of treaties relevant to human rights, social justice, and public health, such as the Kyoto Protocol on Climate Change; the International Covenant on Economic, Social, and Cultural Rights; the Comprehensive Nuclear Test Ban Treaty; the Convention on the Rights of the Child; the Convention on the Elimination of Discrimination Against Women, and the Basel Convention on the Control of Transboundary Movements of Hazardous Wastes. Furthermore, our country's foreign and trade policies have been at odds with the promotion of public health.[8-10,12-15]

Literature and Public Health

Literature (poems, essays, short stories, and novels) has been integrated into many medical curricula. In general, students have responded enthusiastically to the addition of literature to the medical school curriculum.[35]

Literature, medicine, and public health share a fundamental concern with the human condition.[36-40] Through literature, readers can vicariously experience new situations, explore diverse philosophies, and develop empathy with and respect for others whose place in society may be very different from their own. Reading about the experiences of those who suffer the consequences of poverty, racism, stigmatization, and impaired access to health care can help medical students to identify more closely with their patients, whose complex lives they glimpse only during periodic clinic visits. Literature's instructive and evocative powers can be used to introduce basic principles of social medicine and community health; to facilitate discussion between students regarding the social determinants of illness, the health of populations, and the public health responsibilities of physicians; to increase empathy, understanding, and appreciation of alternative viewpoints; and to encourage students to undertake further studies and/or research in public health, and to publicly work towards solutions to sociomedical problems.[37,38]

Curricula covering public health, social justice, and global bioethics might be more interesting and provocative if they incorporated works of literature.[10,37,38]

The following are specific examples:

- George Orwell's essay, "How the Poor Die,"[41] and Anton Chekhov's short story, "Ward No. Six,"[42] offer timeless descriptions of the abysmal conditions which can be found in inadequately funded public hospitals.

- Doris Lessing's, "An Old Woman and Her Cat,"[43] provides a moving fictional entrée into the world of society's dispossessed, through its description of the daily struggles of an aged gypsy and her adopted alley cat trying to cope with life on the streets of London.

- Earnest J. Gaines's short tale, "The Sky Is Gray,"[44] relates the story of a poor, single African-American farm mother trying to obtain dental care for her ill child in a racist Southern farm town.

- Upton Sinclair's novel, *The Jungle*,[45] describes the harrowing experiences of a poor immigrant family. The novel's revolting descriptions of Chicago's meat packing plants spurred public pressure on Congress to pass the Pure Food and Drug Act of 1906 (the precursor to the US Food and Drug Administration). Henrik Ibsen's play, *An Enemy of the People*,[46] portrays a doctor's battle with city officials to clean up the local water supply.

- William Carlos Williams's short story, "The Paid Nurse,"[47] describes a community physician's disdain at the inadequate treatment provided to a victim of an industrial accident by a corrupt company doctor.

- Homeless writer Lars Eighner's autobiographical novel, *Travels with Lizbeth*,[48] addresses his experience of being (inaccurately) labeled a drug user during a hospital admission for phlebitis. Eighner also graphically describes his street survival tactics, including finding safe shelter, hitchhiking, and dumpster diving.

- Grace Paley's short story, "An Interest in Life,"[49] profiles a single mother's search for companionship, struggles raising her children, and difficulties navigating through the often-illogical vagaries of the welfare system.

- In William Carlos Williams's brief tale, "The Insane,"[50] a young pediatrician shares with his physician-father his frustration over the long-term effects on a child's mental health of witnessing violence and of emotional neglect.

- Chekhov's writings on his journey to Sakhalin[51] chronicle the detrimental health consequences of extreme poverty.
- Pastor Niemoller's poem, "First They Came for the Jews,"[52] powerfully exhorts us to speak out on behalf of the disenfranchised, especially since one day we may join their ranks.

Useful selections for sessions relating to war are Mark Twain's posthumously published poem, "The War Prayer," which portrays the horrors of war and excoriates the hypocrisy of those who pray for victory in battle;[53] Dalton Trumbo's novel, *Johnny Got His Gun*,[54] which describes the harrowing experience of a seriously wounded soldier; Walter Miller's apocalyptic novel, *A Canticle for Leibowitz*;[55] Michael Harrison and Christopher Stewart-Clark's collection of poems entitled *Peace and War*;[56] works by Premo Levi[57] and Elie Weisel[58] describing their Holocaust experiences; and poems by Wilfred Owen and Sigfrid Sasson. Jacobo Timmerman powerfully chronicles his experience of torture in the novel, *Prisoner Without a Name, Cell Without a Number*.[59]

Literature can be incorporated into the medical school curriculum in myriad ways. Small group discussion sections constitute an ideal venue for the discussion of literary works, which can be taught alongside articles from the medical and public health literature.[37,60] Using short literary selections on ward rounds to help students and residents better comprehend the sociocultural, economic, religious, and personal factors that contribute to health and affect one's response to illness can improve our insight into patients' lives, and ideally increase our empathy.

Writing assignments can also be valuable, especially when students are able to share their essays with mentors and colleagues.[61] The medical profession has made important contributions to the literary canon, through the works of Francois Rabelais, Thomas Campion, John Keats, Anton Chekhov, Somerset Maugham, William Carlos Williams, and contemporary doctor-writers like Lewis Thomas, Dannie Abse, and Richard Selzer. While not every physician shares these luminaries' narrative abilities, all physicians require solid verbal and written communication skills.

Opportunities for students to write about formative experiences in medical school (e.g., critical incident reports) have been shown to be valuable in facilitating personal growth and development.[62] Some schools require these as part of the medicine clerkship. Others require that students write at least one complete history and physical from the perspective of the patient. Broadening the scope of such writing assignments to include a public health perspective is one way to build on existing pedagogical approaches.

Finally, combining relevant literature with community volunteer work, mentored service-learning projects, or activist-oriented research can broaden students' educational experiences.[38,63] Interdisciplinary learning involving various health professions students should foster lasting cooperation and collaboration.[38]

Photography and Public Health Education

Photography also can be a useful adjunct to teaching about social justice. Space precludes a full discussion of this topic, but a few examples might suffice:

- A session on toxic pollution might include W. Eugene and Aileen Smith's photoessay on the health consequences of methylmercury poisoning in Minamata Bay, Japan.[64]
- Dorothea Lange's poignant pictures of dust bowl migrants evoke the hardscrabble existence of the poor and landless.[65]
- Sebastio Salgado's dramatic photos of laborers illustrate the consequences of our use of planetary resources, along with providing insight into the dangerous nature of many occupations.[66]
- James Nachtwey's photographs allow students to enter war zones and visualize the suffering wrought by human conflicts.[67]

The Call to Service

Physicians have an obligation, borne of their privileged status, the public's investment in their training, and their roles as stewards of the public's health, to be politically active and ensure that our leaders provide for the sickest among us. Unfortunately, while physicians recognize the importance of community participation, political involvement, and collective advocacy,[68] they have lower adjusted voting rates than the general population.[69] When doctors lobby Congress, they focus on issues such as reimbursement and funding for medical research, rather than access to care for the uninsured, tobacco control, women's rights, violence prevention, and other social justice issues.[70] Physician-legislators are rare today compared with past centuries.[71]

Physicians also have a responsibility to oppose, individually and collectively, those forces which contribute to the spread of poverty, over-consumption, the maldistribution of wealth, the economic, political, legal, and educational marginalization of women, environmental degradation, racism, human rights abuses, and militarization and war. This is especially true now, when fewer scientists hold positions of authority than in times past, and when scientific truths have been deliberately obfuscated by the well-funded and sophisticated public relations and lobbying campaigns of those with a vested interest in profiting from the provision of a basic human right like health care.

Doctors as Social Justice Advocates

There are many noteworthy examples of physician-advocates, about whom medical students know too little. For example, pathologist Rudolph Virchow, best known for establishing the cell doctrine in pathology and elucidating the pathophysiology of thrombosis, pulmonary embolism, leukocytosis, and leukemia, made equally valuable contributions to social medicine.[72] Virchow wrote, "Medical education does not exist to provide students with a way of making a living, but to ensure the health of the community."[73] He argued that many diseases result from the unequal distribution of civilization's advantages. He felt that physicians were the natural advocates of the poor, and opined, "If medicine is really to accomplish its great task, it must intervene in political and social life."[74] Virchow served as a legislator and founded a journal entitled *Medical Reform*. He spoke out for public provision of medical care for the indigent, prohibition of child labor, universal education, and free and unlimited democracy. He instituted programs for improving water and sewage systems, stricter food inspection, and improved education and training of health professionals.[72]

Other health professionals have led inspiring lives of social activism, including Dr. Thomas Hodgkin (abolitionist and opponent of British oppression of native populations in South Africa and New Zealand); nurse Margaret Sanger (founder of the family planning movement in the US); Dr. Albert Schweitzer (who won the Nobel Peace Prize in part for developing a missionary hospital for the poor in Gabon, Africa); Florence Nightingale (feminist, founder of the modern nursing profession, and advocate for hygienic hospitals); and Dr. Salvador Allende (assassinated president of Chile and promoter of better living conditions for the poor and working classes). Many individuals labor today, often anonymously, in support of the disenfranchised. Others work through well-known physician-activist organizations, such as Physicians for Human Rights, Doctors Without Borders, Physicians for a National Health Plan, Physicians for Social Responsibility, and the Doctors Reform Society. Increased attention during medical training to social justice and to history and literature relevant to physician activism may encourage students to become more involved in activism throughout their careers.

Conclusions

The importance of economic, social, and cultural contributors to population health demands that physicians' training in these areas be enhanced. One pedagogical approach to augmenting such public health training and to encourage physician activism is through the use of literature. The vicarious experiences afforded by reading the powerful stories of great authors can ideally enhance trainees' attentiveness to their patients' needs and motivate physicians to become more active in addressing the health care needs of their communities and the world.

Acknowledgments

The author thanks Karen Adams, MD, FACOG, for editorial support.

Notes

1. Benatar SR, Daar AS, Singer PA. Global health challenges: The need for an expanded discourse on bioethics. *PLoS Medicine* 2005;2(7):0587–0589.

2. Dwyer J. Teaching global bioethics. *Bioethics* 2003;17(5–6):432–446.

3. Silverberg LI. Survey of medical ethics in US medical schools: A descriptive study. *JAOA.* 2000;100(6):373–378.

4. DuBois JM, Ciesla MA. *Ethics education in US medical schools: A study of syllabi.* Center for Health Care Ethics. Saint Louis University. Presented at the American Society for Bioethics and Humanities meeting, Salt Lake City, Utah, October 2000.

5. El-Nachef W, Chevrier J, Cotter E, et al. *Valuing, vetting and visioning: Advancing health and human rights education in professional health programs.* Program and abstracts of the American Public Health Association 134th Annual Meeting; November 4–8, 2006; Boston, Massachusetts. Abstract 137536. As cited in Evans DP. One world: Global focus. *APHA.* 2006. Posted March 13, 2007. Available at http://www.medscape.com/viewprogram/6761_pnt. Accessed July 18, 2007.

6. Sonis J, Gorenflo DW, Jha P, Williams C. Teaching of human rights in US medical schools. *JAMA.* 1996;276(20):1676–1678.

7. Donohoe MT. Incarceration nation: Health and welfare in the prison system in the United States. *Medscape Ob/Gyn and Women's Health* 2006;11(1). Posted January 20, 2006. Available at http://www.medscape.com/viewarticle/520251. Accessed May 4, 2008.

8. Donohoe MT. Flowers, diamonds, and gold: The destructive human rights and environmental consequences of symbols of love. *Human Rights Quarterly* 2008;30:164–182.

9. Donohoe MT. Causes and health consequences of environmental degradation and social injustice. *Soc Sci and Med.* 2003;56(3):573–587.

10. Donohoe MT. Roles and responsibilities of health professionals in confronting the health consequences of environmental degradation and social injustice: education and activism. *Monash Bioethics Review,* 2008;27(Nos. 1 and 2):65-82.

11. Hansen E, Donohoe MT. Health issues of migrant and seasonal farm workers. *J Health Care for the Poor and Underserved* 2003;14(2):153–164.

12. Donohoe MT. Global warming: A public health crisis demanding immediate action. *World Affairs Journal* 2007;11(2):44–58.

13. Donohoe MT. Obstacles to abortion in the United States. *Medscape Ob/Gyn and Women's Health* 2005;10(2). Posted July 7, 2005. Available at http://www .medscape.com/viewarticle/507404. Accessed May 4, 2008.

14. Donohoe MT. Increase in obstacles to abortion: The American perspective in 2004. *J Am Med Women's Assn.* 2005;60(1)(Winter):16–25. Available at http://www .ncbi.nlm.nih.gov/pubmed/16845763. Accessed May 4, 2008.

15. Donohoe MT. Individual and societal forms of violence against women in the United States and the developing world: An overview. *Curr Women's Hlth Reports* 2002;2(5):313–319.

16. American College of Physicians. The role of the physician and the medical profession in the prevention of international torture and in the treatment of its survivors. *Ann Int Med.* 1995:607–613.

17. Donohoe MT. Internists, epidemics, outbreaks, and bioterrorist attacks. *J Gen Int Med.* 2007;22(9):1380. Available at http://www.springerlink.com/content /v2r74824uv349208/fulltext.pdf. Accessed May 4, 2008.

18. Vergun R, Vergun P, Thomasson C, Donohoe MT. A brief summary of the medical impacts of Hiroshima. In: Okuda ST (with Vergun P), *A Dimly Burning Wick: Memoir from the Ruins of Hiroshima* (New York: Algora Publishing, 2008).

19. Wilson JF. Patient counseling and education: Should doctors be doing more? *Ann Int Med.* 2006;144(8):621–624.

20. Donohoe MT. Corporate front groups and the abuse of science: The saga of the American Council on Science and Health. *Z Magazine* 2007 (October):42–46. Available at http://www.zcommunications.org/corporate-front-groups-and-the -abuse-of-science-by-martin-donohoe. Referenced version available at http://phsj .org/wp-content/uploads/2007/10/corporate-frontgroups-abuse-of-science-acsh-z -mag-with-background-and-refs.doc. Accessed May 4, 2008.

21. Donohoe MT. Genetically modified foods: Health and environmental risks and the corporate agribusiness agenda. *Z Magazine* 2006 (December):35–40. Available at http://zmagsite.zmag.org/Dec2006/donohoe1206.html. Accessed May 4, 2008.

22. Donohoe MT. Unnecessary testing in obstetrics and gynecology and general medicine: Causes and consequences of the unwarranted use of costly and unscientific (yet profitable) screening modalities. *Medscape Ob/Gyn and Women's Health* 2007. Posted April 30, 2007. Available at http://www.medscape.com /viewarticle/552964_print. Accessed May 4, 2008.

23. Chiodo GT, Tolle SW, Donohoe MT. Ethical issues in the acceptance of gifts, part II: Gifts from industry. *J Gen Dentistry* 1999;47:357–360.

24. Donohoe MT, Matthews HA. Wasted paper in pharmaceutical samples. *N Engl J Med.* 1999;340:1600 (brief research study). Available at http://content.nejm .org/cgi/content/full/340/20/1600. Accessed May 4, 2008.

25. Woolhandler S, Himmelstein DU. The high costs of for-profit care. *CMAJ*. 2004; 170(12):1814–1815.

26. Branch WT. Supporting the moral development of medical students. *J Gen Int Med*. 2000;15:503–508.

27. Donohoe MT. Luxury primary care, academic medical centers, and the erosion of science and professional ethics. *J Gen Int Med*. 2004;19:90–94. Available at http://www.blackwell-synergy.com/doi/pdf/10.1111/j.1525–1497.2004.20631.x. Accessed May 4, 2008.

28. Sox HC. Leaving (internal) medicine. *Ann Int Med*. 2006;144:57–58.

29. Donohoe MT. Comparing generalist and specialty care: Discrepancies, deficiencies, and excesses. *Arch Int Med*. 1998;158:1596–1608.

30. Simpson SA, Lang JA. Medical student-run health clinics: Important contributors to patient care and medical education. *J Gen Int Med*. 2007;22:352–356.

31. Cunningham PJ, May JH. A growing hole in the safety net: Physician charity care declines again. *Center for Studying Health System Change* 2006 (March). Available at http://www.hschange.org/CONTENTS/826/. Accessed May 17, 2006.

32. Donohoe MT. Standard vs. luxury care. In: *Ideological Debates in Family Medicine*, S Buetow and T Kenealy, eds. (New York: Nova Science Publishers, Inc., 2007).

33. Donohoe MT. Elements of professionalism for a physician considering the switch to a retainer practice. In *Professionalism in Medicine: The Case-based Guide for Medical Students*, J Spandorfer, CA Pohl, SL Rattner, and TJ Nasca, eds. (New York: Cambridge University Press, 2010).

34. World Health Organization. *World Health Report 2000*. Available at http://www.photius.com/rankings/healthranks.html. Accessed July 26, 2007.

35. Donohoe, MT, Bolger J. Student and faculty responses to the addition of literature to the preclinical curriculum. *J Gen Int Med*. 1998;4(suppl. 1):74.

36. Charon R, Banks JT, Connelly JE, et al. Literature and medicine: Contributions to clinical practice. *Ann Int Med*. 1995;122:599–606.

37. Donohoe MT. Exploring the human condition: Literature and public health issues. In *Teaching Literature and Medicine*, AH Hawkins and MC McEntyre, eds. (New York: Modern Language Association, 2000).

38. Donohoe MT, Danielson S. A community-based approach to the medical humanities. *Medical Education* 2004;38(2):204–217.

39. Donohoe MT. Reflections of physician-authors on death: Literary selections appropriate for teaching rounds, *J Palliative Med*. 2002;5(6):843–848.

40. Donohoe MT. William Carlos Williams, M.D.: Lessons for physicians from his life and writings. *The Pharos* 2004 (Winter):12–17. Available at http://www.alphaomegaalpha.org/PDFs/Pharos/Articles/2004Winter/DonohoeMTWilliamCarlosWilliams.htm. Accessed May 4, 2008.

41. Orwell G. How the poor die. In: *The Collected Essays, Journalism and Letters of George Orwell, IV; In Front of Your Nose, 1945–1950,* Sonia Orwell and Ian Angus, eds. (New York: Harcourt, Brace and World, Inc.): pp. 223–233.

42. Chekhov A. Ward no. six. In: *Seven Short Novels,* Chekhov A. (New York: Bantam, 1976).

43. Lessing D. An old woman and her cat. In: *The Doris Lessing Reader* (New York: Knopf, 1988).

44. Gaines EJ. The sky is gray. In: *Trials, Tribulations, and Celebrations: African-American Perspectives on Health, Illness, Aging and Loss,* Marion Gray Secundy, ed. (Yarmouth, ME: Intercultural Press, 1992).

45. Sinclair U. *The Jungle* (New York: Signet/Penguin, 1990; original 1905).

46. Ibsen H. An enemy of the people. In: *Four Great Plays by Henrik Ibsen,* R Farquharson Sharp, transl. (New York: Bantam, 1959).

47. Williams WC. The paid nurse. In: *The Doctor Stories* (New York: New Directions, 1984).

48. Eighner L. *Travels with Lizbeth* (New York: St. Martin's Press, 1993).

49. Paley G. An Interest in Life. In: *We Are the Stories We Tell: The Best Short Stories by North American Women Since 1945,* Wendy Martin, ed. (New York: Pantheon Books, 1990).

50. Williams WC. The insane. In: *The Doctor Stories* (New York: New Directions, 1984).

51. Chekhov A. Letter to AF Koni (January 26, 1891); Letter to AS survivor (March 9, 1890). In: *The Physician in Literature,* Norman Cousins, ed. (Philadelphia: WB Saunders, 1982).

52. Niemoller P. First they came for the Jews. In: *A Poem a Day,* K McKosker and N Alberry, eds. (South Royalton, VT: Steerforth Press, 1996).

53. Twain M. *The War Prayer* (New York: Harper and Row, 1970; original 1923).

54. Trumbo D. *Johnny Got His Gun* (New York: Bantam, 1939).

55. Miller W. *A Canticle for Leibowitz* (Philadelphia: Lipincott, 1960).

56. Harrison M, Stuart-Clark C, eds. *Peace and War: A Collection of Poems* (Oxford: Oxford University Press, 1989).

57. Levi P. *Survival in Auschwitz* (New York: Touchstone, 1958).

58. Wiesel E. *Night* (New York: Bantam, 1982; original 1958).

59. Timerman J. *Prisoner Without a Name, Cell Without a Number* (New York: Knopf, 1981).

60. Donohoe MT. Literature and social injustice: Stories of the disenfranchised. *Medscape Ob/Gyn and Women's Health* 2005;10(1). Posted January 7, 2005. Available at http://www.medscape.com/viewarticle/496358. Accessed December 19, 2007.

61. Charon R. Personal illness narratives: Using reflective writing to teach empathy. *Academic Medicine* 2004;79(4):351–356.

62. Branch WT. Use of critical incident reports in medical education: A perspective. *J Gen Int Med*. 2005;20(11):1063–1067.

63. Tepper OM, Lurie P, Wolfe SM. Courses in research-based health activism. Virtual Mentor—*Ethics J of the Am Med Assn*. 2004;6(1). Available at http://www .amaassn.org/ama/pub/category/11778.html. Accessed July 18, 2007.

64. Powell PP. Minamata disease: A story of mercury's malevolence. *Southern Med J*. 1991;84(11):1352–1358.

65. Lange D. On-line photos. Available at http://www.freedomvoices.org/pholist.htm. Accessed December 18, 2007.

66. Salgado S. On-line photos. Available at http://www.terra.com.br /sebastiaosalgado/. Accessed December 18, 2007.

67. Natchwey J. On-line photos. Available at http://www.jamesnachtwey.com/. Accessed December 18, 2007.

68. Gruen RL, Campbell EG, Blumenthal D. Public roles of US physicians: Community participation, political involvement, and collective advocacy. *JAMA*. 2006;296: 2467–2475.

69. Grande D, Asch DA, Armstrong K. Do doctors vote? *J Gen Int Med*. 2007;22: 585–589.

70. Landers SH, Sehgal AR. How do physicians lobby their members of Congress. *Arch Int Med*. 2000;160:3248–3251.

71. Kraus CK, Suarez TA. Is there a doctor in the House? Or the Senate? Physicians in US Congress, 1960–2004. *JAMA*. 2004;292:2125–2129.

72. Donohoe MT. Advice for young investigators: Historical perspectives on scientific research. *Adv Hlth Sci Educ*. 2003;8(2)167–171.

73. Wood W. Doctor, advocate, activist. *Public Citizen Health Research Group Health Letter* 2003;19(6):1–3.

74. Nuland SB. *Doctors: The Biography of Medicine* (New York: Vintage Books, 1988).

Index